HANDBOOK OF MEDICAL-SURGICAL NURSING

HANDBOOK OF MEDICAL-SURGICAL NURSING

Edited by

Elizabeth Anne Mahoney, R.N., M.S., Ed.D.

Assistant Professor of Nursing
School of Nursing
Columbia University
New York, New York

and

Jean Pieri Flynn, R.N., B.S., M.A., M.Ed.

Associate in Nursing
School of Nursing
Columbia University
New York, New York

A WILEY MEDICAL PUBLICATION
JOHN WILEY & SONS
New York • Chichester • Brisbane • Toronto • Singapore

FLESCHNER PUBLISHING CO.
Bethany, Connecticut

Editor: R. Craig Percy

Library of Congress Cataloging in Publication Data:

Main entry under title:

Handbook of medical-surgical nursing.
    (A Wiley medical publication) (Wiley red book series)
    Bibliography: p.
    Includes index.
    1. Nursing—Handbooks, manuals, etc. I. Mahoney, Elizabeth Anne.
II. Flynn, Jean P. III. Series.
RT51.H35   1983   610.73'677   83-12377
ISBN 0-471-86982-1

Printed in the United States of America

10 9 8 7 6 5 4 3 2 1

*To the family, friends, and contributors
who made this book possible through their
understanding and support.*

CONTRIBUTORS

Rita M. Bisceglia, RN, MS
Coordinator of Surgical Services
Phelps Memorial Hospital Center
North Tarrytown, New York

Patricia W. Blagman, RN, EdD
Associate Professor
Pace University
Pleasantville, New York

Sharon Brown, RN
Assistant Professor
School of Nursing
University of Texas Health Science Center
Houston, Texas

Caroline Camuñas, RN, MEd
Administrative Nurse Clinician
Presbyterian Hospital
New York, New York

Mary Alice Higgins Donius, RN, BSN, MEd
Clinical Instructor
School of Nursing
Columbia University
New York, New York

Jean P. Flynn, RN, BS, MA, MEd
Associate in Nursing
School of Nursing
Columbia University
New York, New York

Lani Guzman, RN, CCRN, MEd
Cardiovascular Fellow
Louisiana State University Medical Center
New Orleans, Louisiana
Formerly Assistant Professor
Yale University
School of Nursing
New Haven, Connecticut

Marilyn Jaffe-Ruiz, RN, EdD
Chairperson
Lienhard School of Nursing
Pace University
New York, New York

Phyllis Lisanti, RN, BSN, MSN
Associate in Nursing
School of Nursing
Columbia University
New York, New York

Elizabeth A. Mahoney, RN, MS, EdD
Assistant Professor of Nursing
School of Nursing
Columbia University
New York, New York

Marianne Taft Marcus, RN, MEd
Assistant Professor
School of Nursing
University of Texas Health Science Center
Houston, Texas

Harriet R. Nussbaum, RN, EdD
Associate Professor
BSN Program
Felician College
Lodi, New Jersey

Sophie Pasternak, RN
Administrative Nurse Clinician
Presbyterian Hospital
New York, New York

Rita K. Ryan, RN
Administrative Nurse Clinician
Presbyterian Hospital
New York, New York

Marion Oare Smith, RN, BSN, MA
Administrative Nurse Clinician
Presbyterian Hospital
New York, New York

Mary D. Smith, RN, MEd
Assistant Professor
School of Nursing
Columbia University
New York, New York

Laurie Verdisco, RN, BS, MA
Assistant Professor
School of Nursing
Columbia University
New York, New York

Aurora Villafuerte, RN, MSN, MEd
Assistant Professor
School of Nursing
Columbia University
New York, New York

Brenda Salakka Zinamon, RN, BA, MEd
Associate in Nursing
School of Nursing
Columbia University
New York, New York

CONTENTS

Unit I: Homeostatic Mechanisms

1.	Stress and Adaptation	1
2.	Nutrition	9
3.	Fluid and Electrolyte Balance	33
4.	Sensations	71
5.	Temperature Control	101
6.	Immunity	113
7.	Mobility	125
8.	Cellular Growth	139

Unit II: The Perioperative Experience

9.	Preoperative Needs	163
10.	Intraoperative Needs	173
11.	Postoperative Needs	185

Unit III: Major Problems in Medical-Surgical Nursing

12.	Altered Integumentary Functioning	203
13.	Altered Functioning of the Head and Neck	245
14.	Altered Respiratory Functioning	311
15.	Altered Cardiovascular Functioning	383
16.	Altered Gastrointestinal Functioning	435
17.	Altered Urinary Functioning	469
18.	Altered Sexual/Reproductive Functioning	501
19.	Altered Musculoskeletal Functioning	547

20.   Altered Neurologic Functioning   611
21.   Altered Hematopoietic and Hepatic Functioning   683
22.   Altered Endocrine and Metabolic Functioning   727
Appendix A: Abbreviated Outline of a Health History   789
Appendix B: Table of Normal Laboratory Values   791
Bibliography   807
Index   819

PREFACE

Whereas acute care facilities are decreasing in numbers and size and the lengths of hospital stays are becoming shorter, admissions and the use of outpatient and emergency services are escalating. Human longevity and the incidence of chronic disease, regardless of age, are also increasing. These trends in hospital use and the general population place greater demands on the nurse in meeting patient needs. Briefer contact with patients necessitates rapid assessment, identification, intervention, and evaluation by nurses. Because of early discharge, a great need also exists for the provision of continuity of care within and outside the acute care facility and for teaching about the maintenance of health and the prevention of complications and exacerbation of illness. Therefore, nurses need to possess and use a broad knowledge base in the provision of patient care.

Many of the available general and specialized nursing texts focus on the problems and care of the adult patient. Generalized texts are expanding in content but also in size. Although these texts can provide and in-depth study of nursing needs, they can be cumbersome for use on a busy hospital unit. Specialized texts also provide in-depth knowledge in certain areas, but are limited in scope for a general nursing unit.

This handbook, then, is designed to serve as a review and quick reference for nurses in hospital and community settings to help identify and meet the needs of adults who have medical-surgical problems. The manner in which nursing interventions and evaluation criteria are presented can be of interest to inservice educators and nursing audit committees. The book also will be helpful to students preparing for clinical experiences and reviewing for State Board Examinations.

To be consistent with the American Nursing Association standards of care and educational methodologies, the nursing process approach is used. Background data are provided about normal human responses and their deviations, and differences specifically related to the elderly are integrated throughout. Key areas for assessment are indicated; common medical and nursing interventions, including teaching, with their rationales are delineated; and evaluation criteria are identified. Nursing interventions are presented in a format that can be used for performance appraisal. The educational component of nursing interventions can be used for discharge planning. The role of the nurse is emphasized in meeting physical, psychosocial, and educational needs, which include preventive care, discharge planning, and follow-up.

Within the context of the nursing process, a holistic approach to patient care is used to illustrate the interrelationship of mind and body. The mind-body relationship is particularly evident in Unit I, Unit II, and the sections in Unit III that relate to etiology of conditions, health history, and nursing interventions, which, while divided into physical and psychosocial, indicate the importance of considering both the physical and mental needs of the patient. The inclusion of family and/or significant others also shows the relationship of support systems and recovery from physical illness.

The book is organized in three parts that proceed from general to specific considerations. Unit I — Homeostatic Mechanisms — presents concepts that are inherent in many conditions that the nurse encounters in providing care to patients with medical-surgical problems. An in-depth review of these concepts eliminates the necessity for repetition in subsequent chapters. The Table of Contents and Index provide quick references for the location of these data. Unit II — The Perioperative Experience — deals with the general needs of every patient undergoing surgery. Unit III — Major Problems in Medical-Surgical Nursing — deals with modifications for specific procedures. A systems approach is used for organizing content by chapters. Finally, two appendices provide data related to components of the health history and common laboratory values.

EAM and JPF
Columbia University
New York, New York

ABBREVIATIONS AND SYMBOLS

ACTH	adrenocorticotrophic hormone
ADH	antidiuretic hormone
ADP	adenosine diphosphate
AMP	adenosine monophosphate
ANS	autonomic nervous system
ATP	adenosine triphosphate
BCG	Bacillus Calmette-Guérin (vaccine)
bid	2 times a day
BP	blood pressure
bpm	beats per minute
BUN	blood urea nitrogen
CAT	computerized axial tomography
CBC	complete blood count
CHF	congestive heart failure
CNS	central nervous system
CO	cardiac output
COPD	chronic obstructive pulmonary disease
CPR	cardiopulmonary resuscitation
CSF	cerebrospinal fluid
DNA	deoxyribonucleic acid
DW	dextrose in water
ECF	extracellular fluid
ECG	electrocardiogram
EEG	electroencephalogram
ER	emergency room
GFR	glomerular filtration rate
GI	gastrointestinal
GU	genitourinary
Hb	hemoglobin
Hct	hematocrit
ICF	intracellular fluid
ICU	intensive care unit
IgA, etc.	immunoglobulin A, etc.
IM	intramuscular(ly)
IQ	intelligence quotient
IU	international unit(s)

IV	intravenous(ly)
MI	myocardial infarction
NPO	nothing by mouth
OR	operating room
$PaCO_2$	arterial carbon dioxide pressure
$PACO_2$	alveolar carbon dioxide pressure
PaO_2	arterial oxygen pressure
PAO_2	alveolar oxygen pressure
PCO_2	carbon dioxide pressure
PO	oral(ly)
PO_2	oxygen pressure
prn	as needed
q	every
q 4 hr, etc.	every 4 hours, etc.
qid	4 times a day
RBC	red blood cell
RDA	Recommended Daily Allowance(s)
RNA	ribonucleic acid
SC	subcutaneous(ly)
SGOT	scrum glutamic oxaloacetic transaminase
SGPT	serum glutamic pyruvic transaminase
SLE	systemic lupus erythematosus
sp gr	specific gravity
TB	tuberculosis
tid	3 times a day
TPN	total parenteral nutrition
VD	venereal disease
WBC	white blood cell

CHAPTER 1

STRESS AND ADAPTATION
Marilyn Jaffe-Ruiz

OVERVIEW

Humans, from conception until death, in their constant interaction with their environment, are bombarded by a variety of stressors, singly and in combination. In general, the individual maintains wellness through a complex interaction of body systems. When this functioning never begins (e.g., congenital anomalies), ceases to exist (e.g., organ infarcts), and/or accelerates its action (e.g., hyperplasia), the individual can be said to be ill or in a stress state (Fig. 1-1).

Such an individual's adaptive mechanisms are disorganized, and alternative interventions need to be found. It is necessary for nurses to be able to (1) identify and define adaptation and stress in order to help others use their adaptive capacity (including their cognitive abilities), (2) help clients make choices to reduce the amount of stress in their lives and thereby prevent illness, (3) lessen the toll of existing illness, and (4) foster rehabilitation.

Definitions

Adaptation is the capacity of an individual to respond in an active way to stressors in the constantly changing internal and external environment. Adaptation includes a wide range of possible protective behaviors on the part of the person interacting with the current conditions and demands that

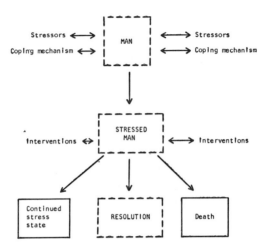

Figure 1-1. Stress adaptation process. Normal stressors are chemical, physical, genetic, sociocultural, ecologic, technologic, and psychologic in nature. The solid boxes indicate a fixed state; the broken boxes indicate the evolving nature of man.

are being imposed. Many factors influence, and are evidence of, human adaptation.

Physiologic factors include those compensatory alterations within the body such as the enlarged hearts of athletes, shivering and sweating in response to temperature changes, and accommodation of pupils to light changes.

Psychologic factors, or coping, include a variety of unconscious defense mechanisms as well as consciously learned behaviors that are used to achieve satisfactory personal and interpersonal relationships. Frequently used defense mechanisms include denial, projection, rationalization, somatization, and repression. In general, the more a person can use cognitive and conscious behaviors (e.g., learning to talk things over with a friend, exercising, identifying sources of stress early) to adapt to a situation, the better off the individual will be.

Sociocultural factors of adaptation include using behaviors of accommodation and assimilation to adapt to prescribed social norms. In our rapidly changing and technologic society this has become increasingly difficult to do. Individual behaviors that help adaptation include learning a foreign language before moving to a foreign country, visiting new locations in advance, establishing contact with a supportive person or network, and making a change gradually, when possible.

Anatomy and physiology review

Human capacity for adaptation depends on a complex neurohormonal communication system that involves the CNS, the ANS, and the endocrine system. A perceived real or imagined stressor stimulates the organism for readiness. The hypothalamus stimulates sympathetic nerve fibers to transmit messages to the adrenal medulla, which releases epinephrine into the bloodstream. Subsequently, the conversion of glycogen to glucose is activated and tissue metabolism is increased, resulting in increased heart rate, BP, body temperature, and O_2 consumption. In addition, there is contraction of smooth muscle, dilation of bronchioles, and flow of blood from internal organs to the musculoskeletal system.

If this state of arousal is prolonged, the hypothalamus stimulates the pituitary to release ACTH, which, in turn, stimulates the adrenal cortex to release glucocorticoids and mineral corticoids into the bloodstream. These corticoids raise blood sugar levels, increase retention of sodium chloride, and decrease retention of potassium. The result of all this is that adequate fluid volume is maintained.

DEVIATIONS

STRESS

Deviations of adaptation are called "stress" — a state whereby the well-being (or integrity) of an individual is endangered. Consequently, the individual must devote energies to protection and adaptation beyond those limits that are usually performed without overt thought.

Theories related to adaptation and stress stem from the original formulations of Hans Selye, who defines stress as "The nonspecific response of the body to any demand made upon it." In other words, any internal or external event that requires a response from the organism is a "stress." How the organism copes with or adapts to the change determines whether illness will result.

Types of stressors

A **stressor** is a stimulus that produces stress. It may be physical, psychologic, sociocultural, technologic, or ecologic in nature, and it may occur singly or in combination with other stressors to produce illness in susceptible individuals. **Physical stressors** include lack of oxygen, trauma, microbial organisms, chemical agents, and genetic factors. **Psychologic stressors** include loss of a significant object (person), injury, threat of physical or emotional injury, developmental milestones, change, frustration of drives, conflicts, and illness in the self or a significant other. **Sociocultural stressors** include immigration, language difficulties, migration, conflicts of norms and customs from one culture to another, ethnicity, deviance, career and job conflicts, poverty, and sexual, racial, or religious prejudice and discrimination. **Technologic stressors** may include jet lag, impersonalization of services (e.g., computers), pollution, additives, radioactive substances, x-rays, overuse of insecticides, medical treatments and medications, and longevity with predisposition to degenerative diseases. **Ecologic stressors** include war, disease, pesticides, and drought.

Signs and symptoms

There are physical and psychologic signs and symptoms of stress. The physical symptoms are dry mouth, palpitations, sweating, nausea, diarrhea, pallor, constricted pupils, shortness of breath, rapid breathing, and urinary urgency. The psychologic symptoms of stress are experienced as anxiety, which is an internal feeling resulting from conflicts, frustrations, and threats to the self (known or unknown). It is an uncanny and unpleasant feeling of dread. Anxiety can vary by degree from mild to severe. It is important for the nurse to identify the degree of anxiety present in the client.

Mild anxiety results in an increased perceptual field and an increased alertness. One can still see connections between events. Mild anxiety can alert one to danger, and it has an energizing effect.

Moderate anxiety results in a narrowed perceptual field and selective inattention. The person can concentrate on only one thing at a time.

Severe anxiety results in reduced perception and a focus on small, irrelevant details. The person is unable to perceive relationships between events. If severe anxiety progresses to panic, personality disorganization occurs. There is a scattered perceptual field. The person is unable to communicate intelligibly, and there is erratic and disorganized behavior. Severe anxiety can immobilize or exhaust a person.

During mild to moderate anxiety, the nurse can help the client mobilize energy in order to effectively cope with the stressful event. If severe anxiety persists or if panic results, more active intervention is needed to help the client reduce anxiety (e.g., remove noxious stimuli, remove client from stimuli, and/or administer medication).

Normal responses

According to Selye, responses by the organism can be either local or general, depending on the type, site, extent, potency, and length of exposure to the stressor.

Local adaptation syndrome refers to the body's response to a stressor that is localized (typified by the inflammatory response to, for example, a splinter, insect sting, or laceration). **General adaptation syndrome** refers to the total response of the whole organism to a stressor that cannot be adapted to locally. There are three stages of the general adaptation syndrome: alarm, resistance, and exhaustion.

Alarm stage. The alarm stage is one of arousal. All systems are "go," ready for a "fight or flight" reaction. The person is alert and attempting to adapt. Initially, intellectual functioning is enhanced; pulse rate, BP, metabolism (temperature), respiratory rate, and muscle tone are increased;

skin is pale, ashen, and cool to the touch; stored energy (glycogen) is converted into usable energy (glucose); pupils are dilated; and the processes of digestion and excretion are diminished, accompanied by the urge to urinate or defecate.

Resistance stage. The resistance stage is one of adaptation in which compensatory efforts are made to preserve life. Body responses eventually return to normal. However, if the stressor continues, the symptoms of the previous alarm stage will also continue, and the person will manifest physical and emotional responses indicative of the stress state. Physically, the vital signs remain elevated, body functioning patterns are irregular, constant fatigue is present, and the person is more susceptible to illness and accidents. Emotionally, the person may be preoccupied, withdrawn, less intellectually able, irritable, and depressed. Stress is cumulative. The organism can usually manage to adapt. When it cannot, the stage of exhaustion ensues.

Exhaustion stage. The exhaustion stage occurs when adaptive responses can no longer be maintained. There is prolonged exposure to stressors and/or cumulative stressors that tax the reserves of adaptability. The entire organism is overcome, and disease and/or death will follow.

Abnormal responses

Pathophysiology (stress response) is the adaptive response gone awry because of a distorted anticipatory response, an excessive response, a deficient response, or an inappropriate response. Psychosomatic illness and chemical substance abuse are also abnormal responses.

A **distorted anticipatory response** produces disease and occurs when one is prepared for "fight or flight" and is in a state of arousal too much of the time. Examples of the result are gastric ulcer, hypertension, worry, and diabetes mellitus.

An **excessive response** is an overreaction in adaptive mechanisms by the organism (e.g., "too much of a good thing"). Examples of an excessive response are scar tissue forming adhesions or keloids, autoimmune responses resulting in allergies, hyperactivity, and acromegaly.

A **deficient response** occurs when there is an inadequate amount of the necessary adaptive mechanisms to allow the organism to effectively interact with the environment. Examples are a low WBC count, low IQ, blindness, and nutritional deficiencies.

An **inappropriate response** is the wrong response at the wrong time, which results in an additional load being placed on an already stressed organism. An example is the retention of salt and water when one is in heart failure.

Psychosomatic illness has been thought to stem from emotional problems that give rise to physical problems. However, if one views the human being as a whole, it would be difficult to say which comes first. With psychophysiologic disorders, structural organic changes may or may not be evident at the time of examination, but the nurse must be cognizant of the fact that the organism is constantly interacting with the environment, with multiple factors operating simultaneously. Therefore, it is not likely that any one factor (e.g., psychologic vulnerability) causes any one particular illness. Disorders typically thought to have a large psychologic component are ulcerative colitis, duodenal ulcer, obesity, skin disorders (e.g., eczema and psoriasis), bronchial asthma, some endocrine disorders, essential hypertension, and heart disease.

Many people use **chemical substances** in an attempt to cope with stress. Both drugs and alcohol can potentially lead to addiction, which would cause an additional physiologic and psychologic stress on the person. Some individuals may be more sensitive to chemical actions and, therefore, more likely to become addicted.

General assessment

A complete **health history** is necessary (*see* Appendix A). Specifically, a careful investigation of recent events (past 6 to 12 mo) needs to be performed. These events need not be unpleasant (e.g., graduation, new job, marriage, and birth of child) to be stressful. However, unpleasant and disturbing events are usually considered more stressful for an individual. Significant events to be attuned to are losses, changes, illnesses, traumas, surgery, developmental crises, and job dissatisfaction. The social readjustment rating scale, developed by Holmes and Rahe, offers a convenient guide for assessment (Table 1-1). As part of the nurse's assessment, a drug and alcohol inventory should also be taken.

Physical examination and **diagnostic tests** should be performed in conformity with common practice. Appropriate diagnostic tests should be performed for specific symptomatology, e.g., CBC, blood chemistries, ECG, and GI series.

TABLE 1-1
The Social Readjustment Rating Scale *

Change	Stress value
Death of a spouse	100
Divorce	73
Marital separation	65
Jail term	63
Death of close family member	63
Personal injury or illness	53
Marriage	50
Fired at work	47
Marital reconciliation	45

Change	Stress value
Retirement	45
Change in health of family member	44
Pregnancy	40
Sex difficulties	39
Gain of new family member	39
Business readjustment	39
Change in financial state	38
Death of close friend	37
Change to different line of work	36
Change in number of arguments with spouse	35
Mortgage >$10,000	31
Foreclosure on mortgage or loan	30
Change in responsibilities at work	29
Son or daughter leaving home	29
Trouble with in-laws	29
Outstanding personal achievement	28
Spouse begins or stops work	26
Begin or end school	26
Change in living conditions	25
Revision of personal habits	24
Trouble with boss	23
Change in work hours or conditions	20
Change in residence	20
Change in schools	20
Change in recreation	19
Change in church activities	19
Change in social activities	18
Mortgage or loan <$10,000	17
Change in sleeping habits	16
Change in number of family get-togethers	15
Change in eating habits	15
Vacation	13
Christmas (holidays)	12
Minor violations of the law	11

*This scale rates the stress of adjusting to various possible life changes. The more change that occurs in an individual's life, the more likely the individual is to become ill. The results of the study by Holmes and Rahe indicate a 90% chance of illness within the next 2 yr for those people who score over 300 life change units during a 12-mo period. A score of 150 to 299 indicates a 50% chance of illness, and there is a 30% chance with a score of 150 or less.
Reprinted with permission from Holmes, T., and R. M. Rahe. The social readjustment rating scale. *Journal of Psychosomatic Research* (August 1967). 215-216.

Common interventions

General interventions would include the following actions: **Educate** patients as to how to pace themselves (e.g., if an individual has just finished a dissertation, married, and moved, it would not be advisable to change jobs). **Plan variety** in the course of a hectic day. Rest periods, diversionary activity, exercise or meditation, and change of environments can be helpful. **Provide anticipatory planning** ("to be forewarned is to be forearmed"). Counsel and teach around specific crises (e.g., preoperative teaching and preparenthood classes). Provide an opportunity for role playing and verbally rehearse feared events. Problem solve conflicts around separation/individuation and independence/dependence. **Counsel** as to how to balance life activities between work/play, family/friends, and managing finances. **Teach health-promoting activities** (e.g., hand washing; proper diet; proper rest, exercise; seat belts; adequate fluid intake; breast and testicular self-examination; and/or modifying smoking, drinking, and overworking habits). Enhance communication with others. **Teach** the patient to tune into the self and be aware of anxiety and somatic symptoms of stress (e.g., shortness of breath, hyperventilation, and insomnia) as a signal to reduce tension. Be aware of common expressions in speech that are indicative of physiologic response to stressful interpersonal situations (e.g., "that really makes my blood boil," "I can't swallow that," "he's a pain in my neck," and "she gets under my skin"). **Help** the patient to learn to identify stressful situations and to change his value system and life-style as appropriate and necessary. **Help** the patient to learn outlets for tension (e.g., catharsis [talking], problem solving, and physical comfort [bath, massage, and warm milk]). **Teach sublimation of tension** through exercise, dance, painting, jogging, singing, or cleaning house. **Teach** the patient to avoid short-term coping mechanisms like overeating, smoking, and abuse of drugs, alcohol, or caffeine. **Teach autohypnotic states** like meditation, relaxation techniques, and imagery. Advise the patient to seek supportive help from friends, clergy, or professionals. **Use biofeedback** and psychotherapy as necessary.

Evaluation criteria.   Stress has been modified or reduced if any of the following results occur: (1) a lessening of symptoms (e.g., less rash or lowered pulse, BP, or respirations); (2) an increased ability to identify potential and actual stressors and to adapt effectively; (3) an increased ability to channel the energy of stress response in order to cope with stressors in a more adaptive way (e.g., problem solving); (4) an increase in walking, talking, or seeking help; (5) a diminution of destructive coping mechanisms (e.g., denial, rationalization, eating, sleeping, or using chemical substances); (6) a decrease in anxiety; and (7) diagnostic data are within normal limits.

CHAPTER 2

NUTRITION
Mary D. Smith

OVERVIEW

Definitions

Nutrition and diet. **Nutrition** is defined as the food one eats and the way in which the body uses it for survival, growth, and the repair of worn-out tissues. The term is also applied to the science that deals with the body's food requirements. Although **diet** is generally considered as a prescribed form of intake that relates to an altered state of health (obesity, diabetes mellitus, high BP, etc.), it also describes the food that is normally consumed in the course of living.

Composition of a normal diet. There are three major categories of **organic** (i.e., carbon-containing) nutrients in foods: *carbohydrates, proteins,* and *fats*. In addition, *vitamins* are organic compounds that appear in very small quantities and help with specific body functions. *Minerals* and *water,* on the other hand, are two **inorganic** nutrients that are bound to the three main nutrients and assist with specific body functions. Inclusion of all six nutrients from a variety of foods constitutes a balanced diet.

Table 2-1 lists the daily requirements of certain nutrients for adults in early, middle, or later maturity.

Basic food groups. In order to ensure adequate intake of all essential nutrients, guides have been developed and recommended numbers of servings from basic food groupings have been determined for specific age groups and for special needs, such as pregnancy and lactation. Table 2-2

TABLE 2-1
*Recommended Daily Allowances ***

	Age	Weight		Height		Protein	Fat-soluble vitamins			Water-soluble vitamins		
							Vitamin A	Vitamin D	Vitamin E	Vitamin C	Thiamin	Riboflavin
	yr	*kg*	*lb*	*cm*	*in*	*g*	*µg RE‡*	*µg§*	*mg α-TE†*	*mg*	*mg*	*mg*
Infants	0.0-0.5	6	13	60	24	kg × 2.2	420	10	3	35	0.3	0.4
	0.5-1.0	9	20	71	28	kg × 2.0	400	10	4	35	0.5	0.6
Children	1-3	13	29	90	35	23	400	10	5	45	0.7	0.8
	4-6	20	44	112	44	30	400	10	6	45	0.9	1.0
	7-10	28	62	132	52	34	700	10	7	45	1.2	1.4
Males	11-14	45	99	157	62	45	1,000	10	8	50	1.4	1.6
	15-18	66	145	176	69	56	1,000	10	10	60	1.4	1.7
	19-22	70	154	177	70	56	1,000	7.5	10	60	1.5	1.7
	23-50	70	154	178	70	56	1,000	5	10	60	1.4	1.6
	51+	70	154	178	70	56	1,000	5	10	60	1.2	1.4
Females	11-14	46	101	157	62	46	800	10	8	50	1.1	1.3
	15-18	55	120	163	64	46	800	10	8	60	1.1	1.3
	19-22	55	120	163	64	44	800	7.5	8	60	1.1	1.3
	23-50	55	120	163	64	44	800	5	8	60	1.0	1.2
	51+	55	120	163	64	44	800	5	8	60	1.0	1.2
Pregnant						+30	+200	+5	+2	+20	+0.4	+0.3
Lactating						+20	+400	+5	+3	+40	+0.5	+0.5

	Water-soluble vitamins				Minerals					
	Niacin	Vitamin B6	Vitamin B12	Folacin	Calcium	Phosphorus	Magnesium	Iron	Zinc	Iodine
	mg NE**	mg	µg	µg	mg	mg	mg	mg	mg	µg
Infants	6	0.3	0.5‡‡	30	360	240	50	10	3	40
	8	0.6	1.5	45	540	360	70	15	5	50
Children	9	0.9	2.0	100	800	800	150	15	10	70
	11	1.3	2.5	200	800	800	200	10	10	90
	16	1.6	3.0	300	800	800	250	10	10	120
Males	18	1.8	3.0	400	1,200	1,200	350	18	15	150
	18	2.0	3.0	400	1,200	1,200	400	18	15	150
	19	2.2	3.0	400	800	800	350	10	15	150
	18	2.2	3.0	400	800	800	350	10	15	150
	16	2.2	3.0	400	800	800	350	10	15	150
Females	15	1.8	3.0	400	1,200	1,200	300	18	15	150
	14	2.0	3.0	400	1,200	1,200	300	18	15	150
	14	2.0	3.0	400	800	800	300	18	15	150
	13	2.0	3.0	400	800	800	300	18	15	150
	13	2.0	3.0	400	800	800	300	10	15	150
Pregnant	+2	+0.6	+1.0	+400	+400	+400	+150	§§	+5	+25
Lactating	+5	+0.5	+1.0	+100	+400	+400	+150	§§	+10	+50

*The allowances are intended to provide for individual variations among most healthy persons in the United States. Diets should be based on a variety of common foods in order to provide other nutrients for which human requirements have been less well defined. See text for detailed discussion of allowances and nutrients.
‡Retinol equivalents. 1 Retinol equivalent = 1 µg retinol or 6 µg β-carotene.
§As cholecalciferol. 10 µg cholecalciferol = 400 IU vitamin D.
†α-Tocopherol equivalents. 1 mg d-α-tocopherol = 1 α-TE.
**Niacin equivalent. 1 NE is equal to 1 mg of niacin or 60 mg of dietary tryptophan.
‡‡The RDA for vitamin B12 in infants is based on average concentration of the vitamin in human milk. The allowances after weaning are based on energy intake (as recommended by the American Academy of Pediatrics) and consideration of other factors, such as intestinal absorption.
§§The increased requirement during pregnancy cannot be met by the iron content of habitual American diets nor by the existing iron stores of many women. Therefore the use of 30 to 60 mg of supplemental iron is recommended. Iron needs during lactation are not substantially different from those of nonpregnant women, but continued supplementation of the mother for 2 to 3 months after parturition is advisable in order to replenish stores depleted by pregnancy.
Reproduced from Recommended Dietary Allowances. National Academy Press, Washington, D. C. 1980. Ninth edition.

provides a comparison of two of the most widely used groupings associated with healthy persons: the "basic four" and the "basic six" (also called the "star of good eating"). The advantage of the basic four is its simplicity, a factor that makes it easy to teach and remember. The basic six, however, has the advantage of taking into account the fat content of foods and, therefore, to some extent, their caloric content. With some minor alterations, the basic six becomes the "food exchange lists" that are widely used for dietary management of diabetes mellitus and, more recently, for successful weight control.

Carbohydrates are composed of carbon, hydrogen, and oxygen, and are found in the form of starches and simple or complex sugars: bread, cereal, potato, table sugar, etc.

Proteins contain nitrogen (and often sulfur and phosphorus) in addition to carbon, hydrogen, and oxygen. Some proteins are considered *complete* because they contain all 8 essential amino acids (threonine, leucine, isoleucine, valine, lysine, methionine, phenylalanine, and tryptophan), whereas the *incomplete* proteins contain only some of these or the 11 nonessential amino acids, which the body itself can manufacture. Because the essential amino acids must be obtained from the foods we eat, and all eight must be present in specific amounts and ratios, sources of complete proteins — such as milk, meat, cheese, and eggs — should be included in a balanced diet. The sources of incomplete proteins — such as grains, legumes, seeds, and nuts — when carefully combined, however, can also provide the essential amino acids needed for tissue building and repair.

Fats, also called **lipids**, are composed of *fatty acids* and *glycerol* in the form of visible fats on, for example, meats, oils, butter, and cream. Fatty acids are classified as saturated or unsaturated, depending on the amount of hydrogen that fills the basic carbon chain of a given fatty acid. Those fats of animal origin are more highly filled with hydrogen and, therefore, are the more *saturated.* Those fats of plant origin are generally less saturated, and those fatty acids having two or more places along the carbon chain without hydrogen are called *polyunsaturated.* A flowing oil of plant origin, such as safflower or corn oil, is an example of the latter. Hydrogenating plant oils, even polyunsaturated ones, to make solid vegetable shortening or margarine will cause them to become saturated.

Vitamins are classified as *water soluble* (B complex and C) or *fat soluble* (A, D, E, and K), depending on whether they dissolve in fat or water to facilitate absorption. Letters and/or names are given to vitamins, with names currently being favored: A or retinol; B1 or thiamin; B2 or riboflavin; niacin or nicotinic acid; B6 or pyridoxine; pantothenic acid; folic acid; B12 or cobalamin; C or ascorbic acid; D or calciferol; E or tocopherol; and K or menadione. In addition, preformed vitamin A (retinol) is found in animal fats and dairy products, whereas provitamin A (carotene) is from plants and is thought to be a precursor of vitamin A. Hypervitaminosis A usually results from excess retinol.

TABLE 2-2

Comparison of Basic Four, Basic Six, and Food Exchange Lists for Adults

Basic four (servings)	Basic six (servings)	Food exchanges (unit)
1. Milk (2) milk, cheese, ice cream	1. Milk (2) same as basic four	1. Milk (1 cup) skimmed low-fat whole
2. Meat (2) beef, veal, lamb, pork, poultry, fish, eggs, nuts, dry peas and beans, peanut butter	2. Meat (2) same as basic four	2. Meat (1 ounce) lean: beef, lamb, fish; shellfish medium fat: beef, pork, cheese higher fat: beef, pork, lamb breast
3. Fruit and vegetables (4) dark yellow, green leafy, citrus, etc. (vitamins A and C)	3. Fat (varies) oil, butter, cream, mayonnaise	3. Fat (1 teaspoon) polyunsaturated: margarine, salad dressing, seeds, walnuts monounsaturated: avocado, nuts, olives, oils saturated: bacon, butter, cheese, cream
4. Bread and cereals (4) bread, rolls, cereal, pasta, rice, crackers	4. Fruit (≥1) same as basic four	4. Fruit (varies) same as basic four
	5. Vegetables (≥1) same as basic four	5. Vegetable A (as desired) asparagus to zucchini
	6. Bread and cereals (4) same as basic four	6. Vegetable B (~½ cup) artichokes, beets, carrots, okra, peas, rutabagas
		7. Bread and cereal (4) same as basic four

Minerals are categorized as 7 essential macronutrients (calcium, phosphorus, sodium, potassium, magnesium, chlorine, and sulfur) and 10 essential micronutrients or trace elements (iron, copper, cobalt, zinc, manganese, iodine, molybdenum, fluorine, selenium, and chromium). (Another four or more trace elements are probably essential, and studies to confirm these as essential continue.) The *macronutrients* must be in the diet at the relatively large level of ≥100 mg/day (e.g., calcium: 800 to 1,200 mg), whereas only a few milligrams or less of *trace elements* are needed (e.g., iron: 10 to 18 mg).

Water is the final nutrient to be considered. Water balance is a very significant aspect of health. The adult body is ~65% water, with a range of from 50 to 80%. The percentage is smaller for the older individual and greater for infants. A normal intake of fluid, including the amount ingested and that synthesized in the body, averages 2,400 ml/day for a healthy adult. Elderly adults are encouraged to ingest sufficient fluids to produce a daily urine output of 1,500 ml.

Approximately two-thirds of our oral fluid intake is in the form of pure water or some other beverage; the rest comes from foods we eat. In addition, a small amount (~150 to 250 ml/day, depending on the rate of metabolism) is synthesized in the body from the oxidation of hydrogen in our foods.

Under normal circumstances, with an atmospheric temperature of 20°C (68°F), an adult who has ingested and synthesized 2,400 ml of water will lose ~1,400 ml in urine, 200 ml in feces, 100 ml in sweat, and another 700 ml as insensible losses through evaporation from the lungs and diffusion through the skin. Situations that alter the environment (such as hot weather or prolonged strenuous exercise) will greatly increase the need for additional intake. With the common knowledge that "a pint's a pound the world around," one can calculate that an average adult with ~40 liters of fluid in the body can attribute >80 lb (~36.3 kg) of body weight to water alone. It is for this reason that "crash" reduction diets focus on inducing water excretion to effect a dramatic "weight loss," and that weight gain can be equally dramatic with water retention.

Anatomy and physiology review

The reader should refer to Chapter 16 for a diagram of the related anatomy and a discussion of the physiology of food movement, secretion of digestive juices, absorption, transportation of digested foods, and excretion of wastes.

Utilization and usual sites of ingestion, digestion, and absorption. The main organs of digestion are the mouth, pharynx, esophagus, stomach, small and large intestines, and rectum. The accessory organs of digestion are the teeth, tongue and taste buds, parotid glands, sublingual and submaxillary salivary glands, gallbladder, liver, and pancreas.

Ingestion is controlled by numerous physiologic, psychologic, and sociocultural factors. Among the physiologic factors is satisfaction of the basic hunger drive, which is controlled by two centers in the hypothalamus: the hunger/feeding center and the satiety center. Another factor is the palatability of specific foods, a result of combined stimulation of the taste buds, the olfactory organs, and receptors in the tongue that are sensitive to the temperature and texture of food.

Digestion is the process by which complex food molecules are broken down into those small enough to travel in the circulation to cells where they can be metabolized. As mentioned previously, vitamins, minerals, and water are broken away from the three main organic nutrients, and these main nutrients themselves are broken down to the simple sugars (e.g., glucose and fructose), amino acids, fatty acids, and glycerol, which are absorbed and circulated to cells for oxidation. The *mechanical* processes of chewing, swallowing, and peristalsis are accompanied by the *chemical* action of enzymes found in salivary, gastric, pancreatic, and small intestinal juices as well as by that of hydrochloric acid and bile (two nonenzyme secretions). Digestion is completed in the small intestine.

Absorption is the passage of simple forms of nutrients to the circulating blood and lymph. This is accomplished primarily in the duodenal and jejunal segments of the small intestine. In the large intestine, most of the water, some B-complex vitamins (especially biotin and folic acid), and much vitamin K are absorbed. These vitamins are produced there by the action of colon bacteria. The process of absorption is assisted through the mechanisms of osmosis, passive diffusion, active transport, and pinocytosis (a process by which a portion of the cellular membrane invaginates to form a saccule to engulf ECF and remains a vaccule, or clear space, within the cell). Bile is necessary for absorption of fatty acids and the fat-soluble vitamins.

Theories

Somewhere between an approach that suggests that the body can and will produce any and all nutrients it lacks, and the megavitamin therapies and prophylactic approach espoused by Linus Pauling and others, lie many hunches, interpretations, and theories related to how one achieves adequate nutrition. Two ideas that have gained wide acceptance and practice in the area of clinical nutrition are (1) **protein complimentarity** and (2) the use of **fiber and bulk** to prevent or treat GI disorders.

Protein complementarity.   Frances Moore Lappé was among the first to articulate on a large scale the concept of combining plant sources of incomplete proteins as an alternative to human dependence on animals for complete protein foods. In 1972 she explained how the proper combinations of grains, legumes, seeds, and dairy products would not only produce a high-quality protein with all eight essential amino acids, but would also provide a much greater variety of foods and help conserve our planet's sources of protein. In addition, one would derive greater advantage from eating lower on the food chain in terms of fewer additives and pollutants, more roughage, less fat, and the much greater variety available.

The **food chain** is thought to be comprised of those aspects of *soil life* (e.g., fungi-algae, rodents, worms, insects, and decomposing bacteria) and *water life* (e.g., oysters, clams, lobsters, fish, algae, plankton, and decomposing bacteria) that, with the help of the sun, produce *plants*. Animals are the primary consumers of soil plants, and birds consume water plants. Both animals and birds are consumed by man — the secondary consumer in this vital chain. In theory, then, by eating the plants, which are lower on the food chain than either animals or birds, man would benefit from availing himself of fresh, unaltered forms of protein. This theory is one of the underlying ideas of protein complementarity.

Fiber and bulk. The daily dietary inclusion of fiber, bulk, or roughage in the form of lettuce, celery, cabbage, raw fruits, nuts, seeds, whole-grain bread and cereal, bran, and vegetables with coverings (such as corn, peas, and beans) has long been accepted as both preventive and therapeutic in the management of bowel functioning and constipation. Among the elderly, for example, the effect of decreased motility of the GI tract can be altered by increasing fibrous food consumption in addition to increasing fluid intake (particularly in the form of natural laxatives, such as fruit juices) and eating meals at regular intervals.

Persons attempting to control dietary intake of calories are advised to increase their intake of the "calorie-free" foods listed in the Vegetable A group of the food exchange lists (*see* Table 2-2). These are bulky, low-calorie foods that provide some satiety during and between meals. The wide variety helps the dieter avoid some of the boredom that often accompanies controlled diets.

Recent evidence regarding the correlation of low-fiber diets and the occurrence of some GI disturbances (such as colorectal cancer) has resulted in the promotion of high-residue intake in the elderly and the general population. Even the management of some GI deviations that are usually treated with low-fiber intake (e.g., diverticulosis and peptic ulcer) has been altered to include more bulk. In theory, the greater bulk prevents a more complete contraction of the intestine, which often produces less pressure and pain.

DEVIATIONS

INADEQUATE FOOD INTAKE

When an individual, through choice or happenstance, consumes fewer calories and nutrients than are required to meet individual needs for basal metabolic processes and activity, a condition of inadequate intake exists. That is, there is insufficient provision of the six basic nutrients to provide energy and promote growth and repair of body tissues.

Etiology

Hunger is a craving for food that is associated with objective sensations, such as rhythmic hunger contractions. (Intense contractions cause tightness or gnawing in the stomach.) In addition, hunger pangs or pains in the stomach, increased restlessness, tension, nervousness, and psychic craving (which results in food-seeking behavior) are considered part of hunger. Absence of hunger, such as that which results from depression or diminished taste and smell sensation in the elderly, can contribute to an inadequate food intake.

Appetite controls the quality of food one eats, and the feeling of satiety or fulfillment controls the quantity of food consumed. When an individual's nutrient storage depots are already filled (e.g., glycogen stores in the liver, or fat stores in adipose tissue) or a filling meal is eaten, the sensation of satiety results. Disturbances of either the satiety or appetite mechanism can result in alterations of specific nutrients: such as an undersupply or deficiency, or an oversupply (as with obesity and hypervitaminosis A).

Lack of food sources.   In some parts of the world, lack of food sources is often due to geographic, economic, or psychosocial barriers. In the USA, the rapidly changing food environment has resulted in new food products in the form of convenience, synthetic, and textured foods. This results in two problems: (1) the basic four food guidelines relate to primary foods rather than these new products, and (2) there is a greater need for nutrition education for the public to better assess advertising claims. Changing population patterns and the greater number of elderly persons in our society have resulted in the discovery that malnutrition is prevalent in the minority poverty areas of large cities, among migrant workers, in rural areas throughout the South, and on Indian reservations. Among the elderly, in particular, malnutrition and chronic health problems result in large measure from our society's youth orientation, lack of economic security among those on fixed incomes, and social isolation.

Disease.   Because they alter the metabolism or absorption of nutrients, diabetes mellitus, hyperthyroidism, and malabsorption syndrome are examples of the numerous diseases or deviations from health that can alter the body's intake, utilization, absorption, and/or digestion of foods. More subtle, but just as capable of altering one's nutrition status, are the various therapies and diagnostic tests employed in the management of illness. For example, drugs (laxatives, antibiotics), controlled diets (low calorie, low sodium, high protein), and diagnostic tests (barium enema, oral cholangiogram) are potential sources of altered GI functioning, particularly when used in combination, in rapid succession, or over long periods of time. Careful monitoring of nutrition status is indicated in these situations.

Nothing by mouth.   During periods of diagnostic study, before surgery, and in the immediate postoperative period, NPO may be prescribed for brief or prolonged periods of time. Unless provision is made to administer nutrients other than through oral intake (e.g., IV or via feeding tube), a state of inadequate nutrition may result.

Other. Biologic aging, decreased caloric need with aging or decreased activity, heredity, environmental factors, chronic disease, periodontal disease, and psychosocial parameters — such as income, inadequate housing, transportation, social interaction, decline of the extended family, lifelong eating habits, and reliance on governmental social programs for solutions to nutrition problems — are other factors that contribute to inadequate intake. These will be discussed in greater detail in subsequent sections of the chapter.

Pathophysiology

Depletion of body reserves. Because tissues prefer to use **carbohydrate** rather than fat or protein for energy, glycogen is stored in the liver and muscles. Although only a few hundred grams in amount, the stores of glycogen can supply enough energy for about half a day. In situations of starvation, there is progressive depletion of tissue fat and protein after the first few hours.

Fat is the next best source of energy to carbohydrates, and bodily fat stores can continue to provide energy for 5 to 8 wk, depending on the individual's stores at the onset of the period of starvation.

When fat stores are nearly depleted, **protein** is used as the energy source if there is a continued lack of nutrient intake. Protein stores are depleted in three phases: rapidly at first; then greatly slowed; and, finally, rapidly again just before death. Death usually occurs when protein stores have been depleted to about half their normal value because maintenance of cellular functioning depends so much on protein. In addition, during the second (slowed) phase of protein depletion, the rate of gluconeogenesis (i.e., the formation of glucose by the liver from noncarbohydrate sources) decreases to the extent that the greatly lessened availability of it induces **ketosis**. Ketones can cross the blood-brain barrier and supply energy to the brain.

As the process of inanition (i.e., weakness and wasting from lack of food or inability to use it) continues, some mild vitamin deficiencies begin to appear. Within a week or more, there are signs of mild deficiencies of water-soluble vitamins in particular, and, over several weeks, the signs and symptoms of severe deficiencies become evident.

Nitrogen balance. The determination of nitrogen balance in the body is a useful reference in indicating a person's state of protein balance. Protein contains ~16% nitrogen — 90% of which is excreted in the urine in the form of urea, uric acid, creatinine, etc., after protein has been metabolized. Therefore, by analyzing the amount of nitrogen excreted in the urine, one can determine the total quantity of protein metabolized in a given period of time.

Nitrogen excretion. Protein replacement may be estimated by analysis of the previous day's excretion of urinary and fecal nitrogen. By adding the grams of nitrogen excreted in the urine over a 24-hr period to the amount excreted in feces (~10% of that in the urine), and dividing the sum by the percentage of nitrogen in protein (16%), one arrives at the total amount of protein (in grams) metabolized that day:

$$\frac{10 \text{ g UN} + 1 \text{ g FN}}{0.16} = 68.75 \text{ g TPM,}$$

where UN is urinary nitrogen excretion, FN is fecal nitrogen excretion (10% of UN), and TPM is total protein metabolized in 24 hr.

Nitrogen balance.   **Negative balance** occurs when the body's loss of protein exceeds its intake of food proteins, as in starvation, a wasting disease, long-term illness, malnutrition, and glucocorticoid hormone activity. **Positive balance** can result from exercise, growth hormone, testosterone, and protein intake that exceeds utilization.

Signs and symptoms

The clinical signs of altered nutrition status are listed in Table 2-3. Possible related deficiencies are also shown.

Vitamins that are stored in the body are in all cells to some extent. Some are stored in the liver (vitamin A for up to 6 mo and vitamin D for 1 to 2 mo, for example). The storage of vitamin K and most water-soluble vitamins is relatively slight, especially those in the B-complex group. As a result, deficiencies of vitamin K and the B-complex group appear within a few days. The signs and symptoms of vitamin C deficiency appear within a few weeks, and death from scurvy will occur within 20 to 30 wk.

Altered intake needs.   The RDA for the aging man or woman are altered in the following ways: there is a decreased need for calories, thiamin, riboflavin, niacin, and iodine. A decrease in the metabolism rate of ~7.5% for each decade beyond the age of 25 yr, a decrease in activity after the active years of adolescent growth and change, and less production of thyroid hormone account for the alteration in metabolism and, therefore, nutrient intake need. Women experience a decreased need for iron with the cessation of menstruation, and men are encouraged to maintain an RDA of 1 mg of thiamin (despite decreased need with aging) because they tend to utilize it poorly. Only those persons who are institutionalized or spend most daylight hours indoors are likely to get less than the recommended 400 IU of vitamin D that is needed.

The need for calories decreases with aging *without* a proportionate decrease in need for other nutrients. Failure to reduce caloric intake results in obesity during the middle and later years.

The nutrition status of a person reflects his current dietary practices, which are influenced by physiologic and psychosocial variables that affect food intake or utilization. The physiologic parameters are influenced by heredity and environment, especially the important aspect of lifelong eating habits. The nutrition status of the elderly is related to the physiologic factors of biologic aging and chronic disease, and the psychosocial factors

TABLE 2-3

Symptoms of Altered Nutrition and Related Deficiencies

Factor	Symptom	Deficiency
General survey and skin		
Appearance	Listlessness, apathy, cachexia.	Carbohydrates, proteins, fats, calories.
Vitality	Easily fatigued, lacks energy, falls asleep in day, looks tired.	Carbohydrates, fat, B-complex vitamins.
Skin	Rough and dry, scaly and irritated, pale or pigmented, bruises or petechiae.	Fat, niacin, ascorbic acid, vitamins A and K.
Weight	Over- or underweight.	Calories, vitamin B1.
Posture	Sagging shoulders, sunken chest, hump back.	Niacin, calcium.
Head and neck		
Hair	Stringy and dull, dry and brittle, grey or depigmented.	Protein.
Glands	Thyroid enlargement.	Iodine.
Eyes	Dryness, signs of infection, thickened conjunctiva, glassiness, increased vascularity.	Vitamins A and C.
Facial skin	Greasy or scaly, discolored.	Vitamin A.
Lips	Dry and scaly, swollen, stomatitis.	B-complex, especially niacin.
Tongue	Glossitis, atrophied papillae, red, beefy, swollen.	B-complex, especially niacin.
Gums	Red at margins, swollen and spongy, receding.	Ascorbic acid.
Teeth	Caries or mottled, absent, worn, malpositioned.	Calcium, vitamin D.
Musculoskeletal		
Muscles	Flaccid and poor tone, underdeveloped, tender.	Protein, niacin, potassium.
Skeleton	Bowed legs, knock-knees, chest deformity and beaded ribs, prominent scapulae.	Calcium, phosphorus, vitamin D.
Legs and feet	Edema, tingling and calf tenderness, weakness.	Protein, vitamin B1.
Abdomen and GI functioning		
Abdomen	Swollen.	Protein, vitamin B1.
GI	Anorexia, indigestion, diarrhea, or constipation.	Calcium, niacin, vitamin B1.
Nervous control	Inattentive, irritable.	Niacin, thiamin, vitamin B1.

Adapted from Williams, S. R. Essentials of Nutrition and Diet Therapy. C. V. Mosby Co., St. Louis. 1978. Second edition. p. 8, 68, and Lewis, C. M. Nutrition: The Basics of Nutrition. Family Nutrition. F. A. Davis Co., Philadelphia. 1978. p. F87-88.

of income, housing, transportation, social interaction, and long-established eating habits.

With the process of biologic aging, the body loses reserve capacity, adaptability, and the capacity to function well under stress. The limited mobility that accompanies many chronic diseases further complicates food intake and utilization. These *complications* may be the result of therapeutic dietary modifications (such as sodium restriction), which contribute to making foods unappetizing or one's nutrition inadequate. In addition, drugs used to treat chronic illnesses may interact with foods and alter the patient's needs for specific nutrients. For example, there is an increased need for folic acid and vitamin D when the anticonvulsant phenytoin sodium (Dilantin) is used, and vitamin C should be present during the full therapeutic course of the urinary antibacterial drug methenamine mandelate (Mandelamine).

The ability to obtain or eat food may be limited by physical conditions such as arthritis, glaucoma, or stroke, and altered nutrient utilization may be associated with the disease itself. Malabsorption secondary to a gastrectomy is a good example of the latter, and it may quickly result in malnutrition, particularly in the elderly.

Any of these psychosocial parameters may affect the availability or acceptability of foods and result in deficiencies. The problems of weakness and social isolation contribute in large measure to the malnutrition of elderly Americans. Their problems are greatly compounded by physical symptoms that are related to the drug therapy that is often used in the management of cardiovascular deviations (e.g., digitalis, diuretics, and antihypertensive agents). Anorexia, nausea, vomiting, confusion, fatigue, GI distress, lethargy, diarrhea, and fluid retention are all examples of these drug-related symptoms. Failure to identify the physical component may lead to the erroneous conclusion that the symptoms are solely psychogenic.

General assessment

Health history. Assessing dietary patterns is an important aspect of collecting a data base about current health status. The assessment can be divided into three parts: weight control, daily food intake, and fluid intake. Specifics related to these three areas may be found in subsequent sections of this chapter. All information collected about these areas should be viewed in terms of the patient's age and activity vis-á-vis his nutritional needs. Patterns and their alterations should be noted and correlated with, or validated through, findings from the physical assessment and laboratory studies portions of data base collection (*see below*). The need for patient education about general or specific aspects of dietary intake should become apparent and documented for intervention at an appropriate time.

Although an actual nursing diagnosis related to dietary adequacy may not be possible until all aspects of the data base have been completed, an excellent start in the process may be initiated through a complete diet history.

Some clinicians include nutrition as one of the systems in taking a patient's history for the review of physiologic systems section of data base collection. Questions should be asked regarding weight patterns, 24-hr diet recall, appetite, who buys and prepares food, social environment of eating, ability to afford food, use of dentures, chewing patterns, and the patient's self-evaluation of nutrition status. In addition, the interviewer should stress information about dietary regulation, special efforts required, and any cultural or religious practices.

The elderly, in particular, are to be questioned about any special diet, appetite pattern, food consumption pattern, weekly or monthly diet recall (if it appears that a 24-hr recall represents an atypical day), daily fluid intake, access to markets and such, and problems of food preparation, chewing, swallowing, choking, or denture use.

Physical examination.   The reader is referred to the section related to signs and symptoms of inadequate nutrient intake and Table 2-3 for assistance in making assessments and conclusions regarding the patient's nutrition status.

A review of the clinical signs of positive and negative nutrition is listed in Table 2-4. This table illustrates that the skin and its appendages (i.e., hair and nails) provide much information about an individual's protein status. Skin turgor is a significant aspect of assessing hydration and water balance, as are the observations of dry skin, a soft or spongy quality upon palpation of the eye, and a lowered BP. There are numerous possibilities, and careful analysis of the data base can yield conclusions and validate nursing diagnoses about nutrition status.

Diagnostic tests.   Routine multiscreening **blood tests** can, in either a general or specific way, reveal alterations in nutrition status. The tests are generally divided into two sections: (1) chemistry and electrolytes, and (2) hematology. The former includes enzymes studies, which indicate the extent of damage to tissues (which release enzymes as cells die). Normal laboratory values are given in Appendix B.

Urinalysis is another multiscreening test that is useful in assessing alterations of nutrition with specific disease processes and deviations from health (such as the glycosuria and ketonuria found in uncontrolled diabetes mellitus). Protein and calcium loss are among the microscopic findings of urine sediment, and these have significance in evaluating nutrition status.

Combinations of test results indicate disease processes, syndromes, and nutrition deficiencies. For example, malabsorption syndrome is indicated by decreased serum values of calcium, phosphorus, and potassium along with noticeable hypoalbuminemia. Starvation is indicated by decreased serum sodium and elevated serum uric acid, and malnutrition and dieting for weight reduction often manifest markedly decreased serum cholesterol and serum potassium levels. In a peripheral smear of blood, macrocytosis and hypersegmented neutrophils indicate a deficiency of vitamin B12 and/or folic acid. An elevation of chloride with a concurrent decrease in potassium and carbon dioxide content can result from an *iatrogenic* cause (as with tube feedings and inappropriate IV fluid administration). GI losses, the use of diuretics, and licorice ingestion can produce elevated carbon dioxide content of the hypochloremic metabolic acidosis type.

It is important to remember when interpreting blood studies that blood *serum* values will be 10 to 15% higher than *whole blood* figures. Values are given in Appendix B.

Blood values of the Hb, RBC count, and circulating blood volume of the active elderly show minimal changes. There are decreased values for these, however, among those elderly persons who are institutionalized. Assessments related to decreased blood values include fatigue, decreased attention span, low Hb levels, low BP, and a decreased circulating blood volume. Little change may occur in the WBC count and the differential WBC count values, but slight leukopenia or relative leukocytosis, hypersegmentation of neutrophils, and monocytosis may develop. The platelet count will show no appreciable difference, but there is somewhat less blood clot retraction ability, which may be due to a rise in the fibrinogen level.

Common interventions

Increased dietary components.   In addition to comparing the RDA of specific nutrients with lists of foods that are rich in these nutrients and providing the appropriate foods in sufficient amounts, it may be necessary to use dietary supplements in the form or tablets, liquids, powders, and prepared formulas to achieve the desired level of diet components. In cases of extreme need, parenteral forms of nutrition may be used.

Dietary needs change some as the adult ages. Some common alterations are presented in Table 2-5. Although there are some obvious discrepancies in the numerical values assigned to the categories of young adulthood, middle age, and elderly, the suggestions presented are related more to the activities and developmental tasks in which the persons are engaged, perhaps, than to the chronologic groupings.

Needs of young adults.   Young adulthood extends from ~20 or 25 to ~40 or 45 yr of age. Nutrition problems often arise as a result of busy lifestyles during this period.

Needs of middle-aged adults.   It has been suggested that for each decade of life beyond the 25th yr, caloric need declines by 7.5%. The decreased basal energy requirements and reduced activity alter the need for calories. Lifelong habits of consuming "empty calories" found in desserts, candy, fatty foods, and beverages contribute to the problem of obesity in these years.

Needs of the elderly.   The special requirements and increased nutrient needs of this age group are discussed throughout the chapter and are presented in Table 2-5. Foods that may be given to the elderly and other individuals who experience problems of biting and chewing are listed in Table 2-6. Suggestions for fortifying foods with protein are also provided.

Supplements.   Whenever lack of appetite, food intolerance, or special dietary restrictions interfere with intake of sufficient nutrients, blenderized

TABLE 2-4

Specific Observations in Assessment of Nutrition Status

Area	Positive nutrition	Negative nutrition
General survey and skin		
Skin	Alert, responsive.	Flat affect, listlessness.
	Smooth, slightly moist with good color; elderly have thicker skin over the abdomen and thin over extremities.	Poor tone and evidence of decreased SC fat and protein; fluid in tissues. Striae may be present; bleeding tendencies with anemia and lack of vitamin C; pale nail beds.
Appearance and vitality	Endurance, energy, and vigor; sleeps well at night; clothing fit.	Muscle wasting; loose clothing or tight clothing may suggest recent weight change.
Weight	Normal for height, age, and body build.	Does not compare favorably with standards for age, sex, and body build; under- or overweight.
Posture	Erect, arms and legs are straight, abdomen is in, chest is out.	Muscular weakness and poor tone, skeletal deformity; immobility or contractures at joints; twitching.
Head and neck		
Hair	Shiny, not easily plucked, appropriate texture and distribution.	Lacks luster, easily plucked, lesions on the scalp, flaky scalp, broken hair.
Glands	No enlargement.	Enlarged thyroid associated with iodine deficiency.
Eyes	Bright, clear, no fatigue or circles.	Dark circles, sunken; poor adjustment to darkness occurs with too little vitamin A; corneal arcus (ring of cholesterol deposits surrounding the iris) may be present.
Mouth	Lips are moist with good color; tongue is pink with surface papillae present, no lesions; gums are pink and firm without swelling or bleeding; teeth are straight without crowding; little odor.	Odor may indicate tooth decay, poor hygiene, or specific diseases; cracked mouth corners with riboflavin deficiency; altered sense of taste; drooling, inability to close mouth completely, excess dryness; very smooth tongue (glossitis) from riboflavin deficiency.

Facial skin and mucous membranes	Reddish-pink mucous membranes (darker in darker complexions); smooth, good color.	Bruising with scurvy; redness with beriberi; dry; lesions; pallor in mucous membranes associated with allergy and anemia.
Musculoskeletal		
Muscles	Well developed, firm.	Atrophied, flabby, twitches.
Skeleton	No deformities.	Bowing, contracture of joints.
Legs and feet	No tenderness, weakness, or swelling; good color.	Weakness and edema, discoloration.
Thorax	No deformities, symmetric.	Skeletal deformities with calcium loss and deficiency of vitamin D; women are particularly affected with osteoporosis after menopause.
Abdomen and GI functioning	Flat, good appetite and digestion; normal, regular elimination.	Enlarged liver and spleen; palpable masses from constipation; anorexia; diarrhea.
Nervous control, mental status, and cognitive functioning	Good attention span for age, does not cry easily, not restless or irritable.	Senile behavior and less ability to reason and recall recent events may be related to vitamin B-complex deficiencies.
Cardiorespiratory	Pulse and respiratory rates within normal limits; no edema.	Elevated pulse and respiratory rates occur with anemia; heart beat irregularities occur with too little potassium; edema can result from excess sodium intake and retention.

Adapted from Williams, S. R. Essentials of Nutrition and Diet Therapy. C. V. Mosby Co., St. Louis. 1978. Second edition. p. 8, and Thompson, J. M., and A. C. Bowers. Clinical Manual of Health Assessment. C. V. Mosby Co, St. Louis. 1980.

TABLE 2-5

Age-Specific Altered Dietary Needs

Age group	Increased need*
Young adult	
Pregnancy	Calories and all nutrients.
Female	Vitamin C.
Male	Protein, vitamin C, riboflavin, vitamin E, and vitamin B6.
Middle-aged male and female	High-nutrient-density foods, such as low-fat forms of milk and cheese, lean meats, etc.; protein, minerals, vitamins, low-cholesterol and low-calorie foods; water and fruit juices.
Elderly male and female	Stress and disease or injury increase the need for high-density-nutrient foods, water, fruit juice, protein, calcium, vitamin D (if no sunshine exposure), B-complex vitamins, low-cholesterol and low-calorie foods.

*Compared with age 18.

or commercially prepared formulas of nutrients may be used to provide any of the following: (1) complete oral or tube feeding intake, (2) fortification of dietary intake, or (3) supplementation of environmental foods eaten.

Elemental diets are those synthetically formulated and chemically defined or molecular diets that are comprised of known chemical nutrients. These may be taken PO, in liquid or reconstituted powder forms, or they may be specially prepared and tailored individually for IV administration as TPN or hyperalimentation.

Hyperalimentation (i.e., oversupplying with nourishment) is an elemental diet form that was developed to promote adequate nutrition and positive nitrogen balance in persons whose conditions (such as intestinal malabsorption or coma) did not permit assimilation of nutrients by more conventional means. Both caloric and specific nutrient requirements are provided in a hypertonic solution for IV administration of TPN.

Administration of **hypertonic IV solutions** with large molecules requires special techniques. Although some success has been attained with peripheral vein administration, the safest way to avoid the pain, swelling, clotting, and phlebitis that often accompany a peripheral placement is through the use of a cutdown into a central vein, such as the right or left subclavian vein, and then threading an IV catheter via the superior vena cava close to the right atrium. This placement permits the large and hypertonic molecules to be immediately diluted with a large volume of blood and to be dispersed quickly throughout the circulation. Although it is

TABLE 2-6

*Food Selection and Protein Fortification for Individuals with
Biting and Chewing Problems*

Category	Foods
Easy to chew	Fish, peanut butter, eggs, legumes, cheese, canned fruits and vegetables, some convenience dinners.
Hard to chew (must be minced, chopped, or cubed)	Whole meat, fresh fruits and vegetables.
Protein fortifiers	Add dry milk powder to cooked cereal, cream soup, and puddings. The following are listed in order of *increasing* cost: dry milk powder (noninstant), cottage cheese, soy flour, soy grits, high-protein baby cereal, eggs, wheat germ, grated cheese, peanut butter, seeds (sunflower, sesame), peanuts, brewers' yeast, nuts (especially pumpkin and squash kernels, cashews, walnuts).

Adapted from Ewald, E. B. Recipes for a Small Planet. Ballantine Books, Inc., New York. 1973. p. 326, and Lewis, C. M. Nutrition: Nutritional Considerations for the Elderly. F. A. Davis Co., Philadelphia. 1978. p. 15.

less often done, it is possible to create an arteriovenous fistula, such as that used for renal dialysis, as a route for hyperalimentation.

Nursing interventions

Measures to increase appetite. The "common sense" approaches consist of providing an attractive environment, serving hot foods hot and cold foods cold, giving smaller portions on a smaller plate, varying colors and textures of food within the same meal, and providing an unhurried and relaxed atmosphere at mealtime. In addition, food selection is important to increase appetite. High-nutrient-density foods, for example, will help provide sufficient nutrients without large portions and are the opposite of "empty calorie" foods, such as sugar and rich desserts. The concept of learning to select nutritionally compact foods is one that has relevance not only throughout the life-span, but also one that seems particularly important for the aged, who tend to prefer sweet things as their taste buds diminish, and for those who have had mobility restricted. Table 2-7 provides a few suggestions for high-nutrient-density vegetarian foods and snacks, which, even for those high in fat content, will help avoid saturated fats and large portions.

TABLE 2-7
High-Nutrient-Density Vegetarian Foods and Snacks

Dips for crackers or raw vegetables:
  1. cheese.
  2. beans.
  3. cottage cheese with herbs.
Sandwiches: whole grain bread with
  1. peanut butter and milk powder (mixed 1:1).
  2. sesame meal blended with honey and milk powder.
Main dish:
  1. bean loaf.
  2. vegetable casserole with cheese.
Snacks:
  1. powdered protein drinks.
  2. mixture of sunflower seeds, peanuts, raisins, and granola.
  3. mixture of cottage cheese, applesauce, nuts, and raisins.

Adapted from Ewald, E. B. Recipes for a Small Planet. Ballantine Books, Inc., New York. 1973. p. 330.

Tube feedings.   When a person cannot chew or swallow a PO diet, administration of nutrients through a nasogastric tube may be required to supplement or replace IV therapy. If the esophagus is obstructed, a gastrostomy or jejunostomy tube can be used to instill nutrients directly into the GI tract. Many of the dietary supplements taken PO can be used successfully for tube feedings, particularly when diluted with water to prevent the diarrhea that can accompany a high concentration of carbohydrates. Formulas are prescribed according to the individual's need and tolerance, beginning with small amounts of solution, which are gradually increased until between 200 and 400 ml are given q 3 or 4 hr. Feedings are given via gravity flow, Murphy drip or disposable bag, or a mechanical feeding pump. There are two types of preparations commonly used: blenderized and commercially prepared formulas.

Blenderized preparations are calculated formulas mixed with water so that fluid levels are kept adequate, sufficient calories are provided, and carbohydrates are minimized. The formula may contain pureed baby foods, meat, milk, vitamins, etc.

Numerous **commercially prepared** formulas are prescribed to meet total needs or very specific ones, such as the need for low-sodium content. Table 2-8 lists products grouped according to formulas that are lactose free, high in protein, or low in protein. This table also presents those formulas with other specific additions or restrictions that make them useful in the management of specific deviations from health.

Tube feeding procedures.   Introducing liquid feedings into the stomach through a tube is also called *gastric gavage.* Surgically placed tubes in

TABLE 2-8
Commercially Prepared Supplements

Type	Brand name
Blenderized (meat base)	Compleat-B
High nitrogen	Precision Moderate or High Nitrogen Vivonex High Nitrogen
High protein	Citrotein Meritene Sustacal Sustagen
Low calorie	Dietene (1,000, 1,200, or 1,400 cal)
Low lactose or lactose free	Ensure Isocal Lolactene
Low or no protein	Contralyte Vivonex Vivonex High Nitrogen
Low residue	Ensure Precision Low Residue

the stomach or jejunum are used for gastrostomy or jejunostomy feedings, respectively.

After ascertaining the type of formula prescribed, the amount ordered, the frequency of administration, and any specific directions, the patient is placed in a comfortable seated or semi-Fowler's position and the procedure is explained. Once the equipment and formula have been obtained, correct placement of the tube must be validated by aspirating contents of the stomach or jejunum, or by injecting a small amount of air into the tube while auscultating over the appropriate area. Aspiration of contents will not only validate placement of the tube, but will also indicate the degree of emptying between feedings. Contents aspirated during this step are to be returned via the tube to avoid depletion of electrolytes. The determination of whether to feed can be based on the volume obtained, with amounts >100 ml being reported and the feeding withheld. The formula, at the correct temperature to prevent cramping or injury, can be allowed to infuse through gravity flow with the help of a catheter tip syringe barrel used as a funnel, or by attaching the feeding tube to the appropriate feeding container.

Precautions during feeding include protecting the patient and the bed from spills; avoiding air entering the tube because it may distend the stomach or jejunum; using room temperature solutions rather than re-frigerated ones to reduce cramping and diarrhea; administering solutions at a rate of ≤60 ml/min at the onset of therapy; observing closely for signs of lactose intolerance (e.g., cramping and diarrhea), stomach cramps, or choking; following intermittent feedings with enough water to clear the tubing of formula (e.g., 10 to 15 ml) before clamping and securing the tube; allowing the patient to remain upright and turned to the right side or seated for ~30 min after the feeding to prevent regurgitation and promote movement through the intestines; and being certain that the equipment is properly cleaned and the formula appropriately stored between feedings.

The patient's safety should be ensured by leaving the call signal cord within reach and by checking the patient at set intervals. Data to be recorded on the patient's chart and appropriate flow sheets include the time, amount, type, and volume of aspirated contents measured and returned before the feeding, and how the patient responded to the feeding.

Hyperalimentation procedure. Expert nursing care is essential in the administration of hyperalimentation solutions for parenteral nutrition in order to avoid the common complications of infection (especially Candida septicemia), hyperglycemia, hypoglycemia, nausea, headache, lassitude, and infiltration of the catheter.

Strict asepsis is critical during catheter insertion, dressing changes, and the changing of bottles, filters, and tubing. The actual timing of dressing changes, filter changes, etc., varies with institutional policies and procedures; however, most hospitals change tubing and filters q 24 to 48 hr, and the dressing around the catheter insertion site q 2 or 3 days. Specially trained personnel using surgical masks and special scrubbing solutions should perform the procedure.

Many institutions prefer to use a pump device in order to ensure adequate flow for good nutrition and to avoid too rapid an infusion with accompanying hyperglycemia.

Keeping air out of the system is another critical aspect of care. Air can enter with thoracic volume changes, such as those resulting from taking a deep breath, when the catheter is in the vena cava. A fatal **air embolus** can be the unfortunate result of air entering the system. Asking the patient to bear down briefly (e.g., performing Valsalva's maneuver) or placing the patient in a slight Trendelenburg's position (i.e., feet higher than head) whenever the tube is open, being changed, or manipulated will prevent air being sucked into the tubing.

Table 2-9 provides the **nursing interventions** and **evaluation criteria** related to tube feeding and hyperalimentation.

TABLE 2-9

Evaluation Criteria for Nursing Interventions Related to Tube Feeding and Hyperalimentation

Interventions	Outcomes
Tube feeding	
Monitor fluid balance.	Balanced intake and output of fluids.
Assess skin turgor.	Good skin turgor.
Take vital signs.	Vital signs within normal range for age.
Estimate level of consciousness.	Alert and responsive.
Evaluate body wt.	Gradual increase in body wt toward normal range.
Assess laboratory values for BUN, serum sodium, and serum osmolarity.	Laboratory test results within normal limits.
Hyperalimentation	
Assess laboratory values for electrolyte balance.	All of the above outcomes *plus* positive signs of tissue repair.
Observe for untoward reactions to solutions.	Absence of signs of infection, untoward reaction to solutions, sugar in the urine, nausea, vomiting, lassitude, convulsions.
Observe for signs and symptoms of infection.	
Monitor weight gain.	
Observe for signs of tissue repair.	
Record intake and output to monitor balance.	
Take vital signs.	
Monitor urinalysis for sugar.	
Observe for nausea, vomiting, lassitude, and convulsions.	

CHAPTER 3

FLUID AND ELECTROLYTE BALANCE

Marianne Taft Marcus

OVERVIEW

The volume and composition of man's body fluid must remain constant in order to support life and maintain normal functions. Man is equipped with homeostatic mechanisms designed to maintain this important balance despite intake of varying amounts of water and solutes.

Many threats to this homeostatic system should concern nurses in all practice settings. Disturbances may occur as a result of (1) inability of individuals in the community to get adequate diet and fluids; (2) lack of understanding of what constitutes adequate diet and fluid intake; (3) potential risk factors, which include vomiting, diarrhea, burns, draining wounds or ulcers, fever, excessive perspiration, heat exposure, and edema; (4) disease states that affect homeostatic mechanisms, such as endocrine disorders, cardiac disease, GI disorders, impaired renal functioning, impaired respiratory functioning, or neurologic damage; and (5) iatrogenic factors, such as IV therapy, low-sodium diet, GI suctioning, paracentesis, thoracentesis, and medications/home remedies (diuretics, laxatives, and sodium bicarbonate).

This chapter is designed to provide the nurse with a review of the normal homeostatic mechanisms for regulating fluid and electrolyte balance, and to provide a reference for identifying specific imbalances with appropriate interventions.

Anatomy and physiology review

Composition and functions. The aqueous medium of the body is comprised of water and dissolved substances known as electrolytes (*see below*). **Water,** which constitutes ~60% of the adult body, is essential as a solvent. Its unique physical properties permit the body to withstand excesses of temperature. Body fluid is divided into **ICF** and **ECF.** Two-thirds of total body water is located within the cells (ICF). The ICF contains nutrients needed by the cells and is the environment for chemical reactions within the cells.

The ECF represents one third of total body water and is located outside of the cells. The ECF is responsible for carrying water, O_2, electrolytes, and nutrients to the cells and removing wastes such as CO_2 and protein breakdown products. The ECF also transports enzymes, hormones, RBCs, and WBCs. The ECF is further divided into interstitial fluid and plasma. **Interstitial fluid** lies outside the vascular space in the spaces between the cells. It constitutes three-fourths of the ECF. Lymph and CSF are considered interstitial fluids. **Plasma,** which lies within the circulatory system and forms the liquid component of blood, makes up approximately one fourth of the ECF. Plasma normally contains a higher percentage of proteins or colloids than interstitial fluid. These proteins and colloids maintain vascular volume by osmotically holding water within the blood vessels and preventing loss into interstitial spaces (Fig. 3-1).

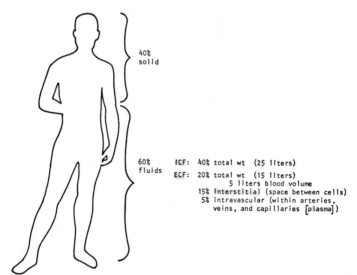

40% solid

60% fluids

ICF: 40% total wt (25 liters)
ECF: 20% total wt (15 liters)
    5 liters blood volume
    15% interstitial (space between cells)
    5% intravascular (within arteries, veins, and capillaries [plasma])

Figure 3-1. Fluid and solid composition of body weight. *See* text for discussion. (Courtesy of Edwin Hord, PhD.)

In addition to the ICF and ECF, there are secretions and excretions derived from ECF and manufactured by the stomach, pancreas, liver, and intestines (e.g., urine, feces, and perspiration).

Water balance depends on maintenance of an equal ratio between gain (intake) and loss (output) over a 24-hr period. Normal amounts and sources of water intake and output are listed in Table 3-1.

Electrolytes.   Body fluids contain two kinds of dissolved substances: those that break down into cations and anions and those that do not (e.g., glucose). Electrolytes are those substances that develop electrical charges (ions) when dissolved in water. Ions may be positively charged **cations**, such as sodium (Na^+), potassium (K^+), calcium (Ca^{++}), and magnesium (Mg^{++}). Other ions develop negative charges (**anions**), as is the case with chloride (Cl^-), bicarbonate (HCO_3^-), and phosphate ($HPO_4^=$).

Each fluid compartment has its own unique composition of water and electrolytes expressed in milliequivalents per liter. The milliequivalent is a measure of the chemical combining power of chemical activity of an ion. The principal ICF electrolytes are Na^+, Mg^{++}, and $HPO_4^=$; whereas the major ECF electrolytes are Na^+, Ca^{++}, and HCO_3^-. Cations and anions are balanced in each fluid compartment to maintain neutrality. The constant by which the variability of electrolyte quantities in secretions and excretions is measured is the normal electrolyte composition of plasma (Fig. 3-2).

Fluid and electrolyte movement.   Water and electrolytes continuously shift to maintain the relative stability of each compartment. The mechanisms by which this transport occurs are discussed below.

Diffusion may be defined as random, incessant movement of ions and molecules in all directions through a solution or gas. Particles move from an area of greater to lesser concentration in order to equalize the concentration in any compartment. Diffusion may be (1) *simple* passage through the pores of semipermeable membrane that separate the fluid compartments, or (2) *facilitated* passage, which occurs slowly and with the aid of certain membrane-bound carrier molecules (lipids), as is the case with large molecules such as protein and amino acids. The rate of diffusion depends on several factors: (1) Permeability of the membrane. The smaller the size of

TABLE 3-1
Normal Amounts and Sources of Water

Intake		Output	
Amount	Source	Amount	Source
ml/day		*ml/day*	
1,200	Beverages	1,500	Kidneys (urine)
1,100	Food	1,000	Skin, lungs (insensible)
300	Metabolic production	100	GI tract (feces)
2,600		2,600	

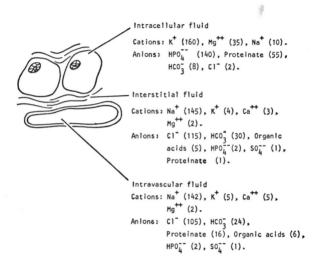

Intracellular fluid

Cations: K$^+$ (160), Mg^{++} (35), Na$^+$ (10).
Anions: HPO$_4^{--}$ (140), Proteinate (55),
HCO$_3^-$ (8), Cl$^-$ (2).

Interstitial fluid

Cations: Na$^+$ (145), K$^+$ (4), Ca^{++} (3),
Mg^{++} (2).
Anions: Cl$^-$ (115), HCO$_3^-$ (30), Organic
acids (5), HPO$_4^{--}$ (2), SO$_4^{--}$ (1),
Proteinate (1).

Intravascular fluid

Cations: Na$^+$ (142), K$^+$ (5), Ca^{++} (5),
Mg^{++} (2).
Anions: Cl$^-$ (105), HCO$_3^-$ (24),
Proteinate (16), Organic acids (6),
HPO$_4^{--}$ (2), SO$_4^{--}$ (1).

Figure 3-2. Electrolyte composition (in milliequivalents per liter) of ICF, interstitial fluid, and intravascular fluid. *See* text for discussion. (Courtesy of Edwin Hord, PhD.)

the diffusing particle, the greater the rate of its passage through the membrane. (2) The electrical charge of the diffusing ion. Membrane pores are lined with positively charged ions, which tend to repel or slow down transport of positive ions. (3) Concentration. The rate of diffusion is directly proportional to concentration. (4) Electrical potential difference. When a difference in electrical potential exists across the membrane, diffusion can occur even without a concentration difference. (5) Pressure gradient. Increased pressure on one side of the membrane increases the force of molecules attempting to diffuse.

Water moves from a lower concentration of solutes to one of higher concentration. This exchange of water through a semipermeable membrane, in order to maintain a concentration balance, is known as **osmosis**. A simple reminder of this mechanism is contained in the phrase "water goes to salt." Osmotic pressure is the drawing power of water based on the number of molecules or the number of dissolved particles per unit of water (expressed as milliosmoles). Normal body fluid osmolarity is 280 to 294 mOsm/kg. The ICF and ECF osmolalities are always equal. Clinically, the nurse should remember the all-important concept of osmosis when administering IV fluids. If a solution of the same electrolyte concentration as plasma (*isotonic*) is added to the bloodstream, the ICF and ECF remain balanced. Normal saline (0.9%) is an isotonic solution. When a solution of lesser concentration than plasma (*hypotonic* — e.g., 0.45% NaCl) is administered, water will go into the cells and cause them to burst. Conversely, if a *hypertonic* solution (e.g., 50% DW) in which the electrolyte concentration is higher than plasma is administered, water leaves the cells and causes them to shrink.

Active transport refers to the movement of ions from an area of lesser to greater concentration with the aid of energy provided by ATP released from the cells. This mechanism is similar to facilitated diffusion except that it always acts against a concentration or electrochemical gradient. The Na^+ pump is an example of active transport. Na^+ and K^+ do not penetrate the cell membrane easily. ATP provides energy to transform a single carrier so that it will transport both Na^+ and K^+.

Filtration refers to the transfer of water and dissolved particles through a permeable membrane from a region of high pressure to one of low pressure. This is accomplished by means of hydrostatic pressure produced by the pumping action of the heart. The passage of water and electrolytes from the arterial end of the capillary beds to the interstitial fluid is an example of filtration. In opposition to hydrostatic pressure, the oncotic pressure (or colloid osmotic pressure) of plasma proteins tends to hold water and electrolytes back. The movement of ECF between intravascular and interstitial compartments is determined by these opposing forces.

Homeostatic mechanisms controlling fluid and electrolyte balance. Despite the wide variation in what humans ingest, the temperatures to which they are subjected, the disease states that occur, and the continuous metabolic processes occurring within the cells, the fluid volume and electrolyte composition of ECF is held relatively constant. Almost every body system and organ is involved in maintaining this homeostasis.

Lungs: The work of the lungs in maintaining homeostasis is principally concerned with acid-base balance. The normal blood pH (hydrogen-ion concentration) is 7.35 to 7.45. When something occurs to alter that value, the lungs act within minutes to correct the situation. This is accomplished through hyperventilation or increased excretion of CO_2 (an acid) in the event of an excess of H^+ in the ECF. If the blood is too alkaline, hypoventilation may occur in an attempt to store CO_2 and raise the H^+ content of the ECF to normal.

Renocardiovascular system: The heart and blood vessels are responsible for adequate perfusion of blood (1,700 liters/day) to the kidneys where the main work of fluid and electrolyte homeostasis occurs. The kidneys themselves perform the following vital functions: (1) Excretory. Excrete products of protein catabolism, strong acids, drugs, and toxins. (2) Regulatory. Regulate concentration of specific electrolytes, volume of water in ECF, and BP (through renin secretion). (3) Regeneration. Produce HCO_3^- to act as a buffer in the event of excess H^+ concentration. (The kidneys take hours or days to respond to acid-base imbalance, whereas the lungs respond within minutes.) (4) Conversion. Change vitamin D to useable form. (5) Manufacturing. Produce erythropoietin required for normal RBC synthesis.

Endocrine system: The adrenals secrete hormones that affect fluid and electrolyte homeostasis. Aldosterone, a product of the adrenal cortex, conserves Na^+, Cl^-, and water, and facilitates the excretion of K^+. Release of aldosterone is increased in Na^+ depletion, pitting edema, dehydration, hemorrhage, stress, constriction of carotid and renal arteries, and administration of large doses of ACTH. Epinephrine and norepinephrine, hormones produced by the adrenal medulla, function in much the same way that the sympathetic nervous system does in times of emergency. They elevate BP, dilate blood vessels perfusing skeletal muscles, constrict blood vessels supplying the GI tract, increase pulmonary ventilation, and inhibit bowel and bladder emptying. The pituitary releases the all-important hormone for water conservation — ADH. Manufactured by the hypothalamus and stored in the pituitary, ADH acts on the pores of the collecting ducts of the kidney nephrons to determine the amount of water reabsorbed from tubular urine and, thus, the amount of water conserved. ADH is released in response to decreased circulating blood volume, pain, morphine sulfate, barbiturates, anesthetics, and emotional and physiologic stress. The parathyroids are also involved in fluid and electrolyte homeostasis. These tiny glands located near or in the thyroid, secrete parathormone, which controls Ca^{++} and $HPO_4^=$ metabolism. Parathormone maintains a normal level of Ca^{++} by promoting absorption of Ca^{++} from the intestine and increasing resorption of Ca^{++} from bone. Parathormone also increases renal excretion of $HPO_4^=$ ions. Thyroid hormone, produced by the thyroid, facilitates normal diuresis and Ca^{++} regulation and releases the hormones triiodothyronine (T_3) and tetraiodothyronine, which increase CO, thereby ensuring adequate kidney perfusion and urinary output.

GI system: The GI tract aids in homeostatic regulation of water by absorbing dietary fluids in addition to 7 to 9 liters of glandular and GI tract secretions each day. This absorption of fluid compensates for fluid loss through the skin, respiration, and kidney excretion.

Nervous system: The brain also aids in the regulation of body water volume. The midbrain has a volumetric monitoring system that receives information from receptors in the walls of the large blood vessels and sends this information to control systems for ADH release, thirst stimulation, and aldosterone release. In addition, the hypothalamus contains a thirst system that responds to changes in body fluid osmolarity.

Pathology

Clinical states that may be accompanied by fluid and electrolyte imbalance include (1) accentuation of the body's response to stress (e.g., pain, anesthesia, acute infections, fear, and trauma); (2) defective regulatory mechanisms (e.g., renal failure or insufficiency, pituitary tumors, obstructive pulmonary diseases, adrenocortical destruction, CNS lesions, metabolic disorders, and parathyroid disorders); (3) defective circulation of body fluids (e.g., CHF and shock); (4) excessive loss of fluid and electrolytes via normal routes (e.g., sweating, vomiting, diarrhea, and diuresis); (5) loss of fluid and electrolytes via abnormal routes (e.g., ostomies, GI fistulas, gastric or intestinal suctioning, burns or exudative skin lesions, hemorrhage, and accumulation of fluid and electrolytes in localized areas); and (6) periods of starvation or prolonged lack of food and/or fluid intake orally (e.g., restricted diets, inability to ingest food and fluids, and food and fluid restrictions required as preparation for surgical procedures, diagnostic tests, etc.).

General assessment

The general assessment of a patient starts with the **health history**, which consists of the following components.

Current health status: (1) Chief concern and duration of illness. (2) Nutrition: (a) Fluid and food intake since onset of illness (anorexia, thirst, changes in diet). (b) Recent weight loss or gain. (3) Medications: prescribed and/or home remedies. (4) Elimination.

Past history: Illnesses, injuries, and/or surgery.

Family history: Renocardiovascular, neuromuscular, and/or endocrine disorders.

Social history: Recent stressful situations.

Review of systems: (1) Body systems: integumentary, GI, GU, neuromuscular, and endocrine. (2) Mental status: perceived changes in mental and emotional status.

A complete **physical exam** should be performed with particular attention to direct inspection, palpation, percussion, and/or auscultation of all the systems identified above. In addition, the clinician should assess the patient's (1) vital signs; (2) breathing patterns (rate and depth); (3) skin and mucous membrane (tissue turgor; presence or absence of moisture in axilla, groin, and oral mucosa; lacrimation; salivation; and appearance of tongue); (4) peripheral veins (distension or inadequate filling); (5) state of sensorium and changes in behavior pattern; (6) neuromuscular status (weakness, paralysis, irritability, or tetany); (7) edema; (8) daily weights; and (9) intake and output measurements.

Finally, the general assessment involves relevant **laboratory data,** which may include any of the following components. (1) *Blood chemistries:* Electrolyte values, pH, PCO_2, CO_2 content, CO_2 combining power, serum osmolality, BUN, plasma proteins, Hct, serum proteins, and serum creatinine. (2) *Urinalysis:* Electrolytes, specific gravity, and pH. (3) *ECG.* (4) *Chest x-ray.*

Common interventions

General treatment consists of replacement of fluid and electrolytes, treatment of the underlying condition, and interventions related to specific entities.

Nursing interventions

Physical 1. Weigh the patient on admission and daily.
2. Measure and record all intake and output accurately.
3. Monitor and record vital signs on admission and as indicated by the condition. Notify the physician of hypotension.
4. Monitor neurologic vital signs on admission and as indicated by the condition. Notify the physician of decreased level of consciousness.
5. Monitor laboratory data closely.
6. Monitor for signs and symptoms of kidney and/or brain disease.
7. Restrict fluids as ordered (clearly indicate restriction at bedside).
8. Manipulate the environment to reduce sensory overstimulation.
9. Ensure safety with side rails if confusion, restlessness, or coma exists.
10. Assist the patient with ambulation when dizziness and hypotension exist.

Psychosocial 11. Reassure the patient. Stress the transient nature of the condition (when possible). Express confidence in therapies instituted to correct imbalance.
12. Notify the physician if the patient fails to respond to therapy as evidenced by continued presence of signs and symptoms of imbalance.

Educational 13. Assess the patient's knowledge of adequate fluid and electrolyte intake.
14. Provide an individualized plan of instruction to include such variables as kidney or brain impairment and mental disease.
15. Teach the patient to monitor intake and output.
16. Teach the patient the correct use of diuretics when applicable.

Evaluation criteria

Risk factors/complications minimized: Diagnostic data within normal limits. Vital signs within normal limits and charted. Neurologic vital signs within normal limits and recorded. Patient conscious. Intake and output values within normal limits and recorded. Daily weights within normal limits and recorded. *Safety measures implemented:* Quiet environment maintained. Side rails in place. IV (when ordered) infusing correct fluid at proper flow rate. IV site is free of signs of infection or infiltration. Notification of fluid restriction is clearly posted at bedside. Abnormal findings reported to physician(s). *Adequate patient knowledge base:* Patient demonstrates ability to (1) describe risk factors for electrolyte imbalance, (2) list sources and amounts of normal intake of water and electrolytes, (3) measure and record intake and output, and (4) state correct ratio of intake and output.

DEVIATIONS

WATER-SODIUM IMBALANCES

Water-sodium imbalances fall into two categories: osmolar imbalances and volume imbalances. **Volume (isotonic) imbalances** are those in which sodium and water increase or decrease together in the same ratio that is normally found in the ECF. **Osmolar imbalances** involve an alteration in the normal relationship of solutes to water in the ECF. Because Na^+ is the most abundant solute in the vascular space, the serum Na^+ level is the best indicator of the osmolality of blood.

HYPEROSMOLAR IMBALANCE

Hyperosmolar imbalance **(hypernatremia)** is a decrease in water relative to solutes or an increase in solutes relative to water in the ECF. Hyperosmolar imbalance may be caused by water deficit or extracellular solute excess. Conditions that may result in hyperosmolar imbalance include impaired thirst sensation (hypothalamic lesions or coma); dysphagia; extreme debility (inability to request or to drink fluids); unavailability of water; profuse diaphoresis; watery diarrhea; polyuria (diabetes insipidus and diabetes mellitus); loss of water from lungs, resulting from deep rapid breathing (tracheobronchitis); excessive IV administration of solutes (hypertonic solutions); and excessive administration of proteins (PO or by tube) without adequate water.

Shrinkage of the cells and dehydration occur as water moves from the ICF to the ECF in an attempt to compensate for the solute excess. Brain cells are particularly responsive to this process.

The following are the *signs and symptoms* of hyperosmolar imbalance: thirst; elevated temperature; increased pulse rate; diminished skin turgor (pinch test: skin remains tented for 20 to 30 sec); dry mucous membranes and rough tongue; soft, sunken eyeballs; difficulty in forming words without frequent moistening of the mouth; apprehension; restlessness; coma; convulsions; weight loss; oliguria; anuria; urine sp gr >1.030; elevated Hb; and serum Na^+ >145 mEq/liter. *Complications* include dehydration, shock, and renal failure.

Diagnosis is based on the health history, physical exam, and diagnostic tests for serum Na^+ level, Hb, and urinalysis.

Common interventions

Treatment consists of correcting the underlying reason for the imbalance and replacing water. PO or IV fluids may be used, depending on the patient's overall condition. The amount of fluids administered is determined by the size and weight of the patient, the presence or absence of fever, and the severity of dehydration.

Nursing interventions

Physical 1. Measure and record all intake and output accurately. Notify the physician of urinary output of <30 ml/hr or <500

ml/24 hr. (Indwelling urinary catheter in place in severe dehydration.)
2. Monitor and record vital signs on admission and q 2 hr (shock may be a complication of dehydration). Notify the physician of temperature >38.3°C (101°F), drop in BP, or elevated pulse or respiratory rate.
3. Monitor for indications of water intoxication (*see below*) or hyperglycemia (thirst, fatigue, polyuria, and glycosuria), which may result from IV therapy administered to correct the imbalance. Notify the physician if symptoms occur.
4. Administer fluids as ordered. Provide and encourage PO fluids when appropriate. Monitor IV fluids. Give prescribed tube feedings with adequate water.
5. Provide scrupulous care of skin and mucous membranes: moisturize, change position, and clean and lubricate mouth, nose, and lips.
6. Manipulate the environment to guard against sensory overstimulation in the event of restlessness.
7. Ensure safety with the use of side rails if restlessness or coma exists.
8. Institute seizure precautions.
Educational 9. Assess the patient's knowledge of adequate fluid and Na$^+$ intake.
10. Provide an individualized plan of instruction. Include risk factors for hyperosmolar imbalance and appropriate sources and amounts of water and Na$^+$.
11. Teach the patient to monitor intake and output.
Prevention 12. Recognize and prevent etiologic factors noted above.

Evaluation criteria. *See* Overview. Risk factors/complications minimized: Skin clean and lubricated. Skin turgor normal. Mucous membranes hydrated. Absence of muscle weakness and/or twitching. Signs of apprehension and restlessness minimal. Patient conscious and alert.

HYPOOSMOLAR IMBALANCE

Hypoosmolar imbalance **(hyponatremia)** is an increase in water relative to solutes in the ECF. Hypoosmolar imbalance may be caused by water excess (water intoxication) or extracellular solute deficit. Conditions that may result in **water excess** include excessive water ingestion by the mentally ill patient; excessive fluid ingestion by alcoholics; inadequate excretion of water (as occurs in renal disease and brain lesions); administration of hypotonic fluids (PO or IV), especially to patients with increased ADH secretion after surgery, trauma, or morphine sulfate injections; and excessive administration of hypotonic solutions by rectum (tap water enemas). **Extracellular solute deficit** may result from insufficient NaCl intake (dietary or therapeutic); diuretic therapy; adrenal insufficiency; and administration of only water to replace water and Na$^+$

lost through diaphoresis, vomiting, or suctioning. Cells become swollen as water moves from the ECF to the ICF in an attempt to compensate for solute deficit. The neuromuscular system is particularly responsive to this process.

The following are the *signs and symptoms* of hypoosmolar imbalance: absence of thirst; depressed body temperature; rapid, weak, and thready pulse; hypotension; extremities cold to the touch (severe Na^+ depletion); neurologic signs (twitching, hyperirritability, disorientation, convulsions, and coma); dizziness when turning in bed; abdominal cramps and diarrhea; polyuria (oliguria in the presence of renal disease); urine sp gr <1.010; decreased Hb; and serum Na^+ <120 mEq/liter. Cerebral edema is a related *complication.*

Diagnosis is based on the health history, physical exam, and tests for the serum Na^+ level, urinalysis, and Hb.

Common interventions

General treatment consists of water restriction, correction of the underlying reason for the imbalance, administration of hypertonic IV solutions when cerebral edema occurs in the absence of renal disease, and prevention of cerebral edema by appropriate replacement of fluids with isotonic solutions.

Nursing interventions

Physical 1. Monitor and record vital signs on admission and as indicated by the condition. Notify the physician of hypotension.
2. Monitor for signs and symptoms of kidney and/or brain disease.
3. Restrict fluids as ordered (clearly indicate restriction at bedside).
4. Manipulate the environment to reduce sensory overstimulation.
5. Ensure safety with side rails if a coma exists.
6. Assist the patient with ambulation when dizziness and hypotension exist.
Educational 7. Assess the patient's knowledge of adequate fluid and Na^+ intake.
8. Provide an individualized plan of instruction to include such variables as kidney or brain impairment and mental disease.
9. Teach the patient to monitor intake and output.
10. Teach the patient the correct use of diuretics when applicable.
Prevention 11. Replace water and Na^+ losses with isotonic solutions: IV or PO (isotonic ice chips, bouillon, or fruit juice, or nasogastric tube irrigations).
12. Avoid excessive tap water enemas.

Evaluation criteria. *See* Overview.

EXTRACELLULAR VOLUME DEPLETION

Extracellular volume depletion **(hypovolemia)** is an isotonic imbalance in which water and electrolytes are lost together in the same proportion as exists normally. Therefore, the serum Na^+ level remains normal. Extracellular volume depletion may be caused by an abrupt decrease in intake, or a rapid or slow loss of fluids, as may occur in hemorrhage, diarrhea, vomiting, kidney disease, fistulous drainage, burns, systemic infection (fever), intestinal obstruction, decreased aldosterone secretion, excessive diaphoresis, abscesses, large open wounds, ascites, and severe uncontrolled diabetes mellitus.

During this process, there is a decrease in the size of the extracellular space and circulatory collapse, leading to eventual depletion of cellular fluid.

The following are the *signs and symptoms* of extracellular volume depletion: thirst, weakness, abdominal pain, nausea, decreased or absent stools (intestinal obstruction), anorexia, weight loss (in excess of 5%), diminished skin turgor (pinch test: skin remains tented for 20 to 30 sec), absence of sweat in axilla and/or groin, decreased tearing and salivation, difficulty in forming words without frequent moistening of the mouth, dry mucous membranes and longitudinal wrinkling of the tongue, decrease in neck vein fullness (when patient is supine), decreased venous pressure, increased venous filling time (>3 to 5 sec), elevated pulse, elevated respiratory rate, decreased body temperature (in the absence of infection), postural hypotension, oliguria progressing to anuria, urine Cl^- excretion <50 mEq/liter, elevated Hct, elevated serum protein, and hard fecal mass. Note that the serum Na^+ level is normal. *Complications* include renal failure and hypovolemic shock.

Diagnosis is based on the health history, physical exam, and tests for urinalysis, urine Cl^- determination, Hct, serum protein, and serum Na^+ level (normal).

Common interventions

Treatment consists of volume replacement without altering the electrolyte composition of the fluid. PO and/or parenteral solutions that are isotonic or balanced in electrolyte composition between the patient's minimal needs and maximal tolerances are given. The underlying reason for the imbalance should also be corrected.

Nursing interventions

Physical 1. Monitor urinary output frequently.
2. Measure and record vital signs on admission and q 2 hr.
3. Observe for signs and symptoms of hypervolemia (*see below*) while the patient is receiving isotonic IV solutions.
4. Administer fluids as ordered. Provide and encourage PO fluids when appropriate. Monitor IV fluids.
5. Provide scrupulous care of skin and mucous membranes: moisturize, change position, and clean and lubricate mouth and lips.
6. Ensure safety if postural hypotension exists.

7. Refer for immediate medical evaluation: urinary output of <30 ml/hr or <500 ml/24 hr, drop in BP below normal for the patient, elevation of pulse and respiratory rate, and signs and symptoms of hypervolemia (*see below*).

Educational 8. Assess the patient's knowledge of adequate fluid intake.

9. Provide an individualized plan of instruction.

10. Teach the patient to monitor intake and output.

Prevention 11. Recognize and prevent the etiologic factors noted above.

Evaluation criteria.   *See* Overview. Risk factors/complications minimized: Skin clean and lubricated. Skin turgor normal. Mucous membranes hydrated. Absence of postural hypotension. Venous filling time <3 sec.

EXTRACELLULAR VOLUME EXCESS

Extracellular volume excess (**hypervolemia**) is an isotonic imbalance in which water and electrolytes are gained together in the same proportion as exists normally in the ECF. Extracellular volume excess may be caused by an inability of the kidneys to rid the body of excess fluid and electrolytes. Conditions that may result in hypervolemia include excessive administration of isotonic solution (particularly at night when renal functioning is diminished); disease states in which homeostatic mechanisms for fluid and electrolyte balance are impaired (e.g., chronic kidney or liver disease, CHF, malnutrition, and hyperaldosteronism); and excessive administration of adrenal glucocortical hormones. During hypervolemia, there is expansion of the extracellular space and circulatory overload.

The following are the *signs and symptoms* of extracellular volume excess: weight gain; dyspnea, cough, moist rales, and pink frothy sputum (when pulmonary edema results); distended abdomen with shifting dullness to percussion (when ascites results); bilateral pitting peripheral edema (mild to severe); neck vein distension (>3 cm above the sternal angle); bounding pulse, which is not easily obliterated; hypertension; and hoarseness. Chest x-ray reveals fluid accumulation (in the presence of pleural effusion or pulmonary edema); and blood chemistries may indicate plasma dilution. Note that skin turgor, inguinal and axillary sweat, and the serum Na^+ level are normal. Pleural effusion, CHF, pulmonary edema, ascites, and generalized edema (anasarca) are related *complications*.

Diagnosis is based on the health history, physical exam, chest x-ray, and tests for BUN and serum K^+ levels.

Common interventions

Treatment consists of removal of excess water and electrolytes without altering the electrolyte composition of the body fluids, restriction of Na^+

and water, administration of diuretics, correction of the underlying reason for the imbalance, and the immediate treatment of pulmonary edema (*see* Chapter 15).

Nursing interventions

Physical 1. Measure and record vital signs on admission and q 2 hr (more frequently in the presence of respiratory or cardiovascular complications). Notify the physician of any elevation of BP, pulse rate, or respiratory rate above normal for the patient.

2. Measure abdominal girth on admission and daily when ascites is suspected or present.
3. Assess for the presence of peripheral edema on admission and daily.
4. Assess respiratory status on admission and daily. Record the specific location of any abnormal findings. Notify the physician of abnormal findings (e.g., moist rales).
5. Restrict fluids and Na^+ as ordered.
6. Schedule fluid intake appropriately to account for a 24-hr period.
7. Clearly indicate fluid restriction at the bedside.
8. Administer diuretics as ordered. Monitor for side effects.
9. Provide scrupulous skin care, particularly in the presence of edema.
10. Elevate any edematous parts.
11. Assist with frequent position changes when ascites and sacral edema are present.

Educational 12. Assess the patient's knowledge of adequate fluid intake.

13. Provide an individualized plan of instruction.
14. Teach the patient to monitor intake and output.
15. Instruct the patient regarding the Na^+-restricted diet.
16. Instruct the patient about the use of diuretics.

Prevention 17. Administer fluids with caution; particularly in the presence of kidney, liver, and/or cardiovascular dysfunction.

18. Closely monitor patients receiving adrenal glucocorticoid hormones.

Evaluation criteria. See Overview. Risk factors/complications minimized: Absence of adventitious breath sounds in all lung fields. Absence of pitting edema and ascites. Absence of hoarseness. Medications (when ordered) administered correctly and charted. Skin clean and intact. Safety measures implemented. IV (when ordered) infusing correct fluid at proper rate. (Despite fluid restriction, IV line may need to be in place to treat underlying disease entity.) IV (when ordered) site is free of signs of infection or infiltration. Notification of fluid restriction is clearly posted at bedside.

HYDROGEN ION IMBALANCE

Homeostatic mechanisms in H^+ balance

The chemical reactions necessary to sustain life are dependent on a delicate balance between **acids** and **alkalies** within body fluids. Millions of H^+ are generated each day, principally as a result of protein metabolism. The concentration of this highly reactive solute determines the relative acidity or alkalinity of body fluids. The pH of body fluids is the measure of this balance. (Normal ECF pH is 7.35 to 7.45.)

Acids contain H^+ and are capable of releasing this ion. Alkalies contain no H^+, but can accept them from acids. The strength or power of each substance is dependent on the number of H^+ it either contains (acids) or can accept (alkalies).

Acid-base balance is maintained by highly efficient control systems that (1) protect the body against changes in pH by releasing or accepting H^+ as the concentration falls or rises (buffers), and (2) remove H^+ permanently from the body (lungs and kidneys).

Bicarbonate-carbonic acid buffer system. The HCO_3^--H_2CO_3 buffer system is responsible for maintaining the H^+ concentration of ECF. The normal HCO_3^-:H_2CO_3 ratio is 20:1.

Protein buffer system. The protein buffer system consists of plasma proteins and Hb. This buffer system is active both in ICF and ECF, and is very powerful and versatile because it can function either as an acid or a base as the condition requires.

Phosphate buffer system. The $HPO_4^=$ buffer system consists of sodium dihydrogen phosphate (Na_2HPO_4) and is responsible for maintaining the H^+ concentration in ICF.

Lungs. The lungs maintain a normal concentration of CO_2 in body fluids ($PCO_2 = 40$ mmHg) by varying the rate and depth of ventilation. A balance is struck so that metabolic production of CO_2 equals pulmonary excretion. When the concentration of H^+ increases in the ECF, the PCO_2 increases (hypercapnia) and hyperventilation may occur. When the concentration of H^+ decreases in the ECF, the PCO_2 decreases (hypocapnia) and hypoventilation may occur.

Kidneys. The kidneys control nonvolatile acid excretion. They respond more slowly (24 to 48 hr) to changes in the pH of body fluids. The kidneys restore HCO_3^- to the body fluids by reabsorbing all filtered HCO_3^- and by regenerating new HCO_3^- to replace that which was consumed by buffering of metabolic H^+.

General considerations in H^+ imbalance

Assessment of H^+ imbalances is complicated by the fact that the regulatory mechanisms described above interact with each other. An imbalance in one of the regulatory processes causes a compensatory response from another process. ECF elevation of HCO_3^- and CO_2 may represent (1) primary imbalance, which occurs as a result of acid or base overload or lung or kidney disease, or (2) secondary imbalance, which occurs in response to compensatory mechanisms aimed at maintaining the normal pH of the ECF. (Table 3-2 illustrates this compensatory process.)

H^+ **imbalances** are classified as follows: (1) Acidosis: a physiologic disturbance that tends to add acid (increase the H^+ concentration) or remove base from body fluids. (2) Alkalosis: a physiologic disturbance that tends to remove acid (decrease the H^+ concentration) or add base to body fluids. (3) Respiratory imbalances: a basic failure in the pulmonary system, or a change in the concentration of CO_2 (H_2CO_3) in the body. (4) Metabolic imbalances: a basic failure in the renal system, or a change in the concentration of plasma HCO_3^-.

METABOLIC ACIDOSIS

Metabolic acidosis **(acidemia)** is a primary deficit of base HCO_3^- in ECF. Metabolic acidosis may be caused by any clinical situation that increases the production of nonvolatile acids or decreases the base HCO_3^- in plasma, causing a decrease in blood pH. Clinical events include (1) overproduction of metabolic acids, as occurs in diabetic ketoacidosis, starvation ketoacidosis, severe infection, hyperthyroidism, alcoholic keto-acidosis, and acid-producing tumors; (2) excessive intake of metabolic acids, which can occur when patients are on ketogenic and high-fat, low-carbohydrate diets, or when patients ingest acidifying drugs (e.g., salicylic acid, boric acid, ammonium chloride, ferrous sulfate, and paraldehyde); (3) inadequate renal functioning, as in uremic acidosis and renal tubular acidosis; (4) excessive loss of alkali, as occurs in severe diarrhea, prolonged vomiting of deep GI contents, and GI or biliary intubation; and (5) severe tissue anoxia (lactic acidosis), as occurs in pulmonary disease, liver disease, and anemias.

The compensatory responses include the following: (1) Respiratory: The decrease in ECF pH stimulates respiration and the release of CO_2 (and, thus, H_2CO_3). (2) Renal: Na^+ and H^+ exchange in the kidneys is increased, causing excretion of H^+ in the form of ammonium (NH_4^+), which results in an acid urine. Excess K^+ is then present in the ECF. Every mole of NH_4^+ excreted results in the addition of a mole of HCO_3^- to the ECF in an attempt to compensate for the acidity of the ECF.

The following are the *signs and symptoms* of metabolic acidosis: apathy, disorientation, delirium, weakness, stupor, coma, hyperventilation (Kussmaul's respiration), cardiac arrhythmias and/or arrest (secondary to excess serum K^+), blood pH <7.35, plasma HCO_3^- <24 mEq/liter, hyperkalemia, PCO_2 <40 mmHg, and urine pH <4.5. Acidosis that results from diarrhea is usually associated with other electrolyte imbalances, such as volume depletion and K^+ imbalance.

Diagnosis is based on the health history, physical exam, and tests for plasma pH, plasma HCO_3^-, PCO_2, serum K^+, and urine pH.

TABLE 3-2
Regulation of Acid-Base Balance

| Parameter | Arterial blood* | | | Compensation factor |
	pH	PCO_2	HCO_3^-	
Normal	7.35–7.45	40 mmHg	24 mEq/liter	$HCO_3^-:PCO_2 = 20:1$, The body attempts to maintain this ratio at all times.
Respiratory acidosis	Decreased	Increased	Increased with compensatory metabolic response	Kidneys retain HCO_3^- during chronic CO_2 elevation.
Respiratory alkalosis	Increased	Decreased	Decreased with compensatory metabolic response	Kidneys excrete HCO_3^- during chronic CO_2 depression.
Metabolic acidosis	Decreased	Decreased with compensatory respiratory response	Decreased	Hyperventilation occurs to reduce the CO_2 level.
Metabolic alkalosis	Increased	Increased with compensatory respiratory response	Increased	Hypoventilation occurs to increase the CO_2 level.

*Changes in HCO_3^- levels take 24 to 48 hr, whereas PCO_2 changes occur immediately.

Common interventions

General treatment consists of recognizing and treating the etiologic factors that precipitated the imbalance. Mild to moderate imbalances will be corrected by the normal compensatory mechanisms (e.g., with chronic renal failure). Examples of specific therapy for moderate imbalances are the administration of insulin to treat diabetic acidosis, and infusion of glucose and saline to treat alcoholic ketoacidosis. Extreme and unresponsive situations will be treated by (1) administering an alkali (e.g., PO alkali such as $NaHCO_3$ or infusions of $NaHCO_3$ or molar sodium lactate); (2) restoring proper blood volume and osmolarity with isotonic solutions, because acidosis frequently results in dehydration secondary to vomiting and diarrhea; and (3) preventing hypokalemia. Complications of therapy include rebound respiratory alkalosis as a result of compensatory mechanisms, and hypocalcemia resulting in neuromuscular irritability and tetany. Calcium gluconate is administered to correct hypocalcemia.

Nursing interventions

Physical 1. Insert an indwelling urinary catheter in severe acidosis to facilitate hourly urine determinations. Notify the physician of a urinary output of <30 ml/hr or <500 ml/24 hr.
2. Measure the rate and depth of respirations.
3. Monitor for CNS depression (delirium and coma).
4. Observe for neuromuscular signs of K^+ excess (weakness, flaccid paralysis, and cardiac arrest). The patient may be placed on a cardiac monitor.
5. Observe for signs of rebound respiratory alkalosis (hypoventilation) and hypocalcemia (tetany) that may result from therapy.
6. Administer fluids and medications as ordered. Provide and encourage PO fluids when appropriate. If IV fluids are given, monitor the type of solution, rate, and site.
7. Institute seizure precautions.
8. Notify the physician if adverse respiratory, cardiovascular, and/or neuromuscular signs or symptoms occur.
Educational 9. Assess the patient's knowledge of the precipitating factors to metabolic acidosis.
10. Provide an individualized plan of instruction.
11. Teach the patient the appropriate management of the underlying disorder.
Prevention 12. Prevent etiologic factors when possible.
13. Provide careful management of clinical conditions (e.g., diabetes mellitus, acid-producing tumors, and renal disease).

Evaluation criteria. See Overview. Risk factors/complications minimized: Absence of CNS signs and symptoms (apathy, disorientation, delirium, weakness, stupor, coma). Absence of signs and symptoms of respiratory alkalosis. Absence of tetany. Absence of signs and symptoms of K^+ excess. Safety measures implemented: Seizure precautions instituted. Constant supervision of delirious patient. Cardiac monitor (when ordered) in place. Crash cart readily available.

METABOLIC ALKALOSIS

Metabolic alkalosis (alkalemia) is a primary excess of base HCO_3^- in the ECF. Metabolic alkalosis may be caused by any clinical situation that increases the base HCO_3^- of the plasma and/or decreases the H^+ concentration of the plasma, causing a rise in blood pH. Clinical events include (1) loss of excessive H^+, as occurs in vomiting, nasogastric tube drainage, lavage, fistulas, and diuresis induced by potent drugs such as furosemide; (2) loss of Cl^-, which leaves Na^+ free to attach to HCO_3^- and cause a rise in serum $NaHCO_3$; (3) excessive intake of alkali, as with ingestion of baking soda and milk of magnesia and excessive $NaHCO_3$ infusion in emergencies; and (4) hyperadrenocorticism, as occurs in Cushing's syndrome and primary aldosteronism.

Compensatory responses include the following: (1) Buffer: Increased HCO_3^- in the ECF reacts with acid buffer salts to decrease the HCO_3^- and increase H_2CO_3. (2) Respiratory: Hypoventilation occurs to conserve CO_2, increasing the PCO_2 and thereby increasing the H^+ concentration of ECF. Secondary respiratory acidosis and hypoxia (leading to lactic acidosis) may result from hypoventilation. (3) Renal: The kidneys attempt to conserve H^+ and excrete large amounts of K^+ and Na^+ with the excess HCO_3^-. This condition can result in severe hypokalemia. With H^+ conservation, NH_4^+ production slows and the urine becomes alkaline.

The following are the *signs and symptoms* of metabolic alkalosis: belligerence, irritability, disorientation, lethargy, tetany, convulsions, cyanosis, depressed respirations, decreased thoracic movements, apnea, irregular pulse, muscle twitching, paralytic ileus, cardiac arrest (secondary to hypokalemia), plasma pH >7.45, plasma $HCO_3^- >24$ mEq/liter, PCO_2 >40 mmHg, and urine pH >7.0.

Diagnosis is based on the health history, physical exam, and tests for plasma pH, plasma HCO_3^-, PCO_2, serum K^+, and urine pH.

Common interventions

The primary aims of therapy are recognition and treatment of the etiologic factors that precipitated the imbalance. Usual treatments include replacement of fluids with isotonic solutions to prevent electrolyte imbalance as a result of vomiting or gastric suction; elimination of excessive alkali ingestion; administration of K^+ if alkalosis results from diuretic therapy; treatment of adrenal hyperfunction (surgery, radiation); administration of KCl when alkalosis and K^+ depletion occur together; and administration of acidifying agents (NH_4Cl or arginine hydrochloride) when alkalosis is *extreme* and unresponsive to compensatory mechanisms or specific therapy. These agents must be administered slowly because they are extremely toxic.

Nursing interventions

Physical 1. Measure the rate and depth of respirations.

2. Monitor for hypotension and tachycardia. The patient may be placed on a cardiac monitor.

3. Monitor for CNS overexcitability.

4. Observe for neuromuscular signs of K^+ depletion (muscle weakness).

5. Observe for Trousseau's sign (carpopedal spasm of the hand when the BP cuff is tightened) and Chvostek's sign (local spasm of the lip, nose, or side of the face in response to a tap below the temple) secondary to Ca^{++} deficiency.

6. Observe for signs of secondary respiratory acidosis and hypoxia due to hypoventilation.

7. Administer replacement fluids and K^+ as ordered. If IV fluids are given, monitor the type of solution, rate, and site.

8. Irrigate gastric tubes with isotonic solutions.

9. Institute seizure precautions.

10. Notify the physician if adverse respiratory, cardiovascular, and/or neuromuscular signs or symptoms occur.

Educational 11. Assess the patient's knowledge of precipitating factors to metabolic alkalosis.

12. Provide an individualized plan of instruction.

Prevention 13. Prevent etiologic factors when possible.

14. Provide careful management of clinical conditions (e.g., Cushing's syndrome and primary aldosteronism).

Evaluation criteria. *See* Overview.

RESPIRATORY ACIDOSIS

Respiratory acidosis **(acidemia)** is an imbalance in which abnormal pulmonary ventilation causes an increase in H^+ concentration of body fluids secondary to excessive retention of CO_2. Respiratory acidosis may be caused by (1) depression of the respiratory center by cerebral disease, drugs (morphine), neuromuscular disorders (poliomyelitis), or cardiopulmonary arrest; (2) chronic pulmonary disorders such as emphysema and pulmonary fibrosis; (3) hypoventilation related to extreme obesity (Pickwickian syndrome); (4) acute pulmonary disorders such as bronchiectasis, pneumothorax, hemothorax, bronchial asthma, bronchial pneumonia, and pulmonary edema; (5) impaired ventilation secondary to CHF, acute alcoholism, and burns of the respiratory tract; (6) inspiration of excessive CO_2 in poorly ventilated spaces; and (7) upper abdominal incision with "splinting."

Respiratory acidosis results in excessive formation of H_2CO_3 from the CO_2 excesses; decreased $HCO_3^-:H_2CO_3$ buffer system ratio; increased H^+ concentration of plasma; lowered serum pH; and elevated or normal PCO_2. Compensatory responses include the following: (1) Buffer defense: Excess H_2CO_3 is neutralized by a Cl^- shift from plasma to RBCs in exchange for HCO_3^-. This corrects the $HCO_3^-:H_2CO_3$ ratio. (2) Respiratory: Hyperventilation occurs in response to increased PCO_2 and lowered serum pH in an attempt to remove excess CO_2. This mechanism is impaired in the presence of pulmonary disorders. (3) Renal: The kidneys attempt to lower H^+ concentration in body fluids by increasing the rate of H^+ and Na^+ exchange, which leads to H^+ excretion and reabsorption of Na^+. Na^+ joins HCO_3^- to form $NaHCO_3$. NH_4^+ formation is increased, which causes increased H^+ excretion in the urine. In the presence of pulmonary disease, renal compensation for this imbalance is crucial. As previously noted, renal compensation is slow compared with respiratory compensation. Consequently, a severe imbalance may result.

The following are the *signs and symptoms* of respiratory acidosis: impaired respiration (dyspnea, wheezing, hyperventilation); CNS changes (disorientation progressing to coma); tachycardia and arrhythmias (inadequate oxygenation secondary to pulmonary impairment); plasma pH <7.35; plasma HCO_3^- >24 mEq/liter; urine pH <4.5; and elevated or normal PCO_2. *Complications* include CO_2 narcosis, ventricular fibrillation, and hyperkalemia.

Diagnosis is based on the health history, physical exam, chest x-ray, and tests for plasma pH, plasma HCO_3^-, PCO_2, serum K^+, and urine pH.

Common interventions

General interventions consist of treating underlying pulmonary disorders by administering antibiotics, bronchodilators, and O_2; assisting with breathing exercises; and performing postural drainage. Uncompensated respiratory acidosis is treated by (1) administering PO or IV $NaHCO_3$ (rapid administration during cardiac arrest), observing for signs of tetany, and administering calcium gluconate if tetany develops, and (2) maintaining fluid and electrolyte balance to prevent dehydration and hyperkalemia. Complications of therapy include CO_2 narcosis when large quantities of O_2 are given to patients with chronic CO_2 retention; rebound respiratory alkalosis; and tetany secondary to sodium bicarbonate administration.

Nursing interventions

Physical 1. Measure the rate and depth of respirations.
2. Monitor the pulse rate and rhythm closely.
3. Observe for neuromuscular signs of K^+ excess (weakness, flaccid paralysis, cardiac arrest). The patient may be placed on a cardiac monitor.

4. Observe for signs and symptoms of CO_2 narcosis (drowsiness, irritability, depression, hallucinations, coma, paralysis, convulsions, facial tremors, poor ventilation, tachycardia, and arrhythmias).
5. Observe for rebound respiratory alkalosis (*see below*).
6. Administer fluids and medications as ordered. Provide and encourage PO fluids when appropriate. If IV fluids are given, monitor the type of solution, rate, and site.
7. Institute safety measures such as constant attendance and/or side rails when disorientation or coma is present.
8. Institute seizure precautions.
9. Administer therapy for correction of respiratory disorders (use O_2 with extreme caution).
10. Notify the physician if respiratory, cardiovascular, and/or neuromuscular signs or symptoms occur.

Educational 11. Assess the patient's knowledge of precipitating factors to respiratory acidosis.
12. Provide an individualized plan of instruction.
13. Teach the patient the appropriate management of the underlying respiratory disorder.

Prevention 14. Limit alkaline substances (e.g., carbonated beverages, bicarbonate of soda) for patients with pulmonary disorders that restrict respiratory excursion.
15. Provide careful management of clinical conditions that result in inadequate oxygenation or CO_2 retention.

Evaluation criteria. See Overview.

RESPIRATORY ALKALOSIS

Respiratory alkalosis (alkalemia) is an imbalance in which hyperventilation accelerates CO_2 loss with a resultant primary deficit of H_2CO_3 in the ECF.

Respiratory alkalosis may be caused by hyperventilation due to anxiety, fever, strenuous exercise, acute hypoxia (high altitudes, pneumonia, acute pulmonary edema, asthma), salicylate intoxication, excessive mechanical ventilation, bacteremia, CNS diseases (tumors, encephalitis, meningitis), chronic hepatic insufficiency, chronic hypoxia (lung disease, cardiovascular diseases), intracranial surgery, and voluntary hyperventilation (overbreathing by a swimmer preparing to go underwater).

Respiratory alkalosis results in increased H^+ concentration in plasma and a decreased PCO_2; an increased $HCO_3^-:H_2CO_3$ ratio in that buffer system; and a rise in serum pH. Compensatory responses include the following: (1) Buffer defense: The plasma content of organic acid is increased and the acids react with excess HCO_3^- to neutralize them and correct the $HCO_3^-:H_2CO_3$ buffer ratio. (2) Respiratory: Hypoventilation occurs in response to decreased PCO_2 levels. By this mechanism the decrease in plasma H_2CO_3 is compensated with a resultant H^+ excess that is excreted by the kidneys. (3) Renal: The kidneys function to stop reabsorption of HCO_3^- and speed up its excretion, and to diminish NH_4^+ production to retain H^+ for restoration of the normal $HCO_3^-:H_2CO_3$ buffer ratio. An alkaline urine results.

The following are the *signs and symptoms* of respiratory alkalosis: increased neuromuscular irritability (hyperreflexia, positive Chvostek's sign, positive Trousseau's sign); convulsions; deep, rapid breathing; light-headedness; circumoral paresthesia; tetany; loss of consciousness; plasma pH >7.45; plasma HCO_3^- <24mEq/liter; PCO_2 <40 mmHg; and urine pH >7.0. Table 3-3 provides a summary of the major signs and symptoms associated with H^+ imbalances. Hypokalemia is a related *complication* when respiratory alkalosis is prolonged.

Diagnosis is based on the health history, physical exam, and tests for plasma pH, plasma HCO_3^-, PCO_2, urine pH, and serum K^+.

Common interventions

General treatment consists of elimination of the cause of hyperventilation and treatment of underlying disorders, such as salicylate intoxication, neurologic diseases, chronic hepatic insufficiency, chronic hypoxia, and anxiety. Severe symptoms may be treated by having the patient rebreathe into a bag. Rebreathing his own CO_2 raises the H^+ concentration of the plasma.

Nursing interventions

Physical 1. Measure the rate and depth of respirations.
    2. Monitor for neuromuscular irritability (reflexes, Chvostek's and Trousseau's signs, convulsions, paresthesias, tetany).
    3. Observe for signs and symptoms of hypokalemia when respiratory alkalosis is prolonged.
    4. Administer fluids, medications, and treatments as ordered to correct the underlying cause of hyperventilation.
    5. Institute seizure precautions.
    6. Provide a rebreathing bag when ordered.
    7. Notify the physician if adverse respiratory, cardiovascular, and/or neuromuscular signs or symptoms occur.
Educational 8. Assess the patient's knowledge of the precipitating factors to respiratory alkalosis.
    9. Provide an individualized plan of instruction.
    10. Teach the patient the appropriate management of underlying disease entities.
    11. Discuss the factors that precipitate anxiety and alternative coping mechanisms.
Prevention 12. Check mechanical ventilators hourly.

TABLE 3-3

Major Signs and Symptoms Associated With Primary Acid-Base Imbalance

Body system	Acidosis		Alkalosis	
	Respiratory	Metabolic	Respiratory	Metabolic
Mental status	Disorientation Coma	Apathy Disorientation Delirium Stupor Coma	Light-headedness Loss of consciousness	Belligerence Irritability Lethargy Disorientation
Respiratory	Dyspnea Wheezing Hyperventilation	Hyperventilation (Kussmaul respirations)	Deep, rapid respirations	Cyanosis Depressed respirations Apnea
Cardiovascular	Tachycardia Arrhythmias	Cardiac arrhythmias Cardiac arrest		Irregular pulse Cardiac arrest
GI		Nausea Vomiting Diarrhea (etiologic factors)		Nausea Vomiting (etiologic factors) Paralytic ileus
Neuromuscular		Weakness	Hyperreflexia Positive Chvostek's and Trousseau's signs Convulsions Circumoral paresthesia Tetany	Tetany Convulsions Muscle twitching Positive Chvostek's and Trousseau's signs
Significant laboratory data	Plasma pH <7.35 Plasma HCO_3^- >24 mEq/liter PCO_2 elevated or normal Urine pH <4.5	Plasma pH <7.35 Plasma HCO_3^- <24 mEq/liter Hyperkalemia PCO_2 <40 mmHg Urine pH <4.5	Plasma pH >7.45 Plasma HCO_3^- <24 mEq/liter PCO_2 <40 mmHg Urine pH >7.0	Plasma pH >7.45 Plasma HCO_3^- >24 mEq/liter Hypokalemia PCO_2 >40 mmHg Urine pH >7.0

13. Educate the public regarding the dangers associated with hyperventilation before underwater swimming.
14. Prevent etiologic factors when possible.

Evaluation criteria. See Overview. Risk factors/complications minimized: Absence of neuromuscular signs and symptoms. Absence of signs and symptoms of hypokalemia. Adequate knowledge base demonstrated: Patient can describe risks for respiratory alkalosis, list factors that precipitate anxiety, and name alternative measures for coping with anxiety.

POTASSIUM IMBALANCES

Potassium (K^+) is the major cation of the ICF. This electrolyte helps to maintain ICF osmotic pressure, aids in transmission of neuromuscular impulses, facilitates carbohydrate and protein metabolism, affects acid-base balance, and affects kidney functioning. The normal serum K^+ level is 3.5 to 5.0 mEq/liter. Serum values of K^+ do not necessarily reflect body stores of this electrolyte because most K^+ is in the ICF.

POTASSIUM DEFICIT

Potassium deficit **(hypokalemia)** is an imbalance in which the serum K^+ level is <3.5 mEq/liter. Potassium deficit may be caused by the following factors: (1) Inadequate intake of K^+, as occurs in extreme dieting, acute alcoholism, anorexia, and NPO status prior to surgery, diagnostic procedures, or as therapy. (2) Excessive loss of K^+, as occurs in diuretic therapy (thiazides, furosemide, ethacrynic acid, mercurials, acetazolamide); primary and secondary aldosteronism and adrenal steroid therapy (stimulate Na^+ retention and excretion in the kidneys); laxative and enema abuse (decreases K^+ absorption time); drainage or suctioning of gastric/GI secretions (richer in K^+ than serum); excessive administration of IV solutions (especially saline) without replacing K^+; prolonged vomiting; diarrhea, ulcerative colitis, intestinal fistulas; excessive diaphoresis without K^+ replacement; renal disease (defective reabsorption or accelerated excretion of K^+); and increased shift of K^+ into cells (treatment of diabetic acidosis and metabolic alkalosis). (3) Increased utilization of K^+ (healing phase of burns).

Potassium deficit results in the following: (1) Increase in resting potential of the cell membrane. Membrane depolarization is stimulated (Na^+ moves into cell and K^+ moves out). Nerve and muscle activity is decreased (neuromuscular, cardiovascular, GI, respiratory, and renal systems experience muscular weakness and atony). (2) Link to acid-base balance (alkalosis enhances renal K^+ secretion).

The following are the *signs and symptoms* of potassium deficit: muscle weakness progressing to total paralysis; shallow respirations progressing to respiratory arrest; lethargy; apathy; irritability; mental confusion and depression; diminished deep tendon reflexes; postural hypotension; arrhythmias; weak, rapid, irregular pulse; ECG changes (low, flat T wave, increased prominence of U wave, sagging ST segment); cardiac arrest; anorexia; nausea and vomiting; abdominal distension progressing to paralytic ileus; increased thirst; polyuria and nocturia (decreased concentration capacity of the kidneys); and serum K^+ <3.5 mEq/liter. Acid-base imbalance and increased incidence of digitalis toxicity (*see* Chapter 15) are related *complications.*

Diagnosis is based on the health history, physical exam, an ECG, and tests for the serum K^+ level.

Common interventions

Treatment consists of PO administration of K^+ via K^+-rich foods (e.g., oranges, bananas, foods high in protein) and/or medications (e.g., KCl, potassium triplex, potassium citrate, potassium gluconate). IV administration of K^+ may be used when the deficit is severe or GI disorders prohibit PO administration. The complications of therapy should be prevented. PO K^+ preparations can cause irritation of gastric mucosa, and should, therefore, be administered with a full glass of water. IV K^+ preparations can cause iatrogenic hyperkalemia (particularly in the presence of inadequate renal functioning), K^+ toxicity with impending cardiac arrest, and pain at the IV site.

Nursing interventions

Physical 1. Monitor vital signs. (Cardiac monitor should be used when severe hypokalemia exists or when the patient is receiving large doses of IV K^+.) Notify the physician of changes in vital signs.
2. Observe for and report signs and symptoms of hyperkalemia (*see below*).
3. Observe for and report signs and symptoms of digitalis toxicity.
4. Administer foods, fluids, and medications as ordered. Provide adequate water with PO K^+ preparations.
5. Do not exceed concentration of 40 to 60 mEq K^+/liter, if IV K^+ is administered. The infusion rate should not exceed 20 mEq/hr unless severe continuous loss indicates more intensive therapy.
6. Institute safety measures, such as constant attendance and/or side rails when mental confusion is present.
7. Assist the patient to ambulate when weakness and hypotension are present.
8. Observe for signs and symptoms of paralytic ileus (abdominal distension, absence of bowel sounds). Maintain NPO status and notify the physician if these symptoms occur.
9. Monitor urinary output closely. Notify the physician if the output is <30 ml/hr or <500 ml/24 hr.
Educational 10. Assess the patient's knowledge of the precipitating factors to hypokalemia.

11. Provide an individualized plan of instruction (e.g., foods rich in K^+, diuretic therapy considerations).
12. Teach the patient the appropriate management of the underlying disorders.
Prevention 13. Prevent etiologic factors when possible (e.g., caution against laxative and enema abuse).
14. Provide instruction concerning diuretic therapy.
15. Provide careful management of clinical conditions (e.g., renal disease, gastric suctioning).

Evaluation criteria. *See* Overview. Risk factors/complications minimized: Absence of signs and symptoms of acid-base imbalance. Absence of signs and symptoms of iatrogenic hyperkalemia (*see below*). Absence of signs and symptoms of paralytic ileus. Absence of signs and symptoms of digitalis toxicity, when appropriate. Safety measures implemented: Cardiac monitor (when ordered) in place. Crash cart readily available. Adequate knowledge base demonstrated: Patient can describe risks for hypokalemia, name signs and symptoms of hypokalemia, name a variety of K^+-rich foods, and discuss risks of diuretic therapy when appropriate.

POTASSIUM EXCESS

Potassium excess **(hyperkalemia)** is an imbalance in which the serum K^+ level is >5.0 mEq/liter. Potassium excess may be caused by any of the three following factors: (1) Inadequate excretion of K^+, as occurs in acute and chronic renal failure, adrenal insufficiency (hypoaldosteronism, Addison's disease), and diuretic therapy with K^+-sparing drugs (spironolactone, triamterone, amiloride). (2) Excessive shift of K^+ from tissues (ICF) to ECF, as occurs in severe tissue damage (burns, crushing injuries, hemolysis, internal bleeding), drugs (succinylcholine, digitalis poisoning), and acidosis. (3) Excessive intake of K^+, as occurs in rapid IV infusions of K^+ and excessive doses of PO K^+ (particularly when renal functioning is impaired).

Potassium excess results in a decrease in resting cell membrane potential. There is initial nerve and muscle irritability. Severe or prolonged K^+ excess results in muscle weakness and flaccid paralysis (neuromuscular, cardiovascular, GI, renal, and respiratory systems affected). Potassium excess is also linked to acid-base balance (acidosis depresses renal K^+ secretion).

The following are the *signs and symptoms* of potassium excess: postural hypotension, bradycardia progressing to cardiac arrest, ECG changes (tall tented T waves, widening QRS, ST segment depression), nausea and vomiting, diarrhea, intestinal colic, oliguria progressing to anuria, muscle twitching progressing to weakness and flaccid paralysis, and serum K^+

level >5 mEq/liter. *Complications* include acid-base imbalance and respiratory arrest.

Diagnosis is based on the health history, physical exam, ECG, and serum K^+ level.

Common interventions

Treatment consists of recognition and treatment of etiologic factors that precipitated the imbalance. Mild K^+ excess imbalance (<6.5 mEq/liter) will be corrected solely by treating the underlying cause, e.g., eliminating all sources of K^+ if excessive intake is the cause. Moderate to severe imbalances are treated by IV infusions of hypertonic solutions (glucose, $NaHCO_3$, Na^+) to promote movement of K^+ into the ICF; insulin therapy to increase glycogen storage and pull K^+ (with glycogen) into the ICF; large amounts of PO fluids to encourage increased urinary output (dialysis may be required with renal impairment); and/or retention enemas of cation exchange resins (sodium polystyrene sulfonate) to remove K^+ through the feces. (Resins are not absorbed, but exchange Na^+ and H^+ for K^+, which is then excreted. PO resins are also available, but the effect is slower.)

Nursing interventions

Physical 1. Monitor vital signs. Notify the physician of changes in vital signs. (Cardiac monitor should be used in severe hyperkalemia.)

2. Administer fluids and medications as ordered.

3. Maintain bed rest until K^+ is normal.

4. Monitor urinary output closely. Notify the physician if the output is <30 ml/hr or <500 ml/24 hr.

5. Assist the patient to ambulate when weakness is present.

Educational 6. Assess the patient's knowledge of the precipitating factors to hyperkalemia.

7. Provide an individualized plan of instruction (e.g., diuretic therapy considerations).

8. Teach the patient the appropriate management of the underlying disorders.

Prevention 9. Prevent etiologic factors when possible (e.g., rapid infusion of K^+).

10. Provide careful management of clinical conditions and/or drug therapy (e.g., hypoaldosteronism, K^+-sparing diuretics).

Evaluation criteria. *See* Overview. Risk factors/complications minimized: Absence of signs and symptoms of acid-base imbalance. Safety measures implemented: Cardiac monitor (when ordered) in place. Crash cart readily available. Adequate knowledge base demonstrated: Patient can describe risks for hyperkalemia, name signs and symptoms of hyperkalemia, and discuss risks of diuretic therapy when appropriate.

CALCIUM IMBALANCES

Body calcium exists in two forms: (1) calcium salts in bone (99%) provide strength for bones and teeth and act as a reservoir for tissue and ECF calcium, and (2) calcium in tissues and ECF (1%). **Serum calcium** exists in several forms: plasma protein bound — unable to leave vascular space (50%); (2) nonionized — combined with citrate, phosphate, and sulfate (5%); and (3) ionized — able to leave vascular space (45%). Ionized calcium is essential for blood coagulation, muscle contractility (including cardiac muscle), transmission of nervous impulses, and maintenance of cell membrane strength. Serum calcium is regulated by the parathyroid glands, dependent on vitamin D and protein for absorption and utilization, and inversely related to serum phosphorus levels. The normal serum calcium level is 4.8 to 5.8 mEq/liter. This value only represents the 1% of bodily calcium that exists in serum in the three forms noted above.

CALCIUM DEFICIT

Calcium deficit **(hypocalcemia)** is an imbalance in ionized Ca^{++} reflected in a serum Ca^{++} level <4.8 mEq/liter. Calcium deficit may be caused by malabsorption of Ca^{++} from the GI tract (e.g., sprue, acute and chronic pancreatitis); excessive loss of Ca^{++} through the wound exudate (e.g.,trauma); excessive loss of Ca^{++} through the kidneys (e.g., renal failure); inadequate dietary intake of Ca^{++} (e.g., with pregnancy and lactation); hypoparathyroidism (e.g., primary, surgically induced); vitamin D deficiency; rapid correction or overcorrection of acidosis (Ca^{++} ionization is increased in acidosis; when balance is restored, hypocalcemia may result); chronic laxative ingestion (alkalosis decreases Ca^{++} ionization); excessive administration of citrated blood (citrate binds with Ca^{++}); and hyperphosphatemia (renal insufficiency, potential complication of hyperalimentation).

Calcium deficit leads to an increase in neuromuscular irritability, which produces hyperreaction of motor and sensory nerves to stimuli, and to decreased cardiac contractility.

The following are the *signs and symptoms* of calcium deficit: tetany; paresthesias, numbness, or tingling; increased peristalsis (nausea, vomiting, diarrhea); convulsions; muscle spasms and cramps; hyperreflexia; circumoral numbness; positive Chvostek's sign; positive Trousseau's sign; laryngospasm; cardiac arrhythmias/arrest; ECG changes (prolonged Q-T interval); serum Ca^{++} <4.8 mEq/liter; elevated serum phosphorus; and 24-hr urine (Sulkowitch's test) shows no precipitation. Osteomalacia and osteoporosis are related *complications.* **Osteomalacia** is a rare condition resulting from severe and prolonged Ca^{++} deficit. In this disorder, bones lose calcium and phosphorus and become soft and pliable. Subsequently, the patient shrinks in height. **Osteoporosis** occurs in 25% of women and

20% of men >70 yr of age. In this disorder, bones become thinner, lighter, and porous. The signs and symptoms include decreased height, frequent painful fractures, and back pain.

Diagnosis is based on the health history, physical exam, ECG, Sulkowitch's test (24-hr urine), and serum Ca^{++} and phosphorus levels.

Common interventions

Treatment consists of recognition and treatment of the causative factors of the imbalance. Mild hypocalcemia, not accompanied by tetany is treated with Ca^{++} salts and vitamin D (to increase absorption): calcium lactate PO, calcium chloride PO or IV, or calcium gluconate PO, IM, or IV. Severe hypocalcemia, accompanied by tetany is treated with IV Ca^{++} (usually 10% Ca^{++} solution) administered slowly until symptoms disappear. The following complications of therapy should be prevented: rebound hypercalcemia (*see below*); tissue hypoxia and sloughing (if IV Ca^{++} infiltrates); and increased incidence of digitalis toxicity and cardiac arrest (when digitalized patients are given IV Ca^{++}).

Nursing interventions

Physical 1. Measure cardiac rate and rhythm. Notify the physician of changes in these measurements. (Cardiac monitor should be used when severe hypocalcemia exists.)
2. Monitor for progression of CNS symptoms (e.g., laryngospasm, convulsions). Notify the physician if these symptoms occur.
3. Administer PO medications as ordered, 30 min before meals or at bedtime to increase absorption.
4. Prevent infiltration if IV Ca^{++} is administered.
5. Do not add Ca^{++} to IV solutions that contain carbonate or phosphate (precipitation will result).
6. Question IV Ca^{++} administration if the patient is receiving a digitalis preparation.
7. Monitor for rebound hypercalcemia (*see below*). Notify the physician if these symptoms occur.
8. Institute seizure precautions and padded side rails.
9. Assist with ambulation and movement when chronic hypocalcemia is present (pathologic fractures may result from demineralized bone).
Educational 10. Assess the patient's knowledge of precipitating factors to hypocalcemia.
11. Provide an individualized plan of instruction (e.g., foods rich in Ca^{++}, vitamin D, and protein).
12. Teach the patient the appropriate management of the underlying disorders.
Prevention 13. Prevent etiologic factors when possible (e.g., caution against laxative abuse).

14. Provide careful management of clinical conditions (e.g., hypoparathyroidism, pancreatitis).
15. Observe patients closely after thyroid surgery for symptoms of hypocalcemia. Calcium gluconate (IV) should be available at the bedside.
16. Prevent osteoporosis by encouraging physical activity and an appropriate diet (high-protein, vitamin D, and Ca^{++} supplements).

Evaluaton criteria. See Overview. Risk factors/complications minimized: Absence of signs and symptoms of hypercalcemia. Absence of signs and symptoms of digitalis toxicity, when appropriate. Safety measures implemented: Cardiac monitor (when ordered) in place. Crash cart readily available. Padded side rails in place. Seizure precautions instituted. Adequate knowledge base demonstrated: Patient can describe risks for hypocalcemia, name signs and symptoms of hypocalcemia, name a variety of Ca^{++}-rich foods, and list measures to prevent osteoporosis.

CALCIUM EXCESS

Calcium excess **(hypercalcemia)** is an imbalance in ionized Ca^{++} reflected in a serum Ca^{++} level >5.8 mEq/liter.

Calcium excess may be caused by (1) excessive mobilization of Ca^{++} from bones, as occurs in prolonged immobility, malignant neoplasms, increased parathyroid hormone levels, excessive vitamin D intake, and acidosis (increases Ca^{++} ionization); (2) decreased renal excretion of Ca^{++}, as occurs with thiazide diuretics (mild hypercalcemia) and renal failure; and (3) excessive intake of Ca^{++}, as occurs in milk-alkali syndrome (patients ingesting milk and alkaline antacids for peptic ulcer symptoms) and dietary excesses.

Calcium excess leads to decreased neuromuscular activity, reabsorption of Ca^{++} from bone, and hypercalciuria, which impairs the ability of the kidneys to concentrate urine.

The following are the *signs and symptoms* of calcium excess: bone pain, flank pain, polyuria, GI symptoms (diarrhea, constipation, anorexia, nausea and vomiting), ECG changes (ventricular arrhythmias), CNS depression (hyporeflexia, lethargy, coma), muscle fatigue, serum Ca^{++} >5.8 mEq/liter, 24-hr urine (Sulkowitch's test) shows increased precipitation, elevated BUN (renal damage), and x-ray (may reveal radiopaque urinary stones/bone cavitation). *Complications* of calcium excess include renal calculi, osteoporosis, osteomalacia, peptic ulcer, renal failure, pathologic fractures, and hypercalcemic crisis. During a hypercalcemic crisis (a medical emergency) the patient will exhibit serum Ca^{++} levels >8 mEq/liter, polyuria, polydipsia, volume depletion, fever, altered levels of consciousness/acute psychosis, azotemia, and/or cardiac arrest.

Diagnosis is based on the health history, physical exam, ECG, x-rays of the kidneys and long bones, Sulkowitch's test (24-hr urine), and BUN and serum Ca^{++} levels.

Common interventions

Treatment consists of recognizing and treating the etiologic factors that precipitated the imbalance. This may involve the administration of diuretics and NaCl (Ca^{++} excretion is promoted by Na^+ excretion), inorganic phosphates when a hypercalcemic crisis occurs, and/or antineoplastic drugs (mithramycin) when hypercalcemia is secondary to neoplasm.

Nursing interventions

Physical 1. Measure cardiac rate and rhythm. Notify the physician of changes in these measurements. (Cardiac monitor should be used.)
   2. Strain urine to detect renal calculi. Notify the physician if calculi are present.
   3. Encourage fluids (3,000 to 4,000 ml/day), unless contraindicated, to decrease formation of renal calculi.
   4. Promote acidification of urine by offering cranberry juice, prune juice, and ascorbic acid (unless contraindicated) to inhibit renal calculi formation.
   5. Monitor GI symptoms closely. Notify the physician if symptoms occur, and take corrective action as ordered (e.g., stool softeners for constipation).
   6. Promote safety by assisting with ambulation, especially if muscle weakness is present.
   7. Exercise extreme caution when turning and moving the patient to prevent pathologic fractures.
   8. Administer medications as ordered.
   9. Provide scrupulous perineal care to discourage urinary infections (increased risk secondary to alkaline urine).
   10. Monitor for rebound hypocalcemia (*see above*). Notify the physician if these symptoms occur.
Educational 11. Assess the patient's knowledge of precipitating factors to hypercalcemia.
   12. Provide an individualized plan of instruction (e.g., dietary information).
   13. Teach the patient the appropriate management of the underlying disorders (e.g., strain urine).
Prevention 14. Prevent etiologic factors when possible (e.g., dietary excesses of Ca^{++}).
   15. Encourage immobilized patients to exercise muscles in uninvolved parts of the body. Tilt tables and trapeze bars may be required to increase muscular activity.

Evaluation criteria. See Overview. Risk factors/complications minimized: Absence of signs and symptoms of hypocalcemia. Absence of renal calculi. Absence of pathologic fractures. Safety measures implemented: Cardiac monitor (when ordered) in place. Crash cart readily available. Patient ambulating with assistance. Adequate knowledge base demonstrated: Patient can describe risks for hypercalcemia, name signs and symptoms of hypercalcemia, and list measures appropriate for discouraging renal calculi formation.

MAGNESIUM IMBALANCES

Magnesium is the fourth most abundant cation in the body. It is found in bones (50%); in the ICF compartment — in specialized cells of the liver, heart, and skeletal muscles (49%); and in the ECF — primarily in the CSF (1%). Magnesium activates enzymatic reactions related to carbohydrate metabolism; vitamin B function; potassium, calcium, and protein utilization; and serum phosphorus regulation. It also promotes neuromuscular integrity. Magnesium is regulated by the parathyroids, is absorbed from the intestine, is excreted in feces and urine, and competes with calcium for absorption. Factors that increase calcium absorption will decrease magnesium absorption. The normal serum Mg^{++} level is 1.5 to 2.5 mEq/liter.

MAGNESIUM DEFICIT

Magnesium deficit (hypomagnesemia) is an imbalance in which the serum Mg^{++} level is <1.5 mEq/liter.

Magnesium deficit may be caused by inadequate intake of Mg^{++} (e.g., prolonged malnutrition, chronic alcoholism); excessive loss of Mg^{++} (e.g., prolonged diuresis, prolonged diarrhea, draining GI fistulas, diabetic ketoacidosis); intestinal malabsorption (e.g., malabsorption syndromes, small bowel bypass); hypoparathyroidism; hypercalcemia (absorption of Mg^{++} from GI tract varies inversely with Ca^{++} absorption); primary hyperaldosteronism; and toxemia of pregnancy.

Magnesium deficit results in an increase in release of acetylcholine at neuromuscular junctions, which produces increased muscular irritability; a decrease in cardiac muscle functioning; and an increase in CNS stimulation.

The following are the *signs and symptoms* of magnesium deficit: tetany, hyperreflexia, positive Chvostek's sign, positive Trousseau's sign, paresthesias, ataxia, convulsions, disorientation, hallucinations, aggressive behavior, irritability, tachycardia, hypertension, cardiac arrhythmias, and serum Mg^{++} <1.5 mEq/liter. Hypercalcemia is a related *complication*.

Diagnosis is based on the health history, physical exam, and serum Mg^{++} level.

Common interventions

Treatment consists of recognizing and treating the etiologic factors that precipitated the imbalance. Mg^{++} replacement is a priority. IM magnesium sulfate provides a therapeutic response in 1 hr. IV magnesium sulfate provides an immediate therapeutic response. Rebound hypermagnesemia (*see below*) may occur, especially in the presence of poor renal functioning. This complication should be prevented. Injectable calcium gluconate is administered to reverse hypermagnesemia.

Nursing interventions

Physical 1. Measure cardiac rate and rhythm. Notify the physician of changes in these measurements.

2. Institute safety measures, such as constant attendance and/or side rails when mental confusion is present.

3. Assist the patient to ambulate when ataxia is present.

4. Institute seizure precautions.

5. Administer foods, fluids, and medications as ordered.

6. Give IM magnesium sulfate (when ordered) deep in the gluteal muscle followed by massage to enhance absorption.

7. Monitor the patient receiving IV magnesium sulfate closely for signs and symptoms of hypermagnesemia. (Have injectable calcium gluconate available.) Discontinue IV immediately and notify the physician if symptoms occur.

8. Question IV administration of magnesium if the patient has diminished renal functioning.

Educational 9. Assess the patient's knowledge of precipitating factors to hypomagnesemia.

10. Provide an individualized plan of instruction (e.g., foods rich in Mg^{++}, diuretic therapy considerations).

11. Teach the patient the appropriate management of the underlying disorders.

Prevention 12. Prevent etiologic factors when possible (e.g., prolonged malnutrition).

13. Provide careful management of clinical conditions (e.g., diabetes, pregnancy, intestinal surgery).

Evaluation criteria. *See* Overview. Risk factors/complications minimized: Absence of hypercalcemia. Absence of rebound hypermagnesemia (*see below*). Safety measures implemented: Seizure precautions instituted. Injectable calcium gluconate available when IV magnesium sulfate is being administered. Adequate knowledge base demonstrated: Patient can describe risks for hypomagnesemia, name signs and symptoms of hypomagnesemia, and name a variety of Mg^{++}-rich foods.

MAGNESIUM EXCESS

Magnesium excess (**hypermagnesemia**) is an imbalance in which the serum Mg^{++} level is $>2.5 mEq/liter$. Magnesium excess may be caused by excessive intake of Mg^{++} (e.g., abuse of Mg^{++}: overdose during replacement therapy or repeated enemas with Mg^{++}) or by impaired Mg^{++} excretion (e.g., chronic renal failure or severe dehydration with oliguria and Mg^{++} retention).

Magnesium excess may lead to a decrease in the release of acetylcholine at the neuromuscular junctions, which produces decreased neuromuscular excitability, and to increased vasodilation.

The following are the *signs and symptoms* of magnesium excess: warm sensation throughout the body; flushing, diaphoresis; drowsiness, lethargy progressing to coma; diminished or absent deep tendon reflexes progressing to flaccid paralysis; respiratory depression; cardiac arrhythmias progressing to arrest; hypotension; ECG changes (increased PR interval, broadening of QRS complex, and elevation of T wave); and serum Mg^{++} >2.5 mEq/liter. Cardiac arrest is a related *complication.*

Diagnosis is based on the health history, physical exam, ECG, and serum Mg^{++} level.

Common interventions

Treatment consists of recognizing and treating the etiologic factors that precipitated the imbalance, using dialysis in renal failure, fluid replacement in dehydration, and eliminating Mg^{++} compounds (enemas, antacids, IV solutions). Mg^{++} excess should be treated with 10% calcium gluconate parenterally.

Nursing interventions

Physical 1. Monitor vital signs closely. (Cardiac monitor should be used.)
2. Institute safety measures, such as side rails in the presence of coma.
3. Administer medications and fluids as ordered.
Educational 4. Assess the patient's knowledge of precipitating factors to hypermagnesemia.
5. Provide an individualized plan of instruction (e.g., adequate fluids and careful management of antacids and cathartics, particularly in the presence of renal impairment).
Prevention 6. Avoid Mg^{++} compounds in the presence of renal disease.
7. Maintain adequate hydration, particularly in the presence of renal disease.

Evaluation criteria.   *See* Overview. Safety measures implemented: Cardiac monitor (when ordered) in place. Crash cart readily available. Injectable calcium gluconate available. Adequate knowledge base demonstrated: Patient can describe risks for hypermagnesemia and name signs and symptoms of hypermagnesemia.

FLUID SHIFTS

ECF exists in plasma (25%) and interstitial fluid (75%). The two fluids are similar in composition except for a wide variation in their protein content (plasma, 18 mEq/liter; interstitial fluid, 1 mEq/liter). Hydrostatic intravascular pressure would force water and electrolytes from plasma into the interstitial space, if it were not for the opposing oncotic pressure created by plasma proteins. When factors occur to alter this balance, potentially dangerous fluid shifts result. The two main fluid shifts are plasma-to-interstitial and interstitial-to-plasma.

PLASMA-TO-INTERSTITIAL FLUID SHIFTS

A plasma-to-interstitial fluid shift is the movement of abnormal quantities of water and electrolytes from the vascular system into the interstitial spaces. This shift may be caused by severe trauma or injury (fluid and electrolytes shift from injured to noninjured areas), as occurs in massive crushing injuries and burns (shift occurs 1st or 2nd day after burn). The shifts may also be caused by perforation of peptic ulcer, intestinal obstruction, surgery (surgical shock), occlusion of a major artery, venous thrombosis, lymphatic obstruction, and depression of plasma albumin (starvation).

The specific causative mechanism is unclear (possibly neurogenic). Plasma-to-interstitial fluid shifts result in decreased fluid in the vascular space (shock), dehydration of injured cells, and/or edema of noninjured areas.

The following are the *signs and symptoms* of plasma-to-interstitial fluid shifts: pallor, tachycardia, hypotension, weak to absent pulse, cold extremities, oliguria, disorientation progressing to coma, and elevated RBC, Hb, and BUN. Irreversible shock and renal failure are related *complications.*

Diagnosis is based on the health history, physical exam, and tests for RBCs, Hb, and BUN.

Common interventions

Treatment involves recognizing and treating the etiologic factors (e.g., obstruction, burn, injury, shock), replacing shifted fluid and electrolytes with PO or IV fluids, correcting protein deficiency when present (high-protein diet and supplements), and preventing complications of therapy. Fluids must be given cautiously (volume overload can result when interstitial-to-plasma shift occurs on 3rd to 5th day after incident or injury).

Nursing interventions

Physical 1. Monitor skin color and temperature closely.
2. Monitor urinary output hourly. Notify the physician of a urinary output of <30 ml/hr or <500 ml/24 hr.
3. Monitor vital signs every hour.
4. Monitor level of consciousness frequently.
5. Institute safety measures when disorientation/coma are present.
6. Turn and position the patient hourly on a regular schedule (edematous tissue in noninjured areas is prone to breakdown).
7. Provide scrupulous skin care.

8. Administer replacement fluids as ordered. If IV fluids are given, monitor type of solution, rate, and site.

Educational 9. Assess the patient's knowledge of precipitating factors to fluid shift.

10. Provide an individualized plan of instruction (e.g., high-protein diet).

Prevention 11. Prevent etiologic factors when possible (e.g., injuries, inadequate diet).

12. Provide careful management of clinical conditions precipitating fluid shift (e.g., surgery, burns, massive trauma).

Evaluation criteria. *See* Overview. Risk factors/complications minimized: Absence of renal failure (e.g., oliguria, anuria, elevated BUN). Absence of irreversible shock (e.g., coma). Absence of circulatory overload after compensatory shift (e.g., pulmonary edema). Absence of skin breakdown. Adequate knowledge base demonstrated: Patient can describe risks for plasma-to-interstitial fluid shift, name signs and symptoms of fluid shift, and name foods high in protein.

INTERSTITIAL-TO-PLASMA FLUID SHIFTS

An interstitial-to-plasma fluid shift is the movement of abnormal quantities of water and electrolytes from interstitial spaces into the vascular system. This type of shift may be caused by remobilization of edema fluid on the 3rd to 5th day after a plasma-to-interstitial fluid shift; compensation after hemorrhage; and excessive administration of hypertonic infusions (plasma, dextran, albumin).

The specific causative mechanism for remobilization of edema fluid on the 3rd to 5th day after an injury is unclear. Osmolality of plasma is increased by excessive hypertonic infusions. (The fluid shifts from interstitial to vascular space to compensate.)

In a shift secondary to hemorrhage (shock), the *signs and symptoms* are pallor, tachycardia, weakness, and hypotension. In a shift secondary to the administration of hypertonic solutions or remobilization of edema (circulatory overload), the signs and symptoms are bounding pulse, engorgement of peripheral veins, moist rales progressing to pulmonary edema, hypertension, cardiac enlargement, decreased Hct, and decreased BUN. Pulmonary edema is a related *complication.*

Diagnosis is based on the health history, physical exam, CBC, and BUN.

Common interventions

Treatment consists of recognizing and treating the etiologic factors (e.g., blood transfusion after hemorrhage) and treating hypervolemia with diuretics, dialysis, or rotating tourniquets in the presence of cardiac or renal impairment.

Nursing interventions

Physical 1. Monitor for shock.

2. Administer therapy to reduce hypervolemia as ordered (e.g., diuretics, rotating tourniquets, dialysis).

3. Observe for signs and symptoms of pulmonary edema (e.g., moist rales, frothy sputum, dyspnea).

Educational 4. Assess the patient's knowledge of precipitating factors to fluid shift.

5 Provide an individualized plan of instruction.

Prevention 6. Prevent etiologic factors when possible (e.g., hemorrhage, excessive administration of hypertonic solutions).

7. Provide careful management of clinical conditions precipitating fluid shift (e.g., remobilization of edema on 3rd to 5th day after trauma).

Evaluation criteria. See Overview. Risk factors/complications minimized: Absence of circulatory overload (pulmonary edema). Absence of irreversible shock (when hemorrhage is precipitating factor). Adequate knowledge base demonstrated: Patient can describe risks for interstitial-to-plasma fluid shift and name signs and symptoms of fluid shift.

CHAPTER 4

SENSATIONS

Patricia W. Blagman

OVERVIEW

Definitions

The stimulation of various areas of the body containing organs of sense (e.g., the skin, joints, muscle, and viscera) results in specific sensations that are brought into conscious awareness. These sensations include the feelings of proprioception, temperature, touch, and various aspects of pain, including paresthesias and visceral pain. (The special senses of sight, hearing, taste, and smell are beyond the scope of this chapter.)

Proprioception. When an individual changes body position (e.g., from sitting to standing), the motion is accomplished with little thought except for the ultimate goal (to stand up). Unless disturbed by pathology, this kinesthetic sense of knowing the location of a body part is always present but is not in the forefront of consciousness. Although there is a vague awareness of body position, there is no need to fix attention on it in order to move. An example of this is the ability to stand without swaying when the eyes are closed (Romberg's sign): no concentration is necessary to hold the position.

Proprioception also involves **stereognosis** (the ability to recognize an object placed in the hand only by its "feel") and **two-point discrimination** (the ability to distinguish between two simultaneous skin contacts). These proprioceptions enhance safety and efficiency without the individual's being particularly alert to these sensations.

Temperature.   The conscious sensations of heat and cold and their gradations result from a temperature stimulus that is applied to receptors in the skin.

Touch.   There are two different forms of touch sensation: simple touch and tactile discrimination. **Simple touch** includes the sensations of light touch (e.g., from a wisp of cotton) and light pressure, as well as an elementary sense of the localization of the touch. **Tactile discrimination** includes the sense of deeper pressure and of spatial localization, such as two-point discrimination. These touch sensations are closely linked with those of proprioception.

Pain.   Pain is an uncomfortable sensation arising from a noxious stimulus. One of the most common nursing diagnoses is the alteration of comfort with relation to some stimulus that results in pain. Therefore, the emphasis in this chapter will be on the phenomenon of pain.

Anatomy and physiology review

The neural pathways for these sensations are similar and at times so closely linked that they are difficult to distinguish anatomically. Nevertheless, some knowledge of the pathways helps the nurse to understand patient symptoms and the mechanisms of effectiveness of the nursing measures taken.

Skin receptors.   All feelings of sensation begin with the application of a stimulus to receptors in the skin. It was traditionally believed that there were separate receptors for pain, touch, warmth, and cold (e.g., the end bulbs of Krause for cold and Ruffini's nerve endings for heat). Newer discoveries indicate a much more intricate network of stimulus-receptor patterns: many skin receptors respond to varied stimuli, and hair movement may also signal temperature change. Many receptors, however, are so specific in their sensitivity that they respond only to specific temperature or touch ranges: so-called "pain receptors" are believed to be receptors with high thresholds to pressure or temperature. Therefore, receptors are considered in terms of their pressure thresholds, their peak temperature senstivity, and the size of their receptive fields rather than in terms of the specific sensations that they trigger.

Nerve fibers.   Impulses from these peripheral somatic receptors are transmitted through peripheral or cranial nerves from the face, ear, etc., through the dorsal root zone and into the spinal cord. Impulses travel at varying rates of speed and over fibers of differing diameters. Because fibers are not specifically or exclusively reserved for one type of impulse, no specific "pain fibers" exist.

Spinal cord.   Nerve fibers enter the dorsal horn from the doral root and synapse. It is at this point that differing sensations become more anatomically differentiated, taking separate paths through the spinal tracts to their end points within the brain. **Proprioception** is conducted from receptors in muscles, tendons, and joints to the spinal cord, where fibers continue uninterrupted by three routes: a reflex arc, spinocerebellar tracts, and fibers that ascend to the medulla, cross, and then continue to the thalamus. Some tough fibers that travel along this third path are responsible for tactile discrimination. Fibers for simple **touch** synapse in the dorsal horn, cross as few as 1 to 2 segments or as many as 10 to 15 segments from the point of entry, and continue in the anterior spinothalamic tract. Fibers that conduct the sensations of **pain** and **temperature** follow each other so closely that they are difficult to identify separately. They synapse in the dorsal horn, cross within two cord sections, and travel in the lateral spinothalamic tract. Fibers of the trigeminal nerve carrying sensations from the face enter the brainstem at the pons and form a descending spinal root to the medulla. There, they synapse, cross, and ascend to the thalamus.

Brain.   Facts are limited in relation to known pathways of pain within the brain. At the level of the thalamus (the terminus of the spinothalamic tract), only crude awareness of pain is established. Nevertheless, emotional reactions, intellectual reasonings, memories of past pain, motor activities, and a sense of the location and intensity of pain all occur as responses to a painful stimulus. These complex activities require an intricate neural network throughout the brain for their integration: there is no one "pain center" in the brain.

Fibers conducting the sensations of touch, pressure, and position from the thalamus are conveyed to a primary sensory receptive area of the cortex, where the sensations are well defined but not comprehended. In the sensory association areas of the parietal lobe, incoming sensations from the primary area and from areas transmitting pain undergo elaborate analysis that leads to full comprehension.

Psychologic dimensions of pain

The pain response involves much more than mere feelings of discomfort of varying intensity. Sensory, affective, and cognitive processes act on motor mechanisms in response to the pain stimulus. **Past experiences with pain** are recalled. Present feelings are evaluated in light of pain experience, and consequences are predicted. The **cognitive response** also includes learned responses. Cultural values (e.g., stoicism or viewing pain as punishment) are pain attitudes acquired in childhood. The **sensory response** involves the identification of the exact site of the body that receives the stimulus. An accompanying classification of the intensity of the feeling (how much it hurts) is made, and the feeling is also categorized by descriptions such as burning, pricking, stabbing, sharp, boring, etc.

A concomitant of pain is behavior motivated by the desire to avoid or escape it. Indeed, the **motivation to avoid pain** is sometimes so strong that it becomes detrimental to health, as when medical treatment is shunned or delayed. When pain occurs and its cause is unknown, considerable **anxiety** or **fear** can be generated. The person contemplates a host of possible explanations, some more frightful than others. An understanding of the cause of the pain, however, may or may not decrease the anxiety.

Suffering is a highly subjective phenomenon. An individual can "suffer" whether the pain is intense or mild, intermittent or constant. Pain that may torment one individual may hardly disturb another because each person's reaction to pain is unique. **Pain verbalization** is partially determined by culture. Some patients need to be questioned closely before they will admit to being in pain, whereas others moan or sigh constantly when they are in pain.

The various dimensions of the response to pain require an enormously complicated interacting neural network. Consider the variety of thoughts and feelings that occur if one picks up a hot pot without using a potholder. To end the stimulus, the pot is immediately dropped — a reflex motor response. The area of injury is localized by examining the fingers. Depending on the degree and size of the redness, one may be overcome with fear or anxiety as a thought of the consequences flashes by. The individual may cry out or make some vocal announcement about the severity of the feeling and its burning quality. Holding, rubbing, and applying cool water or ice may be attempted to decrease the pain. There may be inward anger or mental name-calling for not using a potholder. The individual may be afraid of the reactions of others, who might think him stupid or careless. Some decision about the need for treatment will be made, and some thought about future prevention will occur.

Pain theories

Pain theories give rise to the development of new modalities for pain relief and explain the effectiveness of various treatments. Although a holistic, all-inclusive pain theory is not currently available, there are a variety of theories that attempt to explain certain aspects of pain (Table 4-1). Because nursing is so involved with pain management, a knowledge of these theories can lead to the use of more and varied pain relief measures. In addition, persistent assessment of the pain relief process can contribute to the development of pain theories.

Specificity theory. This theory proposed that specific nerve receptors responded only to pain and that the impulses they received were transmitted directly from the skin to the brain. For centuries, traditional pain theory has explained the mechanism of pain, dominated thinking about pain relief, and caused some present misconceptions about pain.

Pattern theory. Pattern theorists studied fibers in the spinal cord. They advanced pain theory by describing pain transmission in terms of small and large fibers rather than in terms of specific nerve endings responding only to noxious stimuli. The intense stimulation of small fibers was seen to result in pain perception, whereas the large fibers were thought to conduct pain-inhibitory messages.

These two theories (and others, such as **affect theory**) have each contributed important concepts to pain theory but have been inadequate in

TABLE 4-1
Pain Theories

Theory	Physiologic concepts	Major contribution	Current status	Disadvantages
Specificity	"Straight-through" pathway from skin receptors through spinal cord to pain center in brain, assumed to be the thalamus.	Served as origin of development of some surgical procedures for pain relief (e.g., chordotomy).	Skin receptors respond only to a specific range of the stimulus.	Incomplete explanation, responsible for many current misconceptions.
Pattern	Reverberating patterns of neural activity, using large and small fibers in the spinal cord.	Served as basis for development of surgical procedures for relief of phantom pain.	Pain transmission in terms of large and small fibers.	Incomplete explanation; spinal cord surgery does not always alleviate phantom limb pain.
Gate control	Gating mechanism in spinal cord increases or decreases flow of impulses. Action system integrates sensory, affective, and cognitive behaviors to account for diverse pain experiences.	Explains mechanisms of acupuncture, pressure points, Lamaze pain management, massage and touch, and electric stimulators.	Most totally integrated and respected at present; research is continuing.	Not completely holistic.
Specialized Sensory decision	Unknown physiologic sensory discrimination.	Origin of measurement of sensory discrimination.	May help explain difference between strength of stimulus and what the person reports about pain; research is continuing.	Explains a portion of the pain complex.
Endogenous pain control	Endorphin, a morphinelike hormone of the pituitary, inhibits pain-transmitting neurons.	Natural, internal method of pain suppression.	May help explain differences in pain perception; research is continuing.	Explains a portion of the pain complex.

themselves to explain the complex phenomenon of pain. A sufficient pain control theory needs to include such diverse concepts as the specialization of fibers and pathways, the patterning in transfer of information, the impact of psychologic and cognitive processes on pain perception and reactions, the spread of pain, and the persistence of pain after healing.

Gate control theory.   At present, the most integrated and respected theory of pain is the gate control theory, which postulates a gating mechanism in the spinal cord that increases or decreases the flow of nerve impulses from the sensory nerve endings to the CNS. This gating system is modulated by activities within the brain through descending, efferent transmission, which responds to anxiety, past experiences, or other nonsensory activities. The gate control theory has been extensively studied at the physiologic level and is able to explain the mechanisms of various pain puzzles, including referred pain and prolonged pain.

Specialized theories.   There are a few theories that are useful in explaining various aspects of the pain complex. **Sensory decision theory** involves the concept of pain threshold, which maintains that the same painful stimulus evokes varying intensities of pain in different people. The **endogenous pain control theory** involves the analgesic chemicals produced within the brain. Endorphin, a morphinelike hormone produced by the pituitary is a natural pain suppression substance that inhibits pain-transmitting neurons. This and other chemicals contribute to an internal method of pain control.

The complexity and subjectiveness of the pain phenomenon will continue to be studied, and new theories of pain will be proposed or existing ones expanded. The end goal of this research and theorizing, however, will remain the alleviation of suffering for people in pain.

The pain experience

The experiences for patients in pain are probably as varied and diverse as the people themselves. The mystery remains: the same painful stimulus causes one person intense discomfort and another person no discomfort at all. Nurses are continually amazed that their assumptions about pain are so frequently invalid. For example, a patient is expected to have pain after certain procedures, but no pain occurs. Or a patient is not expected to have pain, but pain does occur, and with an intensity never envisioned. An understanding of the anatomic and psychologic dimensions of pain and of current pain theories offers the nurse only a partial view of the pain phenomenon because, in addition, the patient who is experiencing the pain needs to be studied and understood.

The pain experience for the patient

Both the physical and psychologic dimensions are affected in the patient with pain. Although there is a great deal of subjective data about pain, some observable or measurable responses occur but *may* or *may not* be present. Pain itself may be categorized as superficial, deep, or central (Table 4-2).

TABLE 4-2
Pain Syndromes

Syndrome	Origin of stimulus	Characteristics	Associated symptoms	Site perceived
Superficial pain	Skin, tendons, or ligaments.	Burning, sharp.	Restlessness, increased pulse rate, muscle tension.	Localized area.
Deep pain	Internal organs and body cavities (inflammation, alteration in vascular supply, visceral obstruction, or muscle spasm).	Boring, throbbing, crushing.	Nausea, vomiting, decreased pulse rate, decreased BP, pallor, syncope.	Inexact
Central pain syndromes	Autonomic reflex syndromes.	Absence of pathologic process to account for pain.	Incapacitation of varying degrees; fear of next pain episode; depression.	
Phantom limb pain	Site of amputation.	Phantom limb sensation (painful or nonpainful).		Distal to amputation.
Causalgias	Internal, frequently along tract of bullet wound.	Spontaneous bursts of burning pain months after healing; excruciating; set off by even minor stimuli such as bumps, temperature changes, or clothing.		Site of trauma.
Central pain	Insult to afferent neural pathways of CNS.			Site of trauma.

Superficial pain refers to the body area that has been stimulated (e.g., the skin). It does *not* mean that the quality of the experience is shallow or not real. **Deep pain** includes visceral pains, referred pains, and muscle spasms that result from stimuli to the internal organs and body cavities. **Central pain** (e.g., causalgias and phantom limb) occurs without direct relationship to noxious stimuli. Central pain occurs after an insult to any portion of the CNS that directly interrupts neural transmissions or "pain pathways." It is sometimes mistakenly assumed that after spinal cord injury, patients are free of pain. Although this may be true of superficial pain in the affected area, damage to the cord itself will nevertheless produce these central pains.

The **subjective reporting** of pain depends on the linguistic phrases that are available and on the ability to describe such an elusive quality. A toothache is as different from the pain of a sprained ankle as the pain of a heart attack is from that of a burned hand. Words to describe these differences are not precise, nor do they have the same meaning for everyone. Patients usually identify four categories with reference to the pain: its intensity, the type of sensation, an affective dimension, and an evaluative dimension (Table 4-3). Given the wide variety of these pain descriptions, it is understandable that patients may have difficulty with describing these sensations. The diverse nature of the pain experience, and the inadequacy of language to describe it, contribute to the frustration that patients often feel in communicating their unique pain experience to others.

The mental experience. Sociocultural influences play a major role in the way that a patient views and responds to pain. The expression of discomfort is a behavior that is often learned early in life. It is unfortunate that some health care professionals make value judgments about which type of pain expression is "better," regardless of the cultural background of the patient.

A common attitude toward pain that is often culturally transmitted views pain as punishment for past misdeeds. Indeed, the word "pain" is derived from Greek and Latin words that mean "punishment" or "penalty." The infliction of pain has long been a common punishment. Until recent times, the mainstay of child rearing was spanking for misdeeds. Thus, it is important for the nurse to understand the nature of pain expression for each individual.

Anxiety about pain may also vary, depending on an individual's sociocultural background. The avoidance of pain, or of experiences that may cause pain, is a common tendency. Anxiety may be linked to past experiences with pain, to its significance for the person, or to deeper feelings of loneliness, helplessness, and loss of control so often experienced by those in pain. The degree of threat represented by the pain is also a source of anxiety and may further intensify the pain experience. Anxiety, the most powerful, debilitating, and damaging concomitant of pain, always increases suffering. Some of its negative outcomes are listed in Table 4-3.

TABLE 4-3
Subjective Responses to Pain

Physical		Mental	
Dimension	Quality	Influence	Behavior spectrum
Intensity	Mild to severe (scale of 1-10).	Sociocultural	From "moaners" to stoics, and from considering pain part of getting well to considering it punishment for past misdeeds.
Sensation	*Burning:* scalding, searing. *Pressure:* stabbing, cutting, pressing, pinching, cramping, pulling. *Spatial:* jumping, flashing, shooting. *Temporal:* pulsing, throbbing, pounding.	Anxiety	Increases pain perception; interferes with pain relief; increases muscle tension; inhibits post-operative cooperation with coughing, deep breathing, and ambulating; prevents reporting of new symptoms; causes postponement of needed treatment.
Affective	Fearful, frightful, terrifying, cruel, killing, punishing.		
Evaluative	Miserable, horrible, discomforting, distressing, unbearable, or excruciating.	Judgmental	Patient expresses feelings of alienation, isolation, and desertion, and communicates a sense of helplessness and the inability to be in control.

It is now easy to see why it is inaccurate to say that the intensity of a painful stimulus and the intensity of the perceived pain have a one-to-one relationship. The intervening variables discussed above influence each person's pain experience in a unique way.

The pain experience for the nurse

Throughout the entire range of nursing practice settings, almost nowhere is there a patient population free of pain. In the home, in the hospital, and in the clinic, a high percentage of patients are in pain. One would surmise that, with all this experience, nurses must be very adept at diagnosing and alleviating pain, but this is not totally true. At times, certain emotions and values make it difficult for nurses to adequately diagnose and treat the pain response to illness. Ministering to a patient in pain may evoke as intense an experience for the nurse as it does for the patient.

Feelings.   Nurses experience severe discomfort for several reasons when a patient is suffering with pain. Nurses often feel helpless in their inability to increase the patient's comfort, or they become angry that the patient is undergoing such a miserable ordeal. Nurses may even deny the existence of the patient's pain if they are unable to alleviate it. Certain situations may increase a nurse's anxiety: an unsuccessful attempt to have a physician alter an ineffective medication regimen, a harrying assignment that leaves little time for real communication with the patient, or a sense that no measures bring real comfort to the patient. A feeling of not being in control of the situation can be as anxiety provoking for the nurse as it is for the patient. In addition, the anxiety of nurses who provide care to patients in pain may be related to their own fear of pain. As a universal experience, the fear of pain ranks second to the fear of death.

Attitudes.   Some of the most serious handicaps to compassionate care for the patient in pain are certain attitudes and myths that interfere with intelligent and sensitive nursing care. (Table 4-4 presents some of these common misconceptions.)

Intellectual judgments, rather than emotional ones, are needed when providing care to patients in pain. If a patient's pain is different from what is expected, nurses should ascertain whether some new development has occurred (e.g., a postoperative complication or an extension of a heart attack). An emotional judgment to the effect that a patient "shouldn't" be having pain is a presumptive and inappropriate nursing judgment. If pain seems unexpectedly prolonged, it may take considerable interpersonal skill to ferret out the cause (e.g., the patient is afraid, lonely, or depressed).

Nurses often make value judgments about complaining, "Good" (i.e., stoical) patients do not complain too much; "moaners" receive no empathy. Yet, both types of patients are suffering and are probably receiving inappropriate care. The moaner is told to be quiet and the noncomplainer is praised, but neither receives adequate pain relief or any understanding of the meaning of the individualized experiences.

TABLE 4-4

Attitudes Toward Pain: Misconceptions and Realities

Misconceptions	Realities
Men have a higher pain tolerance than women.	Nurses are less responsive to male patients' complaints of pain than to those of female patients.
Women complain about pain more than men do.	Pain tolerance is uniquely individual and not sex related.
Nurses can judge how much pain a patient should have.	Because of the highly subjective nature of the pain experience, only the patient is capable of evaluating the pain. Studies show that staff members frequently infer less pain than the patient's own rating.
Patients should have a high tolerance for pain.	There is no intrinsic value in either high or low pain tolerance.
Real pain has specific organic causes and specific accompanying behaviors.	All pain is real to the patient, even when physiologic and behavioral evidence is lacking.
Administering narcotics sparingly prevents addiction.	Undermedicating with narcotics may lead to craving for a drug for pain relief and, in this way, contribute to the development of addiction.
A "clock watcher" is an addict — or becoming one.	The patient has usually received insufficient pain relief (dose too low or too infrequent). Discomfort forces the patient to keep track of the time and to demand medication on schedule.

All pain is real to the patient even when physiologic and behavioral evidence is lacking. The inability of some nurses to accept this fact undoubtedly stems from their adherence to remnants of the specificity theory, although, as theories become obsolete, nursing is obliged to correct its thinking. Often, nurses think, "This patient's pain isn't real. The patient just wants a pain shot," or "I don't think the patient is having as much pain as is being indicated." Such thoughts have nothing to do with the patient's reality and are not helpful. *The pain is real to the patient.*

Perhaps the most damaging misconception involves the amount of narcotic needed to produce addiction. Because nurses have an inordinate and ungrounded fear of contributing to narcotic addiction or abuse, patients often experience unalleviated suffering. In fact, <1% of hospitalized patients who receive meperidine hydrochloride, 100 mg q 4 hr for 10 days, will become addicted. Furthermore, < 1% of all narcotic addicts in the USA became addicted during hospitalization. Indeed, undermedicating with narcotics may lead to a craving for the drug for pain relief and, in this way, contribute to the development of addiction. The patient is thus required to endure pain because of a nurse's suspiciousness or misinformation.

It is not easy to watch a patient in pain. Yet, nursing practice today often interferes with the provision of pain relief. Old myths and attitudes need to be replaced by facts and by attitudes that are in harmony with the goal — promotion of comfort.

DEVIATIONS

ACUTE PAIN

Acute pain is a description of the *duration* of the pain experience, *not* of its severity. Because acute pain occurs for a brief interlude, an end to the pain is anticipated. Acute pain occurs after surgery or during childbirth, or it may be associated with kidney stones, heart attack, broken bones, ulcers, and a host of other physical ailments. The pain may last for a few weeks (or as long as 6 mo), but it is definitely expected to end. Pain-producing stimuli are the causes of acute pain. Regardless of the pathologic process, pain is produced by relatively few stimuli (Table 4-5).

Any combination of the *signs and symptoms* listed in Table 4-6 may lead to an assumption of pain. However, it is absolutely true that a patient may experience pain and exhibit none of these signs (e.g., a patient with a "splitting headache"). Assessment is not a simple process because patients often report their pain inadequately or inaccurately. (Consider the last time you tried to describe a toothache to a dentist. Sometimes, it is even impossible to pinpoint which tooth is causing the trouble!) Studies also suggest that there is a tendency for patients to be reluctant to discuss their pain. Indeed, nurses often hear of a patient's pain from a visiting relative of the patient, although it had not been reported to the nurse or physician.

TABLE 4-5
Pain-Producing Stimuli

Stimulus	Mechanism	Example
Mechanical	Direct irritation of nerve endings.	Traumas, burns.
Chemical	Lactic acid, histamine, bradykinin.	Substances released in inflammation or ischemia (e.g., intermittent claudication).
Pressure	Substances occupying a confined space.	Tumors, hemorrhage, inflammatory products.
Muscle spasm	Intense, rapid contraction and relaxation of muscle, leading to ischemia or pressure.	Bladder spasms after prostate surgery, uterine contractions in labor.
Overstretching	Distension of a hollow organ with an abnormal amount of a substance.	Air in intestine (gas pains), overdistended bladder.

TABLE 4-6

Acute Pain: Signs and Symptoms

Intensity	ANS responses	Attempts to promote comfort	Communication of discomfort
Mild to moderate (from body surfaces)	Sympathetic response: pallor, elevated BP, increased respiratory rate, increased heart rate.	Protecting the area, rubbing, holding, pressing, splinting, curling up, refraining from any movement.	Restlessness, rocking, moaning or crying out, muscle tension (clenched face or teeth, tight shoulder muscles), guarding, inability to sleep or concentrate.
Severe, deep, or central pain	Parasympathetic response: pallor, decreased BP, decreased heart rate, nausea, vomiting, weakness, fainting.		

Nurses' attitudes and misinformation may also bias pain assessment. A crucial aspect of the nurse's attitude must be to *believe the patient.* When assessing for pain, nurses must try to eliminate any preconceived ideas they may have. To obtain information that is complete and accurate, the nurse must ask necessary specific questions and make specific observations.

Sample assessment tool

The following sample assessment tool is adapted with permission from M. McCaffery, Nursing Management of the Patient with Pain, J. B. Lippincott Co., Philadelphia, 1979, second edition, p. 283-286.

Communication

1. Ability: What is the patient's ability to communicate? Are their limitations on verbal and nonverbal behaviors?
2. Willingness: What is the patient's willingness to discuss pain? Is pain being denied? Does the patient confide only in one person?
3. Resources: What resources (other than the patient interview) are available for pain information?
4. Nonverbal: What nonverbal expression of pain is evident?

Characteristics

1. Stimulus: Does any specific stimulus trigger the pain?
2. Onset, duration, and pattern: What is the onset and duration or persistence of the pain? How long has the patient had the pain? What kind of pattern does the pain have: continuous, periodic, rhythmic, or transient?
3. Location: Is the location of the pain identified precisely or vaguely? Does the location vary?
4. Intensity: What is the intensity of the pain? Is it always of the same intensity? (Sometimes it is helpful to let the patient estimate the intensity on a scale of 1 to 5 or 1 to 10.)
5. Sensation: What is the sensation of the pain? What words describe what the pain feels like? (The patient may have the most difficulty with this question, especially if the sensation is new or rather vague. Offering some words to choose from may be helpful.)
6. Affect: What affective quality does the patient ascribe to the pain: fearful, frightening, grueling, terrifying?
7. Evaluation: What evaluation does the patient make with relation to the pain: discomforting, troublesome, unbearable, excruciating?

Effects of pain on the patient

1. Suffering: To what extent does the pain cause suffering and anguish?
2. Physical signs: What physical signs accompany the pain: diaphoresis, respiratory distress, nausea, or anorexia?
3. Mental image: What mental image of the pain site does the patient have? (Sometimes, misconceptions about the cause of pain can be corrected.)

4. Focus of attention: What is the patient's attention focused on? Does the patient dwell on the pain or disease? Does the patient relate to others in the environment?
5. Activities of daily living: Does the patient exhibit any form of sleep disturbance? (Lack of sleep is a frequent problem related to pain.) How have eating habits changed? (Nausea or anorexia is common.) Has there been a weight loss? How does the pain interfere with work, socializing, or exercise? Are sexual practices interfered with, either from decreased interest or from pain associated with the activity?
6. Social: Have social relationships changed? Does the patient have less time for (and less interest in) friends and relatives?

Emotions

1. Anxiety: What level of anxiety does the patient exhibit? With what is the anxiety associated?
2. Depression: Does the patient act depressed or withdrawn? Does the patient express sadness, helplessness, hopelessness, irritability, powerlessness, or discouragement as signs of underlying depression?
3. Anger: How is anger expressed? Is the patient hostile, aggressive, or passive, and how are these behaviors manifested?

Pain relief attitude

What does the patient *believe* will work best for the pain? What has worked for the patient in the past: imagery, massage, medications, or distraction? What pain relief measures is the patient fearful of (e.g., narcotics)? Greater success with pain relief occurs when the patient and nurse plan pain relief measures together.

Specific situations affecting the pain experience

How much true knowledge and understanding of the situation does the patient have? Is the patient capable of comprehending? Is there misinformation to be corrected?

Level of consciousness

What is the level of consciousness? It is often felt that comatose patients do not feel pain. What is most likely true is that there is the ability to feel pain to some degree but not to respond. After awakening, patients who had been comatose sometimes relate events that were painful (e.g., dressing change, venipuncture, or repositioning). Patients with depressed levels of consciousness must be protected, as much as possible, from pain-producing situations.

Previous pain experience

What are the patient's previous pain experiences? Although previous experiences may leave the patient more fearful and anxious in relation to the current pain, they may also have helped the patient devise pain reduction measures.

Meaning of pain

What is the meaning of pain for the patient? Pain may be viewed in a positive light as a pathway to recovery (i.e., the pain after surgery), or it may be seen as a means of strengthening character. But it may also be interpreted in a negative way as a punishment for misdeeds. Or it may be associated with a threat to life (e.g., the pain after an MI). It is important to understand the meaning of pain for the patient, especially if it is characterized by misinformation.

Level of fatigue

How tiring is the pain experience for the patient? Does it inhibit the ability to be in control or to participate in self-care?

Age

It is thought that the young and the old experience pain less intensely than others.

A pain assessment tool is invaluable in any setting in which pain assessment is a routine part of nursing practice. A published tool can be adopted, or a new tool can be developed by practitioners in the health care setting.

At the completion of assessment, the nurse is ready to formulate the nursing diagnoses, including the patient problem, etiology, and signs and symptoms. The National Conference on Classification of Nursing Diagnoses labels the problem of pain as an "alteration in comfort." The actual diagnosis must also include the causes and symptoms of the problem. Thus, a nursing diagnosis relating to pain may be stated as "alteration in comfort related to 1 day postcholecystectomy, resulting in refusal to cough, fatigue, and sleeplessness."

General interventions

Application of heat and cold.   Both heat and cold can relieve pain. The patient may have a preference for one or need to try both. Because both can cause injury to the skin, heat and cold must be used with caution. Heat should not be used where there is a danger of bleeding; cold should not be used where circulation is impaired. Both heat and cold are dangerous when the sensations of touch, temperature, or pain are diminished. Often, a variety of temperatures or procedures must be tried before one is found that offers the best pain relief.

Analgesics.   Analgesics have long been a common pain relief procedure, used by both laymen and professionals. Although the effectiveness of analgesics is well documented, their side effects can be unpleasant or even dangerous. Analgesics act upon various portions of the CNS to either interfere with the neural transmission of pain or to alter the perception of pain.

Drug usage.   At home, the patient manages the medications for pain relief and may make alterations to suit the situation. When hospitalized, the patient loses this control because the nurse makes the decisions for administering medications. When patients have difficulty obtaining adequate pain relief while hospitalized, they sometimes obtain analgesics from home to supplement those administered by the nurse. (It is interesting to note that neither the nurse nor the physician has a clear line of accountability for pain relief.)

Nonnarcotics.   Nonnarcotic analgesics are usually over-the-counter drugs, the most common being aspirin and acetaminophen, either alone or in combination with other drugs. Patients may have histories of periodic self-medication with these drugs. Although these analgesics are relatively safe, they do produce side effects (Table 4-7).

Other nonnarcotic medications are usually combinations of aspirin or acetaminophen with additives such as caffeine or phenacetin. Although buffers to counteract GI irritation are added to some drugs, the buffering effect of food is cheaper and more effective. Choices between these various drugs and their combinations can be made by expense and by history of effectiveness for the patient. (According to McCaffery, any brand of aspirin that will dissolve in ½ in. of water in 30 sec is adequate.)

Antidepressants, either alone or administered with analgesics, are effective in relieving pain and sleeplessness.

Narcotic analgesics.   Whereas nonnarcotics produce analgesia by blocking pain transmission, narcotics produce analgesia by affecting the CNS and thereby altering the perception of pain. Narcotics are useful in treating severe pain although the hazards of respiratory depression and addiction are well known (*see* Table 4-7). Narcotics may also depress BP while relieving pain, thus giving rise to a dilemma. In the postoperative patient, this dilemma may be dealt with by administering small IV doses and monitoring the effects. This same treatment is effective for another postoperative dilemma: narcotics depress the cough reflex and promote hypoventilation, whereas the lack of pain relief leads to no coughing, hyperventilation, and lung congestion.

There are other times when narcotic administration is controversial, as in the patient with chronic pain and the terminal patient with depressed respirations. In the first patient, the risk is addiction; in the other, it is respiratory arrest. Although such controversies will continue, it is possible that greater dependence on other pain relief therapies will provide a partial solution.

Drug combinations.   Brompton's mixture, used for generations in England, contains a variety of narcotic and nonnarcotic analgesics. In the USA, Brompton's mixture usually contains morphine, alcohol, and some form of aromatic elixir. Other narcotics, antiemetics, or tranquilizers may also be included.

Combining a narcotic and a nonnarcotic analgesic provides a very effective method of pain relief. Because each constituent acts on a different part of the nervous system, their combined use provides more pain relief than does an increase in the dose of narcotic. Thus, aspirin and meperidine, administered together, are more effective than increasing the dose of meperidine.

Placebos.   Myths concerning placebos can be destructive forces in the nurse-patient relationship. The fact that a patient may experience pain relief from placebos is frequently misinterpreted to mean that the patient is faking and that there is no basis for pain. Because of the complexity of the neural network pain system and response patterns, a number of methods relieve pain. About one patient in three may have an effective placebo response, even with cancer, broken bones, or surgery. The response may occur because the patient desperately wants *anything* to relieve the pain. The added effectiveness of telling a patient that a medication will help to relieve pain is well known. Is this not a form of placebo response? It must be kept in mind that placebos cannot be used to diagnose psychogenic pain. (In fact, the overall use of placebos is declining.)

Nursing considerations.   In the hospital setting, nurses are in control of administering the ordered narcotics. Evidence points to the fact that more patients are under- rather than overmedicated. Nurses must accept the fact that withholding or delaying the administration of narcotics is not beneficial to the patient. Pain relief must be a priority nursing goal. When patients and nurses negotiate goals and plan pain relief programs together, a higher degree of pain relief occurs.

Nursing interventions

Pain relief principles.   The following are nine principles of pain relief.

Principle 1: Effective nurse-patient relationships enhance all other pain relief measures.   For optimal effectiveness the nurse and the patient must have optimum communication and understanding with relation to the patient's experience. The patient needs to experience the nurse as a caring, trusting individual who is committed to the goal of pain relief. The nurse needs to experience the patient in pain and discomfort as an individual who is doing everything possible to cope with this stressful situation. This means that most of the work is on the part of the nurse.

There are several attitudes that nurses need to develop. One of the most important and effective is to believe the patient, both with regard to the amount of pain and the degree of pain relief. A second attitude is to respect the patient's own response to pain. This is difficult to do when the patient's behavior differs from the nurse's preconceived idea of what the behavior "should be." Nurses also need to maintain an open mind about which pain relief measures might work. Education in pain relief has been highly slanted toward the use of drugs, though there are many other measures that work effectively and with fewer side effects.

Principle 2: Effective teaching enhances all other pain relief measures.   When the patient has a full understanding of the nature of the pain and the intent of the pain relief measures, there is likely to be much better patient cooperation and participation, as well as better pain relief. The teaching

TABLE 4-7
Common Analgesics

Analgesic	Site of action	Pain relief effect	Onset or duration	Dose	Side effects	Directions for administering	Miscellaneous
Nonnarcotics Aspirin	Peripheral nervous system	Mild to moderate.	30-60 min, peaks in 2 hr	550 mg	GI ulceration.	Administer with food or antacid.	Also used for antiembolic and anti-inflammatory properties.
Acetaminophen	Peripheral nervous system	Mild to moderate.	Peaks in ½ to 2 hr	650 mg	Not well documented; large doses may potentiate oral anti-coagulants.	Better absorption on empty stomach.	Not anti-inflammatory.
Additives Caffeine	Cerebral vaso-constriction	Mood elevation.	Has half-life of 3½ to 4 hr	200 mg	Headache and insomnia.	Avoid at bedtime.	A cup of coffee (100 mg caffeine) may be used instead.
TCAs Amitri-ptyline (Elavil) Imipramine (Tofranil)	Peripheral nervous system and CNS	Used for chronic pain.	Has plasma half-life of 17-40 hr Has plasma half-life of 9-24 hr	25 mg qid	Hypotension, arrhythmias, nausea, and vomiting.	Promotes sleep when administered at bedtime.	Contraindicated in CHF; must be used with caution in elderly patients and those with glaucoma.
Amphetamines	CNS	Strong.	Peak in 30-60 min	5 mg tid	Abuse potential; depress appetite.	Administer after meals; gradually taper dose when discontinuing.	Do not depress respirations or produce sedation; therefore, useful in terminal situations.

Drug	System	Strength/Action	Onset/Absorption	Dose	Effects	Administration	Comments
Narcotics							
Morphine	CNS	Strong.	Slow absorption (20 min IV)	5-20 mg SC	Depress brainstem respiratory center's responsiveness to changes in CO_2; idiosyncratic reactions after first doses; decrease BP.	Monitor respirations closely.	IV morphine maximally depresses respirations in 7 min, SC in 90 min. All narcotics slowly detoxified by liver (>36 hr).
Codeine	CNS	Strong.	Peaks in 30-60 min, SC	30-60 mg		Administer IM or SC.	
Hydrochlorides of opium alkaloids (Pantopon)	CNS	Strong.	Peaks in 30-60 min	5-20 mg			
Synthetic Meperidine (Demerol)	CNS	Strong.	30-50 min, IM	50-150 mg IM			
Narcotic antidote Naloxone (Narcan)	CNS	Reverses respiratory depression.	2 min after IV administration	0.4 mg	Precipitates withdrawal in narcotic-dependent individuals.	Dose may be repeated in 2-3 min	Very short acting.
Combination Brompton's mixture	CNS	Used for pain relief in terminal cancer.		Variable	Effects of constituent drugs.	PO.	Does not depress level of consciousness.
Additives Promethazine (Phenergan)	CNS	Claimed to be antiemetic, sedative, and antihistamine; studies show little effect.	Has prolonged action (18-24 hr)	25 mg	Depresses BP and respirations.	Not recommended.	Does not potentiate narcotic.
Hydroxyzine (Vistaril)	CNS	Decreases anxiety and depresses CNS.	Absorbed in 15-30 min	25 mg	Low incidence of drowsiness.		

TCAs, tricyclic antidepressants.

may range from suggestion and motivation for trying a novel approach (e.g., imagery) to the provision of factual, up-to-date information about specific drugs.

Principle 3: Patients' participation in planning their own pain relief improves results.   Patients in pain often feel a loss of control. Indeed, the entire illness experience usually involves several areas of loss of control. Including the patient in setting up a plan will decrease the feeling of loss of control and enhance the plan.

Principle 4: Incorporating the patient's beliefs about pain relief into the plan improves results.   The patient's belief in the effectiveness of a plan may be quite powerful. Although nurses know the power of this belief when placebos are administered, it must be understood that it applies just as emphatically to other modalities.

Principle 5: Decreasing anxiety decreases pain.   Anxiety accompanies pain and may exacerbate the experience. Anxiety produces many side effects, such as muscle tension and fatigue, that increase the perceived pain. Indeed, a vicious circle is begun: anxiety or the anticipation of pain results in the increased perception of pain, which, in turn, causes more anxiety.

Anxiety may be as powerful in increasing the intensity of pain as the patient's belief from principle 4 is in decreasing it, and perhaps for the same reason: a person's thoughts are capable of inhibiting or exciting the efferent neural transmission from the brain.

Principle 6: Preventing severe pain is easier than relieving it.   Pain relief measures must be planned with regard to prevention as well as relief. If a patient is allowed to reach a very severe pain level, it may take hours (or even days) to decrease the effects. However, if the pain can be relieved before it becomes so severe, a better level of comfort can be maintained.

Principle 7: New pain relief measures require more than one attempt.   Whatever the method, effective pain relief can be expected to increase as the procedure is continued. If the measure is one in which the patient participates, some skill or practice may be needed before it reaches maximum effectiveness.

Principle 8: A combination of methods works better than one method alone.   Whatever combination is chosen, pain relief is much more effective when two or more methods are used, either simultaneously or consecutively.

Principle 9: Pain relief is measured by patient behaviors.   What can be observed by the nurse and what the patient relates are the criteria for judging pain relief.

Pain relief measures.   The following are four pain relief measures.

1. Skin stimulation (pressure and massage):   Rubbing or holding a painful spot is almost a reflex response to some injuries. The soothing effect of massage or pressure may be due to muscle relaxation or to interruption in the neural transmission of impulses. The stimulation is usually applied directly over the painful area, but stimulation to the same area on the *opposite* side of the body or to an adjacent area may be just as effective. Pressure on "trigger" areas (taken from acupuncture sites) may also relieve pain, especially that of headache.

Massage is accomplished by rubbing the hands over a large skin area or by placing the hand on one area and massaging the underlying tissues. Pressure is applied with the heel of the hand, the ball of the thumb, or the fingertips. The Oriental method of massage makes use of the thumb to apply pressure for a few seconds to appropriate sites along the known meridians.

Used in conjunction with other modalities, skin stimulation can be an effective tool in the nurse's repertoire of pain relief methods. (When there is doubt about the existence of phlebitis, these measures should *never* be used.)

2. Relaxation techniques: Back rubs, other forms of massage, and deep breathing have long been used successfully to help patients cope with their pain. Relaxation procedures can help reduce muscle tension and anxiety. They also help alleviate pain by reducing stress, by serving somewhat as a distraction, and by decreasing fatigue. Actual physiologic changes are evident when relaxation procedures are effective: decreased respiratory and heart rates, decreased O_2 consumption, an increase in alpha brain waves, a decrease in BP in cases of hypertension, and muscle relaxation.

Some relaxation techniques (e.g., transcendental meditation and yoga) require special preparation. Two techniques that the nurse can initiate without special study are the repetitive thought process and rhythmic breathing. (The patient must be willing and able to participate in these relaxation techniques with the nurse. Eventually, the patient may be able to manage them alone or with a family member.) The repetitive thought process (Table 4-8) combines reduction of environmental stimuli and concentration on a simple thought or task (repeating words or numbers, or counting breaths or heart rate). Rhythmic breathing (Table 4-9) may be used for brief periods of time, such as during painful procedures. The deep breathe-clench fist-yawn technique effectively produces muscle tension, followed by relaxation and increased oxygenation. Because some degree of concentration is necessary, it can also relieve pain through distraction. It may be used in situations in which the patient is frightened or experiencing unexpected severe pain. There are three steps in this technique: (1) the patient inhales deeply and clenches the fists simultaneously, (2) the patient exhales and is urged to become as "limp as a rag doll," (3) the patient yawns. This technique may be repeated as often as necessary.

Soothing, familiar music can also result in effective relaxation. The patient needs to "experience" the music, to feel it lift away tension and relax the muscles.

Relaxation techniques are used in combination with other pain relief measures. They cannot be expected to relieve pain by themselves.

TABLE 4-8

Repetitive Thought Process

Parameter	Technique
Environment	Quiet, free from interruption.
Position	Maximum comfort: preferably sitting, back well supported, feet flat on floor.
Eyes	Closed.
Examples of process	Repeating a single word, number, or phrase; counting breaths or heart rate; visualizing a calm scene.
Attitude	Patient attempts to "let go" rather than "control," to flow with the experience rather than evaluate it.
Termination	Cleansing breath: deep inhalation followed by deep exhalation.
Time	Up to 20 min each session, bid or tid.

TABLE 4-9

Rhythmic Breathing

Parameter	Technique
Environment	Quiet, free from interruption.
Position	Maximum comfort: preferably sitting, back well supported, feet flat on floor.
Eyes	Closed.
Cleansing breath	Deep inhalation followed by deep exhalation.
Nurse	Repeats: "In: 1, 2; out: 1, 2" (slowly and rhythmically).
Patient Breathing Concentration	Abdominal breathing: slowly and to the count. Should feel air fill nose and lungs; should feel body relax and tension drain out as breath is exhaled.
Termination	Cleansing breath. Patient says, "I now feel relaxed and refreshed."
Time	For several minutes, several times a day.

3. Distraction: Often, becoming involved in a phone call or a television program can temporarily relieve a headache. Such distraction provides effective, welcome relief and should help dispel the myth that if distraction can relieve pain, the pain is neither real nor severe. The following are specific examples of distracters: (1) staring at any fixed point or object while an area near the pain site is massaged, (2) rapid breathing (pant-blow or "he-who"), (3) singing a song, aloud or silently, while tapping out the rhythm with the fingers, toes, or head, (4) storytelling by the patient, nurse, or someone else, and (5) combining massage with any of these techniques.

If one of the rapid breathing distractions is used, the patient must be aware of hyperventilation (exhalation of too much carbon dioxide), which will occur if the patient uses the technique for too long a period of time (as in the third stage of labor) without enough normal breathing. In these rapid-breathing procedures, the respiratory rate should be kept below 1 breath/sec. (Rebreathing carbon dioxide out of a paper bag can easily relieve the symptoms of hyperventilation.)

Distractions can be as simple or complex as necessary, depending on the severity of the pain. In general, the greater the intensity of pain, the less complex the distraction should be. Distraction is such an effective adjunct to pain relief that it may even work when the patient does not think it will.

4. Therapeutic touch: Since the early 1970s an increasing number of nurses have become skilled in using therapeutic touch to facilitate pain relief. Although the mechanism of action is unknown, its effectiveness is highly attested. In essence, the energy field of the nurse's hands interacts with the patient's energy field and restores the patient's imbalance. (*See* Boguslawski in the bibliography.)

CHRONIC PAIN

Chronic pain, either intermittent or relentless, occurs in a variety of illnesses, especially cancer. Arthritis, migraine headache, low back problems, angina, spinal cord injury, phantom limb, myositis, and trigeminal neuralgia are also common sources of chronic pain. Unless it accompanies a terminal illness, chronic pain does not have a foreseeable end. The patient's life is one of constant agony, whether the pain is continuous or occurs for only a part of each day.

With minor modifications, the assessment already described for acute pain is also appropriate for chronic pain. More specific attention, however, must be given to certain aspects of the assessment. In assessing the effects of pain on the patient, the nurse will recognize a dimension that is not apparent in the patient with acute pain: the intensity of upheaval in the patient's life. One's whole life-style may be totally changed and rearranged around the pain pattern. Has the patient had to stop working or been forced into a different kind of employment? Is there a substantial financial change? Other activities of daily living are curtailed, and inadequate nutrition may intensify the side effects of stress. The emotional involvement is severe and chronic. Depression, prolonged anger and resentment, lack of motivation, helplessness, hopelessness, and loneliness are all intensified and debilitating. The patient may be aware of a personality change. Prolonged pain can produce thought disturbances, ranging from confusion to hallucinations.

In assessing situational factors, the nurse must thoroughly investigate the meaning of pain for the patient. Has the patient found a meaning to his suffering? Is it a comfort to him or a burden? Can the patient achieve some form of inner peace amid the turmoil of pain?

Pain relief measures need to be assessed. What measures has the patient used, with what success, and for how long? Which ones does the patient have the most and the least faith in?

Based on this assessment, nursing diagnoses may be developed and an appropriate plan of care instituted.

General interventions

General interventions include transcutaneous electric nerve stimulation (TENS) and invasive procedures such as nerve blocks and surgery.

TENS. Stimulating an area of the skin over or near a painful site with a small amount of electric current can result in pain relief. TENS has been used to treat all types of chronic pain. The stimulation may be intermittent (10 to 30 sec tid or qid) or more continuous. (TENS cannot be used over areas of skin rash, and skin irritation may accompany prolonged use.) Patients may purchase TENS units for home use or receive in- or outpatient treatments. A few patients experience pain relief only during the treatment.

TENS has become a more common means of producing pain relief since the 1970s. Although it is a safe procedure, it should be avoided by pregnant patients or those with pacemakers or arrhythmias. TENS is sometimes used for acute pain, and it has had considerable success with postoperative pain relief. A side effect of TENS is its relief of postoperative ileus.

Nerve blocks. Local anesthetics injected into peripheral, spinal, cranial, or sympathetic nerves can provide pain relief for hours. When neurolytic agents such as alcohol, phenol, or saline are used, the effects can last for months. These procedures are useful when patients are too debilitated to withstand more invasive surgical procedures and when pain is confined to a localized area. Because of the complexity of the neural networks, however, nerve blocks are not always successful.

After these procedures, patients are observed for elevation or depression of BP, toxic or allergic reactions to the drug, respiratory distress, and loss of the sensations of touch and temperature over the affected area.

Surgery. Neurectomy, rhizotomy, chordotomy, and sympathectomy are surgical procedures performed on the afferent network to relieve pain. In a **neurectomy,** a peripheral or cranial nerve is interrupted. This procedure is used infrequently because peripheral nerves tend to regenerate. In addition, because peripheral nerves have sensory and motor fibers, patients could experience a loss of motor functioning. **Rhizotomy** (the interruption of spinal nerve roots as they enter the cord) and **chordotomy** (the interruption of a portion of the spinothalamic tract) are major surgical procedures that require laminectomy and exposure of several segments of the spine. A percutaneous approach that makes use of electric destruction can be performed under x-ray, eliminating the need for major surgery.

After a chordotomy, the sensations of pain and temperature are lost, but not that of touch. Procedures low in the cord may interfere with bowel, bladder, and sexual functioning. Cervical procedures may inhibit respiratory functioning. **Sympathectomy** for pain relief of vascular disease or causalgias is rarely a treatment of choice. The sympathetic nerve chain is interrupted in the thoracic or lumbar region. Postoperatively, the nurse observes for severe fluctuations in BP. With any of these procedures, the level of anesthesia may drop after a few months. In preterminal patients, the duration of analgesia may be sufficient to warrant the surgery.

In **percutaneous or permanent implant electric stimulation,** electrodes are permanently implanted (or needle electrodes inserted) into painful peripheral nerves, often the sciatic. If pain relief is achieved with the needle electrode, the patient is a candidate for a permanent implant. When pain relief is needed, the patient activates the stimulator by means of an external transmitter.

Stereotactic surgery to produce lesions within the brain by coagulation or freezing is reserved for chronic, intractable pain after other methods have failed. Lesions can be produced in the thalamus or frontal lobe in order to modify the pain response and diminish sensation.

All of these invasive procedures are attempts to improve the quality of life of individuals in intense pain. Their use must be carefully considered.

Nursing interventions

In addition to the other interventions already discussed for acute pain, guided imagery and distraction are helpful for chronic pain. However, it should be emphasized that the approach to pain relief needs to be well planned and integrated into the total health care plan. A multiphasic, multidisciplinary approach is needed. In addition, because patients in chronic pain experience considerable muscle tension and other symptoms of prolonged stress, relaxation procedures may have to precede, or be used in conjunction with, all pain relief measures.

Distraction.   With patients in chronic pain, distraction needs to be planned into every day for varying periods of time. Ideally, the distraction should be varied, meaningful (not just taking up time), interesting, and nonfatiguing. A visit from a hospice volunteer, a new book from the library, a mental puzzle such as Rubik's Cube, a new game, and making up stories or songs are a few of the many distracters that can be worked into the patient's life. Providing creative distractions can be a gratifying challenge to nursing ingenuity.

Imagery.   Guided imagery is similar to distraction in that the focus of the patient's thoughts is directed away from the pain. In imagery the patient's imagination is used to conjure up a scenario that provides pain relief. One form of imagery focuses on the pathology causing the pain (e.g., a tumor can be visualized as shrinking or melting away, a stiff joint can be seen exercising and relaxing, or pain can be seen flowing out through the fingers, toes, or incisions). Imagery can be used for momentary pain experiences or for longer ones.

The Simontons, pioneers in the medical use of imagery, have provided cancer patients with tape recordings that help to visualize the healing aspects of their medical treatment and body defenses. The use of this imagery can help reverse the process of the pathology.

Guided imagery can also focus on a pleasurable scene, such as a walk through the woods, a day at the beach, or a drive through the mountains. Attention is paid to as many of the sensations as possible. What did the sea air smell like? How did the wet sand feel on the feet? What sound did the waves make?

Guided imagery requires considerable explanation by the nurse, and the patient needs regular practice. The patient should understand that normal imagination is used in a deliberate way to help relieve pain. As the same image is practiced, more details are included. An account of the images can be tape-recorded. If unwanted drowsiness occurs at the end of the imagery, the patient is instructed to put a deliberate end to the experience by taking a deep breath or two and saying to himself, "I feel awake and refreshed."

Pain clinics

The most exciting and effective development in the field of chronic pain control is the advent of pain clinics, which use a holistic attitude and a comprehensive approach to pain treatment. The goals are to achieve pain relief and to eliminate drugs. The patient is "rehabilitated" through a variety of procedures, including biofeedback, behavior modification, nutrition, meditation, relaxation, psychotherapy (individual, family, and group), acupuncture, and physical and occupational therapy. The patient examines his current existence and his contribution to it and learns "self-help" methods to overcome the crippling effects of pain.

At these clinics, many patients experience for the first time a truly caring attitude on the part of health professionals. The patient is brought into a trusting atmosphere in which every aspect of pain and its relief is considered. The growth of these clinics attests to their successes. Nurses should learn about the clinics in their area for patient referral.

Evaluation criteria

The goals of the care plan for acute or chronic pain relief are used to evaluate the effectiveness of the plan. Because of the subjective nature of the problem, the primary caregiver and patient should work together on the evaluation. The goals of the care plan have been effective if (1) pain is decreased to tolerable levels or totally relieved, (2) autonomic responses are alleviated, (3) a variety of pain relief measures are used, (4) the timing and dosage of pain medication provide pain relief, (5) the side effects of medications are controlled, (6) nurse-patient communication is open and honest, (7) anxiety is diminished, (8) severe pain is prevented, (9) the beliefs of the patient about pain relief are included in the plan, (10) sufficient time and trials are allowed when new measures are introduced, (11) pain stimuli are identified and avoided, (12) the patient carries out activities of daily living and resumes social interactions, and (13) the patient verbalizes an improved quality of life.

HYPESTHESIA

The inability to feel or recognize any of the sensations arising from the skin is a dangerous condition. Such hypesthesia occurs when sensory transmission is blocked or when a person is unable to respond to a stimulus. Spinal cord injury, cerebrovascular accident, nerve blocks, and any condition that leads to a decrease or loss of consciousness are the primary causes of this loss of sensation. Diminished circulation (as in arteriosclerotic changes in the elderly) also produces some degree of hypesthesia.

Nursing assessment of any patient with hypesthesia includes a thorough sensory investigation. In any elderly patient, special attention should be directed to the lower extremities. In patients with any form of paralysis, hypesthesia is to be expected.

Hypesthesia is essentially a safety problem. Because feelings of pressure, heat, or cold and the pain of cuts or bruises cannot be detected, the patient is unaware of an injury that may have occurred. For example, the inside of the cheek may unknowingly be bitten by the stroke patient, or the hands may be burned by hot water from a faucet if temperature sensation is lacking. In a sensory assessment, the nurse (1) inspects the entire body for bruises, sores, and cuts, (2) tests the heat and cold perception of the extremities with tubes of water, (3) tests sharp and dull discrimination with both ends of a safety pin, (4) observes for edema of dependent areas (back of the head, sacrum, legs, paralyzed extremities), (5) questions the patient for awareness of sensory loss, and (6) identifies safety hazards in the environment.

Nursing interventions

Nursing interventions focus on teaching the patient or primary caregiver how to prevent injury and how to perform a daily skin assessment. The patient must understand that the eyes are now the only means of protection for hypesthetic areas. The nurse instructs the patient to do the following:

1. Correct safety hazards in the environment (e.g., slippery floors or ill-fitting shoes and clothing).

2. Use sharp objects with supervision.
3. Be aware of obstacles in ambulating (e.g., chair legs, bedposts, small rugs, or doorknobs).
4. Use the footrest on wheelchairs with care.
5. Lower temperatures in home hot water heaters.
6. Avoid cooling or heating applications to the skin (e.g., hot-water bottles, heating pads, electric blankets, hot packs, or ice packs).
7. Schedule vigilant and meticulous skin inspections, sometimes as frequently as q 2 hr.
8. Use mirrors to assess areas that are hard to visualize.
9. Rinse and inspect the inside of the mouth after every meal, if indicated.
10. Keep the bedding free of wrinkles and crumbs. (Wrinkles cause pressure.)
11. Protect the lower extremities with socks.
12. Buy shoes with extreme care with regard to fit.

For any decrease in level of consciousness, a corresponding decrease in patient attention to sensation will occur. For comatose patients, the responsibility for the prevention of injury rests with the nurse. The same assessment and intervention practices are included in the care plan.

Evaluation criteria

The evaluation of care for the patient with hypesthesia must relate to the goal of preventing injury. Evaluation may be carried out by the nurse, the patient, and/or another primary caregiver. The following questions constitute the evaluation criteria: (1) Can the patient perform a thorough skin inspection, and is the patient committed to doing it? (2) Are there any new areas of skin redness or injury? (3) Can the patient identify environmental safety hazards? (4) Does the patient take appropriate steps to correct any hazards? (5) Does the patient convey an attitude of concern for areas of hypesthesia?

CHAPTER 5

TEMPERATURE CONTROL
Lani Guzman

OVERVIEW

Man is a homoiotherm, or warm-blooded animal, and is thus able to maintain a relatively constant body temperature over a fairly broad range of environmental temperatures. A naked human being can maintain a normal body temperature within an environmental temperature range of 12.8 to 60.0°C (55 to 140°F). Behavioral adaptations, including the use of clothing, allow humans to maintain a normal body temperature over an even broader range of environmental temperatures: in the Arctic, for instance, where temperatures may fall below −60°C (−76°F), or on the moon, where temperatures may exceed 204°C (400°F).

Definition

No single temperature can be considered the "normal" temperature of the body. Instead, there is a range of normal temperatures, depending on the way the temperature is measured and on the condition of the subject at the time of measurement.

In assessment of body temperature, the nurse is most interested in **core body temperature**, that is, the temperature of vital organs such as the brain and heart, which is the least likely to vary with extremes of environmental temperature. However, because it is difficult to directly measure core body temperature, it must be estimated by measuring the temperature of accessible sites that are close to the major arteries. (*See below* for specific information on clinical temperature measurement.)

Even if it were feasible to measure core body temperature, it would demonstrate significant variations over a 24-hr period. This **circadian temperature rhythm** results in highest core body temperatures in the early evening, between 5 and 7 p.m., and lowest core body temperatures in the morning, just before rising.

If the normal circadian rhythm of the body's temperature is taken into account, as well as variations in measurement techniques, the normal body temperature is usually described as being within the range of $37.0\pm0.5\,°C$ ($98.6\pm1.0\,°F$) when measured orally. Rectal temperatures are normally $0.5\,°C$ ($1.0\,°F$) higher than the oral temperature; axillary temperatures are normally $0.5\,°C$ ($1.0\,°F$) lower.

Anatomy and physiology review

Heat is continually being produced as a by-product of metabolism and continually being lost to the environment. The core body temperature is the result of the dynamic balancing of heat production and loss. The controlling organ in this balance is the hypothalamus.

Heat production.   At rest, the metabolic production of energy is ~ 1 kcal/kg body wt/hr. On the average, 75% of the energy in food is directly transformed into heat; the remaining 25% is mainly used to fuel muscle movement. However, because the movement of muscles against the friction of surrounding tissues also generates heat, almost all of the energy in the food we consume is eventually transformed into heat.

Energy production, and thus heat production, can be increased in several ways, the most important of which is **muscular contraction.** Through muscular contraction, trained athletes can raise their heat production by up to 20 times their basal rate. (Not all of this energy is turned into heat, however, since some of it is turned into mechanical energy to propel the body.) **Shivering** is a form of muscular contraction that generates heat without generating any mechanical energy. Shivering can increase heat production by up to five times the basal rate. Shivering can occur in almost all the muscles of the body. Heat can also be produced through **nonshivering thermogenesis,** which results from the heat-producing effects of hormones, including thyroxine, epinephrine, and norepinephrine.

Heat loss.   There are four main ways in which heat is lost from the body: radiation, conduction, convection, and evaporation.

Radiation is the loss of heat through the emission of heat waves from the body. It accounts for $\sim 60\%$ of the body's heat loss under normal circumstances. The amount of heat lost through radiation depends on the difference between the environmental temperature and the temperature of the skin surface. If the environment is warmer than the skin surface, radiant heat will be transferred *to* the body.

Skin temperature can be altered physiologically by the circulation of more or less blood through peripheral vessels. To increase heat loss, the body increases blood circulation through the periphery, by means of peripheral vasodilation. To decrease heat loss, the body initiates peripheral vasoconstriction.

Conduction is the transfer of heat from a warmer to a cooler body by direct contact. Conduction to the air in contact with the body represents a minor source of heat loss under normal circumstances. However, if the surrounding air is continually circulating, conductive heat loss can be significant (e.g., on windy days, or if the body is moving rapidly through stationary air, as when traveling in a convertible).

Conductive heat loss can also be significant if the body is in contact with water (e.g., during swimming). Conduction to solid objects with which the body is in contact is usually a minor source of heat loss.

Convection is the movement of warmed air away from the body by means of air currents. Together, conduction and convection account for ~12% of heat loss under normal circumstances.

Evaporation is the loss of heat through the vaporization of body water. Normally, ~600 ml/H_2O/day are vaporized by the body. Although heat is lost in the process, the amount of this insensible fluid loss cannot be regulated to control body temperature.

Sweating is the mechanism by which the body regulates heat loss through vaporization. In hot environments, it is the *only* available mechanism for heat loss. In humid environments, however, even sweating may be ineffective. Because women sweat less than men, they are less able to tolerate hot, humid environments.

CNS control of body temperature.   The temperature of the body is regulated by the CNS via the temperature-regulating center in the hypothalamus. The hypothalamus receives information on core body temperature from temperature receptors in the hypothalamus itself, from skin receptors, and from receptors in the spine and abdomen.

If the hypothalamus senses that the body is cooler than it should be, it sets heat-conserving and heat-producing mechanisms into action. Heat production is increased mainly through the initiation of shivering and nonshivering thermogenesis. Heat loss is decreased by peripheral vasoconstriction and diminished sweating. Vasoconstriction lowers the skin surface temperature and thus also lowers conductive, convective, and radiant heat losses. Behavioral responses are also triggered, in addition to the automatic physiologic responses to the hypothalamic sensation of cold. The person attempts to get warm by putting on additional clothes, by flexing and contracting large muscle masses, and by trying to find a warmer environment.

If the hypothalamus senses a body temperature that is too warm, it initiates mechanisms that decrease heat production and increase heat loss (i.e., peripheral vasodilation and increased sweating). The behavioral response consists of decreasing both activity and food intake.

Theories of disordered thermoregulation

In health, the body temperature is maintained within a narrow range, despite wide ranges in environmental temperatures. Disordered thermoregulation, however, may occur in a variety of situations: abnormal heat production, abnormal heat loss, and impaired central thermoregulation.

Abnormal heat production can result in either hyper- or hypothermia. Abnormally decreased heat production occurs in conditions such as starvation, immobility, and hypothyroidism. Conversely, abnormally increased heat production can occur in disorders such as hyperthyroidism and malignant hyperpyrexia.

Abnormal heat loss can also result in either hyper- or hypothermia. Abnormally increased heat loss can occur with burns, excessive alcohol intake, atherosclerosis, or when the individual is unable to tolerate an abnormally low ambient temperature. Abnormally decreased heat loss can occur with disorders of the sweat glands, dehydration, certain skin disorders such as scleroderma, or as the result of an inability to tolerate an abnormally hot, humid environment.

Impaired central thermoregulation can result from an abnormal setting of the hypothalamic thermostat, altered behavioral responses to temperature variations, or the inability of the hypothalamus to sense peripheral body temperature.

Normally, the hypothalamus is set within the normal body temperature range. If the sensed core temperature varies from the set temperature of the hypothalamic thermostat, thermoregulatory mechanisms are initiated. However, the set temperature of the hypothalamic thermostat can be altered by substances called endogenous pyrogens. If the hypothalamic thermostat is set at a higher than normal temperature, heat-loss mechanisms will not be set into effect until the core temperature exceeds the hypothalamic thermostat set point. Conversely, if the set point is lower than normal, heat-loss mechanisms will be initiated earlier than normal.

Altered behavioral adaptation to altered body temperature can occur at the extremes of age, because of psychoactive medications, or because of mental illness. In health, humans sense heat or cold and dress appropriately. In the conditions listed above, however, either inappropriate behavior or none at all is manifested in response to these sensations.

Finally, in conditions such as spinal cord injury, the hypothalamus may be unable to sense core body temperature or to activate appropriate thermoregulatory mechanisms. Thus, inappropriate sweating is frequently seen in spinal cord injury.

General assessment

Nursing assessment of the individual at risk for significant alteration in body temperature falls into two main categories: (1) health history for risk factors and (2) physical assessment for indicators of present alterations in body temperature. Risk factors for significant alteration in body temperature depend on etiology (Table 5-1).

TABLE 5-1

*Risk Factors for the Development of
Significant Alteration in Body Temperature*

Alteration	Risk factors
Fever	Similar to risk factors for the development of an infection, including malnutrition, chronic disease, steroid therapy, and exposure to communicable disease
Heat injury	Hot, humid environment Newness (and nonacclimatization) to environment Old age Diabetes mellitus Atherosclerosis Dehydration Abnormalities of sweating mechanism
Systemic cold injury	Cold or cool environment Old age Use of alcohol Use of tobacco Atherosclerosis Diabetes mellitus Altered skin integrity

Clinical measurement of body temperature remains controversial despite the voluminous literature on the subject. Accurate measurement depends on the use of an appropriate measuring instrument, on the use of the appropriate measurement site, and on allowing adequate time for the thermometer to register the temperature of the measurement site.

Three types of clinical thermometers that are in use today are the mercury, electronic, and disposable thermometers. Electronic thermometers provide an optimal combination of accuracy and speed of measurement. (Mercury thermometers are slow, and disposable thermometers may not provide an accurate measurement.)

Three common **measurement sites** are the mouth, rectum, and axilla. The routes, norms, and contraindications for each site are listed in Table 5-2.

The *mouth* is used for estimation of core body temperature because it is in close proximity to the carotid arteries. Optimal placement of an oral thermometer requires that the bulb of the thermometer be placed in the posterior sublingual pocket. It does not seem to matter which side of the mouth is used, nor if the mouth is closed or left open.

The *rectum* may also be used to measure body temperature because the nearby arteries supplying the colon allow rectal temperatures to approximate core body temperature. Because rectal temperature measurement is

TABLE 5-2
Clinical Temperature Measurement

Route	Normal temperature	Duration of mercury thermometer insertion	Contraindications
		min	
Oral	36.5-37.5°C 97.6-99.6°F	8	Recent ingestion of hot or cold liquids Recent smoking Recent therapeutic application of heat or cold Mouth injuries Likely to bite on thermometer O_2 therapy
Rectal	37.0-38.0°C 98.6-100.6°F	2	Bleeding disorders Rectal disease Fecal impaction
Axillary	36.0-37.0°C 96.6-98.6°F	10	None

less convenient and pleasant than oral measurement, it should only be used when oral measurement is contraindicated. There is no evidence to support the belief that rectal measurements are more accurate than oral temperatures, even in people with fever, provided that optimal technique is used. The well-lubricated thermometer should be inserted 4 cm (1.5 in.) into the rectum.

Axillary temperature measurements allow the estimation of core body temperature because of the axilla's proximity to the arteries of the upper arm and shoulder. The axillary site is usually used only when oral and rectal temperature measurements are both contraindicated. Again, there is no reason to believe that axillary temperatures are less accurate than oral or rectal temperatures, provided that optimal technique is used.

Allowing adequate time for the thermometer to reach the temperature of the measurement site is generally only a problem with mercury thermometers. (*See* Table 5-2 for guidelines on clinical temperature measurement.) Physical assessment can also detect the specific signs of altered body temperature that are listed above in the section on deviations from normal body temperature. Laboratory tests that may aid in the determination of the cause of altered body temperature are listed in Table 5-3.

Common interventions

Because alterations in body temperature are due to abnormal heat production, abnormal heat loss, or impaired central thermoregulation, initial interventions must be directed at identifying and treating the underlying abnormality, whenever possible. Symptomatic or supportive treatment can only help the patient survive the acute crisis. Symptomatic therapies are listed in Table 5-4.

Evaluation criteria

The effectiveness of the measures taken in the care of the individual with altered body temperature is demonstrated by (1) normal body temperature, (2) the absence of other signs and symptoms, such as tachy- or bradycardia, altered level of consciousness, and alteration in skin color and temperature, and (3) the absence of complications.

DEVIATIONS

FEVER

Fever is defined as an abnormally high body temperature. Although the term is nonspecific, it generally refers to elevations in temperature that are the result of endogenous diseases that reset the hypothalamic thermostat rather than to conditions in which the elevated body temperature results from a failure to tolerate a stressful environment. An oral temperature >37.5°C (99.6°F) is usually considered to indicate fever.

TABLE 5-3
Laboratory Tests in Altered Body Temperature

Alteration	Laboratory test	Characteristic abnormalities
Fever	CBC	Elevated WBC
	ESR	Elevated ESR
	Cultures (blood, urine, sputum, wound, etc.)	Positive for organism
Heat injury	CBC	Elevated WBC
	Blood chemistry	Elevated BUN
		Hypokalemia
	Arterial blood gases	Respiratory alkalosis
	ECG	Tachycardia
		ST and T wave changes
	Clotting parameters	Prolonged
Systemic cold injury	Arterial blood gases	Metabolic acidosis
	Blood chemistry	Hemoconcentration
		Hypoglycemia
	ECG	Bradycardia
		Arrhythmias

ESR, erythrocyte sedimentation rate.

TABLE 5-4

Interventions for Alterations in Body Temperature

Abnormality	Example	Interventions
Abnormal heat production		
Increased	Excessive activity, stress	Relaxation therapy
	Hyperthyroidism	Drugs, surgery
	Shivering	Phenothiazines
Decreased	Hypothyroidism	Thyroid supplements
	Immobility	Exercise (even mild exercise like active range of motion)
		Provision of exogenous heat:*
		Warm fluids
		Oral or IV
		Hemodialysis
		Peritoneal dialysis
		Warm baths
		Heating pads
Abnormal heat loss		
Increased	Cold ambient temperatures	Warmed environment
	Burns	Body insulation
		Education about prevention of systemic cold injuries
Decreased	Hot, humid environment	Cooled environment
		Fluids
		Tepid baths (water or alcohol)
		Hypothermia
		Education about prevention of heat injuries
Impaired central thermoregulation	Infection	Antipyretics: aspirin or acetaminophen
		Antibiotics as indicated

*Rewarming should proceed slowly: rapid rewarming is associated with increased mortality from systemic cold injuries.

Acute fevers are usually the result of infections. In an infection, exogenous pyrogens, released by the infecting organism, and endogenous pyrogens, released by phagocytic lymphocytes, reset the hypothalamic thermostat, thus initiating all of the mechanisms that increase body temperature to the new set level. Prolonged fevers can be the result of untreated or unresolved infections. However, they can also result from conditions such as neoplasms and tissue infarctions. Prolonged fevers are usually the result of prolonged release of endogenous pyrogens.

The *signs and symptoms* of fever are manifested in four phases: the prodromal phase, the chill phase, the flush phase, and defervescence. During the prodromal phase, there are only nonspecific complaints: malaise, headache, nausea, and aches and pains. The body temperature is usually normal.

In the chill phase, the hypothalamic thermostat is reset to a higher level, and mechanisms are initiated to decrease heat loss and increase heat production. In this phase, peripheral vasoconstriction and shivering occur, and the patient usually complains of being cold. Behavioral responses may include turning up the room thermostat or using extra blankets.

The next phase, the flush phase, occurs when the body's temperature approximately equals the hypothalamic thermostat temperature. Although the body temperature is high, the patient usually feels better than during the chill phase.

Eventually, the patient will defervesce, when the set point of the hypothalamic thermostat returns to more normal levels. Mechanisms to increase heat loss and decrease heat production are set into effect: peripheral vasodilation, removing excess bedclothes, diaphoresis, etc.

When the temperature is elevated, particularly during the flush phase, associated changes occur in other systems of the body: tachycardia, tachypnea, headache, nausea, delirium, dehydration, and anorexia. The CO increases, allowing increased supply of nutrients and oxygen to the infected tissues. Although fever is thought to be an adaptive mechanism in lower animals, fever in humans outweighs any benefits. (For laboratory tests used in cases of fever, *see* Table 5-3; for common interventions, *see* Table 5-4.)

HEAT INJURIES

Heat injuries, including heat exhaustion and heatstroke, are elevations in body temperature that are due to an inability to tolerate high ambient temperatures. Heatstroke, the more severe type of heat injury, can be life threatening. Heat exhaustion, also known as heat collapse or heat prostration, is a less serious form of heat injury.

Heat injuries are the result of the body's inability to lose heat in a hot, humid environment. This may involve a failure of heat-losing mechanisms, particularly of the ability to sweat normally and/or to regulate temperature. At body temperatures $>41.7°C$ ($107°F$), the body is unable to further attempt the regulation of body temperature.

Heat exhaustion is the more common form of heat injury. It often occurs in the elderly and the physically active. Prodromal *symptoms* include weakness, vertigo, headache, nausea, anorexia, and dizziness. In the acute stage, the patient collapses, looks ashen gray, and has cold, clammy skin. The BP is usually low, and the body temperature is usually normal.

In **heatstroke**, the body temperature becomes elevated, often >41.1 °C (106 °F). Heatstroke most commonly occurs when the ambient temperature is >32.2°C (90°F) and when the humidity is high. It is most often seen in the elderly and in individuals with atherosclerosis, diabetes, alcoholism, and certain skin diseases. There are few prodromal signs of heatstroke, although they may be preceded by heat exhaustion. During the acute stage, the body's temperature becomes acutely elevated, and associated *signs and symptoms* occur: hot, dry skin; absence of sweating; tachycardia; rapid, shallow respirations; elevated BP; and a depressed level of consciousness. (For laboratory tests used in cases of heat injuries, *see* Table 5-3; for common interventions, *see* Table 5-4.)

SYSTEMIC COLD INJURIES

Cold injuries, like heat injuries, are the result of the body's inability to tolerate a thermally stressful environment. Cold injuries can be local (e.g., frostbite) or systemic. This section will deal only with systemic cold injuries.

Systemic hypothermia occurs when the body temperature falls <35 °C (95°F). At body temperatures <34.4°C (94°F), the hypothalamus becomes less able to regulate body temperature; at temperatures <29.4°C (85°F), it loses this ability completely.

Systemic cold injuries are most common in two distinct groups of people: (1) relatively healthy, active people who are exposed to low ambient temperatures for extended periods of time, and (2) older people, often in poor health, who are exposed to moderately low ambient temperatures for a prolonged period of time. In this second group of people, systemic hypothermia is often called "urban" hypothermia.

Urban hypothermia is more common in men, alcoholics, the mentally ill, the elderly, and people with other medical problems. It is common in the elderly because of their decreased ability to adapt to extremes of temperature and because they tend to be less physically active, have lower resting metabolic rates, and may have vascular or neurologic problems. They may also be unable to afford a well-heated living space.

Systemic cold injuries are the result of increased heat loss, usually in a cold environment. In an attempt to conserve body heat, peripheral blood vessels constrict. At close to normal ambient temperatures, blood vessels constrict only in the extreme periphery. At colder ambient temperatures, however, deeper vessels also constrict, thus potentially causing widespread tissue damage.

When blood vessels constrict as a response to a cold environment, the tissues may not obtain enough oxygen and nutrients to survive. The result is anoxic damage, with destruction of the vessel walls. Plasma leaks out of the damaged vessels into the interstitium. The remaining blood becomes concentrated and thus more prone to clotting. Clotting further reduces the blood supply to the constricted area, and a vicious cycle of anoxic injury is initiated. Muscles, nerves, and blood vessels are most susceptible to cold injury.

Signs of moderate hypothermia include cold, cyanotic skin; slowed respiratory rate; slowed, irregular heart rate; shivering; and a depressed level of consciousness (disorientation, apathy, drowsiness, confusion, and impaired judgment).

As hypothermia progresses and the body temperature drops further, the person may seem dead; however, a victim of hypothermia cannot be considered dead unless serious resuscitation efforts are maintained until the body's core temperature is >30°C (86°F). Signs of severe hypothermia include pulselessness, apnea, absence of shivering, and unresponsiveness to any stimuli. (For laboratory tests used in cases of systemic cold injuries, *see* Table 5-3; for common interventions, *see* Table 5-4.)

CHAPTER 6

IMMUNITY

Rita K. Ryan and Marion Oare Smith

OVERVIEW

Definitions

Immunity is the mechanism by which the human body recognizes the existence of foreign substances and resists their harmful effects. "How man interacts with his environment" is a broad definition.

Immunity occurs as man interacts with the environment. For example, (1) exposure to bacteria, such as mumps and chicken pox, leads to disease and/or immunity; (2) exposure to foreign proteins leads to allergic responses, such as hay fever and drug allergies; and (3) transplantation of foreign tissue, such as a kidney or a heart, leads to rejection mechanisms. Immunity is based on the ability to distinguish between "self" (the body's own cells) and "non-self" (other cells); is characterized by specificity of response and highly selective reactions to specific stimuli; and performs a defense function and the more diverse functions of homeostasis and surveillance.

Natural immunity, defined as those immune responses that are innately present, is characterized by the existence of antibodies without apparent exposure to a triggering immunogen. It is inherited genetically; is characteristic for individuals, races, and species; and may occur in varying degrees, as in varied resistances of individuals to colds or influenza. Natural immunity accounts for species-specific resistance to organisms (e.g., distemper affects dogs but not humans), and can be altered by modifying such factors as environment, age, and nutritional, physical, and psychologic status. It is poorly understood in terms of the mechanisms involved in its operation.

Acquired immunity, which is defined as the body's ability to protect itself against foreign substances for which it does not have natural immunity, involves survival of individuals rather than species. It is not inherited, but results from the development of specific immune responses. It may be due to humoral or cell-mediated immunity. Humoral immunity involves the production and release of antibodies to destroy foreign antigens (phagocytosis), and is produced by (1) active production of antibodies or sensitized lymphocytes in response to a foreign substance, or (2) passive acquisition of antibodies that have been produced in the bodies of other persons or animals. Cell-mediated immunity involves responses in which specifically sensitized lymphocytes are responsible for mediating the immune reactions (e.g., hypersensitivity, transplant rejection, and resistance to pathogens).

Passive immunity results in an immediate ability to rescue the body from invading antigens. It is temporary, lasting for a few weeks to months. For example, immunity from a mother to her child in utero lasts longest (up to 6 mo); a human source lasts from a few weeks to a few months; and an animal source lasts from several days to 2 wk.

Active immunity is produced by natural or artificial stimulation, so that the body produces its own antibodies and sensitized lymphocytes. It involves the development of a "memory" such that the immune response persists for years or even a lifetime. Active immunity does not occur immediately in life, but requires time for the body to develop its immune response. It can be produced by (1) the initial attack of a causative organism, with or without full symptoms of a disease, or (2) a vaccination or inoculation with killed organisms, live attenuated organisms, or toxoids. A comparison of active and passive immunity is provided in Table 6-1.

TABLE 6-1
Comparison of Active and Passive Immunity

Factor	Active	Passive
Genesis	Host participation. Exposure to immunogen through natural exposure or immunization.	No host participation. Transfer of antibody from an actively immunized host.
Components	Cell-mediated and humoral immunity.	Humoral immunity.
Onset of action	Only after a latent period.	Immediate.
Duration	Long lived.	Transitory.

Anatomy and physiology of immune responses

Human immune responses develop as important functions of the lymphoreticular system and constitute an important homeostatic characteristic of host resistance. The essential functions of immune responses are protection from infections, removal of abnormal neoplastic cells, and acceptance or rejection of cells and tissues (as in organ transplants and blood transfusions). However, a damaged or pathologic immune system may direct its powerful abilities against the body itself and cause disease.

The **lymphoreticular system** consists of bone marrow; the spleen, thymus, lymph nodes, and tonsils; and various groups of lymphocytes and macrophages throughout the body. The system, which originates with bone marrow stem cells that differentiate into RBCs, granulocytes, and uncommitted lymphocytes, includes primary organs that develop immunologically competent lymphocytes: the thymus develops T cells, and the mammalian equivalent of the bursa of Fabricius (postulated to be lymphoid tissue of the GI tract) develops B cells. In addition, it includes lymph tissue and the bloodstream, where lymphocytes migrate, proliferate, and mature in response to stimulation of antigens.

Antigens are substances (not normally present in the body) that stimulate the production of specific antibodies. Antigens are usually large protein molecules, which include bacteria, viruses, and their toxins. Antigens can consist of (1) proteins, such as those of transplanted human organs, blood cells of donors, and serums used for immunizations; (2) allergens, such as ragweed and grass pollens, that only cause disease in susceptible individuals; and (3) small molecules (called haptens) that combine with a protein to act as an antigen. Examples of haptens are drugs such as penicillin and sulfa, and the chemical constituents in dust, animal danders, and industrial chemicals.

Two functional divisions of the immune system are cellular immunity and humoral immunity. **Cellular immunity** is thymus-dependent (T cell) in embryonic development and includes all immunologic responses of sensitized lymphoid cells. It is an important defense mechanism against intrinsic neoplastic growths and is important in the rejection of transplanted tissue by the host. Cellular immunity is a major component of certain autoimmune diseases. **Humoral immunity** is developed by follicular lymphoid tissue and is responsible for the synthesis of immunoglobulins (antibodies). It is thymus-independent (B cell) in embryonic development and an important defense mechanism against invading microorganisms. Humoral immunity plays an active role in the inflammatory response.

The immune system consists of several different kinds of cells. The **T cell,** which is produced by the thymus, is transported (when immunologically competent) to the peripheral lymphoid organs (spleen, lymph nodes). It is identified by surface receptors to antigens that develop during maturation, and it constitutes ~65% of all lymphocytes in the circulation. T cells play a major role in cell-mediated immune responses. The **B cell,** which differentiates under bone-marrow control, has, as its primary role, development into a cell that secretes immunoglobulins. It is a primary responder to bacterial invasion and is responsible for humoral immunity. **Macrophages,** which differentiate from monocytes under bone-marrow control, are mononuclear cells found in many body organs and tissues. Macrophages remove and destroy bacteria, neoplastic cells, and colloidal material by the process of phagocytosis. They play an important role in the immune responses of both the cellular and humoral types.

Antibodies, another major component of the immune system, are proteins that are synthesized within plasma cells of the lymphoreticular tissues. Produced after the introduction of an antigen that combines with B cells to form plasma cells, antibodies have the ability to combine with the specific antigen that stimulated their production. They are part of the body's natural resistance to foreign antigens (such as viruses) and are all immunoglobulins.

Major immunoglobulin antibodies include IgG, IgA, IgM, IgD, and IgE. The most important and most abundant in man, **IgG** plays a crucial role in host defenses against infection. **IgA,** the principal immunoglobulin found in seromucous secretions, is important in the resistance to respiratory, GI, and GU infections. **IgM,** the largest immunoglobulin molecule, functions as a specific antitoxin against bacteria and the promotion of phagocytosis. The function of **IgD,** which is present in all serums, is not known. **IgE,** which has the lowest level in normal serums, is a mediator of allergic reactions.

An antigen-antibody reaction, a response of the body to the entrance of antigens, can continue for weeks to years after the body starts to produce antibodies. The reaction is highly specific (each antibody is effective only against the particular antigen that stimulated its production), and results in modes of action in which antibodies operate as (1) agglutinins, causing bacteria to clump together and, therefore, be harmless; (2) antienzymes, to inhibit enzymatic activity; (3) antitoxins, e.g., tetanus antitoxin antibodies; (4) bacteriolysins, to dissolve or liquefy the invading organism; (5) cytotoxins, to have a specific destructive effect on the cells; (6) hemolysins, to destroy RBCs by liberating Hb; (7) opsonins, to coat bacteria and render them more susceptible to phagocytosis; (8) precipitins, to precipitate from a solution the antigen producing the solution; and (9) blood group antibodies. (The ABO and Rh blood group antigens play a major role in transfusion reactions.)

Two theories of antibody formation are the clonal selection theory and the instructive theory. The clonal selection theory, widely accepted today, holds that an immunologically competent cell (T or B) has the ability to respond to only one antigen or to a very closely related group of antigens. It maintains that lymphocytes are genetically endowed with these specific abilities. It further states that each individual has a large pool of lympho- cytes, each of which is capable of reacting with specific antigens. Finally, it claims that the initiation of the immune response occurs when the antigen interacts with a particular cell that is receptive to it, resulting in (1) cell proliferation to form a clone of cells that can bind the antigen, or (2) cell differentiation, which produces T and B "memory" cells. The instructive theory, which is no longer accepted, holds that the specificity of the antibody is determined by the antigen.

DEVIATIONS

HYPO- OR AGAMMAGLOBULINEMIA

Hypo- or agammaglobulinemia is a severe deficiency or absence of immunoglobulins. It was the first immunodeficiency disorder to be recognized. There are three main forms of this disorder: **Transient**, which occurs in early infancy, involves no production of immunoglobulin in the fetus and the depletion of immunoglobulins transferred from maternal blood. It is a temporary deficiency that lasts until the infant synthesizes his own immunoglobulins. The **congenital** form of this disorder consists of two types: a more common X-linked recessive disorder observed only in males, and an autosomal recessive type that can occur in both sexes. Both types become evident early in infancy and are characterized by the absence of B cells. The third form of this immunodeficiency disorder is **acquired,** which is categorized as primary (no known cause) or secondary (associated with leukemia, myeloma, lymphoma, nephrosis, and liver disease). Acquired occurs in both sexes and can become evident at any age (usually between 15 and 35 yr). The patient presents with the normal number of B cells, which suggests a possible etiology of (1) malignant B cells that are unable to synthesize immunoglobulins, (2) an increased loss of immunoglobulins via the GI or urinary tract, or (3) an increased breakdown of immunoglobulins.

Hypo- or agammaglobulinemia is a disorder of the humoral components (B cells, plasma cells, and immunoglobulins). The cellular components (T cells) are normal. In the congenital form, there is an apparent failure in the differentiation of stem cells. In the acquired form, there is an apparent failure in the differentiation of B cells from plasma cells. Immunoglobulins (antibodies) defend against invasion of microorganisms, especially bacterial agents. Lack of immunoglobulins leads to susceptibility to infections (particularly bacterial) and/or to severe recurrent upper and lower respiratory infections. Because cellular immunity is intact, recovery from viral infections such as mumps and chicken pox is not impaired.

Signs and symptoms include recurrent bacterial infections, absence of serum immunoglobulins, diarrhea and malabsorption (in acquired), and a high incidence of rheumatoid arthritis symptoms and autoimmune diseases.

The general assessment consists of the patient's health history, a physical exam, and diagnostic tests. The patient will most likely have a pattern of recurrent bacterial infections, normal recovery from viral infections, and normal responses to immunizations. It should be remembered that congenital may be distinguished from acquired based on the family history and the age of onset. *Diagnostic tests* include measurement (by immunochemical methods) of serum levels of immunoglobulins (compared with age-adjusted standards). In addition, serum antibody responses should be normal after administration of diphtheria, poliovirus, and tetanus vaccines; serum lymphocyte counts should be normal; and a lymph node biopsy should reveal an absence of plasma cells.

Common interventions

General interventions include IM injections of gamma globulin q 3 to 4 wk and the administration of antibiotics to treat infections. **Nursing** interventions are aimed at guarding against infection and bolstering normal defenses. Patient and family teaching are essential in order to guard against dangerous infections. Protective isolation should be instituted if the patient is hospitalized. To bolster the patient's defenses, the nurse should perform the following actions:

1. Provide adequate nutrition, rest, and meticulous hygiene.
2. Maintain the patient's normal respiratory functioning.
3. Encourage the avoidance of smoking and alcohol, which can destroy lymphocytes.
4. Recognize promptly signs and symptoms of infection or illness.

Evaluation criteria. The frequency of injections is reduced. The patient and family verbalize an understanding of the condition, and there is compliance with the gamma globulin injection regimen.

PLASMA CELL MYELOMA

Plasma cell myeloma, a multifocal malignant neoplasm of bone marrow, is one of the major plasma cell dyscrasias. (Other dyscrasias include Waldenström's macroglobulinemia, heavy-chain disease, and primary amyloidosis.) Plasma cell myeloma, which has been increasing in frequency in recent years, usually occurs in persons >40 yr old. It affects men more often than women (2:1 ratio) and has a median survival expectancy of 2 yr; however, a patient can live for many years after the initial presentation of the disease. Although its etiology is unknown, epidemiologic studies suggest that chronic stimulation of the immune system may be related to myeloma: There is an increased incidence after exposure to low-dose radiation, and there is an increased incidence of gallstones and liver disease in myeloma patients.

The pathophysiology of the disease is as follows. A plasma cell of the bone marrow undergoes neoplastic transformation and proliferates to form a clone of malignant cells. Uncontrolled proliferation of these malignant cells continues, and multiple parts of the skeletal system become involved. Plasma cells extend beyond the marrow to the cortex of the bone, resulting in (1) multiple patchy "punched out" areas on x-ray; (2) frequent bone pain when flat bones (ribs, sternum, spine, skull, shoulder, and pelvis) are involved; (3) possible pathologic fracture when skeletal bones are involved;

and (4) bony destruction, leading to hypercalcemia, hypercalcuria, reduction in height as vertebral bones "collapse" into each other, and nerve root or spinal cord compression (which results in pain, neuropathy, and paresthesias). Plasma cells produce excess amounts of one type of immunoglobulin (monoclonal), leading to (1) a decrease in the production of normal immunoglobulins (resulting in increased susceptibility to infections or poor antibody response to primary immune stimulation) or (2) a decrease in erythropoietic capacity of the bone marrow (resulting in anemia). An excessive amount of specific (usually IgG or IgA) immunoglobulin, called M (myeloma) protein, is secreted into the bloodstream, leading to Bence Jones proteinuria or hematologic abnormalities. **Bence Jones proteinuria** results in an impairment of renal functioning that can be acute or chronic, can be complicated by hypercalcemia and amyloid deposits, and is exacerbated by the presence of dehydration. The **hematologic abnormalities** are related to the ability of the M proteins to bind with fibrinogen, prothrombin, and clotting factors V and VII (resulting in coagulation disturbances) and with RBCs (resulting in a decrease in RBC life-span, complications in blood-typing and cross-matching procedures, a rapid sedimentation rate, and normochromic anemia).

Gradual and insidious onset is typical, with evidence of a chronic progressive systemic disease and a history of increased susceptibility to infections. Common complaints include fatigue, anorexia, weakness, and weight loss. *Signs* of advanced involvement include bone pain, anemia, renal insufficiency, neurologic deficits, and repeated bacterial infections.

General assessment involves the health history, a physical exam, and the following *diagnostic tests:* Blood tests should be performed to determine the patient's CBC, Hb/Hct, RBC, WBC, platelet, and calcium levels; serum globulin concentration; and rouleaux formations (a characteristic clumping of RBCs like a roll of pennies). Urine tests are used to determine Bence Jones protein and calcium levels, and a bone marrow examination may reveal myeloma plasma cells. Finally, x-rays of bones in painful areas may identify characteristic "punched out" areas and pathologic fractures.

Common interventions

General interventions to reduce cell tumor mass include the use of radiation, chemotherapy, interferon, and plasmapheresis. **Radiation** therapy (tumors are mildly radiosensitive) can provide palliation of bone pain. It is used with orthopedic procedures to treat potential or actual pathologic fractures in order to allow for rapid reambulation. **Chemotherapy** involves the combination of predinisone with alkylating agents (cyclophosphamide [Cytoxan] and melphalon [Alkeran]). It is currently being investigated in clinical trials with combination chemotherapy, high doses, and varying schedules. Major side effects of the chemotherapeutic agents include pancytopenia, leukopenia, alopecia, and hemorrhagic cystitis. Combination and high-dose regimens often intensify toxicity and require careful preventive measures. The use of **interferon** as an immunotherapy is limited by availability and expense. It is administered as an SC injection q 12 hr. Its major side effects are malaise and leukopenia. It is currently the subject of a major research effort funded by the American Cancer Society. **Plasmapheresis** is used to remove plasma cells from the blood, thereby allowing for the return of other elements. Its use is also in the investigation stage, and current use is limited.

Among the *complications* of myelomas are progressive renal failure, bone marrow failure, bone pain, and structural skeletal defects. Renal failure is treated with adequate hydration (priority), peritoneal or hemodialysis, and rarely, renal transplantation. For bone marrow failure, RBC and platelet transfusions are used to treat anemia and thrombocytopenia, and antibiotics are used to treat bacterial infections. Bone pain is treated with ambulation and weight bearing (to promote reabsorption of calcium) and identification and treatment of potential fractures. Normal saline IV hydration, mithramycin (Mithracin), and corticosteroids are used to treat hypercalcemia. Paralysis is prevented by identification and prompt treatment of spinal cord compression, and analgesics are used to reduce pain.

Nursing care is centered on patient education, the promotion of ambulation and hydration, and the prevention of recurrent bacterial infections.

1. Teach the patient and family about the importance of preventing hypercalcemia.
2. Control pain via creative and persistent use of analgesics and other measures.
3. Encourage the use of walkers, canes, etc.
4. Encourage a fluid intake of 3,000 to 4,000 ml/day to ensure a minimum urine output of 1,500 ml/day.
5. Encourage body mechanics, bed boards, and supportive chairs.
6. Engage a physical and occupational therapist to provide consultations and treatment.
7. Encourage weight bearing and/or walking.
8. Monitor and encourage patient awareness of his WBC count.
9. Teach the patient to take his temperature daily and to report it if it is >37.8°C (100°F).
10. Make efforts to identify potential sources of infection.
11. Take measures to protect the patient from infection and facilitate his immune defenses.

Evaluation criteria. Response to treatment is indicated by normal or improved blood cell counts (Hb/Hct, WBC, and platelets); a decrease in Bence Jones proteinuria; a decrease in serum protein abnormalities (IgG or IgA); and a reduction in bone pain and osteolytic lesions. The patient and family verbalize (1) rationale, side effects, and precautions to take regarding the treatment program, and (2) the importance of ambulation, weight bearing, and fluid intake.

HYPERSENSITIVITY (ALLERGY)

Sensitization to environmental allergens is seen in 1 out of every 10 persons in the USA. Although certain individuals have a genetic predisposition to allergy, the mechanism is still not completely understood. Common allergens include **inhalants** (animal dander, house dust, plant pollen, and fungal spores), **ingestants** (food, drugs, and food additives), and **contactants** (direct skin exposure to food or pollen, causing urticaria or systemic allergic symptoms).

The discovery of the IgE class of immunoglobulins and its association with reaginic activity has helped clinicians to understand some aspects of the allergic reaction. **IgE antibodies** have a cytophilic affinity for the membranes of mast cells, neutrophils, and basophils, and can sensitize these cells to allergens. They cause the release of vasoactive substances secondary to the contact of these sensitized cells with provoking allergens, and produce the symptomatology of allergic response. **Reagin** is an antibody found in serum from allergic individuals that can transfer sensitivity to specific allergens from an allergic individual to a normal person. It can be tested by the Prausnitz-Kustner (PK) reaction, and is called PK antibody or skin-sensitizing antibody.

The primary role of the mediators of allergic reactions is defense against injury by causing inflammation and stimulating tissue repair. **Histamine** is formed by the decarboxylation of histadine, which is stored in the granules of mast cells. It exerts major pharmacologic effects on its release: increased vascular permeability, contraction of smooth muscle, and increased gastric, nasal, and lacrimal secretions. **Slow reactive substance of anaphylaxis** is a substance of unknown composition that can produce a slow contraction of smooth muscle, which is inhibited by antihistamines. It may be responsible for the prolonged bronchospasm seen in asthma. **Serotonin,** a preformed vasoconstrictor held in mast cells, is released secondary to an antigen-antibody reaction similar to histamine. It produces contraction of smooth muscle and increased vascular permeability. **Prostaglandins** include a variety of naturally occurring aliphatic acids that are widely distributed in tissues and released during anaphylactic reactions. They may play a role in asthma and urticaria in man.

The clinical *symptoms* of the allergic response are dependent on the route of exposure and the distribution of sensitized tissues in the body. The allergic individual may exhibit any one of the following reactions alone or in combination. **Anaphylactic shock** is sudden vasomotor collapse and shock after contact with the offending antigen. It is common after IV injections, but can also occur after PO, SC, or IM administration. **Allergic (extrinsic) asthma** is bronchospasm with excessive secretion after inhalation of the specific antigen. **Allergic rhinitis** is characterized by sneezing, watery rhinorrhea, and red and irritated conjunctiva in response to exposure of the nasal mucous membrane to an allergen. **Urticaria (hives)** may occur after ingestion of the offending allergens. Erythematous skin areas cause severe pruritus and discomfort. Local edema may accompany urticaria and become life threatening when the mucosa of the pharynx or larynx is affected, causing respiratory obstruction. **Atopic dermatitis (eczema)** is most frequently seen in children with a family history of allergy. It may present in infancy as a pruritic dermatitis involving the head, neck, and flexor aspects of the trunk and extremities. In many cases the provoking allergen is not identified. Many patients react to animal products and foods in the diet.

The basis of therapy in allergic disease is the historical data provided by the patient. The history should include family incidence of allergy, course of the individual's allergic condition (e.g., seasonal or during pregnancy), and related social or environmental factors (e.g., pets, foods, and drugs). The physical exam should focus on the symptomatology described in the history (e.g., rash, food intolerance, respiratory problems). In addition to the general laboratory work-up (CBC, urinalysis, serology, etc.), the following specific *diagnostic tests* should be performed: a differential WBC to detect eosinophilia, which occurs in allergic reactions; a serum IgE level, which is elevated in allergic conditions; and an absolute lymphocyte count, which can detect immune deficiency. Finally, the following skin tests should be performed: a cutaneous prick or scratch test, followed by an intracutaneous test if the former is negative. Although it is a more sensitive technique, the danger with the intracutaneous test is the possibility of a systemic reaction in a highly sensitive individual.

Common interventions

General treatment of allergic disease requires a long-term commitment to a regimen that is structured specifically for the allergic individual. Three modalities are widely practiced today: (1) avoidance of offending allergens (dust control, pet removal, dehumidifier to inhibit molds); (2) drug therapy (antihistamines, corticosteroids, and sympathomimetics); and (3) immunotherapy (desensitization to allergens by injection of the same allergens in increasing dosages over time). Immunotherapy is believed to stimulate the production of IgG (blocking) antibodies to the antigen.

Nursing treatment consists of education and prevention. The allergic individual is at risk in any situation in which his history is not communicated. Preventing the emergency anaphylactic episode is a much easier task than responding to one. The following are educational and preventive nursing actions:

1. Ask the patient the right questions about allergies.
2. Be aware of the patient's previous response to drugs or contrast media.
3. Label the chart and Kardex accurately.
4. Have emergency drugs and equipment available when administering parenteral drugs.

5. Encourage the patient to wear a medical alert bracelet that lists his allergies.

If anaphylactic shock occurs, the nurse should keep in mind that it is a medical emergency. A calm, cool, and professional demeanor should be maintained while the following actions are performed:

1. Establish an adequate airway (a bedside tracheostomy may be required).
2. Have an emergency cart with appropriate drugs available (epine-phrine, aminophylline) to correct the specific organ failure.
3. Initiate O_2 therapy.
4. Monitor IV fluids and medications.
5. Provide support to the anxious patient and family.

Evaluation criteria.   The patient verbalizes the potential dangers of not making the allergy history known. The patient avoids the offending allergens, follows the medical regimen for his particular allergic condition, and wears appropriate medical alert identification.

AUTOIMMUNE DISEASES

Autoimmunity is the development of antibodies to one's own antigens. These antibodies, which are capable of reacting against a person's own cells, have been observed in many diseases that are manifestations of immune reactions against the self. The etiology of the autoimmune phenomena is unknown. An autoimmune response may be seen in the presence of infectious diseases; however, no evidence exists indicating that this response results in a self-perpetuating autoimmune disease. Tolerance to the components of one's own body prevents the occurrence of the autoimmune phenomena in the healthy individual. Several theories have been proposed to explain the breakdown of this self-tolerance. The **altered antigen theory** maintains that some physical, chemical, or microbiologic event may alter an antigen so that it is no longer recognized as part of the self by the lymphoid system. The **sequestered antigen theory** states that an autologous antigen might never contact antigen-receptive lymphoid cells until after the period of embryologic development in which tolerance to the self normally develops. The **heterophile antigen theory** holds that an infecting organism might contain an antigenic determinant similar to some component of the host. In response, the host might produce antibodies that cross-react with its own tissues. The **release of forbidden clone theory** maintains that a mutation might occur in lymphoid cells, resulting in failure to recognize normal tissue antigen as part of the self. (This theory is less popular today.)

The disorders that have been classified as autoimmune occur as either systemic or organ-specific entities. The common feature of all autoimmune disorders is tissue injury caused by an apparent immunologic reaction of the host with its own tissues. Some of the pathogenic mechanisms that occur include damage to the cell membrane from the action of autoantibodies and complement, the development of inflammatory reactions by autoantigen-antibody-complement complexes, cytotoxicity from the reactions of sensitized lymphocytes with the autoantigen of the cell membrane, the existence of a vaculitis, and the preponderance of the autoimmune phenomena in females. **Systemic disorders** are those in which major involvement is in more than one organ: rheumatoid arthritis (*see* Chapter 19), polyarteritis nodosa, SLE, scleroderma (*see* Chapter 12), and polymyositis and dermamyositis. **Organ-specific disorders** are those in which major involvement is in a single organ: hemolytic anemia in blood (*see* Chapter 21), demyelinating diseases in the CNS (*see* Chapter 20), poststreptococcal nephritis in the kidney (*see* Chapter 17), rheumatic heart disease (*see* Chapter 15), and myasthenia gravis in muscle (*see* Chapter 20).

Autoimmune diseases have an insidious onset and slow progression. *Signs and symptoms* include inflammation and vasculitis. The disease tends to be specific to the organ and/or system involved, resulting in diminished functioning.

Common interventions

General treatment includes the avoidance of those factors that precipitate exacerbation of symptoms (e.g., sun, cold, stress, smoking), the administration of medications (e.g., steroids, sedatives, analgesics), and symptomatic treatment. **Nursing** interventions are as follows:

1. Provide for frequent rest periods in order to avoid fatigue.
2. Avoid stressful situations and other factors that precipitate symptoms.
3. Maintain adequate nutrition and hydration, and prevent infection.
4. Provide supportive therapy (e.g., comfort measures, range-of-motion exercises, pulmonary toilet, etc.) as appropriate.
5. Encourage verbalization of feelings and concerns related to the chronic nature of the condition.
6. Teach the patient and family about the nature, progression, and therapeutic regimen related to the disease, and about the need for follow-up care.
7. Suggest a means of adapting life-style.
8. Advise the patient about specific organizations and community agencies that provide information and/or peer support related to the condition.
9. Refer the patient to other health team members as necessary.

Evaluation criteria.   The patient verbalizes an understanding of the signs and symptoms of the disease progression and of the therapeutic regimen. The patient maximizes functional capacities for health. Complications are avoided, or recognized and treated early.

CHAPTER 7

MOBILITY

Phyllis Lisanti

OVERVIEW

Definition

Mobility is defined as the state or quality of being mobile; the facility of movement. Mobility is relevant to all dimensions of an individual's life: physical, social, economic, psychologic, and spiritual. **Immobility** has been described as the prescribed or unavoidable restriction of movement in any area of the individual's life.

Mobility is frequently used to define one's health and physical fitness. If mobility is altered, numerous problems and complications can result. Each body system responds in its own way to alterations in mobility. The individual who has altered mobility requires careful and skillfull assessment by the nurse along with creative intervention in order to prevent complications from occurring. The reader is referred to the appropriate chapters for an anatomy and physiology review specific to each body system. General and nursing interventions related to each body system are included in this chapter.

Theories

The theoretic bases relevant to the concept of immobility are the disuse phenomena and physiologic deconditioning. **Disuse** was summarized by Kottke and Blanchard as, "The physiological basis of the development of functional ability by any tissue or organ of the body is use . . . . Inactivity or nonuse results in regression of the organ with loss of ability to function." **Deconditioning,** the loss of physiologic conditioning or the capacity to function, occurs secondary to lack of use and occurs because all or part of the body is not used.

Research has demonstrated that alterations in mobility can lead to physiologic and psychologic disability. Much of the disability can be prevented if the functioning of unaffected body systems is maintained.

General assessment

The general assessment of all patients with impaired mobility consists of the following three basic components. The patient's **health history** should be collected with attention directed to (1) the reason for contact, (2) current health status (including mental status, activity level, nutrition, intake and output, past medical problems, allergies, and concurrent medical problems), and (3) a review of the patient's body systems. The **physical examination** of the patient should (1) involve an assessment of vital signs (BP, pulses, etc.), (2) elicit data specific to the structure and functioning of the affected area, and (3) involve inspection, palpation, and auscultation of the affected area as appropriate. **Diagnostic tests** (x-rays, cultures, urinalyses, environmental studies, etc.) should be performed as appropriate for the specific body system affected. (The reader is referred to the appropriate chapters for a complete discussion of the assessment of each specific body system.)

DEVIATIONS

The following discussion focuses on **immobility** and its effects on the various body systems.

INTEGUMENTARY SYSTEM

Decubitus ulcer (pressure sore or bedsore) is defined as a localized area of cellular necrosis. Individuals who are at risk for developing decubiti include those who are elderly, malnourished (obese or emaciated), edematous, lacking bowel and bladder control, lacking adequate circulation, or immobilized due to neurologic dysfunction, coma, restraints, bed rest, wheelchair, traction, or casts.

Pressure usually destroys surface tissue and disturbs the nerve impulses to and from the involved area. An accompanying **decreased blood supply,** in turn, diminishes nutrition of the area involved, leading to tissue anoxia. The localized area of tissue necrosis tends to occur between underlying bony prominences and overlying compressing surfaces, such as a bed, chair, brace, cast, etc. Extreme elevations of capillary pressure (above the normal range of 16 to 33 mmHg) that result from prolonged tissue ischemia can lead to cell death and ulceration. **Cell death** is manifested by an inflammatory process, vasodilation, and reactive hyperemia. The *signs and symptoms* of decubitus formation are erythema, edema, and bluish to black discoloration with sloughing of tissue.

Common interventions

General **medical** interventions include meticulous skin care, relief of pressure, daily visual exam of the skin, education of the patient and family, and improvement of the patient's general physical condition. General **surgical** interventions include local wound care, surgical debridement and skin grafting on more extensive ulcers, and prevention of infection (which can lead to osteomyelitis).

Nursing interventions

1. Identify high-risk individuals.
2. Institute a regimen of care.
3. Make a daily visual exam of the patient's skin.
4. Use water, air, or eggcrate mattress and/or some other device for pressure relief and equalization.
5. Turn the patient at least q 2 hr, and during each position change visually assess the skin.
6. Use a footboard to counteract shearing force.
7. Use a bed cradle to relieve weight and pressure of bedclothes from legs and feet.
8. Keep the patient flat in bed (if tolerated) while providing care to reduce shearing force.
9. Use foam rubber boots to protect the patient's heels.
10. Avoid the use of doughnuts and rubber rings.
11. Avoid the use of alcohol for skin massage.
12. Avoid overuse of sedatives and tranquilizers, which may decrease the patient's desire and ability for movement.
13. Institute a regular toilet schedule to cope with bowel and bladder problems.
14. Provide adequate fluids and a nutritious diet.
15. Keep the patient's skin clean, dry, and well lubricated (use soap sparingly, rinse well after use, and dry well after bathing with a patting motion).
16. Keep bed linens clean, dry, and wrinkle free.
17. Educate the patient and his family about the need for adquate nutrition and fluids, routine skin inspection, frequent movement, and skin care.

Despite faithful execution of a preventive regimen, the patient, in many instances, will develop decubitus ulcers due to concurrent pathologies. The three stages of decubitus formation and the appropriate nursing measures are as follows:

Stage I (redness)

1 Cleanse the area carefully and gently.
2. Gently massage around the area to increase the circulation. (Vigorous massage should be avoided because it may be irritating and cause additional damage.)
3. Apply a drying medication, such as an antiseptic powder. (Powders decrease friction, absorb moisture, have a cooling and protective effect, and are mildly antibacterial.)
4. Avoid any pressure to the area.

Stage II (redness and edema)

1. Cleanse the area carefully by gently lathering with a surgical soap.
2. Rinse and dry gently.
3. Apply silver sulfadiazine cream to the area as ordered. The use of heat lamps is now controversial. If a heat lamp is used, it should be placed no closer than 18 in. and no further than 24 in. for 10 min to the dry area.
4. Avoid any pressure to the area.

Stage III (redness, edema, and necrosis)

1. Gently cleanse the ulcer with surgical soap, and thoroughly rinse at least q 8 hr.
2. Use wet-to-dry dressings as ordered to debride necrotic tissue.
3. Avoid any pressure to the area.

Evaluation criteria. Skin integrity has been maintained. Formed ulcers have healed. Infection has been prevented in formed ulcers.

MUSCULOSKELETAL SYSTEM

The major effects of immobility on the musculoskeletal system are atrophy, weakness, joint stiffness, and disuse osteoporosis.

When a muscle is not used, a wasting process (atrophy) occurs, which leads to weakness of the muscle. The process of atrophy and weakness begins within a few days of immobilization or bed rest.

When a joint is immobilized, severe deterioration occurs: loss of the joint space with proliferation of intracapsular fatty connective tissue and growth of adhesions between tissue, ligaments, and bones leads to joint stiffness.

Osteoporosis (increased porosity or softening of the bones) is a response to immobility. It always occurs and is considered physiologic rather than pathologic. It is believed that during periods of immobility there is normal to excess osteoblastic activity and a greater increase in osteoclastic activity.

This imbalance of production vs. destruction leads to the development of osteoporosis. Complications of osteoporosis, such as fractures and renal calculi, are pathologic.

The *signs and symptoms* of musculoskeletal involvement include muscle weakness, pain and difficulty with joint movement, pain with weight bearing, and fractures.

Common interventions

Interventions are aimed at preventing the complications that occur from musculoskeletal disuse: contractures, deformities, pathologic fractures, and osteoarthropathy. General interventions include a supervised exercise program by the physical therapy department.

Nursing interventions

1. Encourage self-care within the limits of safety.
2. Provide a firm mattress.
3. Provide a padded footboard.
4. Provide a trapeze to encourage movement and self-care.
5. Reposition the patient q 2 hr.
6. Provide skin care.
7. Schedule range-of-motion exercises of nonaffected parts or areas.
8. Avoid the use of a knee gatch.
9. Encourage standing and weight bearing as soon as possible.
10. Use a tilt table.
11. Encourage exercise against resistance.
12. Encourage walking between parallel bars.
13. Educate the patient and family.
14. Avoid calcium supplements or increased calcium intake because these measures do not prevent osteoporosis but merely add to the increased amounts of calcium in the blood and urine.

Evaluation criteria.   A planned program of exercise has been executed. Muscle size and strength has been maintained. Structure and functioning of the musculoskeletal system has been maintained.

CARDIOVASCULAR SYSTEM

The major effects of immobility on the cardiovascular system include an increased work load of the heart, the development of orthostatic hypotension, and an increased incidence of thrombus formation. **Orthostatic** (or postural) **hypotension** is a decrease in BP when a person rises. **Thrombus** is a blood clot that obstructs a blood vessel or a cavity of the heart.

Loss of the influence of gravity, venous stasis, trauma (pressure) to vessel walls, and dehydration are all causes of the cardiovascular *complications* of immobility.

Pathophysiology

Increased cardiac work load.   The increased work load of the heart is due to a 25 to 30% increase in CO, a 40% increase in the stroke volume, and a 30% increase in the total work of the heart when a person lies down.

Orthostatic hypotension.   The recumbent position removes the influence of gravity on the circulatory system, with a resultant decrease in peripheral resistance. On reclining, there is a sudden inflow of blood to the central areas of the body, with a resultant increased work load of the heart (CO and stroke volume increase in the lying position). Dilation of the blood vessels also occurs due to a diminished neurovascular response. If an individual is immobilized for a long period of time, the blood vessels (in response to the diminished neurovascular reflex) develop a decreased ability to respond to position change or to constrict in the standing position. In the upright position, a failure of vasoconstriction with a resultant pooling of blood in the lower portion of the body, can lead to a drop in BP, mild cerebral anoxia manifested by dizziness, and possibly syncope.

Thrombus formation.   The incidence of thrombus formation appears to increase during immobility (possibly) due to venous stasis, trauma to the vessel walls, and hypercoagulability of the blood. **Venous stasis** can result from a lack of muscular activity (which aids venous return). Positions that restrict circulation are the lateral recumbent and those that use the knee gatch. **Trauma** to the blood vessels can be induced by placing the patient in positions that tend to damage blood vessels; for example, the lateral recumbent position, in which the upper leg rests heavily upon the lower leg. When the intima of the blood vessel wall is damaged, a layer of platelets covers the damaged area, resulting in **clot formation. Hypercoagulability** may be induced posttrauma (e.g., surgery, accidents), by dehydration, or by the increased calcium levels seen in the immobile state.

Valsalva maneuver

The Valsalva maneuver is the act of forcibly exhaling with the glottis, nose, and mouth closed. This action causes increased intrathoracic pressure, slowing of the pulse, decreased return of blood to the heart, and increased venous pressure. The Valsalva maneuver is performed quite frequently by patients who are on bed rest but who are freely mobile. Although the normal heart can withstand the sudden changes in pressure that occur with the Valsalva maneuver, the compromised heart may not tolerate changes in pressure and blood flow. In addition, the changes in pressure that occur may be responsible for dislodging a thrombus, which may then cause a pulmonary embolus.

The *signs and symptoms* of cardiovascular involvement are (1) easy fatigue and elevated pulse rate secondary to an increased work load of the heart; (2) lowered BP, elevated pulse rate, and dizziness and syncope in an upright position secondary to orthostatic hypotension; and (3) pain, swelling, heat, and tenderness in the calf secondary to thrombus formation.

Nursing interventions

Increased work load of the heart

1. Allow self-care within safe limits to the maximum allowed.
2. Increase the patient's activity gradually.
3. Promote measures to conserve energy.

Orthostatic hypotension

1. Change the patient's position frequently.
2. Encourage the patient to dangle his feet before he gets out of bed.
3. Change the patient's position from horizontal to vertical.
4. Place the patient upright while he is in bed.
5. Allow the patient out of bed to the chair as permitted.
6. Ambulate the patient as early as permitted.
7. Apply a pressure bandage to the patient's legs and abdominal binder as indicated.

Thrombus formation

1. Provide fluids as ordered.
2. Avoid trauma to the patient's extremities.
3. Encourage the patient to avoid crossing his legs while he is in a chair.
4. Position the patient properly while he is in bed.
5. Encourage the patient to avoid any position with one leg atop the other.
6. Provide active or passive leg exercises and elevate the patient's legs.
7. Apply antiemboli stockings.
8. Avoid rubbing the patient's legs.
9. Avoid the use of a knee gatch.
10. Administer heparin therapy as ordered.

Valsalva maneuver

1. Teach the patient to exhale while changing his position and moving in bed.
2. Provide a diet with adequate fluids and high fiber.
3. Administer stool softeners and laxatives as ordered.
4. Provide a position of comfort when the patient is using the bedpan.
5. Avoid patient constipation.

Evaluation criteria.   The patient's vital signs remain relatively stable. The patient demonstrates no dizziness or syncope on ambulation. The patient assumes self-care and an exercise schedule that is within safe limits. The patient has soft, formed bowel movements with regular frequency.

RESPIRATORY SYSTEM

The major effects of immobility on the respiratory system are decreased chest expansion, stasis of secretions, CO_2 narcosis, and respiratory acidosis.

It is harder to breathe when lying down because the intraesophageal pressure increases and the tidal volume is slightly reduced. The mechanics of respiration may be affected by the muscle atrophy and weakness previously discussed. Chest expansion may be decreased due to positioning, pressure of the mattress, or, with some patients, chest binders and/or pain. These factors may lead to stasis of secretions, which, when combined with interference in normal ciliary action, can predispose the patient to hypostatic pneumonia. In the recumbent position, the ciliary action is less effective because mucous distribution shifts. Mucus pools on the lower surface of the bronchioles, leading to drying of the upper surface as opposed to an equal distribution of mucus around the bronchioles in the upright position (Fig. 7-1). These changes make the patient more susceptible to bacterial growth and the subsequent development of pneumonia.

Decreased chest movements and diminished cough reflex may affect O_2-CO_2 exchange in the lungs. The resulting accumulation of CO_2 in the blood along with a decrease in O_2 tension leads to tissue hypoxia. The body's compensatory mechanisms can temporarily correct the imbalance, but without correction of the underlying pathology, the patient will rapidly progress to CO_2 narcosis and respiratory acidosis, eventually leading to respiratory and cardiac failure, coma, and death.

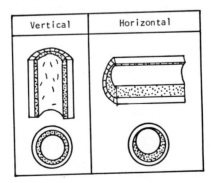

Figure 7-1.   Gravity's effect on mucous distribution in a bronchiole. *See* text for discussion. *Reprinted with permission from* Browse, N. The Physiology and Pathology of Bedrest. Charles C. Thomas, Publisher, Springfield, Ill. 1965.

The *signs and symptoms* of respiratory involvement are weakened cough, rapid respiratory rate, shallow-labored breathing, and moist-wet respirations secondary to stasis of secretions; rapid pulse, elevated temperature, altered mental status, irritability, confusion, disorientation, use of auxiliary muscles to breathe, pain on respiration, purulent sputum, and elevated leukocytes secondary to bronchopneumonia; drowsiness, irritability, hallucinations, depression, coma, poor ventilation, tachycardia, arrhythmias, paralysis of extremities, facial tremors, and convulsions secondary to CO_2 narcosis; hyperventilation at rest, wheezing, tachycardia, cyanosis, mental disorientation, plasma pH <7.35, plasma bicarbonate of 29 mEq/liter, acid urine pH of 6.0, shallow-rapid respirations, dyspnea, and suprasternal retraction secondary to respiratory acidosis.

Nursing interventions

1. Monitor temperature, pulse, and respirations q 4 hr, or more frequently as indicated. Monitor blood gases.
2. Change the patient's position at least q 2 hr.
3. Encourage deep breathing and coughing exercises q 2 hr.
4. Provide adequate fluid intake.
5. Position the patient to avoid pressure on his chest and facilitate chest expansion.
6. Provide pulmonary toilet as indicated.
7. Administer antibiotics as ordered.
8. Assist with any measures necessary to correct O_2-CO_2 imbalances and improve ventilation (such as drug therapy or mechanical ventilation).

Evaluation criteria. The temperature, pulse, and respirations remain within normal limits. The patient expectorates secretions. The arterial blood gases are within normal limits.

RENAL SYSTEM

The major effects of immobility on the renal system are difficult urination, stasis of urine in the kidney, and renal calculi.

The supine position, which is associated with immobility, increases the blood flow to the kidneys with a resultant increase in urine volume. The postural effect dilutes the plasma, which leads to a decrease in ADH secretion, a decrease in tubular reabsorption, and an increase in urine volume. Increase in plasma volume without changes in osmotic pressure leads to increased renal plasma flow and increased diuresis. The patient who is immobilized, possibly in the recumbent position, frequently experiences difficult urination (which may be due to a variety of reasons, such as embarrassment, positional discomfort, and/or inability to relax the muscles necessary for voiding). Sitting upright facilitates urination by virtue of gravity. Without the benefit of gravity, urine tends to pool in a greater number of calyces, leading to stasis (stagnation) (Fig. 7-2).

Stasis, increased excretion of calcium and phosphorus, and elevated urine pH predispose 15 to 30% of immobilized patients to develop renal calculi.

The *signs and symptoms* of renal involvement are difficult voiding; pain, hematuria, backache, and nausea and vomiting secondary to urinary calculi; and any signs of infection secondary to stasis.

Nursing interventions

1. Change the patient's position at least q 2 hr.
2. Place the patient in an upright position to void whenever possible.
3. Provide early ambulation as indicated.
4. Encourage and provide adequate fluid intake.
5. Monitor intake and output, specific gravity, and characteristics of urine.
6. Provide acid-ash foods and fluids.
7. Avoid unnecessary catheterization.
8. Provide all measures to induce and encourage spontaneous voiding.

Evaluation criteria.   The patient has maintained preimmobility patterns of voiding. Infection has been prevented. Calculi formation has been prevented.

GI SYSTEM

Immobility does not appear to have a direct effect on the GI tract, but patients who are immobilized do develop constipation and anorexia.

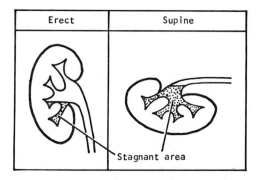

Figure 7-2.   Gravity's effect on the outflow of urine from the renal pelvis. *See* text for discussion. *Reprinted with permission from* Browse, N. The Physiology and Pathology of Bedrest. Charles C. Thomas, Publisher, Springfield, Ill. 1965.

The development of constipation (a decreased ability to respond to and perform the act of defecating) can result from such factors as a change in diet, change in schedule, position, discomfort, change in level of activity, embarrassment regarding the use of a bedpan, lack of privacy, and/or generalized loss of muscle tone. A *complication* of constipation is fecal impaction, which may be removed manually, but in rare situations, will require surgical removal.

Anorexia, frequently encountered with immobilized patients, may result from a change in diet, dislike of hospital food, inactivity, and/or boredom. Prolonged anorexia may contribute to a negative nitrogen balance.

The *signs and symptoms* of GI involvement include headache, dizziness, malaise, loss of appetite, abdominal distension, no stool, and hard stool secondary to constipation; and abdominal distension, oozing of watery stool, and hard mass on digital exam secondary to fecal impaction.

Nursing interventions

Constipation

1. Provide adequate fluids, prunes, high fiber, fruits, and vegetables.
2. Administer laxatives and stool softeners.
3. Provide a position of comfort.
4. Encourage a regimen of good bowel habits.
5. Promote exercise of abdominal muscles.
6. Provide for privacy.
7. Monitor bowel movements so constipation is prevented.
8. Prevent impaction.

Anorexia

1. Provide small, frequent meals that are high in protein; food from home that is attractively arranged; and a room that is free of odors.

Evaluation criteria.   Intake of nutritious diet has been adequate. The diet has included high-fiber foods. Usual bowel patterns have been maintained. Constipation and impaction have been prevented.

METABOLIC SYSTEM

The major effects of immobility on the metabolic system include a slight decrease in the basal metabolic rate (BMR), negative calcium and nitrogen balance, and decreased aldosterone and ADH secretion and ACTH production.

The lowered BMR may be related to diminished overall activity of the body during immobilization. The negative nitrogen balance results from increased muscle breakdown, and the negative calcium balance is due to bone resorption. Decreased aldosterone and ADH secretion is related to the postural effect of recumbency. Decreased ACTH secretion occurs with the supine position (the exact mechanism is not known).

The *signs and symptoms* of metabolic system involvement include decreased appetite and sluggishness secondary to decreased BMR; bone softening secondary to negative calcium balance; decreased appetite and muscle weakness secondary to negative nitrogen balance; increased urine output secondary to decreased aldosterone and/or ADH secretion; and decreased ability to cope with stress secondary to decreased ACTH secretion.

Nursing interventions

1. Provide a high-protein diet, high fluid intake, and acid-ash foods and fluids.
2. Elevate the head of the bed.
3. Promote active and passive exercises.
4. Promote weight bearing as indicated and tolerated.
5. Provide all measures to reduce stress.
6. Ambulate the patient as early as possible.

Evaluation criteria. The patient demonstrates adequate dietary intake and maintenance of muscle and bone strength. The patient has a urinary output within normal limits. Blood and urine studies remain within normal limits. The patient demonstrates appropriate responses to stress.

PSYCHOLOGIC EFFECTS

Patients who are immobilized or on bed rest due to a pathologic process frequently become bored, depressed, or anxious. These emotional responses are related to life changes that occur secondarily to the pathologic process. A patient who is also deprived of meaningful stimuli may suffer from **sensory deprivation,** which has been described by Chodil and Williams as "a situation in which reception or perception of stimuli is blocked or altered, or in which the environmental stimuli are blocked or altered."

Altered psychologic responses may be related to (1) poorly functioning receptors (e.g., eyes, ears, nose, etc.) or decreased perception, (2) environmental stimuli that are diminished or lack relevance or meaning, and/or (3) alterations in the reticular activating system, which is responsible for arousal and alertness.

The *signs and symptoms* of psychologic involvement are boredom, difficulty in concentration or coherent thinking, hallucinations (auditory, visual, kinesthetic, or somatesthetic), daydreaming, anxiety, fear, depression, lability of mood, noncompliant behavior, increased pain sensitivity, introspection, feelings of helplessness and inadequacy, and rebellion and hostility.

Nursing interventions
Sensorially impaired

1. Provide protection and security.
2. Provide eyeglasses as needed.
3. Provide hearing aids as needed.
4. Provide herbs and seasonings for food.

Environmentally deprived

1. Provide reality orientation.
2. Provide a clock, radio, television, etc.
3. Increase the patient's contact with the environment.
4. Increase meaningful stimuli and social contacts.
5. Allow the patient to become involved in planning of care.

Evaluation criteria.   The patient has been protected from accidents. The patient is oriented to time, place, and person. The patient has been provided with meaningful environmental stimuli.

CHAPTER 8

CELLULAR GROWTH

Marion Oare Smith

OVERVIEW

Definition

The powers of generation and regeneration are basic and universal among living organisms. Cells, the physiologic structural units of all life, are continually growing and reproducing. The adult human being is composed of billions of cells that have a multitude of specialized functions.

Cellular growth may be considered in the following three categories: (1) growth in relation to development, such as the progressive growth and differentiation that is characteristic of the human being as he or she matures from infancy to adulthood; (2) growth in relation to renewal of cell populations, such as the replacement of cell groups that are lost due to normal wear and tear; and (3) growth in response to the organism's mutual interaction with its environment, such as the replacement of cells after trauma (e.g., wound healing), controlled overgrowth in response to stress (e.g., hyperplasia and hypertrophy), or uncontrolled growth (e.g., neoplasia).

Composition of the cell

Protoplasm, the viscid colloidal material of the cell, is 70 to 85% water; its other constituents are proteins, carbohydrates, lipids, and electrolytes. The cell's ability to function is due to the complex combinations and relationships of these chemical elements.

Proteins. Proteins, which constitute 10 to 20% of the cell mass, are important in the molecular organization of protoplasm, and are indispensable to the vital processes of the cell. Proteins exist as *structural proteins,* which form the membranes of the cell and of the various elements within the cell, or *enzymes,* which lie within the cell and function as catalysts for biochemical reactions (e.g., oxidations, reductions, and phosphorylations). Alkaline phosphatase, for example, is an enzyme found in the brush border of the proximal convoluted tubule cells of the kidney, in the striated border of the columnar absorbing cells of the intestine, and in the nuclei of many cells, particularly of endothelium.

Carbohydrates. Carbohydrates constitute ~1% of protoplasm and serve as energy sources for the cell. There are three classes of carbohydrates: *monosaccharides,* or simple sugars (e.g., glucose), *disaccharides,* or double sugars (e.g., glycogen), and *polysaccharides,* or multiple sugars (e.g., the mucopolysaccharide hyaluronic acid, which is a component of intercellular material such as synovial fluid, connective tissue, and the humors of the eye, and which has important influences on the exchange of substances between blood plasma and tissue cells). The nucleic acids RNA and DNA are polysaccharides that are composed of ribose or deoxyribose (monosaccharides), in addition to phosphoric acid and purine and pyrimidine bases. The nucleic acids RNA and DNA function in the replication of cells and in the metabolism and synthesis of proteins that are necessary for growth and development.

Lipids. Lipids are fatlike substances that constitute 2 to 3% of protoplasm. Lipids (1) combine with structural proteins to form the membranes of the cell and of various elements within the cell, (2) allow for selective transport of substances through membranes because of their solubility characteristics, (3) can function as a storage medium for excess carbohydrate that has been changed into fat, and (4) are insoluble or only partially soluble in water. Phospholipids and cholesterol are examples of lipids.

Electrolytes. The major intracellular electrolytes are potassium, magnesium, phosphate, sulfate, and bicarbonate (*see* Chapter 3).

Structure and function of the cell

Although human cells vary greatly in size and shape as they differentiate for varied functions, they all have the same basic structure. The three major parts of the cell are an outer covering (*the cell membrane*), a main colloidal solution (*the cytoplasm*), and a control center (*the nucleus*). The other organelles of the cell include mitochondria, lysosomes, endoplasmic reticula, Golgi apparatus, centrioles, and cilia.

Cell membrane. The cell membrane (1) lines all cells, as well as the physical structures (e.g., the nucleus) within the cell, (2) is composed of a thin, elastic membrane that is 60% proteins and 40% lipids, and (3) has minute pores that allow for free diffusion of molecules between the cell and its environment. This membrane controls the passage of substances into and out of the cell by *diffusion* through the pores or the matrix of the membrane, by *active transport* through the membranes (facilitated by enzymes and other special carrier substances), and by *pinocytosis,* a mechanism in which the cell membrane surrounds and engulfs certain substances in response to their coming into contact with it. The cell membrane is also involved in *phagocytosis* (a process similar to pinocytosis but on a larger scale), in which the membrane spreads to encompass large particles such as bacteria or necrotic debris.

Although the cell membrane can be repaired after rupture, this process may be impeded by an insufficient number of calcium ions in the ECF. The mechanism of repair is not entirely clear. It is presumed that the lipids and proteins of the cytoplasm precipitate to form a new membrane. The process may also involve endoplasmic reticulum (a network of tubular and vesicular structures).

Cell membranes may be governed by the receptor theory, which proposes that cell membrane substances called "receptors" are capable of interacting with specific stimuli (e.g., epinephrine) to effect an exchange of information. This theory accounts for information passing through the cell membrane without an actual movement of substances.

Cytoplasm.   Cytoplasm consists of small and large particles within a clear fluid portion. Dispersed particles, such as dissolved proteins, electrolytes, glucose, lipids, and specialized structures (organelles) are also found in cytoplasm. By virtue of its structure, cytoplasm allows for physical and chemical reactions within the cell and for metabolism, which is essential to the life of the cell.

Mitochondria.   Mitochondria are the most important organelles and can vary in number (a few hundred to several thousand), depending on the energy requirement of each cell. Within the mitochondria, nutrients and oxygen come into contact with enzymes to form carbon dioxide and water. By means of this oxidation, mitochondria are involved in the synthesis of ATP, which then becomes an energy source throughout the cell for important functions such as protein synthesis.

Nucleus.   The nucleus, the control center of the cell, is surrounded by a double-layered membrane. The nucleus influences growth, repair, and reproduction. Its contents include *nucleoli,* which contain RNA (a substance that acts as a messenger carrying information to control protein synthesis) and *chromosomes,* composed of DNA, which carries the code of genetic information. Chromosomes are capable of self-reproduction and of controlling the production of RNA. The understanding of DNA has been the key to unraveling the mystery of heredity.

The cell cycle

The life cycle of the cell is controlled by DNA. All cells progress in an orderly sequence through the cell **life cycle,** which consists of five distinct phases. (1) G_0 (G = "gap") is called the resting phase because no cells are in the process of division, although all other cell activities are taking place. (2) G_1 is the phase in which RNA and proteins are synthesized to prepare for DNA synthesis. The cell is now committed to undergo mitosis. (3) In the S (synthetic) phase, DNA is synthesized and two identical sets of chromosomes are formed. (4) G_2 is the phase in which DNA synthesis ceases, although RNA and protein synthesis continue. (5) In the M (mitosis) phase, genetic material separates (chromosomes), the cell undergoes division, and two daughter cells are created.

In terms of **cell division**, there are three variations of progression through the cell cycle. (1) Cells may continually progress through the cell cycle (continuous growth and reproduction). Some examples are the blood-forming cells of bone marrow, the germinal layer of skin, and the epithelium of the GI tract. (2) Cells may normally remain in G_0 but are capable of progressing through the cell cycle under the proper circumstances. These cells may not reproduce for long periods of time, and reproduction only occurs in response to an appropriate stimulus (e.g., muscle cells). (3) Cells may be permanently in G_0. These cells have permanently left the cell cycle and will die without reproducing (e.g., nerve cells).

Cell growth is normally a controlled and regulated process whose exact mechanisms, however, remain unknown. Four essential facts to remember are (1) the characteristics of growth are different for different cell types, (2) genetic information (DNA) in the nucleus regulates reproduction, (3) insufficient numbers of a given type of cell can stimulate rapid reproduction, and (4) general body growth is controlled by growth hormone.

Growth hormone, secreted by the pituitary, influences metabolism by increasing the rate of protein synthesis, decreasing the rate of carbohydrate utilization, and increasing the mobilization of fats and their use for energy. Although growth hormone is secreted from birth to death, its concentration in children is 1.5 times that in adults. It particularly controls skeletal growth. (In adults, after the epiphyses of long bones unite and further growth becomes impossible, soft-tissue growth is still stimulated.)

Special cell units

Tissues. Tissues, groupings of specialized cells that perform special functions, unite to form organs, the structural units of the body.

Epithelial tissue is found in the epidermis and in the linings of body cavities and vessels (e.g., the peritoneal cavity, blood and lymph vessels, liver, gallbladder, respiratory tract, and GU tract). The regeneration of epithelial tissue occurs rapidly under favorable conditions.

Nervous tissue is found in the brain, spinal cord, and in nerves throughout the body. It consists of highly specialized cells that have the ability to carry messages in the form of electric charges and chemical changes. Adult nerve cells do not regenerate by dividing; however, they do grow axons.

Muscle tissue is of three types: involuntary, voluntary, and cardiac. *Involuntary (smooth) muscle tissue* is found in (1) the muscles of the internal organs, (2) the digestive tract, (3) the walls of respiratory passages, blood vessels, large lymphatic trunks, and GU ducts, and (4) the pupils of the eye. Regeneration of involuntary muscle is possible, but healing occurs mainly by scar tissue formation. *Voluntary (striated skeletal) muscle tissue* is found in the muscles of the body wall and the extremities. Three facts with regard to its regeneration are (1) the enlargement of existing muscle fibers can occur by an increase in cytoplasm, (2) its embryonic cells (sarcoblasts) can multiply, and (3) large defects are usually replaced by a connective tissue scar. *Cardiac muscle tissue* is found in the wall of the heart and in portions of the pulmonary vein. Its regenerative capacity is insignificant: existing fibers increase in thickness, and healing takes place by the formation of scar tissue.

Connective tissue is found in blood cells, cartilage, bone, and throughout the body. It has relatively few cells and a large amount of intercellular substance. The fibroblasts of loose connective tissue reproduce rapidly and form networks of fibers that aid in the healing of defects in other tissues with little regenerative power.

DEVIATIONS

ATROPHY

Atrophy is an acquired decrease in the size of a normally developed tissue or organ. Physiologic processes often lead to a decrease in size within a normal range (e.g., the thymus gland atrophies as a child matures, and the ovaries and breast tissue decrease in size in postmenopausal women). Atrophy, however, can also be a pathologic decrease in size beyond the normal range of variability. Examples of **disuse atrophy** are (1) the muscular atrophy after denervation or immobilization (1 to 2 mo of disuse can decrease muscle size by 50%), and (2) the decreased size of adrenal glands with large doses of corticosteroid drugs over an extended period of time. **Atrophy after disease or circulatory disorders** occurs in (1) atherosclerosis, which interferes with blood supply and causes atrophy of brain tissue, (2) arteriolar nephrosclerosis and pyelonephritis, which cause kidney atrophy, and (3) optic nerve atrophy in late glaucoma.

Disease, the compression of a part, denervation, or a change in hormonal feedback signals leads to deficient blood and lymphatic circulation. This decreased circulation plus increased metabolic activity can cause the accumulation of metabolic waste products, which leads to the increased activity of catabolic intracellular enzymes and destruction of protoplasm. This leads to a reduction in cell volume and/or in the number of cells, resulting in an adaptation of organ size to the blood and lymph supply.

The *signs and symptoms* of atrophy include a decrease in the size of the tissue or organ, as noted by palpation or physical observation, and in a decrease in cellular functions, indicated by a gradual or abrupt change in the functioning of body organs such as the brain, kidneys, optic nerve, or adrenal glands.

Diagnosis is based on a health history, physical exam, laboratory tests to detect changes in functioning, and x-rays and scans to detect changes in size.

Common interventions

Treatment consists of prompt and continued treatment of disease entities such as glaucoma, atherosclerotic plaques in carotid arteries, or pyelonephritis. It may also involve stimulation of denervated muscles with strong electric impulses (until reinnervation occurs) in Guillain-Barré syndrome, spinal cord injury, or nerve trauma.

Nursing interventions

1. Avoid prolonged pressure or constant trauma that could reduce circulation to a part. (Use frequent turning and positioning of bedridden patients, and rotate injection sites.)
2. Institute active range-of-motion exercises, whenever possible, to ensure muscular contraction. (Muscle fibers tend to shorten without continual movement.)
3. Provide passive range-of-motion exercises on a regular daily schedule (usually qid) to provide stretching.
4. Use positioning devices such as splints and hand rolls to keep body parts in extended (as opposed to contracted) positions.

HYPERTROPHY

Hypertrophy is an increase in the size of a tissue that occurs as a result of the enlargement of existing cells. Forceful muscular activity causes muscle fibers to enlarge, as in the increased muscle size of ballet dancers, weight lifters, and persons engaged in heavy physical labor. (Weak muscular activity, even over long periods of time, will not result in hypertrophy.) Increases in size occur most often in the skeletal muscles, heart, kidneys, endocrine organs, and in smooth musculature if there is an obstruction of a hollow viscus or duct. Ventricular hypertrophy occurs as a compensatory measure to increase CO. The etiology of benign prostatic hypertrophy is unknown. Endocrine disturbances, chronic infections, and hereditary predispositions may play a role (*see* Chapter 17).

Both hypertrophy and hyperplasia (an increase in the size of tissues occurring as a result of the formation and growth of new cells) may occur in the same tissue at the same time. Hypertrophy may initially succeed in improving organ functioning (e.g., the increased CO and tremendous physical ability of the weight lifter): muscle fibers increase their quantity of contractile protein and of various nutrient and metabolic substances such as glycogen and ATP. Thus, the power of muscle and the nutrient mechanisms for maintaining power are increased.

In cardiac hypertrophy, coronary blood flow does not increase in proportion to the mass of cardiac muscle. This can result in hypoxia, a decrease in contractile power, coronary insufficiency, and anginal pain due to relative ischemia. In other instances of hypertrophy, the obstruction of a hollow viscus or duct (such as of a ureter by an enlarged prostate gland) may lead to the enlargement of smooth muscle, such as the bladder wall, in an attempt to compensate.

The *signs and symptoms* of skeletal muscle hypertrophy are easily visible on physical examination. The health history may provide evidence of hypertrophic changes that have become dysfunctional (e.g., angina with cardiac hypertrophy, or urinary dysfunction with prostatic hypertrophy). Palpation or diagnostic studies such as x-ray and scanning may provide evidence of enlarged glands or smooth muscle.

Diagnosis involves a health history and physical exam. For detailed assessment of organ functions, as well as common interventions, *see* the relevant portions of Chapters 15, 16, 17, and 19.

CANCER

Cancer is a general term that refers to over 200 types of neoplastic diseases. These diseases can occur in many forms and affect many organs (Fig. 8-1). Neoplasia refers to a pathologic overgrowth of tissues. Neoplasms can be benign or malignant. *Benign neoplasms* have cells that reproduce to form a mass of tissue known as a "tumor," can vary in size and may grow to obstruct organs, causing pressure or bleeding; can be surgically removed; and do not metastasize. *Malignant neoplasms* have cells that reproduce in a disorganized pattern; contain cells that are morphologically different from those of the normal tissue from which they arose; are characterized by the presence of undifferentiated cells, atypical cells, and evident changes in the cytoplasm and nucleus; and may spread to other parts of the body. Neoplasms are classified according to their parent tissue (Table 8-1). *Carcinomas* are cancers of epithelial tissue, such as the skin and the lining of the lung. *Sarcomas* are cancers of connective tissue, bone, and muscle. *Leukemias* are cancers of blood-forming organs. *Lymphomas* are cancers of the lymphatic system.

Cancer is the second most common cause of death in the USA. It tends to evoke fear and dread, and is often considered a taboo topic, a stigma, or a deviance. Nevertheless, cancer is a group of chronic diseases in which much progress has been made in treatment and in improving the quality of life.

Etiology

The exact etiology of human cancers has not been determined. Cellular changes with regard to mitosis, arrangement of nuclei, and general architecture of the cells definitely suggest that relevant mechanisms operate at the molecular level. It appears that carcinogenesis (the process by which

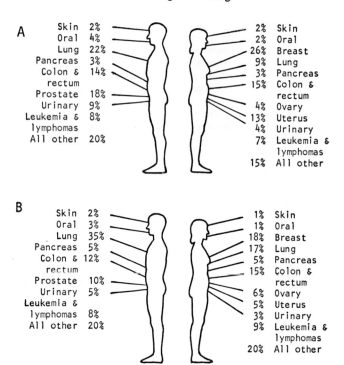

Figure 8-1. (A) Estimated cancer incidence (1983) by site and sex. These estimates are based on data from the National Cancer Institute's Surveillance, Epidemiology, and End Results (SEER) Program (1973-1978). Nonmelanoma skin cancer and carcinoma *in situ* have not been included in the statistics. The incidence of nonmelanoma skin cancer is estimated to be ~400,000. (B) Estimated cancer deaths (1983) by site and sex. *Reprinted with permission from* Silverberg, E. Cancer Statistics, 1983. *Cancer* (January-February 1983). 9.

cancer is produced) is a complex, multistage phenomenon that is characterized by the combined action of several etiologic factors.

Epidemiologic studies have played an important role in identifying etiologic factors. These studies are a major activity of many organizations: the National Cancer Institute has a SEER program (Surveillance, Epidemiology, and End Results), the American Cancer Society publishes yearly volumes of *Cancer Statistics* and *Cancer Facts and Figures,* and state tumor registries maintain data regarding cancer incidence and survival. Epidemiologic studies have retrospectively analyzed relationships that were suggested by clusters of cases of cancer (e.g., the study that linked intrauterine exposure to diethylstilbestrol with adenocarcinoma of the vagina in young women) and have demonstrated the effects of cocarcinogens (such as the studies that showed a greatly increased incidence of lung cancer in workers who were exposed to asbestos and who were also cigarette smokers). Specific risk factors have been associated with specific cancers. Some of the important epidemiologic features of cancer are the marked differences in incidence and mortality in different geographic areas, the differences with relation to genetic backgrounds, and the increase in incidence of cancer with increasing age. This last fact suggests that cancer (1) is a disease that does not typically occur until after the reproductive years, (2) has replaced infections and parasitic diseases as a major cause of death, and (3) generally requires long periods of exposure to carcinogenic agents before it occurs.

Two basic etiologic concepts have been considered: (1) healthy cells are transformed into cancer cells by events at the molecular level that operate to change cell structure and function and by environmental factors that impinge on the human body; (2) malignant cells are not being destroyed. The "Surveillance Theory" suggests that each individual normally has malignant cells that are kept in control by his own immune system (*see* Chapter 6). Indeed, the competence of immune systems, endogenous hormonal influences, and psychophysiologic well-being are important host factors. The etiology of most cancers appears to be a complex interplay between environmental influences and factors of host resistance. **Environmental factors** that have been identified include demographic and geographic variables, dietary factors, tobacco, radiation, viruses, alcohol, occupational carcinogens, air pollution, and drugs. **Host factors** that have been identified include genetic factors, immunologic factors, endogenous hormonal states, and psychologic variables.

Pathophysiology

Formation of a tumor. A tumor mass is formed as the result of a complex interaction of many factors that alters DNA and, thus, impairs the mechanisms controlling cellular growth. When a malignant cell is produced, it begins to reproduce itself. Multiple doublings of the malignant cell lead to the formation of a detectable tumor mass. Tumor doubling time (the average length of time for cells to reproduce themselves) varies according to the type and site of the neoplasm and affects the rate of tumor growth. In general, hematopoietic cancers (e.g., leukemia) have a faster doubling time than solid tumors (e.g., breast). Since many doublings must occur before a cancer becomes clinically detectable, cancer may be present for many months or years before it is discovered or is damaging to the individual.

Tumor growth may also be due to a decreased rate of cell death in malignant tissues. Well-differentiated cells tend to perform functions, die,

TABLE 8-1

Classification of Neoplasms

Parent tissue	Benign	Malignant
Epithelium		
Skin and mucous membrane	Papilloma	Squamous cell carcinoma
Glands	Polyp	Basal cell carcinoma
		Transitional cell carcinoma
	Adenoma	Adenocarcinoma
	Cystadenoma	
Endothelium		Endothelioma
Blood vessels	Hemangioma	Hemangioendothelioma
		Angiosarcoma
Lymph vessels	Lymphangioma	Lymphangiosarcoma
		Lymphangioendothelioma
Bone marrow		Multiple myeloma
		Ewing's sarcoma
		Leukemia
Lymphoid tissue		Malignant lymphoma
		Lymphosarcoma
		Reticulum cell sarcoma
		Lymphatic leukemia
Connective tissues		
Embryonic fibrous tissue	Myxoma	Myxosarcoma
Fibrous tissue	Fibroma	Fibrosarcoma
Adipose tissue	Lipoma	Liposarcoma
Cartilage	Chondroma	Chondrosarcoma
Bone	Osteoma	Osteogenic sarcoma
Synovial membrane	Synovioma	Synovial sarcoma
Muscle tissue		
Smooth muscle	Leiomyoma	Leiomyosarcoma
Striated muscle	Rhabdomyoma	Rhabdomyosarcoma
Nerve tissue		
Nerve fibers and sheaths	Neuroma	Neurogenic sarcoma
	Neurinoma (neurilemoma)	
	Neurofibroma	Neurofibrosarcoma
Ganglion cells	Ganglioneuroma	Neuroblastoma
Glia cells	Glioma	Glioblastoma
		Spongioblastoma
Meninges	Meningioma	
Pigmented neoplasms		
Melanoblasts	Pigmented nevus	Malignant melanoma
		Melanocarcinoma

Parent tissue	Benign	Malignant
Miscellaneous		
Placenta	Hydatidiform mole	Chorionepithelioma (choriocarcinoma)
Gonads	Dermoid cyst	Embryonal carcinoma
		Embryonal sarcoma
		Teratocarcinoma

Reprinted with permission from Bouchard-Kurtz, R., and N. Speese-Owens. Nursing Care of the Cancer Patient. C. V. Mosby Co., St. Louis. 1981. Fourth edition. p. 13.

and lack the ability to reproduce. Since malignant cells are not well differentiated, they live longer and cause hyperplasia even if the rate of mitosis is constant.

Spread of a tumor.   Malignant cells are spread to other local tissues (*invasion*) or distant tissues (*metastasis*) in four ways: (1) By direct extension into surrounding structures. (2) By travel in the lymphatic system or bloodstream. In the lymphatic system, spread will occur in a regular pattern along the lymph nodes (e.g., the most proximal node will be affected first). Lymph nodes may serve as deterrents to spread. In the bloodstream, malignant cells will invade the venous system first (which accounts for the frequent initial spread to the liver and lungs). Eventually, they enter the arterial system, where they spread to all body organs. (3) By serosal spread. Detached cancer cells diffuse into serous cavities (e.g., the pleural or peritoneal) and produce ascitic fluid. (4) By embolization and thrombosis. Cancer cells become trapped in the microcirculation. (In experiments, anticoagulants have decreased metastasis.)

The biochemical qualities of cancer cells may also account for their ability to spread. Because cancer cells have fewer calcium ions in their cell membrane, they have greater negative surface charges. Therefore, the cells tend to repel one another, resulting in an increased ease of separation. In addition, (1) some cancer cells produce lytic substances that may ease invasion through tissues, (2) the motility of malignant cells may be a factor because of their amoeboid activity, and (3) the cells have lost the "growth restraint" of surrounding tissues. (The location of metastasis and the characteristics of spread vary with the type of cancer.)

Effects of a tumor.   The growth of tumor masses can lead to physical alterations in adjacent organs and tissues and, depending on location, can produce obvious lumps or nodules; ulceration or bleeding; bone destruction; CNS or peripheral nervous system involvement, leading to seizures, paralysis, or pain; obstruction of a hollow viscus (e.g., GI tract, bronchus, or ureter) and consequent problems; and obstruction of mediastinal structures and consequent problems. Tumor enlargement can lead to insufficient nutrition and consequent devitalization of a portion of the lesion. This necrosis can result in ulceration and bleeding or pain, if sensory nerves are involved. In addition, tumor cells may produce increased amounts of physiologically active substances, such as hormones, leading to symptoms such as hypercalcemia from increased parathyroid-like hormone, hyperadrenocorticism from the ACTH-like secretions of bronchogenic cancer, and syndrome of inappropriate ADH.

The growth of tumor cells may also interfere with normal tissue function or compensatory mechanisms. For example, the invasion of marrow by leukemic cells leads to a decreased production of normal blood cells. This results in anemia, with consequent cellular O_2 depletion; leukopenia, with increased susceptibility to infection; and thrombocytopenia, with increased tendency to bleed. In addition, life-threatening medical emergencies can result from tumor growth: massive hemorrhage from a GI tumor, major infectious processes such as pneumococcal meningitis, or profound neurologic symptoms from spinal cord compression.

Signs and symptoms

In situ lesions occur in the earliest recognizable stage of cancer. Malignant cells are present only on surface epithelial tissue and are evident only from cytologic examination of surface cells (e.g., Pap smear or sputum cytology). **Quiescent cancers** produce few or no symptoms. They may be detected by changes during a routine medical survey. Quiescent cancers, unrelated to the cause of death, are often discovered during autopsy. **Invasive cancers** produce symptoms that are clinical abnormalities stemming directly or indirectly from the presence of the tumor (e.g., physiologic derangements that are produced indirectly).

It is important for lay persons and health professionals to know the seven warning signs of cancer: (1) Change in bowel or bladder habits. (2) A sore that does not heal. (3) Unusual bleeding or discharge. (4) Thickening or lump in the breast or elsewhere. (5) Indigestion or difficulty in swallowing. (6) Obvious change in a wart or mole. (7) Nagging cough or hoarseness. Techniques that have been developed to aid in cancer detection include self-examination techniques (breast or testicular); programs to teach self-exam techniques (which, to be successful, mandate a one-to-one contact with a health care professional and a regular monthly performance of the technique); and identification of high-risk groups and specific screening recommendations. The diagnostic tools used in the detection of cancer are (1) cytologic examinations by Pap smear of cervical scrapings, bronchial secretions, urine sediment, sputum, gastric secretions, and any other body secretions or fluids; (2) histologic tissue examination by incision-excision biopsy, needle aspiration biopsy, and scraping or brush techniques; (3) radiologic techniques, including x-rays, radioisotope scans, ultrasound procedures, and CAT scans; (4) tests of blood, urine, and stool samples; and (5) endoscopic studies.

General assessment

The history must include the familial history of malignancies, the environmental history for life-style risk factors and for exposure to potential carcinogens, and the assessment of psychologic variables. The physical examination must emphasize the detection of precancerous lesions and sources of infections. *Diagnostic* testing consists of two phases: (1) diagnosis of the cancer, and (2) a staging work-up for definition of its extent in terms of three components: primary tumor, lymph nodes, and metastases. Diagnostic testing also identifies histopathology: the type of cancer (e.g., ovarian, lung, or breast) and the grading (e.g., well differentiated, moderately differentiated, or poorly differentiated).

Common interventions

The goal of treatment is to reduce the total number of cancer cells to a point where natural body defenses can keep them under control. Neoplastic cells are the offending agents, and treatment is directed at their removal or destruction. The basic principle is to cure the patient while causing minimal functional and structural alteration. **Local treatment modalities** include surgery and radiation therapy. *Surgery* was the earliest successful treatment and remains the current main curative therapy. Its effectiveness is limited by the location and extent of the cancer, however, and it often results in functional or structural alteration. *Radiation therapy* is most successful with relatively small, localized cancers. (Tumor cells vary in their sensitivity to ionizing radiation.) Two important facts must be considered before radiation therapy is administered: (1) the accessibility of the location and anatomic extent of the tumor, and (2) the tolerance of adjacent normal tissues to ionizing radiation. In some cases, complete tumor cell destruction can be achieved without functional or structural alteration.

Systemic modalities include chemotherapy and immunotherapy. *Chemotherapy,* first used in the late 1940s, is particularly important for cancers that are known to disseminate in early stages (e.g., leukemia), as well as for advanced disseminated cancer. It is considered curative in certain cancers (e.g., choriocarcinoma, acute lymphatic leukemia, and Hodgkin's disease) and can produce significant periods of remission or amelioration in other cases. The drugs used in chemotherapy are effective because of their action at the cellular level to inhibit growth or destroy susceptible cells. Normal cells can be affected, however, because the drugs lack tumor specificity and are toxic to vital organ systems (bone marrow, liver, kidneys, nervous system, and lungs). *Immunotherapy* is a newer method of treatment with variable and controversial results. Current methods have not yet been consistently effective. The goals of immunotherapy are to stimulate the immunologic system in an anergic person, to strengthen the immune response to specific tumor cells, and to augment the effectiveness of an already functional immune system. Immunotherapy has the prospect of assisting in the destruction of cancer cells, as do other therapies, but also of ultimately preventing cancer through immunization.

Its side effects range from mild to severe local and systemic reactions and from mild to life-threatening anaphylaxis. The selection of treatment modalities is ideally done on a multidisciplinary basis. (Combinations of treatment have been shown to be more effective.) A careful consideration of the characteristics of the specific individual and of the specific disease process is important for projecting long-range treatment plans. **Adjuvant therapy** combines modalities to (1) reduce the total number of cancer cells by surgical removal and (2) destroy cells that might be present in other parts of the body by chemotherapy in order to delay and possibly prevent the recurrence of cancer. Cooperative controlled clinical studies are developed by multidisciplinary and multi-institutional medical groups to answer complex questions with regard to treatment options.

Effective treatment includes programs of **rehabilitation and psychologic support** that assist patients, families, and health care staff to cope effectively and that assist in the restoration of abilities, physical appearance, and quality of life by means of physical, occupational, and rehabilitation services. Sophisticated services are required to support patients through complex and intensive therapeutic programs with regard to intensive alimentation, access to blood component transfusions, and control of infections. Therapeutic measures should be used to provide effective palliation when care or total control is not feasible: surgery, radiation, and chemotherapy can provide relief of distressing symptoms such as obstruction, pain, and hemorrhage; health care interactions can assist the patient to maintain self-esteem, autonomy, and hope.

Interventions are influenced by four features of cancer and its treatment: (1) the modalities of treatment may be handicapping as well as beneficial to patients and often lead to changes in bodily function and appearance; (2) the general metabolic effect of the cancer process may produce profound alterations in energy levels, nutritional status, fluid and electrolyte balance, and endocrine functioning; (3) the chronic nature of most forms of cancer often requires that the patient, family, and health personnel change their goals from (a) complete care or total rehabilitation to (b) control or remission to (c) successful coping and palliation to (d) a "healthy" dignified death; (4) the implications of the relative uncertainty and research nature of many treatment programs must be taken into account.

Nursing interventions

During surgical treatment 1. Help the patient and family to be physically and emotionally prepared.

2. Help the patient to work through anticipatory and postoperative grief over changes in appearance and function.

3. Administer general pre- and postoperative care (*see* Chapters 9 and 11).

During chemotherapeutic treatment 1. Ensure that informed consent is obtained.

2. Monitor dosage safety by checking doses against individual body surface area (m^2) or weight. The physician will adjust dosages for factors such as ascites and edema, which obscure "real weight," previous severe toxicity, recent treatment (e.g., radiotherapy), and impaired critical organ functioning (e.g., liver or renal failure).

3. Administer chemotherapeutic agents carefully to avoid extravasation into tissue, which can cause skin irritation and necrosis. The following precautions are essential:
   a. Wear gloves to protect self.
   b. Assess needle placement carefully by checking for good blood return. Do not use the site if function is questionable. Ideally, IV needles should be changed q 24 hr.
   c. Administer vesicant drugs through the sidearm of a running IV.
   d. Discontinue administering the drug if the patient complains of burning, pain, or other discomfort (Table 8-2).

4. Time the administration of drugs in relation to the following factors:
   a. Premedication of the patient to reduce GI symptoms, allergic reactions, and anxiety.
   b. Hydration of the patient to ensure a large fluid output after administering drugs such as cis-platinum (to prevent tubule damage), methotrexate (to ensure drug excretion), and cyclophosphamide ([Cytoxan] to prevent cystitis, if drugs stayed in the bladder).
   c. Patient's energy levels, biorhythms, and preferences.

5. Teach the patient and family to relate treatment routines to symptoms and to possible side effects.

6. Teach the patient and family to use resources (e.g., chemotherapy booklets from the American Cancer Society and the NIH).

7. Facilitate acceptance and participation so that the patient is alert to expectations and knowledge and feels in control rather than intimidated.

8. Before initiating treatment, carefully assess the health status of the patient with regard to potential sources of infection, nutritional

TABLE 8-2

Nursing Actions for Suspected Infiltration of Vesicant Drugs *

1. Discontinue administration of drug immediately.
2. Maintain open IV line with slow infusion of nondrug solution.
3. Seek medical intervention for steroid and/or sodium bicarbonate administration.
4. Retard absorption by applying ice packs for at least 24 hr and by keeping patient's arm at rest.
5. Consider plastic surgery consultation.

*E.g., doxorubicin (Adriamycin), Daunorubicin, vinblastine (Velban), vincristine, actinomycin D, mitomycin, and nitrogen mustard.

status, fluid and electrolyte balance, energy level, mobility, emotional status, and specific organ functioning (especially as related to potential side effects of drugs).

9. Know the significance of chemotherapeutic drug side effects (which ones are expected and tolerable and which ones indicate undue toxicity).

10. Consider how the side effects will manifest themselves to the nurse and to the patient.

11. Know the drug excretion route and be aware of the expected nadir of the drug (when the maximum bone marrow depression is expected).

12. Be fully aware of the patient's past drug treatments because toxic effects may be related to cumulative dosages of the same drug and because prior treatment with other drugs may increase side effects (e.g., vincristine sulfate, if administered soon before asparaginase).

13. Identify and institute measures to minimize the untoward reactions of specific drugs (Table 8-3).

During external radiation therapy 1. Teach the patient and family about skin, diet, and bone marrow depression.

2. Alleviate fears of radiation therapy (Table 8-4).

3. Use creative interventions for localized reactions related to the site of treatment (e.g., for head and neck sites, anticipate dysphagia, sore throat, reduced production of saliva, and decreased ability to smell and taste).

4. Assess for any late complications of therapy (e.g., radiation pneumonitis, CNS damage, and secondary cancers).

During internal radiation therapy 1. Obtain clarification (by radiation safety officer) of the radiation safety precautions that are needed. (The three principles of controlling radiation exposure are time, distance, and shielding.)

2 Ensure safety for personnel, adequate care for the patient, and reassurance and knowledge for the patient and family.

Evaluation criteria.   The Oncology Nursing Society and the American Nurses' Association Division on Medical-Surgical Nursing Practice have established the following 10 outcome standards for cancer nursing practice: prevention and early detection, information, coping, comfort, nutrition, protective mechanisms, mobility, elimination, sexuality, and ventilation. More specifically, they state that effective cancer nursing practice should ensure that the patient and family possess adequate information regarding the disease and its prevention, detection, and therapy in order to be able to participate in therapy, self-management, optimal living, and peaceful death. During the course of the disease, the patient and family should learn to manage the resultant physical and psychologic stress and be able to identify and utilize those factors that aid in their comfort.

Finally, the patient and family should be able to maintain adequate nutrition, hydration, elimination status, mobility, sexual identity, ventilatory capacity, and a knowledge of preventive health measures. (A brochure on these outcome standards may be obtained by writing the ANA, 2420 Pershing Road, Kansas City, Mo. 64108.)

CELLULAR DEATH AND NECROSIS

Cellular death occurs when the metabolism and vital functions of the cell cease. **Cellular necrosis,** the process that follows cellular death, is defined as the progressive disintegration of a dead cell. The normal **life-span of cells** varies greatly: *nerve cells* usually live as long as the body; *RBCs* have a normal life-span of 120 days; *active secretory cells* have a brief life-span (mitosis is common). **Cytomorphosis,** the developmental changes through which the cells pass, has three states: *embryonal*(cells are unspecialized and divide rapidly), *differentiated* (changes in form and structure allow for specialized functioning), and *degenerative*(changes lead to death). Other influences can also injure cells and hasten cellular death. The effect of these influences is determined by the vulnerability of the cell, the duration of the stress, and the strength of the stressor. Agents that can cause cellular injury or disease include microorganisms, physical agents, chemical agents, factors that interfere with blood flow (leading to ischemia), and genetic disturbances.

The normal processes of cellular development (or those of cellular injury) lead to cellular death. Morphologic changes follow, which, at times, may be too swift to be observed. These changes can be recognized by the altered structure of the cell, leading to coagulation of proteins in the cytoplasm and obliteration of cell boundaries. The cell may also liquefy, swell, and burst (lysis) as intracellular enzymes are liberated. (The higher the specialization of the tissue, the less likely is it to replace itself with cells similar to the original cells.)

The *signs and symptoms* of cellular death are inflammation, infection, blackened and avascular areas of tissue, pain (initially), wound healing and/or scar tissue, and changes in organ functioning (e.g., neurologic deficits).

Diagnosis is based on the health history, physical exam, and diagnostic tests. Pathologic specimens may not differentiate immediately between a normal cell and a dead or injured cell unless signs of cellular necrosis are present. Tests of major organ functioning may not evidence change until progressive and extensive damage has occurred (e.g., in kidney functioning).

Common interventions

Debridement, removal of all foreign matter and the excision of dead and necrotic tissue, is a necessary process to stimulate the regeneration of cells. Debridement may be accomplished by surgical or physical means or by the

TABLE 8-3

Nursing Management of Common Side Effects of Chemotherapy

Side effect	Detection	Nursing measures
Bone marrow depression Leukopenia	WBC below normal 5,000 to 10,000/mm2, with granulocytes 55 to 65% and lymphocytes 25 to 35%. (If fewer than 4,000/mm2, use care and caution; if fewer than 2,000/mm2, follow measures strictly.) Decrease in WBC may be expected sign of effective ant:tumor dosage. Normal signs of infection may be absent because of marked decrease in granulocytes.	Observe WBC, especially at expected time of nadir. Plan for environment that does not expose patient to sources of infection. Inspect routinely for possible infection and teach patient to do so and report promptly (e.g., eye, rectum, skin, and mucous membranes). Because infections may be due to patient's own bacterial flora, encourage meticulous personal hygiene, encourage good respiratory functioning, and identify and treat potential sources of infection *before* therapy. Do not take rectal temperatures. Promptly start nystatin (Mycostatin) for suspected *Candida* infections for greatest effectiveness. Institute protective isolation when counts are below 1,000 to 2,000/mm2. Use special skin preparation before any venipuncture. Change IV sites q 72 hr. Consider an elevated temperature in leukopenia patient a medical emergency: initiate antibiotic therapy promptly.
Thrombocytopenia	Counts below normal (300,000 to 500,000/mm2). Bleeding may occur at variable levels, depending on the individual. Be alert if counts	Observe counts and consider the expected nadir in order to predict continued decline or recovery.

	are below 100,000/mm². Some may tolerate counts below 20,000/mm². Nadir of drug and expected actions must be considered in taking precautionary action. Signs and symptoms: skin changes (petechiae, bruising, and purpura), nosebleeds, hematuria, heme-positive stools or emesis, and joint pains.	Consider platelet transfusions for bleeding or if count is below 20,000/mm². Avoid IM or SC injections and minimize number of venipunctures for blood samples. (Apply site pressure.) Keep temperature normal with acetaminophen (Tylenol) and sponging. (High temperatures shorten platelet life.) Do not administer aspirin or drugs containing aspirin. Consider energy demands placed on patient. (Provide for rest periods.)
Anemia	Reduction in pretreatment Hb levels. If below 8 mg, expect marked symptoms. Signs and symptoms: fatigue, shortness of breath, depression, pallor, tachycardia, dizziness, and weakness.	Administer RBC transfusions as ordered. (Dangers of transfusion reactions and hepatitis need to be considered.)
GI Stomatitis	Dry mouth or intolerance of acidic foods may be initial complaint. Erythema, pain, and ulceration of the mucosa.	Inspect mouth daily and teach patient to do so. (Initial signs may indicate that drug should be stopped. Symptoms will increase even after drug is discontinued.) Provide meticulous oral hygiene qid. Avoid commercial mouthwashes.
Nausea and vomiting	May appear directly after administration or may be delayed up to 8 hr, depending on drug.	Administer preventive antiemetics and drug combinations at regular intervals before and after treatment. Promote a quiet, restful environment with no noxious stimuli. Reduce or avoid food intake before drug administration. Provide consistent support. Assist patient with relaxation measures.

Side effect	Detection	Nursing measures
Diarrhea		Use antidiarrheal agents as preventive premedication if diarrhea has been a past problem. Provide diet low in roughage but high in constipating foods (e.g., cheese and apples). Avoid rectal temperatures if breakdown of GI mucosa is a potential effect. Provide fluid replacement if diarrhea, nausea, and vomiting occur.
Alopecia	Hair loss usually occurs 3 to 4 wk after administration. Almost certain to occur with certain drugs in high dosages (e.g., doxorubicin [Adriamycin] and Daunorubicin). Other drugs and dosages cause partial to total hair loss (e.g., cyclophosphamide [Cytoxan], vinblastine [Velban], and vincristine). Hair loss can include scalp and all other areas of body hair.	Plan to support patient for profound psychologic impact: (1) arrange for a wig before hair loss occurs, and (2) assist patient to verbalize anticipatory grief and grieving. Reassure patient that regrowth will occur after drug is stopped. Apply scalp hypothermia to minimize hair loss.
Neuromuscular	May go unnoticed if patient and nurse are not alert for them. Signs and symptoms: acute jaw pain (should be noted immediately); constipation progressing to paralytic ileus; peripheral neuropathy indicated by burning, tingling, numbness in extremities, loss of deep reflexes, or actual motor changes; and temporary depression and/or subtle changes in affect and personality.	Use stool softeners and/or laxatives prophylactically to prevent constipation.

Hormonal

Women may experience temporary cessation of menstrual periods or, if menopausal, may have uterine bleeding. Breast enlargement in men and decreased libido and virilization in women are side effects with certain drugs.

Plan for support. (These effects can be particularly destructive to self-esteem if patient is unaware of relationship to treatment regimen. Most effects subside after drugs are stopped.) Advise about conception. Although infertility can result from drug therapy, conception often continues to be possible. However, the uncertain effects of drugs on germ cells make most authorities recommend against conception. The issue should be discussed so that informed decisions are made. Genetic counseling *before* therapy is initiated may be suggested.

Cutaneous changes

Color changes over veins, rashes, changes in color and texture of nails. Severe cutaneous reactions can occur from bleomycin. Extravasation of vesicant drugs causes local tissue necrosis.

Plan for support and patient education. (*See* Table 8-2 for treatment of vesicant drug extravasation.)

Renal toxicity

Changes in urine and blood tests of renal functioning: creatinine clearance, serum creatinine, and BUN.

Assess renal functioning and hydration. This is essential.
Eliminate drugs promptly and dilute them in a good urine output.
Medications may be used with certain drugs to decrease incidence of damaging side effects: a mannitol diuresis decreases potential toxicity of cis-platinum; allopurinol is administered to prevent hyperuricemia; sodium bicarbonate or other medications are used to alkalinize the urine (pH>7.0) before administration of high doses of methotrexate, which dissolves better in an alkaline urine.

Side effect	Detection	Nursing measures
Anaphylactic reactions	*See* Chapter 6.	Be especially alert if drug is administered for first time and/or is relatively new. Be alert to drugs that are more likely to cause an anaphylactic reaction after repeated doses. Be sure that emergency drugs are nearby. Be prepared to discontinue drug and maintain *open* IV line (*see* Chapter 6).

TABLE 8-4

General Patient Teaching Before External Radiation Therapy

Area of concern	Patient teaching
Skin	Do not wash away skin markings that indicate the treatment area.
	Keep the treatment area dry (check with physician regarding baths or showers).
	Wear 100% cotton garments close to the skin.
	Avoid wearing tight-fitting garments.
	Do not apply soaps, creams, ointments, or cosmetics to the treatment area unless they are allowed by the physician.
	Protect the skin from direct sunlight (check with physician regarding length of time).
	Do not use a hot-water bottle, heating pad, or sunlamp on the treated area.
Diet and fluid intake	Encourage foods high in protein and calories.
	Drink at least 2 to 3 quarts of liquid each day.
	Eat small meals frequently.
	If ordered by the physician, take an antiemetic 30 min before treatment and before meals.
Bone marrow depression anemia	Remember that some lethargy, general weakness, and shortness of breath are not uncommon.
	Plan frequent rest periods as part of the day's schedule.
Leukopenia	Maintain good personal hygiene.
	Avoid sources of infection.
Thrombocytopenia	Notify the physician if there are signs of bleeding in body wastes or from mucous membranes.
	Avoid potentially injurious situations (contact sports) if thrombocytopenia is severe.
Fear of radiation therapy	Remember that external radiation therapy does not cause the patient to become radioactive.
	Stress that the treatment is not painful.
	Remain very still during treatment.
	Rememember that only the patient is in the room during treatment.
	Remember that a closed-circuit TV system monitors the patient during treatment.

Adapted with permission from Dietz, K. A. Programmed instruction: radiation therapy. *Cancer Nursing* (April 1979). p. 129.

use of proteolytic or fibrinolytic enzymes. The use of *drains and packing* in wound care encourages the escape (and prevents the accumulation) of products of cellular necrosis.

Nursing interventions

1. Protect vulnerable individuals from stressors that can cause cellular injury.
2. Maintain continuous and unwavering medical and surgical asepsis.
3. Maintain surveillance with regard to infectious diseases, especially hospital-acquired infections.
4. Institute protective measures for immobile patients or those with reduced mobility (e.g., measures in OR and for bedfast and/or paraplegic patients to decrease prolonged pressure over bony prominences). (*See* Chapter 7.)
5. Identify and control harmful physical and chemical agents by preventing exposure to extreme heat or cold, by using protective shielding during radiation therapy and diagnostic x-rays, and by controlling toxic chemicals.
6. Institute measures that aid excretion of the products of cellular necrosis and that facilitate wound healing (provide adequate nutrition, high in protein and vitamin C; administer RBC transfusions if Hb is low; and ensure adequate blood supply by positioning and the avoidance of tight, constricting clothing or bandages).
7. Administer allopurinol as ordered. (Allopurinol, which inhibits uric acid production, is often administered when extensive cellular destruction is expected, as when chemotherapy is used for rapidly growing cancer.)
8. Increase the patient's fluid intake to ensure adequate hydration and a large urine output.

Evaluation criteria.   Interventions have been successful if there is wound healing, proper organ functioning, and a decreased incidence of hospital-acquired infections.

CHAPTER 9

PREOPERATIVE NEEDS

Elizabeth Anne Mahoney and Jean Pieri Flynn

The preoperative period extends from the time of notification that surgery is to be performed and/or admission to the acute care facility until the patient arrives in the OR. The focus of the preoperative period is to prepare the patient to be in the best possible physical and psychologic state for surgery.

Emergency vs. elective surgery

Patient preparation and readiness for surgery will vary with the nature of surgery (emergency or elective). **Elective surgery** implies that although the surgery may be necessary, the individual has some flexibility in determining when the surgery will be performed. This allows more time for physical and psychologic preparation of the patient and his family/significant others.

By its very nature, **emergency surgery** denotes that there is little time between the decision for surgery and the actual procedure. Thus, the patient may not be in an optimal physical or psychologic state for surgery. In emergency situations, preparation may be more directed toward physical needs, such as skin preparation or blood transfusions, in order to minimize operative risks. There may be little or no time for preoperative teaching, which will have implications for the postoperative period. In an emergency situation, the psychologic needs of both the patient and his family must be considered, and measures must be taken to provide information and decrease anxiety.

163

General assessment

A complete **health history** should be collected. Especially relevant data include the reason for contact, current health status (chief concern, nutrition, tobacco, and drugs), past health history (restorative interventions, allergies), relevant family history, and a review of systems (the specific system requiring surgical intervention; the cardiovascular, respiratory, GU, hematopoietic, and autoimmune systems; and the patient's mental status, with special attention given to the level of anxiety).

A complete **physical exam** should be performed. Particular attention should be given to the direct inspection, palpation, percussion, and/or auscultation of all areas listed under the health history review of systems above.

Most patients routinely have a basic battery of **diagnostic tests** performed: chest x-ray, ECG for anyone >35 yr or with previous cardiac disease, CBC, and urinalysis. Other commonly ordered blood tests are serum electrolytes; prothrombin and clotting times; and blood type and cross-match. In many institutions, these tests are performed as part of a "transadmission" procedure and are completed before the patient arrives on the unit. Preoperative work-up may include diagnostic tests specifically related to the surgical or other medical problems. For example, the patient with a peptic ulcer may need a gastric analysis, an upper GI series, and/or gastroscopy to document the lesion.

Anesthesia assessment

The anesthesiologist or nurse anesthetist should visit the patient the evening before or the morning of surgery to evaluate the individual's general health status and to determine the kind of anesthesia to be given.

Risk factors

Physical and psychologic status.   Factors that relate to the patient's physical and psychologic status include age, nutritional status, general state of health, and level of anxiety. In general, older patients are more prone to surgical risks because they have other chronic illnesses, such as hypertension and other cardiovascular diseases, respiratory diseases, and/or diabetes mellitus. The elderly's tolerance of drugs, including anesthetic agents, can be decreased because of decreased metabolic and circulatory rates, and because of the number of medications being taken. The latter factor also increases the potential for incompatibility.

Nutritional inadequacies can be manifested in any age group and can be caused by such factors as decreased activity, decreased economic base, loneliness, and illness. Obesity, decreased weight, or lack of specific dietary components can predispose individuals to poor healing, susceptibility to infection, and delayed recovery from surgery. Fluid and electrolyte balance is also of particular concern because of anticipated blood loss during surgery, stress response, and restricted intake before and after surgery.

A person in any optimal state of health can withstand the stress of surgery more than one who has a chronic illness, infection, recent weight change, or malaise. Impairment of any major body system (e.g., cardiovascular, pulmonary, GU, or hematopoietic) predisposes the patient to intra- or postoperative complications.

An individual's mental status plays a key role in successful recovery. Anxiety and fear negatively influence the patient's response to surgery. Anxiety and fear of the unknown are usual reactions, and increased levels of either will intensify the patient's stress response and the potential for complications during or after surgery. If the patient expresses an unusual degree of anxiety and/or verbalizes a fear of dying during the procedure, surgery should be postponed or cancelled.

Surgical procedure.   Operative risk is influenced by the body area involved and the extent of the procedure. Intrusion into body cavities (chest, abdomen, or brain), prolonged operating time, or surgery on more than one body organ creates greater operative risk by extending the anesthesia time and increasing the potential for fluid and electrolyte imbalance and infection.

Anesthesia.   The duration and type (general vs. local or regional) of anesthesia affect operative risk. Persons with debilitating conditions do not tolerate lengthy anesthesia well. Because general anesthesia depresses all body systems, individuals with impaired cardiac, respiratory, and renal functioning are greater surgical risks.

Other factors

Understanding of surgery.   It is important to assess what the patient thinks is going to happen to him during surgery and also what will be expected of him pre- and postoperatively. This information will be especially important to the physician and the nurse in determining what the patient wishes to know and what he must be taught (*see below*).

Anxiety level.   All patients fear surgery. The extent to which an individual is afraid will depend on his basic psychologic makeup, his past experience with surgical procedures, and his method of handling stress. Anxiety usually centers around fear of postoperative pain; a diagnosis (e.g., cancer); loss of body parts, with resulting disfigurement; loss of consciousness and control because of anesthesia; an imposed change in life-style postoperatively; and death. Anxiety can be manifested in a number of ways: withdrawn silence, demanding behavior, crying, or continuous talking or laughing. Observations and assessments made concerning the patient's level of anxiety can be useful in planning preoperative teaching to help decrease the patient's fear of surgery.

Consults.   If abnormalities in body functioning are found through various components of the preoperative assessment, a consult should be requested to determine the extent to which the abnormality will affect the outcome of surgery. For example, an abnormal ECG tracing should be followed with a cardiology consult to clear the patient for surgery.

Medical interventions

Explanation of surgery and outcomes. The surgeon is responsible for fully explaining the nature of the operation and the possible complications or disfigurements that may result from the procedure. The physician should also tell the patient if any part of his body is to be removed. In some instances, pictures or diagrams may be necessary to help the patient visualize essential outcomes of the procedure.

Consents. Before surgery can be performed, two consents must be obtained: permission for anesthesia and permission for the actual procedure. The consent is a legal document that protects the patient from undergoing operative procedures he does not want or know about. The hospital and staff are also protected by the consent, which documents that the patient was informed of surgery and consented to have surgery. The consent is signed by the physician, patient, and a witness, who is verifying the patient's signature.

In general, any person >18 yr may sign an operative consent. Occasionally, because of unconsciousness or mental incompetence of a patient, a family member or guardian may need to sign the form. Once signed, the consent becomes a permanent part of the patient's chart.

The consent is only valid for the designated surgery. A consent becomes invalid if a patient decides not to have the surgery. This change should be documented in the chart, and the phyician should be notified. If the patient again agrees to have surgery, a new consent must be obtained.

Orders for preoperative preparation. On the eve of surgery, the following measures should be ordered: anesthesia premedications, skin preparation, restriction of oral intake, and preparation specific to certain surgical procedures. The latter three areas are discussed under nursing interventions (*see below*).

There are basically three types of preoperative anesthesia premedication: narcotics, sedatives/tranquilizers, and anticholinergics. Narcotics, usually meperidine (Demerol) or morphine sulfate, are used preoperatively to decrease anxiety, to relax the patient, and to potentiate the effects of anesthesia. Narcotics may cause nausea and vomiting and depress respiratory functioning or BP. Sedatives or tranquilizers (secobarbital [Seconal], diazepam [Valium], or hydroxyzine hydrochloride [Vistaril]) are also used to allay anxiety and relax the patient. They also lower BP and pulse, potentiate the action of narcotics, and act to reduce the amount of anesthetic agent necessary for surgery. Although tranquilizers can cause severe hypotension, respiratory status will not be impaired. Because trachebronchial secretions usually increase during surgery as a result of cells being irritated by anesthetic agents, anticholinergics (atropine or scopolamine) may be administered as "drying agents" to minimize the chances of postoperative atelectasis and pneumonia. Thus, pre- or postoperatively, patients may complain of dry mouth. Both atropine and scopolamine have undesirable effects: atropine can cause tachycardia; scopolamine can cause confusion, restlessness, and hallucinations. Preoperative medications must be administered on time to prevent problems during the induction of anesthesia. Other medications for preparation of the patient may be ordered for specific surgical procedures. For example, cathartics may be ordered before bowel surgery.

Nursing interventions (days before surgery)

Perioperative teaching.   Perioperative teaching, a major nursing responsibility, can begin as soon as a data base has been collected and the patient knows about the impending surgery. Key areas for teaching include anxiety, clarification and reinforcement of the patient's understanding of surgery and anesthesia, and pre- and postoperative expectations. (Table 9-1 provides an overview of the nursing interventions presented in this section.)

Most patients will want at least some basic information about the nature of the surgical experience. The ability to understand the data provided will be influenced by the patient's anxiety level, past experiences, and intellectual capacity. Because an anxious patient will not be able to comprehend what is being taught, anxiety must be reduced before teaching can begin. First, anxiety must be recognized. Then the nurse must communicate an interest in the patient and a sensitivity to what he is experiencing.

The individual should be made comfortable in his new environment. Verbalization of concerns should be encouraged so that they can be dealt with. Wearing one's own clothes, handling personal belongings, having family or significant others present, and having other diversional activities can alleviate stress. Whenever possible, the individual's past ability to cope should be applied to the current situation. Discussing concerns frankly will acknowledge their reality to the patient and provide opportunities for clarifying misconceptions. Information about what to expect is another means of decreasing anxiety. Simple definitions and explanations should be given; few people want to know the details of surgery. Major areas to be covered with the patient are discussed below. When more information is desired, it should be provided. If necessary, the physician can be contacted for more explicit data. The nurse must not assume knowledge a person may not possess, which is particularly true when health-related personnel are patients. Not all of these patients may be familiar with the surgery and, as patients, their understanding may be blocked by anxiety. The nurse should carefully review with each person what to expect.

A variety of personnel may be involved in the teaching process: nurses from the hospital unit, OR, and/or recovery room; the private physician, anesthesiologist, and/or house staff; and/or a respiratory therapist. Therefore, coordination of activities and similarity of information are essential to prevent conflicting information and overwhelming the patient by the

TABLE 9-1

Overview of Preoperative Nursing Interventions

Day(s) before surgery	Morning/day of surgery
1. Minimize anxiety	1. Prepare skin
2. Clarify and reinforce understanding of surgery and anesthesia	2. Provide hygiene care
3. Teach about preoperative expectations	3. Review chart
Diagnostic tests	Diagnostic test results
Sleeping medication night before surgery	Consents signed and witnessed
NPO after midnight	Preoperative medication orders
Skin preparation	4. Check patient for anxiety level
4. Teach about postoperative expectations	5. Ensure name band in place
Recovery room	6. Remove dentures, other prostheses, jewelry, bobby pins, etc.
Pain management	7. Remove cosmetics and nail polish
Coughing and deep breathing	8. Send valuables home or to hospital safe
Positioning	9. Record vital signs
Ambulation	10. Report untoward signs or missing data to physician or OR
IV solutions	11. Have patient void before premedication
Vital signs	12. Apply OR cap, support stockings, etc.
Intake and output	13. Administer and record preoperative medications
Dressings	14. Raise side rails
Tubes	15. Write nurse's note
	16. Assist with transfer of patient onto stretcher and any ordered medications or equipment
	17. Send chart, x-rays, with patient to OR

number of teachers. The nurse should ask the patient if he has any questions and answer those to reinforce previous teaching rather than repeat it.

Preoperative preparation (skin preparation, sleeping medication, NPO after midnight [*see below*]) and postoperative expectations should be explained to the patient. The following is a discussion of postoperative expectations.

Patients undergoing general and regional (axillary or spinal) anesthesia will be transferred to the **recovery room.** This adds a minimum of 30 min before the return to the unit. Individuals should know that level of consciousness (calling by name), airway (oxygen), vital signs, dressings, tubes, control of movement (arms, legs), and other patient parameters will be closely monitored. The patient should be returned to his room only when he is oriented and stable.

The patient should be informed that **pain** is expected, although it will diminish after the first 24 to 48 hr. Medications should be ordered and taken when pain is present. The principles of pain relief should be stressed and applied (*sée* Chapter 4).

The patient should be taught the need for **coughing** and **deep breathing** for a few minutes at least q 2 hr to improve lung expansion and remove secretions. Slow, deep breaths followed by a deep cough should be advised. The patient can place his hands at the sides of his ribs or on his abdomen to feel the appropriate movement. Because this procedure can cause pain, especially after abdominal or thoracic surgery, the patient should be told that medications will be given before such activity. Also, the placement of hands or a pillow over the incisional area can serve as a splint, thus minimizing discomfort. Many patients are afraid that coughing or moving will cause the "stitches to pop;" they should be informed that this is very unlikely.

Patients should be told that they will be turned q 2 hr while on bed rest to promote respiratory expansion and drainage and to prevent pressure on any one area.

Depending on the patient's level of consciousness and the nature of the surgery, **mobilization** should begin in the evening or morning after surgery. The individual should be cautioned to obtain assistance in getting out of bed until he is no longer dizzy while sitting or standing and until his gait is steady. Because ambulation can be painful, the patient should know about splinting and the availability of medications. The benefits of early ambulation — increased muscle tone and functioning of all body systems and shortened recovery time — should be reviewed.

Most patients have an **IV** started for surgery and usually return to the unit with an IV in place. Infusions should continue until the individual is able to tolerate fluids. For some this is a matter of hours, for others days, depending on the type of surgery. An estimate of the time that the IVs will continue should be given to the patient.

The patient's **vital signs** (BP, pulse, respirations, and temperature) are usually monitored q 4 hr for the first 24 to 48 hr after the patient's return to the unit. These signs provide information about the cardiovascular, respiratory, and heat regulatory responses and serve as early signals of complications. The patient should be told that this frequent monitoring is routine postoperatively.

Intake, output, and specific gravity of urine are measured for the first 24 to 48 hr to determine hydration. The patient should be told that all fluid intake (oral and parenteral) and loss (urine and tubes) will be monitored. If the patient is using the bathroom, he must be told to void into a container (urinal, bedpan) and to save the output for measuring.

Patients should be told that **dressings** are used to cover the incision for protection and to absorb drainage. Dressings are usually larger than incisions, and patients should not be alarmed by their size. When the suture line is clean and dry, the wound is frequently uncovered after the first postoperative day. The staff should check the dressing and wound site to monitor healing.

Based on the nature of the surgery, **tubes** may be present that require additional monitoring. These include nasogastric or intestinal tubes (GI surgery), chest tubes and oxygen (chest surgery), or Foley catheters or other urinary tubes (GU surgery). The patient should be informed about what tubes to expect and that the nurses will be checking the tubes frequently to ascertain their patency and proper functioning.

Skin preparation. Traditionally, preparation of the patient's skin has been performed on the day or evening before surgery; however, at present, the preferred time is 1 hr before surgery. The patient should know when to expect the skin preparation and that it is done to prevent wound contamination. Skin preparation is discussed in detail below.

Sleeping medication. The patient should be offered and encouraged to take the medication as necessary to ensure rest the night before surgery. Rationales should be given to those who are hesitant to take unfamiliar drugs.

NPO after midnight. Unless specifically ordered by the physician to be taken with sips of water, all oral medications should be discontinued. If a patient is not scheduled for surgery until late in the afternoon, a light or fluid breakfast may be ordered. The following nursing measures are important for the patient who is NPO: The patient should be informed that he must not eat or drink, and explained why; all food and fluid should be removed from the bedside; an NPO sign should be placed over the bedside and/or on the door; and the diet kitchen and other personnel should be informed.

Diagnostic tests completed. All diagnostic tests should be completed and their results indicated on the chart. Omission of test results can cause delay of surgery and unnecessary stress for the patient and staff.

Other considerations for specific procedures. Surgery on the GI tract requires certain specific preparation, such as enemas and/or cathartics to minimize the possibility of fecal spillage into the peritoneal cavity during the procedure. In the case of bowel or cardiac surgery, antibiotics may be ordered to decrease the potential for postoperative infection.

Nursing interventions (morning of surgery)

The preparation of the patient on the morning of surgery should be accomplished as early as possible to detect and rectify omissions and to prevent undue rushing, which can result in increased anxiety and/or potential errors. (1) Skin preparation should be done to remove hair and bacteria from the operative area and to minimize wound contamination. Two methods are commonly used: shaving and cleansing with an iodide-base agent, or depilatory. Both preparations can cause allergic reactions, and, therefore, skin testing should be done before their use. Shaving can result in abrasions or cuts, and some hair may not be removed. The literature reports an increased preference for depilatories because of their ease in application and more uniform results. Less extensive areas of skin are being prepped by each method without an increased incidence of infections. (2) Hygiene measures should include mouth care and a clean hospital gown. An OR cap and elastic or other stockings that are ordered should be at the bedside. (3) The patient's chart should be reviewed to ascertain that diagnostic test results are recorded, that consents are signed and witnessed, and that preoperative medications have been ordered. (4) The patient should be checked for the following: (a) Minimized level of anxiety and preoperative reinforced teaching. (b) Name band in place for proper identification. (c) Dentures, other prostheses, and jewelry removed to prevent their loss or damage. Some institutions allow the patient to wear a wedding band that is secured with tape. However, if cautery is used and grounding is not uniform, the skin can be burned under the ring. (d) Cosmetics and nail polish removed to allow for adequate assessment of color and tissue perfusion. (e) Valuables sent home or placed in the hospital safe to prevent loss. (f) Vital signs stable and recorded for base-line data. (5) Any untoward signs or missing data should be reported to the physician or OR staff. (6) The patient should void before being medicated to prevent incontinence during surgery. A catheter may be inserted in patients who are to have lower abdominal or pelvic surgery. (7) Preoperative medications should be administered 30 to 60 min before surgery and recorded on the medication record and physician's order sheet. Side rails should be raised to promote patient safety. (8) A nurse's note should be written to reflect the patient's general state and the preoperative measures that have been implemented. The chart, and any medications or equipment that have been requested, should be sent with the patient to the OR.

Evaluation criteria

Risk factors/complications minimized: Signs of anxiety minimal, patient verbalizes anxiety. Diagnostic data within normal limits. Skin clean, hair removed. NPO since midnight. Vital signs stable and recorded.

Voided before being medicated. Premedications administered and charted. Nurse's notes written, describe patient's status. *Understanding, acceptance of surgery demonstrated:* Patient describes (generally) reason for and nature of surgery; has no further questions. Consent signed. *Safety measures implemented:* Identification band on wrist. Dentures, other prostheses, jewelry, cosmetics, nail polish removed. Side rails raised after medication. Abnormal results, missing data, high anxiety level reported to physician(s).

CHAPTER 10

INTRAOPERATIVE NEEDS

Rita M. Bisceglia

OVERVIEW

The intraoperative period extends from the time that the patient arrives in the OR until he or she is admitted to the recovery room or returned directly to the unit. The focus of the intraoperative period is on providing a safe environment and on minimizing the hazards of anesthesia and surgery for the patient who requires surgical intervention.

General assessment
Environment. Providing and maintaining a safe environment for the patient undergoing surgery consists of several components.

Cleanliness of room and equipment: Although each hospital has its own cleaning policies and procedures, the OR nurse is responsible for checking that these procedures have been carried out and that the floor, furniture, and equipment in the room are clean and free from dust before surgery begins.

Providing necessary equipment in proper working order: All equipment to be used during a procedure (e.g., overhead lights, suction, microscope, etc.) should be checked for proper functioning to ensure patient safety. Malfunctioning equipment (e.g., cracked suction caps) can create a threat to patient safety by causing unnecessary delays in surgery and by increasing anesthesia time. Checking the apparatus before the start of surgery prevents such problems.

Fire and explosion hazards: Fire and explosions occur because of a combination of factors: flammable material, oxygen, a source of ignition, and the carelessness of personnel. If any one of these factors is absent, no problem will exist. Although few flammable anesthetics are used today, those that are must be considered potential problems and precautions must be implemented. Oxygen is always present, in the OR it may be found in higher concentrations. The source of ignition is usually a spark, static electricity, or faulty electrical equipment. Because of these facts, it is incumbent on all OR personnel to be aware of and adhere to certain general safety regulations, which may include the following: (1) Prohibiting smoking and the use of any equipment that produces open flames. (2) Requiring explosion-proof switches and outlets or three-pronged grounded outlets. The latter should be at least 5 ft above the floor. (3) Maintaining distance between the anesthetic equipment and electrical devices. (4) Inspecting all electrical equipment for safety and proper functioning on a regular basis and before use. (5) Having all personnel be familiar with procedures for the prompt repair of defective equipment. (6) Maintaining a relative humidity of $\geq 50\%$. (7) Using conductive flooring, footwear, and static-electricity-free material when flammable anesthetic agents are available in the OR suite.

Patient.   Patient needs vary depending on the surgical procedure, type of anesthesia, and preoperative condition of the patient.

Surgical procedure: The OR nurse must be aware that both the physical and the psychologic needs of the patient will vary depending on the surgical procedure to be performed and should plan for the patient's care accordingly.

Although all patients have some basic fear related to surgery, many procedures have greater emotional significance than others (*see* Chapter 9). The OR nurse should anticipate the necessity of providing additional emotional support, understanding, and/or explanations to those patients who still require them upon entering the OR suite.

Type of anesthesia: The type of anesthesia to be used depends on the patient's condition, his or her age, the medication taken by the patient, the surgical procedure (type and duration), the use or nonuse of electrosurgical units, and the patient's preference. The choice is made by the anesthesiologist and the surgeon.

Preoperative condition: Information regarding the patient's preoperative condition may be obtained by the OR nurse in different ways, depending on the structure of the institution providing the care. For example, the nurse on the unit may collect data and develop a nursing care plan that the OR nurse will use, or the OR nurse may make use of a preoperative visit for the development of an OR nursing care plan. Whichever method is used, it is imperative for the OR nurse to be aware of the following information: general physical condition; any chronic diseases; physical handicaps; sensory deficits; allergies to medication, antiseptic agents, or adhesive; and emotional status.

Common interventions

Monitoring of vital signs. During the patient's stay in the OR, various signs are monitored depending on the type of surgery and anesthesia. When the surgery to be performed requires the services of an anesthetist and/or anesthesiologist, he or she is responsible for monitoring such signs as pulse, respirations, BP (including arterial, when necessary), ECG, and temperature. (In some institutions, temperature is monitored in all patients; in others, it is only monitored when needed.) It is the OR nurse's responsibility to assist the anesthesiologist and to be alert for any changes that necessitate rapid intervention. If the surgery is being performed without the assistance of anesthesia personnel, it is the responsibility of the OR nurse to monitor and record such signs as pulse, respiration, and BP, as indicated by hospital policy.

IV infusion. Almost all patients coming to the OR will have an IV started either before arriving or during their stay in the OR suite. The nurse must be aware of the principles of fluid and electrolyte balance and must know how to set up an IV and how to provide care to a patient who has one.

Anesthesia. Anesthesia may be defined as a diminished or lost sense of feelings, especially the sense of pain, with or without the loss of consciousness. Anesthesia may be general, regional, or local.

General anesthetics block the awareness centers of the brain and may be administered by inhalation, IV, or rectally. When adequate amounts of the anesthetic agent reach the brain, the patient loses consciousness. In order to assist the anesthesiologist intelligently and to provide optimum care for the patient, the nurse should know the agents that will be used, the method of administration, the length of induction, the associated hazards, and the advantages and disadvantages (Table 10-1). The OR nurse must be familiar with the following four stages of anesthesia. **Stage I** starts with the administration of the agent and lasts until loss of consciousness. The patient may appear drowsy or dizzy, and speech is usually slurred. **Stage II** starts with the loss of consciousness and lasts until there is relaxation. This stage is sometimes referred to as the excitement stage because the patient may appear excited, breathe irregularly, and move the arms and legs or the whole body. During this stage, the patient is very susceptible to external stimuli (noise or a sudden touch). It is therefore vital for the nurse to remain at the patient's side, maintain a quiet atmosphere, be ready to restrain the patient, if necessary, and assist the anesthesiologist as indicated. With the advent of fast-acting agents, the excitement is not frequently seen, but the patient *does* go through this stage, and the nurse must be prepared to act quickly if symptoms are observed. **Stage III** starts with relaxation and lasts until the loss of reflexes and the depression of vital functions. This is also known as the surgical stage because it is the stage at which most surgery is performed. The patient's respirations are regular, the pupils contract, the eyelid reflexes disappear, the jaw relaxes, and auditory sensation is lost. Positioning, prepping, draping, and surgery may now begin. **Stage IV** is the

TABLE 10-1
Commonly Used Anesthetic Agents

Agent	Administration	Induction	Explosion hazards	Advantages	Disadvantages
Ether	Open drop inhalation	Slow	Explosive	Good relaxation; wide margin of safety; inexpensive; nontoxic.	Long recovery; irritating, pungent odor; irritating to skin, mucous membranes, lungs, and kidneys; causes nausea, vomiting, and urinary retention.
Nitrous oxide	Inhalation	Rapid	Nonflammable	Rapid induction and recovery; no odor or taste; few aftereffects.	Poor relaxation; may produce hypoxia, except in brief procedures.
Halothane (Fluothane)	Inhalation	Rapid, smooth	Nonflammable	Nonirritating; pleasant, sweet odor; little excitement; rapid induction and recovery; seldom causes nausea or vomiting.	Requires special vaporizer; narrow margin of safety; may depress cardiovascular system; limited relaxation; expensive; may cause liver damage.
Methoxyflurane (Penthrane)	Inhalation	Slow	Nonflammable, nonexplosive	Excellent muscle relaxation; seldom causes nausea or vomiting.	Requires special vaporizer; may cause kidney or liver damage.
Enflurane (Ethrane)	Inhalation	Rapid	Nonflammable	Easy maintenance; rapid recovery; fair muscle relaxation; marked cardiovascular stability; good operative analgesia; pleasant odor.	Contraindicated in patients with seizure disorders and diabetes mellitus.
Cyclopropane	Inhalation	Rapid	Explosive	Rapid induction and recovery; wide margin of safety; good relaxation; well tolerated; pleasant, sweet odor.	May cause cardiac arrhythmias, shock, bronchospasm, postanesthesia nausea and vomiting.
Isoflurane (Forane)	Inhalation	Rapid	Nonexplosive	Rapid induction and recovery; strong analgesia; good muscle relaxation.	Expensive.
Thiopental sodium (Pentothal)	IV	Rapid, pleasant	None	Rapid induction and recovery; little equipment needed; nonirritating; low incidence of postoperative nausea or vomiting.	Powerful respiratory depressant; poor relaxation.

Drug	Route	Onset		Description	Side Effects
Ketamine (Ketalar)	IV, IM	Rapid	None	Short action; good for short procedures; may be used to supplement weaker agents.	May cause respiratory depression; induces BP rise; patient may act irrationally when recovering from anesthesia; may produce hallucinations.
Fentanyl (Sublimaze)	IV, IM	Rapid	None	Short duration; 80 times more potent than morphine.	May cause respiratory depression, nausea and vomiting, bradycardia, or muscle rigidity.
Fentanyl and droperidol (Innovar)	IM, IV	Rapid	None	Produces calmness and decreases responsiveness to painful stimuli; good premedication for anesthesia.	May cause respiratory depression, laryngospasm, bronchospasm, and hallucinations.
Cocaine	Topical	Rapid	None	Rapid action; patient is conscious.	High toxicity; may be fatal if injected.
Lidocaine hydrochloride (Xylocaine)	Infiltration, topical, block, spinal	Rapid	None	Longer duration of action than procaine; does not produce local irritation effect.	Occasional idiosyncrasy.
Tetracaine (Pontocaine)	Topical, spinal	Rapid	None	Long duration; good spinal anesthetic for operations lasting 2-3 hr.	Possible idiosyncrasy.
Procaine hydrochloride (Novocain)	SC, IV, spinal	Rapid	None	Low toxicity; nonirritating to tissues.	Possible idiosyncrasy.
Bupivacaine hydrochloride (Marcaine)	Infiltration, block, epidural	Rapid	None	Long duration (up to several hr); nonirritating.	Allergic reaction possible; cardiac arrhythmias may occur.

danger stage. Respiratory and cardiac functioning are too depressed: the patient is not breathing, and there is little or no heartbeat. Because this is not a desired stage of anesthesia, the nurse must be prepared to assist with emergency resuscitation measures.

Regional anesthetics block pain sensation at the nerve trunk or roots and affect a region of the body without inducing loss of consciousness. Regional anesthesia may be *spinal* (the drug is injected into the subarachnoid space, usually between L3 and L4) or *epidural* (the drug is injected into the caudal canal epidurally). The main agents used are tetracaine hydrochloride (Pontocaine) and lidocaine hydrochloride (Xylocaine) (*see* Table 10-1). The drugs are often mixed with glucose to make them heavier than CSF. The nurse should know that there is no control over the drug once it is injected, that respirations may become depressed because of paralysis of the intercostal muscles, and that hypotension may result. Therefore, the nurse should be prepared to assist the anesthesiologist if a problem arises.

Local anesthetics block pain sensation in a relatively small and specific area of the body, either by topical application or infiltration. Some common local anesthetic agents are Xylocaine, bupivacaine hydrochloride (Marcaine), and Pontocaine. These medications are usually administered by the surgeon.

The OR nurse is responsible for having the correct drug available and for observing, reporting, and recording the patient's response to it. An IV is usually started before arrival in the OR or by the surgeon immediately before the procedure. The circulating nurse is responsible for monitoring the IV.

Nursing interventions

Anxiety reduction. Although measures to reduce patient anxiety have already been taken (*see* Chapter 9), the OR nurse must nevertheless assess their effectiveness and reinforce and/or implement additional measures as indicated. An ideal time for this assessment occurs when the nurse greets the patient and makes a final check on the preoperative preparation.

When the patient has been taken into the OR and transferred to the operating table, the nurse should stay near the patient until anesthesia is administered, not only as a safety precaution but also to reduce anxiety. By holding the patient's hand or gently touching the arm or shoulder, the nurse communicates that a caring person is nearby.

Safety factors. Some safety factors have already been mentioned (e.g., the proper functioning of equipment and assistance with the administration of anesthesia). This section will focus on the factors that are frequently associated with physical safety.

Preparation and maintenance of a sterile operative area: This is essential to reducing the risk of infection. Each person in the OR during the procedure must have a good knowledge of sterile technique. The circulating nurse is generally considered responsible for carefully watching for any break in technique by any member of the surgical team and for taking appropriate action.

All OR personnel are expected to have a general knowledge of the fundamental principles of sterilization, as well as specific knowledge of any sterilizing equipment used in the OR. The OR nurse must also be aware of the various sterilization indicators that are used and must make sure that they are checked before he or she dispenses supplies considered sterile.

An approved surgical scrub, gowning, and gloving procedure must be properly carried out by all members of the scrub team before surgery.

Preparation of the operative site: The "prep" is done immediately before draping the patient and starting the surgical procedure. The purposes of the prep are to reduce the number of bacteria on the skin to a minimum and to leave an antimicrobial residual on the skin to prevent microbial growth during the procedure.

The prep is usually performed by the nurse or the surgeon's assistant. The nurse is usually responsible for setting up the prepping material. (Each institution, however, establishes its own procedures and OR routines.) Solutions for washing frequently contain hexachlorophene or have an iodine base. The choice of solution is generally determined by hospital policy, the preference of the surgeon, and any allergies that the patient may have. The following are general guidelines for prepping:

1. Prep the operative site and a wide surrounding area.
2. Cleanse outward from the operative site.
3. Use a new sponge when returning to the operative site.
4. Do not allow the prepping solution to pool under the patient and remain there during the operative procedure because this may be irritating to the skin and cause a reaction.
5. Dry the area carefully by placing a towel over the prepped area and patting it dry.
6. As the towel is removed, be sure to avoid contaminating the operative site with its edge.
7. For the final preparation ("painting"), use an antiseptic solution, generally an iodophor or one with an alcohol base.

Draping: Draping is a procedure that helps to isolate the incisional area from contamination. The surgical drapes used in different institutions will vary in material, quantity, and manner of application. Nevertheless, the following basic principles should be adhered to:

1. Drape the entire patient area, including the foot of the table, the arm boards, and the screen at the head of the table.
2. Use at least two layers of linen or a waterproof material. (A double amount should be used at the incision site.)
3. Protect sterile gloves with the sterile drapes.
4. Handle the drapes as little as possible.

5. Keep sterile drapes higher than waist level until they are put in place.
6. Never reach across the operating table (an unsterile area) to drape the opposite side; go around the table.
7. Leave the drape as placed, unless moving it away from (never *toward*) the incisional site.
8. Do not handle a drape that becomes contaminated; discard it without contaminating your gloves.

Anticipation of needs: This is an important nursing function in the OR. Quick, aseptic, and efficient provision of every item necessary for the procedure decreases anesthesia time and the amount of time that the sterile field and incisional area are open and susceptible to microbial contamination.

Sponge, needle, and instrument counts: The surgical team is responsible for taking all reasonable measures to prevent foreign objects from inadvertently being left in the patient. Although each institution has its own policy and procedure, the written policy usually includes what procedures require counts, what materials are to be counted, when counts are to be taken, and what documentation is required.

Positioning: The patient's position is determined by the operative procedure, the surgical approach preferred by the surgeon, and the patient's general condition, age, and size. (The anesthesiologist may make adjustments as necessary.) The time for positioning usually depends on the type of anesthesia used. Most patients receiving general or regional anesthesia are positioned after they are anesthetized, when the anesthesiologist states that the patient is ready to be moved. Patients receiving local anesthesia are usually positioned before the injection. Guidelines for determining an ideal position include good exposure and accessibility of the operative field, good access for the administration and observation of the effects of the anesthetic agents, the maintenance of adequate respiratory and circulatory functioning, and the absence of pressure on muscles and nerves.

The circulating nurse is usually responsible for positioning, or assisting with positioning, the patient. Therefore, the nurse must know the mechanics of the operating table and how to achieve a good operative position. The following are important points for the circulating nurse to remember when positioning a patient:

1. Do not move the anesthetized patient until the anesthesiologist indicates that it may be done.
2. Move the anesthetized patient gently and slowly.
3. Protect the patient from unnecessary exposure.
4. Avoid quick, jerky movements when removing the gown or sheet. (Lint and bacteria can be dispersed into the air and can then settle on the sterile field.)
5. Never place the arm board so that the angle of abduction is >90 degrees.

6. Pad the braces, headrest, straps, etc., to prevent pressure on nerves or blood vessels.
7. Make sure that the following items are available in the room when required for support: pillows, sandbags, rolled sheets, blankets, doughnuts, and tape.

After positioning has been completed, the nurse should make sure of the following factors:

1. No pressure points exist.
2. There is no constriction that will cause damage to nerves and blood vessels.
3. There is no interference with the proper functioning of tubing (e.g., IV or urinary drainage).
4. Supports or straps used to maintain the position are properly placed and secured.

Care of specimens.   Proper care and handling of operative specimens is essential to good patient care in the OR. Most patients undergoing surgery will need to have some type of specimen sent to the laboratory for examination. In some instances, the diagnosis and future treatment depend on the results of the pathology examination. Therefore, the nurse must be aware of what is required by hospital policy for the handling of specimens. The following are some general guidelines:

1. Label the specimen with the patient's name and hospital number, the date, surgeon's name, and type of specimen.
2. Preserve tissue specimens by placing them in a dry container (for immediate examination or frozen section) in an approved fixative solution and/or on ice.
3. Preserve cultures by placing them in a container without media or with approved media.
4. Record specimens on the patient's OR record sheet, in a specimen book, and in the OR log.

Dressings and transferring from the OR.   At the completion of surgery, the circulating nurse usually assists with the application of the dressing. The sterile dressing is applied and held in place by a member of the scrub team, drapes are then removed; and the circulating nurse checks to see that the surrounding area is clean and dry before tape or bandages are applied. If necessary, a clean gown is provided, and the patient is then covered before being moved to a stretcher or bed for transportation to the recovery room or directly to the unit.

Documentation.   Maintaining records is an important responsibility of the OR nurse. In order to ensure quality care, there must be proper and adequate documentation of the care provided to the patient during the intraoperative period. The circulating nurse should complete the OR record sheet and include all required information about the patient's condition for the use of the recovery room or unit nurses. Any other required records should also be completed.

DEVIATIONS

VOMITING AND/OR ASPIRATION

Vomiting can occur at any time and without warning in the anesthetized patient. Because general anesthesia causes depression or suppression of the gag reflex, measures to prevent aspiration are essential. Suctioning equipment must be available at the head of the OR table, and it should be ready for use as soon as the patient enters the OR. Nursing measures for a patient who is vomiting include assisting with suctioning, putting the OR table in Trendelenburg's position, and tilting the patient's head to the side or as directed by the anesthesiologist.

The possibility of vomiting is greatly reduced by the patient's being kept NPO for at least 6 to 8 hr before surgery. For elective procedures, the patient is routinely kept NPO after midnight. Emergency surgery is usually delayed, if possible, for 4 to 6 hr after the patient has had any food or fluids. If delay is impossible, measures are taken to empty the stomach, or a general anesthetic is not used.

LARYNGOSPASM

Laryngospasm, a sudden complete or incomplete contracture of the laryngeal muscle tissue, prevents adequate ventilation of the patient. The treatment consists of mask ventilation with sustained moderate pressure and IV administration of a muscle relaxant such as succinylcholine chloride. The nurse should be prepared to assist the anesthesiologist with the treatment.

HYPOVOLEMIC SHOCK

Hypovolemic shock is the most common type of shock encountered in the OR. A diminished blood volume leads to decreased filling pressure and, consequently, to decreased return and CO. The treatment consists of improving blood volume status by the administration of whole blood as soon as possible or by the use of plasma blood expanders or serum albumin until whole blood is available. The nurse should assist with obtaining, setting up, and administering these products as quickly as possible.

CARDIAC ARREST

Cardiac arrest (standstill or fibrillation) is a sudden and unexpected cessation of respirations and functional circulation. In patients undergoing surgery, it may occur because of blood loss and shock or as a reaction to anesthesia. CPR should be instituted immediately according to established hospital policy. All OR personnel should participate in an annual review of this procedure.

MALIGNANT HYPERTHERMIA

Malignant hyperthermia (hyperpyrexia) is a syndrome that occurs in apparently healthy children or young adults. The incidence is estimated to be from 1 in 50,000 to 1 in 100,000, with a mortality rate of 30 to 40%. This condition is associated with a hereditary predisposition, muscle relaxants such as succinylcholine, and inhalation anesthetic agents such as halothane or enflurane. Patients must be questioned carefully about anesthetic problems that they or their relatives have had. Although the etiology is still unknown, it is generally agreed that the previously mentioned agents trigger the release of calcium via defective calcium-storing mechanisms of the muscle cells. Heat is then liberated by other chemical changes, which account for the sudden rise in temperature. Early recognition of the *signs and symptoms* of malignant hyperthermia is critical to the patient's survival. Signs and symptoms include any or all of the following: tachycardia and/or arrhythmia, unstable BP, dark blood in the surgical field despite adequate inspired O_2, rapidly developing increase in body temperature (as high as 42.2°C [108°F], skeletal muscle rigidity, cyanotic mottling of the skin, metabolic and respiratory acidosis, hyperkalemia, and hypercapnia.

Common interventions

Immediate therapy must be initiated:

1. Stop anesthesia,   muscle relaxants, and surgery immediately. Change any equipment (e.g., IV tubing and anesthesia masks, tubing, or machine) that might have been in contact with the causative agent.
2. Hyperventilate the patient with 100% O_2.
3. Initiate cooling (administer IV iced saline solution rapidly; provide surface cooling with ice and/or hypothermia blanket; and lavage the stomach, rectum, and peritoneal cavities with iced saline solution).
4. Administer dantrolene sodium (Dantrium) by rapid IV infusion.
5. Administer procainamide hydrochloride (Pronestyl) if required for arrhythmias, either by drip or in bolus form.
6. Secure monitoring lines: ECG, temperature, Foley catheter, arterial pressure, and central venous pressure.
7. Monitor ECG, temperature, urinary output, arterial pressure, blood gases, central venous pressure, and electrolytes (potassium and sodium).
8. Administer sodium bicarbonate for acidosis.
9. Maintain urinary output of $\geq$ 2 ml/kg/hr; administer mannitol and furosemide, as ordered by the physician.

10. Maintain serum potassium within normal range:
    a. If high, correct with 10 to 30 U of insulin and 50 ml of 50% glucose.
    b. If low, correct with appropriate potassium chloride infusion.
11. Monitor the patient until the danger of a subsequent episode has passed.

All OR nurses must be aware of the signs, symptoms, and treatment of this crisis situation and must be prepared to act quickly. An annual review of malignant hyperthermia protocol is advisable.

Evaluation criteria

Before surgery.   The OR is clean and free from dirt and dust. Necessary equipment, in proper working order, is available in the room. Sterilization indicators have been checked before an article is considered sterile. The sterile team has carried out the approved scrub, gowning, and gloving procedures. Sterile instrument tables, with all necessary instruments, have been set up. The patient's preoperative work-up is complete and checked. The patient is anesthetized without complication, and positioned, prepped, and draped properly.

During surgery.   The patient is observed for any complication of surgery or anesthesia. Sterile supplies are delivered to the sterile field as needed and without any unnecessary delay. The sterile field has been maintained. Sponge, needle, and instrument counts are correct, and specimens have been properly handled.

After surgery.   The dressing is applied. The patient is cleaned (new gown if necessary), covered, and transferred safely from the OR table to the stretcher or bed. All necessary documentation has been completed. The patient is transported to the recovery room or returned directly to the unit.

CHAPTER 11

POSTOPERATIVE NEEDS

Brenda Salakka Zinamon

OVERVIEW

The postoperative period encompasses the time from admission to the Recovery Room (RR), ICU, or direct return from the OR to the clinical unit until normal body functioning has returned. The focus of the postoperative period is to return the patient to normal functioning and to prevent or minimize postoperative discomforts and complications.

The patient's destination (RR, ICU, or direct return to the unit) is determined by the kind of anesthetic used, the nature of the surgery, the condition of the patient, the expected postoperative course, and whether the RR is open 24 hr/day. Patients who have had local anesthesia or have an infected (contaminated or "dirty") wound are usually returned directly to the hospital unit where the staff is responsible for the postanesthesia assessment and intervention.

RECOVERY ROOM

General assessment

The patient is brought to the RR by the anesthesiologist or nurse anesthetist. The RR nurse should tell the patient that the operation is over, address the patient by name to help orient him to person, and begin baseline assessments immediately. Priorities include assessment and care of airway, breathing, circulatory status, level of consciousness, operative site, drains and other tubes, fluid and electrolyte balance, and safety. These priorities and methods of assessment are listed in Table 11-1. Assessment data are recorded along with the time of admission to the RR.

After these immediate needs have been assessed, the nurse should receive a report from the surgeon or anesthesiologist. Pertinent information includes condition of the patient; type, details, and findings of surgery; significant preoperative history (e.g., seizures, arrhythmias); specific drugs used preoperatively or during surgery (e.g., steroids, insulin); type of anesthetic agent, narcotic, muscle relaxant, and/or reversal agent used, and the patient's response to them; complications during surgery that might affect the postoperative course; estimated blood loss and replacement, any reaction, and last Hct value; IV fluid given during surgery and what to follow in RR; urine output during surgery (presence or absence of Foley catheter and whether clamped or unclamped); type and number of drains or catheters used and left in by surgeon; pressure readings of any specific

TABLE 11-1

Immediate Assessment in the Recovery Room

Parameter	Method
Airway	Check for adequate airway. Note absence or presence of prosthetic airway.
Breathing	Cup patient's chin in fingers with palm over nose. Count respiratory rate and depth. Note quality of oxygen exchange. Assess chest expansion.
Circulation	Assess and note BP; pulse rate, volume, and regularity; temperature; and skin color. Check capillary filling in finger and toenails for tissue perfusion. Check apical pulse for 1 full min, especially on elderly patients or patients taking cardiac medications. Check peripheral pulses when patient has had vascular surgery.
Level of consciousness	Assess and note response to stimuli, light, touch, his name, or a command. Assess if patient is moving voluntarily or making audible or intelligible sounds.
Operative site	Check operative site for amount, color, odor, and consistency of any wound drainage. Check bed linens for any bloody drainage.
Drains and other tubes	Assess if patient has drainage tubes in place and whether these are patent and draining (e.g., catheters, chest tubes, etc.). Check that monitoring parameters (e.g., central venous pressure, arterial lines) are functioning properly.
Fluid and electrolyte balance	Check and record all types of IV solution used. Check IV for patency and drip rate, and regulate prn. Record output accurately.
Safety	Prevent harm to patient by keeping side rails up, locking stretcher brakes, and remaining with patient.

monitoring equipment; and knowledge of the patient and family concerning the outcome of surgery. After the postoperative report has been received, frequent monitorings ($\sim$q 15 min) are made until the patient is stabilized. Normal and abnormal findings are listed in Table 11-2.

Common interventions

Oxygen. Adequate oxygenation is important in the postoperative patient to lessen the impact of vasoconstriction caused by hypothermic states in the OR and to promote adequate tissue perfusion and thus enhance wound repair. Adequate pain medication is necessary to facilitate proper coughing and deep breathing.

IV infusion. IV therapy is determined by the physician and is based on such factors as the patient's electrolyte status, amount and kind of fluids lost during surgery, and the patient's cardiopulmonary and renal status. IV fluid orders should include the type of fluid, the rate of administration, and any additives.

Common postoperative orders

1. Record vital signs and neurologic signs q 15 min $\times$ 8 or until stable, then q 30 min $\times$ 4, then q 1 to 4 hr. Notify the physician if BP is <90 to 100 or >150 to 160 systolic, or <50 or >90 diastolic; pulse is >120/min or <60/min; or temperature is >38.3°C (101°F).
2. Keep the patient NPO until he is fully alert and bowel sounds return. Then use ice chips as tolerated (unless contraindicated by surgery, e.g., bowel surgery).
3. Administer Demerol, 75 mg IM, q 3 to 4 hr prn for pain.
4. Administer Phenergan, 12.5 mg IM, prn for nausea and vomiting when vital signs are stable.
5. Give an IV solution and/or discontinue it when the patient is tolerating fluids.
6. Monitor input and output every shift for the first few days postoperatively.
7. Suction the oropharyngeal area prn.
8. Assist the patient to turn, cough, and deep breathe q 2 hr.
9. Notify the physician if the patient has not voided within 8 hr postoperatively or has a distended bladder.
10. Reinforce the dressing prn.
11. Note orders for tubes and catheters (e.g., suction, kind and amount; T-tube to gravity drainage).
12. Obtain Hct and electrolytes in the a.m.
13. Notify the physician of increased agitation and restlessness.

Additional orders are written for specific types of surgery (e.g., neurosurgery, elevate the head of the bed at all times; cataract surgery, have the patient lie on the unoperated side only) or for patients with specific health problems (e.g., diabetes: sugar, acetone, diacetic acid q 4 hr, etc.).

TABLE 11-2

Assessment Findings of the Postanesthesia Patient

Area of assessment	Findings	
	Normal	Abnormal
Airway	Clear, noiseless breathing.	Snoring sounds. No sound at all. Flaring nostrils. Crowing respirations. Stridor. Wheezing sounds. Moist, rattling sounds (indicative of secretions).
Breathing	Slow, deep, but regular. Effortless. Air moving through mouth or nose. Chest movement equal bilaterally. Chest movement painless.	Rapid, difficult. Shallow, quiet, slow. Shallow, difficult respirations with patient using neck and diaphragmatic muscle. Retractions at intercostal spaces and suprasternal notch. No air moving through mouth or nose. Chest movement unequal, unilateral, painful.
Circulation		
BP	Within normal range as determined by preoperative stable status.	Fall of systolic reading >20 mmHg. Systolic BP <80 mmHg. BP continuously dropping 5-10 mmHg over several readings.
Pulse	Slightly rapid immediately after surgery.	Bradycardia or tachycardia. Irregular, thready, or quivery pulse.
Apical pulse	Regular,	Irregular. Arrhythmias, particularly premature ventricular contractions.
Peripheral pulse	Palpable, regular,	Diminished or absent. Irregular,
Temperature	First 12 hr after surgery, possible hypothermia. First 24-48 hr after surgery, 37.7°C (99.8°F).	Elevated or subnormal.
Skin	Pink, warm, dry.	Cool, moist, clammy (shock). Dusky, pale. Blueness of nailbeds or lips (use inner lip for detection in dark-skinned persons). Flushed, warm face.

Level of consciousness	Normal sequence postanesthesia includes muscular irritability, restlessness and/or delirium, ability to recognize pain, ability to reason and control behavior. Initial drowsiness is followed by increased mental alertness.	Altered loss of consciousness due to shock will start by apprehensiveness, followed by confusion or mental clouding, and then listlessness.
Operative site	Dressing in place and dry or with small amount of slightly bloody drainage.	Bleeding or drainage that has soiled or saturated the dressing.
Drains	In place, patent. Drainage devices, if ordered, working properly.	Dislodged. Not patent. Not draining.
Fluid status	IV infusing as ordered. Urinary catheter draining ≥30 ml/hr. Ability to void within 8 hr. Jugular veins fill to anterior border of sternocleidomastoid muscle when patient is supine. Venous distension extends 3 cm above sternal angle when patient is at 45-degree angle. Pinched skin falls back to its normal position when released. In elderly patients, tongue turgor more reliable. Mucous membranes wet and moist. Normal skin turgor.	IV not infusing. Urine output <30 ml/hr (hypovolemia or renal failure). No urine output. Jugular veins flat when patient is supine (decreased plasma volume). Venous distension >3 cm indicates elevated venous pressure (fluid volume excess or CHF). Skin remains raised for many seconds (severe fluid volume deficit). Skin taut (edema). Longitudinal furrows (fluid volume deficit). Mucous membranes dry and sticky (hypernatremia). Edema (fluid volume excess).

Pain medications

Immediately after surgery, pain medications are withheld until each stage of anesthesia has been fully reversed. In the RR, pain medications are frequently administered IV by the anesthesiologist who specifically orders the drug and dose.

Nursing interventions

Vital signs. BP, pulse, and respirations are monitored q 15 min until stable, then q 4 hr for the first 48 hr postoperatively. Preoperative values should be used for base-line comparisons. Discrepancies in values indicate the need for more frequent monitoring and intervention. Abnormal findings (*see* Table 11-2) should be reported. A weak, thready pulse and decreased BP may indicate volume deficit and require increasing IV fluids; a full, bounding pulse and elevated BP may indicate volume overload and require decreasing IV fluids.

Respiratory changes may indicate the need for continued oxygen therapy, coughing and deep breathing, and/or position changes. Snoring may indicate partial airway obstruction. The patient's jaw should be pulled forward, or an oral airway (Fig. 11-1) should be inserted to prevent the tongue from occluding the pharyngeal area.

Temperature is usually monitored q 4 hr postoperatively. Warm blankets are used to treat hypothermia. Shaking chills can result from some anesthetic agents or may be related to fever. The onset and duration of a

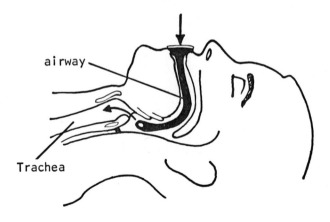

Figure 11-1.   Artificial airway. An airway functions by preventing the tongue from falling back to obstruct the patient's airway. *Adapted with permission from* Sutton, A. L. Bedside Nursing Techniques in Medicine and Surgery. W. B. Saunders Co., Philadelphia. 1969. p. 135.

chill should be noted and assessments made regarding skin color and temperature. (*See* Table 11-2 for abnormal skin color implication.) Comfort (warmth) and protection against injury against side rails, etc., should be provided. Rectal temperature should be taken during (if possible) and after a chill. Elevations should be reported immediately.

Level of consciousness. In general, it takes from 2 to 6 hr before postoperative patients have reacted from anesthesia or are able to respond to stimuli around them. Careful monitoring of the level of consciousness is important in order to detect signs of hypoxia, shock, or neurologic deficits postoperatively.

Positioning. Two positions that promote an adequate airway are Sims's position and semi-Fowler's with the head of the bed elevated 30 degrees. The semiconscious or unconscious patient must always be positioned with his head to the side and his chin extended forward in order to prevent airway obstruction by the tongue and decrease the chance of aspiration of mucus and/or vomitus. If these positions are contraindicated by surgery (e.g., cervical fusion) the nurse must observe for excessive oral secretions and suction the patient as necessary.

Environment. The nurse can provide a safe environment by constantly observing the patient, keeping side rails raised, keeping the bed in the low position (if adjustable), and locking stretcher brakes.

Psychologic care. Frequent orientation to the RR environment, reminders that surgery is over, and the nurse's presence and attention help to decrease the patient's anxiety. Simultaneously, the family needs to be informed of the patient's condition by the physician. The RR nurse should communicate the patient's progress to the staff on the unit.

Discharge from the RR

In most institutions, the anesthesiologist is responsible for discharging the patient from the RR. **Criteria** for discharge include stable vital signs; patient alert and oriented to person, place, and time after general anesthesia, or patient controls limbs after regional anesthesia; satisfactory respiratory status; and normal reflexes. The discharge **procedure** includes notifying the unit of the patient's status and impending return, summarizing the RR progress on the chart, and accompanying the patient to his room. On the unit, the RR assistant or nurse helps the staff in transferring the patient from the OR stretcher to the bed; positioning the patient safely (e.g., on his side, with side rails up, and bed in low position); placing a call bell within reach; and attaching drainage tubing.

RETURN TO UNIT

General assessment

When the postoperative patient is readmitted to the unit, the staff nurse's assessments include assessment of airway, circulation, level of consciousness, operative site, fluid status, GU status, GI status, kinds and patency of tubes (attachment to drainage), and complaints of pain (Table 11-3). This is a more complete assessment over time than is the RR general assessment (*see above*).

Common interventions

Postoperative orders are written by the surgeon to readmit the patient back to the floor. The postoperative orders would be the same as for the RR (*see above*).

Nursing interventions

The following interventions are important with the postoperative patient. (Table 11-3 shows typical findings of an uncomplicated postoperative patient on admission to the unit.)

1. Monitor level of consciousness q 4 hr. Monitor more frequently for patients with craniotomy, etc.
2. Monitor vital signs q 4 hr for the first 48 hr. Monitor more frequently if there is a change from base line. Notify the physician if temperature is elevated to >38.3°C (101°F), if pulse is >120/min or <60/min, or if BP is <90 to 100 or >150 to 160 systolic or <50 or >90 diastolic.
3. Assist the patient with coughing and deep breathing q 1 hr. Encourage the patient to use assistive devices (e.g., incentive spirometer, compressed pressurized nebulization). Assist the patient to splint his incision while coughing. Encourage the use of intercostal and abdominal muscles to prevent atelectasis.

TABLE 11-3
Typical Findings of an Uncomplicated Postoperative Patient on Admission to the Unit

Area of assessment	Observations
Respiratory	Respirations slow, deep, even at rate of 18-20/min.
Circulatory	Skin pink, warm, dry; BP within base-line range; apical pulse within base-line range; temperature 37.2°C (99°F).
Neurologic	Groggy conversation; gross muscular coordination intact.
Wound	Dressing dry and intact. No drainage.
Fluid status	IV infusing at 125 ml/hr. Elecrolytes within normal limits.
GU	No bladder distension.
GI	No nausea or bowel sounds. Abdomen soft, not distended.
Tubes (if present)	Drainage tube(s) patent and draining; connected to suction/gravity as ordered.

4. Assist the patient with positioning and turning q 2 hr. Position the patient on his side with a pillow at the back, knees flexed, and chin extended, when possible.

5. Monitor fluid and electrolyte status. Monitor IV rate and solution. Observe for signs of electrolyte imbalance (hyponatremia, hypokalemia), fluid overload, dehydration, and infiltration.

6. Monitor the dressing or operative site. Observe for proper functioning of drainage devices. Milk tubes prn and notify the physician if malfunctioning occurs. Observe the dressing. Is it intact? Dry? Note the amount, nature, etc., of any drainage.

7. Change the dressing. Have the physician perform the first postoperative dressing change. Maintain aseptic technique. Observe the condition of the wound/suture line for edema, induration, color, and skin tearing.

8. Use the following guidelines for various types of wound healing.
   a. For primary intention without drainage: remove the dressing and leave the wound exposed to air after the first 24 to 48 hr, protect the wound from trauma, and avoid tight clothing etc., over the suture line.
   b. For primary intention with drainage: keep the wound covered, note the extension of drainage, and soak the soiled dressing with saline before removing (to prevent removing healing dermis).
   c. For secondary intention or debridement: use gauze with large interstices to promote removal of necrotic tissue/debris with the dressing, and use wet-to-dry dressings as ordered.
   d. For secondary drainage sites with stab wounds: isolate secretions from the major wound to prevent deterioration of the wound, and change the dressing prn with care not to dislodge any drains.

9. Monitor for complications of wound healing.
   a. For infection: notify the physician, culture the wound, initiate isolation precautions, if drainage is present, and administer antibiotics, as ordered.
   b. For dehiscence (6 to 8 days postoperatively): return the patient to bed, cover/reinforce the suture line with dressing, notify the physician immediately, and remain with and calm the patient.
   c. For evisceration (6 to 8 days postoperatively): treat the patient as for dehiscence, and cover abdominal contents with sterile saline dressings.

10. Maintain patient safety by keeping the bed in a low position, raising side rails padded with pillows or blankets, changing the patient's position to a more comfortable one, maintaining proper body alignment, and obtaining an order for an analgesic, sedative, or restraints if necessary.

11. Keep the patient NPO until he has recovered from the effects of anesthesia (as indicated by alertness, presence of normal gag reflex,

and swallowing without difficulty) and until bowel activity is present. (Patients who have had spinal or other forms of regional anesthesia are generally allowed PO fluids when the reason for surgery does not contraindicate. For patients maintained NPO, administer mouth care.)

12. Provide pain relief. Differentiate incisional pain from that caused by a full bladder, faulty positioning, etc. Administer pain medication prn before such activities as coughing, deep breathing, and ambulation are begun. Administer fractional doses of pain medication for 8 to 12 hr when drugs such as droperidol (Inapsine) have been used intraoperatively. (Additional pain management is presented in Chapter 4.)

13. Ambulate early. Begin ambulation the evening of or the day after surgery to prevent complications of immobility (see Chapter 7). Instruct the patient to rise slowly, dangle, stand, then walk with assistance until balance and gait are steady. Increase the frequency of ambulation as tolerated.

14. Reinforce preoperative teaching and provide additional explanation to patient/family when emergency surgery has been performed.

15. Assist the patient/family to deal with psychologic factors related to stress of surgery, including fear of malignancy, isolation, lack of sleep, and pain.

16. Continuously assess pulmonary and respiratory status, circulatory status, level of consciousness, wound/operative site, pain management, and fluid and electrolyte status.

Evaluation criteria

The treatments and interventions have been effective if the following results are obtained. Vital signs are stable. Patient is alert and oriented. Airway is patent, and there is adequate coughing and deep breathing. Circulation is adequate as evidenced by the presence and quality of pulses, skin color, and temperature. Hydration is maintained. Wound is clear, and the dressing is dry and intact (or expected drainage). Pain is minimized or relieved. Drains and tubing are in place and patent. Normal GI and GU functioning returns. Environmental safety is maintained. Ambulation is effective. Absence or minimal signs of stress (patient and family). The patient and family verbalize postoperative regimen and follow-up. Absence or early detection and treatment of postoperative complications.

DEVIATIONS

Postoperative complications may involve single organs, organ systems, or all systems. The nurse should have a thorough knowledge of the status of each organ system preoperatively in order to assess postoperative complications. Careful monitoring of the postoperative patient is necessary to detect early signs of postoperative complications. In this section, various complications, their treatment, and nursing interventions to prevent them are discussed.

WOUND INFECTION

Infections are caused by beta-hemolytic streptococci or clostridia and can occur within hours after an operation. Later wound infections are caused by bacterial infections. Aerobic infections occur about the 5th postoperative day. Anaerobic infections occur about the 6th to 8th postoperative day. The incidence of infections is increased in individuals who are malnourished, alcoholic, have vascular insufficiency, and/or have impaired functioning of their immune system. Infections are caused by the presence of organisms, a lengthy exposure of the wound in the OR, and contamination during surgery and/or later in wound management. The organisms most commonly responsible for wound infections include staphylococci, streptococci, enteric bacilli, *Pseudomonas aeruginosa*, clostridia, and bacteroides.

The *signs and symptoms* of wound infection include redness, tenderness, and heat in the area of the wound/incision; wound drainage (purulent exudate); deep pain in the incision; fever (with aerobic infections, the patient's temperature spikes during the afternoon or evening and returns to normal by morning); elevated pulse; chills; malaise; drainage odor (aerobic, musty; anaerobic, acrid/putrid); and increased WBC in the presence of an erythematous wound.

Common interventions

General treatment involves culturing the wound, drainage, and other draining areas. A wound with identifiable zones of necrosis, infection, and inflammation should be cultured at several sites, not a single site only. Correct technique must be used in obtaining specimens for anaerobic culture, because these organisms are short-lived when exposed to oxygen. Treatment also involves irrigation of the wound with sterile normal saline, insertion of drains or suction tubing to remove waste products, administration of antibiotics as ordered based on culture findings, frequent vital signs (especially temperature), and a CBC.

Nursing interventions

1. Apply a nonocclusive dressing once the wound infection is identified.
2. Pack the wound as ordered to keep it open.
3. Change the dressing of an open wound to rid it of infectious material and to debride it.
4. Apply sterile saline to loosen the dressing, and avoid pulling newly formed tissue off with the dressing if healthy granulation tissue (deep pink) is present.
5. Keep the dressing dry if necrotic tissue develops, and remove it quickly so that debridement occurs.

6. Use strict aseptic technique to avoid further contamination.
7. Frequently change the dressing ($\geq$q 4 hr) if excessive drainage is present.

WOUND DEHISCENCE

Wound dehiscence is a partial or total splitting or separation of the wound edges that usually occurs 6 to 8 days postoperatively. Predisposing factors include malnutrition, elderly age, obesity, unusual strain on the abdominal wall from coughing and vomiting, infection secondary to faulty closure of the wound during surgery, midline abdominal incisions, and circulatory and pulmonary difficulties (e.g., hypovolemia, hypoxemia).

The *signs and symptoms* include patient complaints of "something suddenly giving away" in the wound; a gush of serosanguineous drainage (major symptom); and separation of the wound edges.

Nursing interventions

1. Report dehiscence *immediately* to the surgeon.
2. Alert another nurse or physician.
3. Remain with the patient.
4. Have the patient lie in bed.
5. Minimize anxiety.
6. Instruct the patient to bend his knees.
7. Check vital signs for any indication of shock.
8. Have IV, nasogastric tube, and suction ready.
9. Notify the OR that the patient is returning for resuturing of the wound.
10. Apply an abdominal binder for heavy/older patients or those with weak or pendulous abdominal walls.
11. Encourage proper nutrition with adequate amounts of protein and vitamin C.
12. Splint/support the incision during coughing and ambulation.

WOUND EVISCERATION

Wound evisceration, the protrusion of abdominal viscera through the abdominal incision, is a surgical emergency that occurs 6 to 8 days postoperatively. The etiology, signs and symptoms, and interventions are the same as for wound dehiscence, except that the extruded contents should be *immediately* covered with a sterile, moistened towel or gauze until the patient is returned to the OR.

RESPIRATORY

Pulmonary complications generally develop in the first 48 hr postoperatively. Atelectasis and pneumonia are the most common pulmonary complications. Risk factors include heavy smoking, preexisting respiratory problems (e.g., COPD, chronic emphysema, asthma, bronchitis), obesity, polycythemia, hypertension, prolonged general anesthesia, and thoracic, abdominal, and emergency operations. (*See* Chapter 14 for an in-depth discussion of atelectasis and pneumonia.)

CARDIOVASCULAR

The cardiovascular system is placed under great stress by surgery. Major cardiovascular postoperative complications include hemorrhage, shock, and clot formation: thrombophlebitis (*see* Chapter 15), and embolism (*see* Chapters 14, 15, 17, and 20). Factors predisposing the patient to cardiovascular complications include coronary artery disease (as evidenced by the history or preoperative ECG), elevated blood lipid levels, preoperative enlarged heart (on x-ray or clinical exam), preoperative cardiac arrhythmias (e.g., atrial fibrillation, which can lead to postoperative arterial emboli), hypertension, heavy use of nicotine, diabetes, obesity, preoperative pulse deficits in extremities, phlebitis, preoperative evidence of past venous disease, chronic arterial insufficiency (which predisposes the patient to venous stasis), presence of visceral malignancy, and prolonged surgery.

HEMORRHAGE

Hemorrhage is an abnormal internal or external discharge of blood. Primary hemorrhage occurs at the time of surgery. Intermediary hemorrhage occurs within the first few hours after surgery. Secondary hemorrhage occurs some time after surgery. Hemorrhage may be caused by slipping of a suture, a dislodged clot, wound evisceration, and hemostatic defects.

Bleeding is the cardinal *symptom* of hemorrhage. Bleeding at the capillary level is slow, general, and oozing. Bleeding at the venous level is dark and bubbles out. Bleeding at the arterial level is bright red and spurts. Other signs and symptoms include apprehension and restlessness, progressing to lethargy; cold, clammy skin; drop in BP; bounding or thready pulse; rapid and deep respirations; temperature drop; and decreased Hb.

Nursing interventions

1. Treat the patient as described for shock (*see below*).
2. Inspect the wound site for bleeding.
3. Apply a gauze pad as a pressure dressing to wounds where possible.
4. Administer blood (typed) or blood substitute as ordered until blood is available.
5. Ligate any bleeding vessel immediately prn. If superficial, the vessel could be cauterized.

SHOCK

Shock is the failure of the circulatory system to perfuse tissues, leading to tissue hypoxia and lactic acidosis. It usually occurs during the first few postoperative days. Table 11-4 lists the causes, *signs and symptoms,* and treatment modalities for the various kinds of shock.

Regardless of the cause of shock, the general effects are anoxia, anoxemia, altered temperature, oliguria, anuria, thrombosis with subsequent emboli due to blood stasis, increased pulse and respirations, and decreased BP. If observations indicate impending shock, help should be summoned and the physician notified immediately. Shock must first be evaluated and its cause determined before adequate and effective therapy can be carried out.

Nursing interventions

1. Keep the patient warm.
2. Keep the patient flat (especially after spinal anesthesia or head surgery) or raise the patient's legs above the level of the heart.
3. Prepare IV equipment, if not already in place.
4. Closely observe the patient's vital signs until he has recovered from shock.

VOMITING

Vomiting, the ejection of gastric contents through the mouth, results from an accumulation of fluid or food in the stomach before peristalsis returns. It is common in many postoperative patients immediately after surgery. Vomiting may be a side effect of anesthesia or of interference with peristalsis after manipulation of the GI tract.

Nursing interventions

1. Keep the patient NPO before surgery.
2. Keep the patient NPO until bowel sounds actively return (or if he is nauseated).
3. Assess distension.
4. Listen for bowel sounds.
5. Check for passage of flatus or bowel movement.
6. Medicate the patient with antiemetic prn.
7. Support the wound during retching and vomiting.
8. Position the patient on his side or prone to help prevent aspiration of vomitus.
9. Have suction apparatus available.
10. Suction oral cavity prn to keep vomited material out of the airway.
11. Save the specimen for examination.
12. Refresh the patient with mouthwash, clean linens, etc.
13. Note the amount and odor (ammonia, fetid, etc.) of vomitus.

14. Prepare the patient for nasogastric intubation.
15. Administer antiemetic medication as ordered.
16. Report excessive or prolonged vomiting.
17. Offer hot tea if tolerated.

PARALYTIC ILEUS

Paralytic ileus is a lack of or ineffective coordination of peristalsis. If its duration is >3 days, problems such as occult wound dehiscence or intra-abdominal sepsis may arise. Paralytic ileus follows most major surgical procedures, especially intestinal operations. Temporary ileus may be caused by a reaction to the anesthesia, trauma, or abdominal operations. Prolonged ileus may be caused by electrolyte imbalance, wound infection, or metabolic diseases.

The *signs and symptoms* of paralytic ileus are absence of peristalsis, gastric and bowel distension, vomiting, absent or high-pitched bowel sounds, and hyperactive bowel sounds on abdominal percussion.

Nursing interventions

1. Keep the patient NPO.
2. Attach an intestinal tube to suction.
3. Monitor the GI tube function, drainage, etc.
4. Monitor IV fluids and hydration status.
5. Assess the abdomen for bowel sounds, flatus, bowel movement, and decreased distension.
6. Check the wound frequently for signs of dehiscence or deep sepsis.
7. Check for elevated temperature and WBC with the presence of persistent ileus for intra-abdominal sepsis.
8. Use colon lavage as ordered.

CONSTIPATION

Constipation is the retention of fecal material, delay in excretion, or deviation from usual elimination habits. Constipation most frequently occurs after abdominal surgery and/or with immobility. It may be caused by limitation of PO fluids, dehydration (encourages absorption of fluid from colonic contents and results in desiccated stools), incisional pain, immobility, opiates and antacids containing calcium or aluminum, some narcotic analgesics (e.g., codeine), attempts to defecate on bedpan, and lack of privacy.

The *signs and symptoms* of constipation are complaints of abdominal distension, cramping pain, and the sensation of pain in the rectum. Fecal impaction, a *complication* of constipation, may be evidenced by frequent passage of small amounts of liquid stool around a mass of feces in the rectum, the absence of a bowel movement within the usual habit time, a hard stool with painful defecation, or severe rectal pain.

TABLE 11-4

Postoperative Shock: Differentiation of Causes, Signs and Symptoms, and Treatment

Type	Causes	Signs and symptoms	Treatment
Hypovolemic	Reduction in intravascular volume relative to patient's vascular capacity.	Decreased BP. Elevated HR. Thready pulse. Increased respiratory rate. Decreased level of consciousness. Cool, moist skin. Decreased temperature.	Raise legs to increase venous return of pooled blood from extremities to the heart. Speed up IV infusion to further increase blood volume. Carefully record fluid volume replacement to avoid fluid overload. Administer O_2 to facilitate adequate oxygenation of cells. Notify physician for administration of proper medication (e.g., vasoconstrictors, steroids, antibiotics, or bicarbonate). Monitor VS q 15 min. Record I and O. Stay with patient to assess and decrease anxiety.
Septic (most common cause of postoperative shock)	A change in capillary endothelium, permitting loss of blood and plasma through capillary walls into surrounding tissues. *Causes:* Gram-negative septicemia (most common). *Predisposing factors:* Diabetes mellitus, hematologic diseases, corticosteroid therapy, immunosuppressive drugs, and radiation therapy.	Apprehension, confusion, and restlessness (early symptoms). Warm skin. High fever. Pulses full initially, later vasoconstriction. Urine output normal at first, then slows rapidly. Hyperventilation. Pulmonary hypertension.	Administer balanced salt solution for volume replacement. Administer massive doses of antibiotics IV. Drain abscess/other source of infection. Start corticosteroids (physician preference due to deleterious effects). Support additional failing body systems. Implement additional measures cited under hypovolemic shock.

	Precipitating events: Often, operations on urinary, biliary, or gynecologic systems.	
Cardiogenic	Failure of heart to pump adequately (e.g., MI, cardiac tamponade, pulmonary edema, or arrhythmias and arrest).	First sign: fast pulse rate (>110). Diminished urine output (<20 ml/hr). Impaired mental functioning. Cool, moist, pallid skin. Systolic BP drops to ≤90, or if patient is hypertensive, 30 mmHg below patient's own norm. Decreased/absent peripheral pulses. On auscultation, ventricular diastolic gallop and S_3. Jugular venous distension. Elevated CVP,	1. Mild left ventricular failure: Administer O_2 and PO diuretics. Limit salt intake. 2. Severe left ventricular failure: Monitor arterial pressure, pulmonary wedge pressures, and CO. Administer pressor agents (e.g., norepinephrine, dopamine, or dobutamine). Maintain 5% DW IV with a microdrip. Insert urinary catheter and monitor hourly urine output. Monitor VS q 15 min. Monitor blood levels of PO_2, PCO_2, and Hct. Monitor cardiovascular parameters and lung sounds to detect signs of impending cardiac failure (e.g., increasing CVP, distended neck veins, and pulmonary rales).

CVP, central venous pressure; HR, heart rate; I and O, input and output; S_3, third heart sound; VS, vital signs,

Nursing interventions

1. Ambulate the patient early to aid in promoting peristalsis.
2. Maintain adequate fluid intake to keep the stools soft.
3. Maintain proper diet to promote peristalsis.
4. Provide privacy when the patient is using the toilet/commode.
5. Administer a stool softener.
6. Administer bulk agent added to diet, as ordered, as soon as the patient can eat.
7. Perform a digital rectal examination to detect fecal impaction. Extract digitally or give oil-retention enema as ordered.
8. Avoid laxatives in patients with recent colonic anastomosis. Never give laxatives until a rectal examination has been done to exclude impaction.
9. Administer laxatives and/or enemas as ordered.
10. Continue to implement preventive measures.

ACUTE STRESS ULCER

Acute stress ulcer is sudden and massive GI bleeding that can follow any major operation, particularly in a septic or toxic patient. Acute stress ulcers occur one to several days postoperatively with no warning and usually follow major trauma, sepsis, and massive burns.

Early *signs and symptoms* of acute stress ulcer include pallor, restlessness, tachycardia, and tachypnea. If the ulcer worsens, the patient will vomit large amounts of bright red blood and rapidly go into shock.

Nursing interventions

1. Minimize stress and/or its reactions.
2. Administer antacids and inhibitors of gastric acid secretions.
3. Monitor the patient closely.
4. Refer to treatment of shock and hemorrhage (*see above*).
5. Prepare the patient for nasogastric intubation with iced saline irrigation.
6. Prepare the patient for blood transfusion.
7. Monitor for shock.
8. Administer antacid and drugs to inhibit gastric acid secretions as ordered.
9. Prepare the patient for surgery, if he is unresponsive to medical treatment.

[The two most common postoperative urinary complications are retention and renal failure. *See* Chapter 17 for an in-depth discussion of these problems.]

CHAPTER 12

ALTERED INTEGUMENTARY FUNCTIONING

Phyllis Lisanti

OVERVIEW

Skin, the largest organ of the human body, is a barrier between the internal organs and the external environment. It is composed of tissue that grows and renews itself continuously.

As the most readily accessible body system, the skin is a sensitive indicator of various physical and emotional states. Adequate nutrition and fluid status are indicated by skin that is smooth, even in color, elastic, and slightly moist. Healthy feelings toward oneself are often reflected in good personal hygiene and skin care. Poor nutrition and fluid status are indicated by skin that is dry and lacking in turgor. In addition, poor personal hygiene is readily detected by the condition of the skin, which may be an indication of personal values or a depressed mental state.

Many kinds of skin alterations are called lesions and may be classified as primary and secondary lesions. Primary lesions, which may initially appear from previously normal skin, include macules, papules, nodules, wheals, vesicles, and pustules. Secondary lesions result from modifications in primary lesions and include plaques, scales, crusts, erosions, ulcers, and fissures. Definitions of these lesions are listed in Table 12-1.

Anatomy and physiology review

The skin serves as a sense organ for temperature, pain, and touch; acts as a barrier to prevent loss of body fluids and electrolytes; and acts as a barrier

TABLE 12-1

Primary and Secondary Skin Lesions

Lesion	Definition
Primary	
Macule	A flat, nonpalpable, circumscribed change in skin color (e.g., freckle).
Papule	A solid, elevated, palpable area, usually ≤0.5 cm in diameter.
Nodule	A small, solid, palpable mass (usally firmer than a papule) that may be located in the dermis or subcutaneous tissue.
Wheal	A firm elevated, irregular, superficial, usually short-lived area of localized skin edema (e.g., hive, mosquito bite).
Vesicle	An elevated, circumscribed lesion filled with serous fluid, usually ≤0.5 cm (e.g., blister).
Pustule	An elevated, circumscribed lesion (vesicle) filled with purulent material.
Secondary	
Plaque	A raised but flat, solid lesion formed from papules or nodules, usually >1 cm.
Scale	A thin flake of dry epidermis (e.g., dry skin).
Crust	A covering formed from the dried remains of serum, pus, or blood.
Erosion	A circumscribed area where there is loss of the epidermis. The area is usually moist but does not bleed or drain.
Ulcer	A deep loss of skin surface that may bleed, drain, or develop scar tissue (e.g., decubitus).
Fissure	A linear crack in the skin that extends into the dermis (e.g., athlete's foot).

to protect the internal environment from injurious elements in the external environment. The skin consists of the epidermis, the dermis, and subcutaneous tissue (Fig. 12-1).

The outermost layer of the skin, the **epidermis**, is thin, avascular, and divided into the horny and the inner layers. The horny layer is composed mostly of keratin. The inner layer is where melanin and keratin are formed. Keratin is the major component of hair and nails, and melanin is the pigment that provides color to the hair and skin. The inner layer relies on the dermis for nutrition. The **dermis** is highly vascular, tough, connective tissue; contains nerves, lymphatics, sebaceous glands, and hair follicles; and merges with the lower level subcutaneous tissue. **Subcutaneous tissue** stores fat for temperature regulation and contains the remainder of the hair follicles and the sweat glands.

At this point in man's evolution, **hair** and **nails** mainly have a cosmetic function. There are two kinds of sweat glands: eccrine and apocrine.

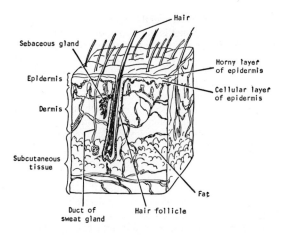

Figure 12-1. Anatomy of the skin. *Reprinted with permission from* Bates, B. A Guide to Physical Examination. J. B. Lippincott Co., Philadelphia. 1979. Second edition. p. 43.

Eccrine glands cool the body by producing sweat, which eventually evaporates. **Apocrine glands** are located in axillary and genital areas, secrete sweat that provides the characteristic body odor, and are stimulated by emotional stress. **Sebaceous glands** secrete sebum (released through the hair follicles), which is a fatty substance that has a protective lubricating effect on the outer layer of the epidermis.

Bacteria are normally present on the surface of the skin and serve a protective function. The resident bacteria serve to prevent excessive growth of fungi on the skin.

Variations in skin **pigmentation** and texture and hair characteristics will be observed in the elderly, dark-skinned, and black patient. The elderly may demonstrate various changes that are considered normal and age related: (1) a tendency to increased freckling or patches of hypopigmentation; (2) thinner and less elastic skin, with a tendency toward dryness, flaking, and scaling; (3) increased wrinkle patterns, especially in sun-exposed areas; (4) a decrease in body and scalp hair, with a tendency to greying. In addition, there is increased growth of facial hair in women, and coarse hair growth in the ears, nose, and eyebrows in men.

Skin color changes are more difficult to assess in the dark-skinned or black individual. Healthy dark skin has a red undertone that is readily recognizable. Color should be assessed in the sclera, conjunctiva, buccal mucosa, tongue, lips, nail beds, palms, and soles. The oral mucosa of the black patient may have freckling in the gums, lining of the cheeks, and borders of the tongue. Pallor and cyanosis may be observed by examining the buccal mucosa and palpebral conjunctiva of the eye. In addition, certain skin conditions occur more frequently in black people: A **keloid** is a raised, firm, thickened, red scar that is out of proportion for the amount of scar tissue needed for repair and healing. **Vitiligo,** common to all people, is especially distressing to dark-skinned people because of its greater visibility. Vitiligo presents as areas of hypopigmentation surrounded by normally pigmented skin. **Pseudofolliculitis** may occur as a result of shaving. An inflammatory reaction occurs when the cut hairs emerging from the curved follicle become embedded in the skin. Hair problems or traction **alopecia** may develop related to hair trauma frequently encountered in the tightly pinned or elaborate corn-row hairstyles. Pick combing and hot combing can also produce hair damage.

General assessment

A general assessment of the skin requires the collection of a thorough history, careful inspection and palpation of the skin over the entire body, and information from various procedures performed on the skin.

A thorough **health history** should include information regarding skin care habits (facial and hair care, fingernails and toenails, and body care); any past history of skin disorders (family history of skin disorders); allergies with skin response (family history of allergies); skin response to emotional situations; and the present skin problem (onset, duration, characteristics, and predisposing factors). Characteristics to be asked about include color; the presence of redness, heat, pain, burning, itching, swelling, tenderness, and tingling; the area of involvement (size and location); the type of lesion (primary or secondary); and the distribution of the lesion (linear, angular, or unilateral). The nurse should also note whether the predisposing factors are occupational, environmental, geographical, seasonal, emotional, or situational in nature, or whether they are caused by foods or medications. The relieving and aggravating factors, treatment (present, past, home remedies), and psychosocial effect of the skin disorder (coping mechanism, effect on self-image, effect on life-style/job, and emotional response to the disorder) should also be noted.

During the **physical examination** of the skin, the patient must be fully undressed and the examiner must have good lighting. The observation of the skin begins with a general survey and continues throughout the entire physical exam. All skinfolds, the bottom of the feet, and areas between toes must be carefully examined. The skin is assessed through inspection and palpation with notation of color, vascularity (evidence of bruising and bleeding), lesions (color, type, grouping, distribution), edema, moisture (dryness, oiliness, perspiration), temperature, texture, thickness, mobility, and turgor. Inspection and palpation of the fingernails and toenails include notation of color, shape, lesions, configuration, consistency, and adherence to nail bed. Inspection and palpation of the scalp and hair focus on surface characteristics, nodules, color, texture, quantity, distribution, configuration, and the presence of parasites.

The Wood's light and diascope are two tools used to further assess the skin. The **Wood's light** is a lamp designed to transmit only long-wave ultraviolet wavelengths. These wavelengths cause specific substances to emit fluorescence and make possible the determination of some fungal and bacterial infections. **Diascopy** is a procedure in which a diascope or translucent object is used to apply pressure on the skin to ascertain noncongestive skin changes.

Common interventions

General interventions for the treatment of skin conditions include surgery and curettage, cryosurgery, ultraviolet therapy, and x-ray therapy. Therapies used in dermatologic conditions are aimed at cleansing the skin (removing debris and preventing infection), reducing inflammation, relieving dryness and itching, deodorizing, and protecting the skin by lubricating, retarding fluid loss, or decreasing friction.

Specific therapies include wet dressings and compresses, baths, and topical and systemic medications. **Wet dressings** and/or **wet compresses** are used to cleanse the skin, reduce inflammation, and maintain drainage. Commonly used solutions/preparations include cool tap water, normal saline, Burow's solution, and potassium permanganate solution. The clinician should be careful to avoid burns and maceration of the patient's skin. When a large area of the body is affected, **baths** are used to cleanse the skin and reduce inflammation and itching. Commonly used solutions include water, normal saline, colloids (Aveeno), medicated tar (various coal tar preparations), corn starch, and bath oil (Lubriderm, Alpha Keri). The clinician should avoid leaving the elderly individual unattended for prolonged baths because the elderly are prone to dizziness due to age-related changes in the neurovascular reflexes. The clinician should also monitor the water temperature carefully in order to avoid burns or chilling, and ensure patient safety from slipping by using hand-rails or non-skid strips in the tub. **Topical medications** are used to deliver a specific medication, lubricate, cool, protect, retard water loss, and/or decrease inflammation. Commonly used preparations include lotions (calamine, etc.), ointments and creams (petroleum jelly, lanolin, corticosteroids, etc.), and powders. Ointments and pastes are not suitable for use on hairy or oozing surfaces. Topical steroid preparations are relatively safe in that little of the drug is likely to be absorbed and cushingoid-type steroid toxicity rarely occurs. **Systemic medications** for skin disorders include adrenocorticosteroids, analgesics, antibiotics, sedatives, antifungals, etc. The reader should refer to a pharmacology text for specific details regarding dosage and precautions for systemic drugs.

Nursing interventions

Nursing support is ongoing, may be long-term, and requires understanding, patience, and encouragement by the nurse.

Dry skin, which is a contributing factor to special skin care problems, is caused by loss of water. Those with fair skin and advanced age are predisposed to dry skin. Other factors contributing to the problem include excessive bathing, exposure to ultraviolet light, swimming, excessive use of strong soaps, and long exposure to low humidity. *Physical* nursing interventions include the following actions:

1. Limit bathing to once per week in winter and twice per week in summer.
2. Provide humidification.
3. Apply lubricating creams or lotions.
4. Avoid excessive exposure to sun.

Pruritus, an unpleasant cutaneous sensation that produces the desire to scratch, is a prevalent problem among individuals with skin disorders. *Physical* nursing interventions include the following:

1. Maintain a cool environment.
2. Provide diversionary activities.
3. Alleviate anxiety and stress.
4. Avoid trauma to skin by clipping nails short.
5. Administer treatments, baths, compresses, or soaks as prescribed.
6. Apply antipruritic lotions, creams, or ointments as prescribed.
7. Administer antipruritic medications as prescribed.
8. Administer tranquilizers or sedatives as prescribed.
9. Continue assessment of itching and the success of measures to alleviate.

Society places much value on unblemished skin. The skin is an important part of the self-image and the image presented to the world. The relevant **psychologic** considerations that the health team must be aware of for the individual with a skin disorder include general attitudes toward people with skin disorders (prejudice of others, and the patient's perception of the disorder), the attitude of the health team (listening, talking, touching, observing, respect, concern, and patience), and the skin's response to emotions (physiologic response of the skin to emotional stress). *Psychosocial* nursing interventions include the following:

1. Maintain an open mind about the individual's behavior.
2. Encourage and support compliance with the therapeutic regimen.
3. Provide an accepting and empathetic attitude.
4. Provide and promote all measures to relieve anxiety and reduce stress (e.g., a room that is cool with proper humidity, sufficient bedcovers, maintain usual sleep patterns, provide television and reading materials, etc.).
5. Provide adequate staffing to support the patient if disfigurement is a problem and if the patient seeks isolation.
6. Provide a therapeutic milieu.
7. Refer the patient for group therapy or psychiatric counseling.
8. Advise the use of cosmetics, if appropriate.

Effective **education** of the patient with a skin disorder requires that the nurse carefully assess and realistically deal with the patient's needs.

1. Teach the patient about the skin disorder.
2. In detail, clearly teach the treatment and medication regimen.
3. Explain the rationale for treatments, medications, and any special procedures.
4. Foster independence and participation in the plan of care.
5. Explain the time frame and expected results for the treatment.
6. Instruct the patient to refrain from self-medication.
7. Encourage and promote maximum self-care.

Evaluation criteria

The patient's anxiety and stress are minimized. The patient's itching is alleviated. The skin lesions are diminished or absent. The patient and/or significant others demonstrate knowledge of the condition and the ability to give treatments and take medications. The patient demonstrates maximal self-care. No infection, scar formation, or other sequelae occur. Vital signs remain within normal range. Cross-contamination and infection are prevented. Recurrence of problem is minimized or eliminated.

DEVIATIONS

BURNS

A burn is tissue injury resulting from excessive exposure to thermal, chemical, electric, or radioactive agents. Complete worldwide statistics on the incidence of burns are unavailable. In the USA, burns rank as the 3rd leading cause of accidental deaths.

Burns may be caused by heat from flames, hot liquids, hot surfaces, electrical current, chemicals, or radiation. Predisposing factors include age (very young and elderly), poverty, and substance abusers (individuals who smoke, drink, and/or use drugs).

Burn assessment requires information about age, past medical history, cause of the burn, part of the body burned, size of the burn, and depth of the burn. The **age** of the patient is important to determine severity and outcome. The very young and the elderly (<2 and >60 yr) have a higher mortality. A **past medical history** is needed to determine allergies, drug or alcohol addiction, and the presence of chronic diseases such as cardiovascular, renal, pulmonary, metabolic, or neurologic. These factors all place the patient at greater risk. Determining the **cause** of the burn is necessary because some types of burns require different initial care and continuing observation. The part of the body (**area**) is important when considering mortality and complications (e.g., burns of the perineum are especially prone to infection from contamination by urine and feces). Determining the **size** of the burn is necessary in the overall plan of care required. Burn size may be determined by the rule of nines or Berkow's method. The **depth** is usually classified at first, second, third, or fourth degree, depending on the skin layers involved in the injury.

A **first-degree** (partial thickness) burn involves the epidermis only, and is usually a minor trauma. If the patient is an infant or elderly, medical assistance may be required. First-degree burns are caused by sunburn, hot objects, and scalding. The *signs and symptoms* include skin that is pink or red in color, pain on touch, blanching with pressure, sensitivity to temperature change, and the presence of some edema and blisters. The prognosis is good, although infection may develop. The clinician should apply cold water to stop the burning process and apply a dry dressing if needed.

A **second-degree** (partial thickness) burn involves the epidermis and part of the dermis. It is caused by deep sunburn, flash fire, and scalding liquids. The *signs and symptoms* include extreme pain, pink to red-colored skin, large blisters, surface moisture (fluid loss), and firmness at the burned area. Second-degree burns normally heal within 10 to 21 days. *Complications* include scarring and infection. The clinician should cool the burn with cold water immersion, administer analgesia for pain, not disturb or rupture blisters, cover the area with a clean or sterile dressing, and seek medical treatment.

A **third-degree** (full-thickness) burn involves the epidermis and the dermis. It is caused by flame, ignited clothing, immersion in scalding water or liquid, electricity, and chemicals. The *signs and symptoms* include waxy white and/or red to brown color at the burned area; no pain at the site, but pain around the area; no blanching; and a leathery, dry, and hard area with pronounced subcutaneous edema. An eschar normally develops, and large areas require grafting. Infection, loss of mobility, and scarring are associated *complications*. The clinician should not disturb charring or clothing, and provide immediate medical care.

Fourth-degree burns cause deep destruction to fascia, muscles, and bones. They are caused by prolonged contact with a flame or an electric or chemical source. The *signs and symptoms* of fourth-degree burns are charring, absence of pain, and possible lack of pressure sensation. They require grafting and may necessitate amputation. Infection, scarring, and loss of mobility are related *complications*. The clinician should provide emergency measures (e.g., CPR) and emergency medical care.

Common interventions

Emergency treatments and priorities of burn care include providing ongoing emotional support, stopping the burning process (cold water immersion), establishing and maintaining a patent airway (an endotracheal tube or tracheostomy may be necessary; oxygen, humidification, and ventilatory assistance may also be required), meeting fluid needs (establishing an IV route with a large-bore needle), and providing wound care. The various methods of caring for the wound are all aimed at maintaining a stable general condition, preventing infection, and promoting healing.

Some of these methods include exposure to air with daily cleansing, hydrotherapy, occlusive dry dressings, wet dressings, and topical anti-microbials. Grafting is necessary in full-thickness wounds. The four basic types of grafts are as follows: **autografts**, which are obtained from the patient's own body; **isografts**, which are histocompatible tissue obtained from an identical twin; **allografts**, which are disease-free tissue obtained from bodies of living or dead individuals; and **zenografts**, which are from animal sources or man-made substances.

Nursing interventions

Physical 1. Maintain isolation.
2. Monitor IV therapy (to prevent and treat shock).
3. Administer pain medication as ordered.
4. Maintain the patient NPO as ordered, monitor the nasogastric tube, and meet nutritional needs.
5. Insert a Foley catheter and monitor intake and output carefully.
6. Weigh the patient.
7. Administer prophylactic tetanus toxoid.
8. Obtain specimens and wound cultures.
9. Administer antibiotics as prescribed.
10. Monitor vital signs as indicated.
11. Administer O_2.
12. Provide wound care as prescribed.
13. Prevent complications.
Psychosocial 14. Provide emotional support.
15. Accept the patient's behavior without judgment.
16. Communicate genuine caring and concern.
17. Encourage the expression of feelings: stress, anxiety, grief, anger, guilt, etc.
18. Prepare for discharge (develop a plan with the family and educate the family).
19. Provide for follow-up care.
20. Contact available community resources.
Educational 21. Teach the patient about skin care, wound care, prescribed exercises, use of elastic garments and splints, care of blisters, skin discoloration, and itching and flaking of skin.
Prevention 22. Educate the patient and family about all preventive measures, such as using care with cigarettes, wearing fire-retardant clothing, avoiding alcohol use and smoking, making stoves child-proof, using self-closing extension cords, and avoiding the use of space heaters.

Evaluation criteria. *See* Overview. Intake and output within normal limits. Patient receives adequate nutrition (weight becomes stable). Patient communicates and expresses feelings freely. Patient returns for follow-up care.

[For a discussion of wound dehiscence and evisceration, see Chapter 11.]

SEBORRHEA

Seborrhea is a functional disorder of the sebaceous glands marked by an increase in the amount and an alteration in the quality of the sebaceous secretion. Seborrheic dermatitis is a commonly occurring chronic inflammatory disorder of the skin with a tendency to lifelong recurrences. It occurs more frequently in areas that are well supplied with sebaceous glands or in skinfold areas where bacterial count may be high. The cause of this disorder is unknown. A constitutional predisposition exists for some individuals throughout postpubertal life. Emotional and physical stress may precipitate recurrences.

Symptoms of seborrheic lesions vary from fine, dry, yellowish scales with erythema of the skin to yellowish, greasy patches that include macules and scaly papules with a typical yellowish color. Seborrhea starts on the scalp and may extend to the eyebrows, ears, nasolabial area, chest, axillae, and inguinal/scrotal area. Seborrhea is a condition of the skin, rather than a disease. Consequently, various diseases must be ruled out (e.g., psoriasis, neurodermatitis, tinea capitis, atopic eczema, SLE and discoid lupus erythematosus, tinea corporis pityriasis rosea, and tinea versicolor). Infections, hair loss, and lichenification are related *complications. Diagnosis* is based on the health history and physical exam.

Common interventions

The main objective of care is to control the disorder without overtreatment and to allow for skin repair. Treatment is symptomatic and includes topical medications containing sulfurs, salicylic acid, resorcinol, and tars in various preparations to the scalp; topical steroids to control extensive inflammation; and topical medications combined with detergent shampoos 2 to 3 times a week.

Nursing interventions

Physical 1. Advise the patient to avoid excess heat and perspiration.
2. Advise the patient to avoid rubbing and scratching.
3. Advise removal of any external irritants.
4. Suggest remedies to control scalp itching and flaking.
5. Administer topical medications as prescribed.
6. Observe for the occurrence of secondary infections.
Educational 7. Educate the patient so that maximum self-care is achieved.
8. Advise and encourage a nutritious diet.
9. Advise the patient to avoid overwork, stress, infection, and lack of rest and sleep.

Evaluation criteria.   *See* Overview.

ACNE VULGARIS

Acne vulgaris is an inflammatory disease involving the pilosebaceous follicle. Acne usually begins at puberty and primarily affects young adults. The incidence is considered to be 100% because only rarely do individuals make the adolescent transition without a few comedones (blackheads) or pustules. Predisposing factors to acne vulgaris include genetic predisposition, anxiety, stress, and emotional tension. The basic cause remains hypothetical, but the prime defect is an abnormal response of the pilosebaceous apparatus to androgenic stimulation. Sebum, an irritant to the skin, will cause papule development.

The *characteristic* lesions of acne may be whiteheads and blackheads (comedones), papules, pustules, nodules, and cysts. The lesions occur primarily on the face, neck, and trunk. Acne may be mild, transient and self-limited, or it may be severe, persistent, and disfiguring. Infection, scarring, and psychologic disturbances are related *complications*. *Diagnosis* is based on the health history and physical exam.

Common interventions

Treatment is individualized according to the severity of the condition. **Medical** care includes advising a nutritious diet and eliminating foods believed to worsen the condition, adequate skin and scalp care, antibiotic therapy (in severe pustular conditions), PO corticosteroids, estrogenic hormones, ultraviolet light, exfoliants, and abrasives. **Surgical** interventions include comedo extraction, incision and drainage of cysts and pustular lesions, intralesional injection of corticosteroids, dermabrasion, chemosurgery, and cryosurgery.

Nursing interventions

Physical 1. Give instructions regarding skin care (advocate frequent washings with special soaps, advise frequent shampooing with medicated shampoo, keep skin free of external occlusion, and advise abrasive soaps).
2. Advise a nutritious diet with adequate fluids. Eliminate foods that aggravate the condition.
3. Administer topical keratolytics as prescribed. (Keratolytic agents cause loosening of the horny layers of the skin.)
4. Apply vitamin A topically.
5. Administer antibiotics and PO estrogens as prescribed.
Psychosocial 6. Provide emotional support and allow for verbalization of feelings. (Acne causes embarrassment and self-consciousness at a time when identity development is critical. Anxiety is present in every acne client. Feelings of guilt, anger, and depression are prominent.)
Educational 7. Educate the patient about the disorder.
8. Teach skin and hair care (diet, medications, and special treatments).

9. Promote and encourage active participation in the therapeutic regimen.
10. Dispel myths. (Acne is not related to sexual activity. Acne is not caused by diet.)
11. Advise continued medical care even when the skin is clear.
Prevention 12. Keep hands away from, and hair off of, the face.
13. Do not squeeze pimples or blackheads.
14. Avoid friction and trauma to the face and neck.
15. Avoid cosmetics.
16. Avoid perspiration around the face.
17. Talk over problems and feelings with an understanding friend.
18. Continue treatment.

Evaluation criteria.   *See* Overview.

PEDICULOSIS CAPITIS

Pediculosis capitis is the infestation of the head with lice. Transmission occurs by direct contact with contaminated articles, combs, brushes, wigs, hats, bedding. School epidemics are common.

The *symptoms* of pediculosis capitis are tiny, oval, white eggs that are attached to the hair shaft by a gluey substance — usually on the scalp, hair at back of head, and behind the ears. The insect bite causes itching and scratching, and may lead to infection.

Nursing interventions

Physical 1. Shampoo the patient with gamma-benzene hexachloride as directed (hair need not be cut).
2. Remove nits with a fine-toothed comb.
3. Examine and treat (as needed) all other individuals in close contact with the patient.
4. Disinfect or boil combs and brushes.
5. Treat complications as necessary.
Psychosocial 6. If there is a school epidemic, advise all students to shampoo with gamma-benzene hexachloride shampoo as directed on the same night.
Educational 7. Teach about transmission and control.
8. Dispel myths (not a sign of being dirty).

Evaluation criteria.   *See* Overview. Patient's hair is free of pediculosis capitis.

PEDICULOSIS CORPORIS

Pediculosis corporis is the infestation of the body with lice. This form of pediculosis is usually associated with unhygienic living conditions. It is transmitted by direct contact with the individual, clothing, outer garments, bedding, or towels.

The *symptoms* of pediculosis corporis may be detected by pruritus and infection secondary to scratching. The louse lives in the clothing and can even feed off the skin while clinging to the clothing.

Nursing interventions

    Physical 1. Have the patient first bathe well with soap and water and then apply gamma-benzene hexachloride cream or lotion as directed.
    2. Launder and/or sterilize all clothing, linens, and bedding.
    3. Fumigate mattresses, pillows, etc., with a spray containing gamma-benzene hexachloride.
    4. Spray room and air thoroughly before use.
    5. Spray all items that cannot be washed.

    Evaluation criteria.   *See* Overview. Patient and contacts are free of pediculosis corporis.

PEDICULOSIS PUBIS

Pediculosis pubis is the infestation of the pubic hair region with lice. Pediculosis pubis is usually spread by sexual contact, but may also be transmitted by infested clothing, bedding, towels, and toilet seats.

The *symptoms* of pediculosis pubis may be detected in pruritus ani and vulvae. It may also be detected from a reddish brown dust (dried insect excreta) in the underwear. The insect saliva may produce a macule, which may be located on the thighs, axilla, and trunk. These areas may become infested along with the patients eyebrows and eyelashes.

Nursing interventions

    Physical 1. Have the patient bathe well with soap and water.
    2. Apply gamma-benzene hexachloride shampoo, lotion, or cream to the affected area as directed. (Gamma-benzene hexachloride should *not* be applied around the eyes.)
    3. Apply ophthalmic preparations as available to treat eyelash infestation.
    4. Machine wash all clothing and linens.
    5. Treat all sexual contacts and family.

    Evaluation criteria.   *See* Overview. Patient and contacts are free of pediculosis pubis.

ADENITIS

Adenitis is an inflammation of a lymph node or gland. Hidradenitis suppurativa (HS) is a bacterial infection of the apocrine glands, occurring most often in the axillae and anogenital regions. HS is rare, occurring in ~2% of the population. The predisposing factors include individuals with tendency to acne vulgaris, women, obesity, and a family history of HS. The cause of HS is an initial bacterial infection of the follicle, leading to invasion and blockage of the apocrine duct.

HS is *characterized* by a chronic, suppurative, scarring process that begins with painful, red nodules in body areas where apocrine glands are present. These nodules progress to tender, diffuse, lumpy, indurated areas that eventually rupture and drain purulent, malodorous material. Scarring and destruction of the apocrine glands are associated *complications*.

HS may be *diagnosed* with the health history and physical exam. The clinician should rule out furuncles. On assessment, the HS lesion presents as deeper, more painful, and more purulent. The HS nodule often displays a sinus tract beneath the skin.

Common interventions

Medical treatment involves the administration of systemic antibiotics, steroids for inflammation (after the antibiotics are initiated), and moist heat (hot compresses, sitz baths, and wet-to-dry dressings). **Surgical** interventions include drainage and surgical excision of the affected area, with skin grafting in extreme chronic cases.

Nursing interventions

Physical 1. Administer antibiotics as prescribed.
2. Administer steroids as prescribed.
3. Apply compresses or dressings.
4. Assist with sitz baths.
Psychosocial 5. Provide emotional support.
6. Facilitate sexual and family counseling.
7. Facilitate group conferences.
Educational 8. Teach about the nature and chronicity of the disease.
9. Advise the avoidance of tight clothing, obesity, and irritating chemicals.
10. Promote and foster maximum participation in the therapeutic regimen.

Evaluation criteria.   *See* Overview.

PARONYCHIA

Paronychia is an acute or chronic infection of the marginal structures around the fingernail. The predisposing factors to paronychia include trauma to the nail fold and repeated or prolonged exposure to moisture. It can be caused by infection or trauma.

The *symptoms* of paronychia include redness, swelling, pain, tenderness, and suppuration. Related *complications* are cellulitis and lymphangitis. Paronychia can be *diagnosed* by the health history, physical exam, and a culture of the site.

Nursing interventions

Physical 1. Investigate and eliminate precipitating factors.

2. Initiate drying procedures (loose clothing, air conditioning, powders, and topical dehydrating medications).

3. Avoid all conditions that lead to constant or repeated moisture or maceration of the skin.

4. Administer prescribed antibiotic and/or antifungal medications if infection is present.

Educational 5. Teach the patient to seek medical attention for injury around the fingernail.

6. Stress gentleness in manicuring.

Evaluation criteria. *See* Overview.

CELLULITIS

Cellulitis is inflammation of the dermis and subcutaneous tissue. The predisposing factors to cellulitis include wounds, preexisting infections, and poor constitutional condition. Any pathogen may cause cellulitis; the most frequent is the hemolytic *Streptococcus*.

The *signs and symptoms* of cellulitis include red streaks in the area, regional node involvement, tenderness, swelling, and constitutional symptoms. Permanent lymphedema, central suppuration, hemorrhage, necrosis, and gangrene are related *complications*. *Diagnosis* is made by the health history and physical exam.

Common interventions

Cellulitis is normally treated with bed rest, immobilization of the affected part, administration of systemic antibiotics and soaks, and hospitalization, if indicated.

Nursing interventions

Physical 1. Provide bed rest.

2. Prevent hazards of immobility.

3. Administer antibiotics as ordered.

Evaluation criteria. *See* Overview. No complications of bed rest evidenced.

FURUNCLE

A furuncle (or boil) is an acute, localized, deep-seated inflammation of the skin that arises from within a hair follicle and usually ends in suppuration and necrosis. The predisposing factors include occlusion, friction, overhydration of skin, traction of hair, exposure to oil or grease, a diet rich in sugars and fats, acne, obesity, diabetes, chronic illness, and poor hygiene. *Staphylococcus aureus* is a common cause.

The *signs and symptoms* of a furuncle include tenderness, pain, heat, and cellulitis around the hair follicle; a boggy and yellow center with a core of pus; and malaise, regional adenopathy, and temperature elevation may develop with extension furunculosis. The vast majority of furuncles heal without *complications.* Occasionally, however, bacteriemia and (rarely) osteomyelitis and thrombophlebitis occur. *Diagnosis* is made by the health history, physical exam, and culture of the lesion.

Common interventions

1. Rule out underlying diseases.
2. Use broad-spectrum antibiotics if necessary.
3. Reduce weight in obese patients.
4. Cleanse the area with antiseptic soap.
5. Apply hot, wet compresses as indicated.
6. Administer topical antibiotics or lotions as indicated.
7. Incise and drain as indicated.
8. Use isolation techniques to prevent spread to other individuals.

Nursing interventions

Physical 1. Administer antibiotics as ordered.
2. Apply hot, wet compresses as ordered.
3. Cleanse the area with an antibacterial soap.
4. Apply dressings for drainage collection.
5. Protect the area from irritation, squeezing, and trauma.
6. Apply antibacterial ointment as ordered.
7. Take precautions to prevent spread of infection.
8. Discard razor blades after use and soak the razor in alcohol.
9. Keep the area dry with antiperspirant or alcohol (if located where moisture collects).

Psychosocial 10. Explain all procedures to the patient.

Educational 11. Instruct the patient to do the following:
   a. Avoid squeezing pimples near the nose.
   b. Keep the draining lesion covered with a dressing.
   c. Place soiled dressings in a paper bag and burn.
   d. Wash hands thoroughly after care of the lesion.
   e. Bathe with bacteriostatic soap.
   f. Discard razor blades after use and cleanse razor with alcohol between shaves.
   g. Take medications as ordered.
   h. Lose weight, if indicated.
   i. Treat underlying chronic disorders as indicated.
   j. Eat a nutritious diet.
   k. Practice good personal hygiene.

Evaluation criteria.   *See* Overview.

HERPES SIMPLEX

Herpes simplex is an acute viral eruption of the skin. The virus of herpes simplex may be one of the most widespread pathogens of human beings. Fifty percent of humans have evidence of having been infected at some time. The sites most commonly affected are about the lips, but lesions can appear on skin and mucous membranes. There is a tendency for recurrence on an involved area. The precipitating factors to herpes simplex include fever, common cold, wind, sunlight, psychic influences, implicated foods, stomach upsets, and trauma. Herpes virus hominis I is associated with nongenital infections. Herpes virus hominis II is associated with genital infections.

The onset of herpes simplex is acute, with *symptoms* of burning and itching followed by the development of vesicles, either singly or in groups, on an erythematous base. The vesicles are filled with a clear fluid, which adsorbs and leaves a thin crust after several days. *Complications* include erosions, secondary infection, and infection of newborn. Herpes simplex can be *diagnosed* by the health history, physical exam, biopsy, and blood antibody titer.

Common interventions

Treatment is symptomatic and involves eliminating the precipitating factors, applying cold, wet compresses during the acute stage, and administering topical steroids (avoid applying near eyes) and a drying agent (e.g., idoxuridine).

Nursing interventions

Physical 1. Apply cold, wet compresses during the acute stages.
2. Administer topical steroids as ordered.
3. Administer a drying agent as ordered.
Educational 4. Instruct the patient to eliminate precipitating factors.
5. Advise the patient that the disease can be spread through intimate contact.
6. Advise the patient to avoid irritating mouthwash and toothpaste and to correct dental deformities.

Evaluation criteria. See Overview.

HERPES ZOSTER

Herpes zoster (shingles) is an acute viral infection of the nervous system causing cutaneous lesions. It often occurs in older individuals. The predisposing factors to herpes zoster are exposure to chicken pox, trauma, and other underlying conditions (e.g., leukemia, lymphoma). It is caused by the varicella or varicella-zoster virus.

Characteristically, skin lesions are vesicles that unilaterally follow the course of one of the spinal or cranial nerves. The intercostal nerves in the area of the waist are more common sites of involvement. Oculomotor functioning may become impaired due to involvement of the 5th cranial nerve. Before the eruption of the vesicles, many patients will experience itching, pain, and tenderness in the area where the eruptions will occur. The infection can be mild and uneventful, lasting 2 to 3 wk, or severe with persistent neuralgia. *Complications* include bacterial infection with pustules, gangrenous ulcers, scarring, scarring keratoconjunctivitis (if zoster is on the face and the eyes become involved), and postherpetic neuralgia (increases with advancing age).

In addition to the health history and physical exam, herpes zoster can be *diagnosed* by a smear and biopsy from the vesicle base.

Common interventions

1. Methods of treatment are nonspecific and directed toward relief of symptoms.
2. Rule out concomitant malignancy.
3. Provide emotional support.
4. Administer analgesia.
5. Consult with an ophthalmologist as indicated.
6. Administer corticosteroids, antihistamines, and sedatives as indicated.
7. Apply wet compresses.
8. Inject locally mixtures of lidocaine and insoluble corticosteroid.
9. Spray ethyl chloride locally for pain relief.
10. Apply drying and antipruritic lotions.

Nursing interventions

Physical 1. Apply local treatment to the skin as ordered.
2. Apply wet compresses.
3. Prevent infection.
4. Administer medications as outlined above.
Psychosocial 5. Provide emotional support for those patients undergoing diagnostic tests to rule out underlying diseases.
6. Reassure the patient that shingles is usually not a serious disease.
7. Reassure the patient that medication for pain relief will be administered.
Educational 8. Instruct the patient about the disease process.
9. Instruct the patient about all procedures and therapies.
10. Instruct the patient to take medications as prescribed.
11. Promote maximal participation by the patient in the therapeutic regimen.
12. Encourage follow-up medical care.

Prevention 13. Educate the patient to all signs and symptoms that indicate secondary infections or complications.

Evaluation criteria. *See* Overview.

WARTS

Warts (verrucae) are benign intraepidermal tumors of the skin. It is doubtful that any human escapes this viral infection. Warts are slightly contagious and autoinoculable. They are caused by the papovavirus hominis.

Characteristically, the common wart is a small, elevated circumscribed, painless, flesh-colored, hyperkeratotic papule. Black dots, caused by hemosiderin, may be seen scattered throughout the lesion. The surface of the wart is rough. Plantar warts are simply warts, on the plantar surface of the foot, grown inward due to pressure or standing. Plantar warts are painful on pressure and do not appear spontaneously as does the common wart. Venereal warts (condyloma acumminata) are fleshy, nonhorny, cauliflower-like epidermal growths that have an affinity for moist areas. General *complications* of warts include pain and veneral complications (interference with intercourse, urination, or defecation; spread by sexual intercourse; and scarring). *Diagnosis* is based on the health history and physical exam.

Common interventions

Medical treatment of warts includes the use of cantharidin, keratolytic agents, podophyllin, psychotherapy, and suggestion therapy. **Surgical** treatment includes surgery, electrodesiccation, and cryosurgery with liquid nitrogen.

Common warts frequently do not require treatment because they may disappear spontaneously. Preparations of salicylic acid, silver nitrate, and/or podophyllin may be used for their caustic/keratolytic properties in wart removal. **Plantar warts** are more resistant to therapy. Success has been achieved with electrosurgery, acid, podophyllin and cantharidin preparations, liquid nitrogen therapy, and suggestion therapy. Simple excision may produce a painful scar. **Venereal warts** may be treated with podophyllin. All contacts should have warts treated at the same time. If new warts appear, the patient should seek treatment immediately.

Nursing interventions

Physical 1. Administer treatments/preparations to warts as prescribed.
2. Assist with procedures as needed.
Psychosocial 3. Explain all procedures and treatments to the patient.
4. Provide suggestion therapy.

5. Advise contacts (as necessary) to seek medical care.
6. Provide emotional support.
Educational 7. Instruct the patient in all aspects of the disease process and therapeutic regimen.
8. Advise the patient to treat all warts, because remaining lesions may cause recurrences.
9. Treat all contacts (as needed).

Evaluation criteria. *See* Overview. Contacts have received medical care.

FUNGAL INFECTIONS

Fungi are parasitic or saprophytic organisms that feed off the skin. Ringworm is a general term applied to mycotic infections of keratinized areas of the body. **Tinea capitis** has worldwide distribution. **Tinea pedis** is the most common of the superficial fungal infections and probably affects half of the adult population at some time during their lives. The predisposing factors include poor hygiene, poor nutrition, debilitating diseases, and a tropical climate.

TINEA CAPITIS

Tinea capitis, a contagious fungal disease of the scalp, usually affects children before puberty. It is caused by the fungi, *Microsporum* and *Trichophyton*.

The clinical *symptoms* are scalp lesions, which appear as round, gray, scaly patches. The lesions may be accompanied by boggy swelling that is followed by permanent scarring and some permanent hair loss. *Complications* include scarring, hair loss, and secondary infections.

In addition to the health history and physical exam, tinea capitis may be *diagnosed* with a Wood's light in a darkened room or with direct microscopic examination and culture of the hair stumps for fungi.

Common interventions

1. Administer griseofulvin PO.
2. Shampoo 2 to 3 times/wk.
3. Apply topical antifungal preparations.
4. Treat all family members and pets.

Nursing interventions

Physical 1. Administer griseofulvin as prescribed.
2. Shampoo the patient as prescribed.
3. Apply topical antifungal preparations as prescribed.
4. Avoid exchanging combs, brushes, and headgear.
5. Treat all family members and pets.
Psychosocial 6. Provide emotional support and understanding.

Educational 7. Teach the patient all facets of the disease process and therapeutic regimen.

   8. Teach the patient medication administration.
   9. Explain the shampoo rationale.
   10. Advise the patient to use his own comb, brush, and headgear.

Prevention 11. Avoid environmental factors that enhance heat, moisture, maceration, and trauma.

Evaluation criteria. *See* tinea unguium *below.*

TINEA PEDIS

Tinea pedis (ringworm of the feet or athlete's foot) is a very common skin infection. Many individuals have the disease and are not even aware of it. Tinea pedis probably affects half of the adult population at some time in their lives. The predisposing factors include the summer season, moisture, tropical climates, and individual susceptibility. It is caused by fungi.

Symptoms of tinea pedis include an acute, inflammatory vesicular process that affects the soles and interdigital webs. Hyperpigmentation, scaling, and fissuring of the webs may be present. Moisture, pruritus, and burning may also be present. *Complications* include bacterial infection of the blisters, cellulitis, maceration, fissures, and lymphangitis. In addition to the health history and physical exam, tinea pedis may be *diagnosed* with lab tests (microscopic exam, and scrapings and culture).

Common interventions

   1. Administer PO corticosteroids for cases with severe inflammation.
   2. Administer broad-spectrum antibiotics if cellulitis and/or lymphangitis and lymphadenitis are present.
   3. Administer griseofulvin as indicated.
   4. Use wet soaks to remove scales and crusts.
   5. Apply nonocclusive topical agents.
   6. Keep feet clean, dry, and well-aerated.
   7. Elevate feet if edema is present.

Nursing interventions

Physical 1. Administer medications as prescribed.

   2. Apply wet soaks as ordered.
   3. Keep feet clean, dry, and well-aerated (elevate if necessary).

Psychosocial 4. Explain the incidence and prevalence of the disease.

   5. Explain susceptibility factor.
   6. Provide emotional support.

Educational 7. Advise the patient to do the following:

   a. Keep feet clean, dry, and well-aerated at all times.
   b. Alternate shoes between wearings to allow for airing and drying.
   c. Wear light cotton socks and change them frequently.

   d. Wear open or perforated shoes to allow for aeration of feet.
   e. Apply foot powder daily to keep feet dry.
   f. Use cotton pledgets between toes at night to absorb moisture.
   g. Wear clogs in public pools or showers.

Evaluation criteria. *See* tinea unguium *below.*

TINEA UNGUIUM

Tinea unguium (ringworm of the nails) is a chronic infection of the nails of the hands or feet. One or more nails may be involved. Tinea of the fingernails is rare. Tinea of the toenails is very common and almost inevitable in patients with recurrent attacks of tinea of the feet. Predisposing factors include tinea of feet and injury to nail. It is caused by *Trichophyton rubrum.*

Characteristically, the nail develops a white or yellow discoloration of the lateral border. Formation of a thickened, elevated, brittle and deformed nail then occurs. Finally, a cheesy substance under the nail and disintegration of the nail may occur in later stages. *Complications* include bacterial infection and loss of the nail.

Tinea unguium may be *diagnosed* by the health history, physical exam, and lab tests (scrapings and culture, microscopic exam, and Wood's light).

Common interventions

1. Administer PO griseofulvin for tinea of finernails (ineffective for tinea of toenails).
2. Administer topical fungistatic agents.
3. Debride and/or surgically evulse the nail.

Nursing interventions

Physical 1. Administer medications and topical agents as prescribed.
2. Assist with surgical procedures as needed.
Psychosocial 3. Explain all procedures to the patient.
4. Explain the course and treatment of the disease.
5. Reassure and support the patient.
Educational 6. Instruct the patient in all aspects of treatment.
Prevention 7. Provide care for tinea of feet.
8. Protect nails from injury.

Evaluation criteria. *See* Overview. Family members are free of infection.

ECZEMA AND DERMATITIS

Eczema (synonymous with chronic dermatitis) is caused by one or more internal and external factors. Acute or chronic conditions are characterized by erythema, papules, vesicles, pustules, scales, or crusts, alone or in combination. The lesions may be dry or with a watery discharge, and there may be thickening, infiltration, itching, and burning. **Atopic dermatitis** is an eczematous disease with a characteristic distribution occurring in persons with a family history of allergic diseases. It is a commonly occurring skin disorder seen in infants after 2 mo of age, adolescents, and adults. Predisposing factors include a family history of allergy, dryness of skin, wool and lanolin as irritants, food allergy, emotional stress, nervousness, and a childhood history of the condition.

The disease may vary from a mild single episode to severe and chronic with recurrent episodes. Adolescent and adult *symptoms* include marked dryness and thickening of skin, excoriation, pruritus, and sweat retention. Adult lesions appear most commonly on the antecubital and popliteal areas. *Complications* include secondary infection and scarring. *Diagnosis* is based on the health history and physical exam.

Common interventions

1. Reduce pruritus and scratching.
2. Administer sedation and antihistamines.
3. Administer corticosteroids in severe cases.
4. Administer broad-spectrum antibiotics for secondary infection.
5. Apply topical steroids.
6. Prescribe bland baths.

Nursing interventions

Physical 1. Administer systemic and topical medications as prescribed.
2. Provide soothing baths.
Psychosocial 3. Alleviate stress.
4. Provide emotional support to the patient and family.
Educational 5. Instruct the patient and/or family to avoid the following:
   a. Anything that irritates the skin (e.g., woolen clothing, rough fabrics).
   b. Excessive bathing (bathe only axillae, anogenital areas, fingers, and toes).
   c. Overheating or chilling.
   d. Soaps, household detergents, and cleaners.
   e. Smallpox vaccination and/or any person with vaccination or herpes simplex.
   f. Precipitating and/or any irritating factors.
Prevention 6. Advise the patient and family to do the following:
   a. Get adequate rest.
   b. Eat a nutritious diet.
   c. Take medications as prescribed.
   d. Carry out the therapeutic plan as ordered.

Evaluation criteria.   *See* Overview.

CONTACT DERMATITIS

Contact dermatitis or dermatitis venenata is a common inflammatory condition of the skin due to contact with irritating or allergenic materials. Predisposing factors include a preexisting skin condition, frequent immersion in soap and water, and extremes of heat and cold. Causes include cosmetics, poison ivy, soaps, detergents, industrial chemicals, hair dye, nickel, rubber, and chemicals. Reactions may be primary (caused by exposure to an irritating agent) or allergic (from exposure to a substance by a sensitive individual).

Characteristic skin manifestations include redness, swelling, vesicle or bullae formation, itching, burning, weeping, crusting, drying, and fissuring in well-defined patches. Lesions usually appear at the point or area of contact with the causative agent. *Complications* include secondary bacterial infection and scarring. *Diagnosis* is based on the health history and physical exam.

Common interventions

1. Remove the cause.
2. Relieve the inflammation with topical steroids.
3. Apply cool compresses for the itching.
4. Cleanse and protect the skin.
5. Administer sedatives and/or antihistamines.

Nursing interventions

Physical 1. Remove the causative agent.
2. Administer systemic and topical medications as ordered.
3. Apply cool compresses.
4. Cleanse and protect the skin.
5. Explain all procedures and reassure the patient.
Educational 6. Instruct the patient to do the following:
    a. Take medications.
    b. Protect and cleanse the skin.
    c. Avoid heat, soap, and rubbing.
    d. Avoid any home remedies.
    e. Avoid touching uninvolved body areas with involved areas.
    f. Wash thoroughly after exposure to irritating agents.
    g. Avoid causative agents.

Evaluation criteria.   *See* Overview.

PSORIASIS

Psoriasis is a noninfectious chronic, proliferative, inflammatory disease. It affects 5% of the population and is uncommon in the elderly. Predisposing factors include stressful situations, fatigue, hormonal factors, environmental changes, trauma to skin, and heredity. Psoriasis ranges from a mild, benign skin disorder to a severe disease with disabling complications. It is characterized by periods of remission and exacerbation.

Symptoms include circumscribed erythematous patches covered with heavy, dry, silvery scales of varying size. Coalescence of patches occurs over time to form large, irregular patches. Bilateral symmetry is present. It occurs at the following sites: bony prominences (knees, elbows, sacrum), scalp, external ears, genitalia, perianal area, nails, and dorsa of the hands. *Complications* include arthritis, exfoliative erythroderma, excoriation, and thickening (lichenification). *Diagnosis* is based on the health history, physical exam, and lab tests.

Common interventions

Methods of treatment are aimed at controlling the disease, preventing complications, and reducing scaling and itching. No cure is known.

1. Encourage daily bathing to soften and remove scales.
2. Apply topical corticosteroids and coal tar preparations followed by occlusive dressings.
3. Encourage gradual and regular exposure to sunlight and/or ultraviolet light.
4. Avoid erythema and burning.
5. Administer systemic antimetabolites (methotrexate) in severe cases of psoriasis. (Monitor liver values and platelet, WBC, and RBC counts, routinely.)

Nursing interventions

Physical 1. Administer systemic and topical medications as prescribed.
2. Cleanse skin as needed.
3. Apply dressings as needed.
Psychosocial 4. Provide support related to chronicity and cure.
5. Reassure the patient that the disease is not contagious.
Educational 6. Instruct the patient to cleanse his skin daily and take medications as prescribed.
7. Explain the disease process and therapeutic regimen.
Prevention 8. Advise the patient to avoid scratching.
9. Teach the patient ways to protect his skin.

Evaluation criteria. See Overview.

SEBACEOUS CYSTS

Sebaceous cysts, or "wens," are rounded, benign neoplastic growths of variable size that contain sebum. True sebaceous cysts are relatively uncommon. The predisposing factors include impaired local circulation and occlusion of a sebaceous duct or gland. They are caused by retention of sebaceous gland excretion.

Characteristically, the lesions are soft, elevated, cystic growths covered by normal skin, often with a central comedo; contain a milky-cheesy, foul-smelling material; and are located on the scalp, face, back, and scrotum. *Complications* include secondary infection and scarring. *Diagnosis* is made by the health history, physical exam, and biopsy of the lesion.

Common interventions

1. Excise surgically for permanent cures. (If drained there is a tendency for recurrence.)

Nursing interventions

Physical 1. Prepare the patient for surgery (*see* Chapter 9).
2. Monitor vital signs.
3. Administer medications as ordered.
Psychosocial 4. Explain surgical procedures.
5. Provide support and reassurance.
Educational 6. Instruct the patient about the need for follow-up visits, postoperative care, and the signs and symptoms of infection.
Prevention 7. Avoid occlusion of areas prone to cyst development.

Evaluation criteria. See Overview.

BASAL CELL EPITHELIOMA

Basal cell epithelioma is a malignant neoplastic cancer of the basal cells of the epidermis. It is probably the most common human malignancy and the most frequently encountered of the skin cancers. Predisposing factors include excessive exposure to the sun, fair skin, occupational exposure to coal tar, pitch, creosote, arsenic compounds, and radium. Its main cause is sunlight.

In general, lesions occur on sun-exposed areas (the face, upper lip, scalp, neck, and ears). Lesions may invade and erode contiguous tissue but rarely metastasize. The cure rate is 95% with early diagnosis, effective treatment, and slow growth of cancer.

Symptoms include crusting, ulceration, and single or multiple elevated, waxy nodules, with pearly, rolled borders, central depression, and telangiectasia. *Complications* include destruction of underlying tissue and recurrence of lesions. *Diagnosis* is made by the health history, physical exam, and biopsy and histologic examination of the cells.

Common interventions

X-rays, excision, chemosurgery, electrosurgery and curettage, and cryosurgery are the usual forms of treatment.

Nursing interventions

Physical 1. Prepare the patient for surgery or therapy.
2. Administer medications as prescribed.
3. Administer treatments as ordered.
4. Provide postoperative care as needed.

Psychosocial 5. Provide reassurance.
6. Explain the method of treatment.

Educational 7. Teach the patient about warning signs such as change in color, shape, or size of skin lesion (moles) and to seek immediate treatment.
8. Advise the patient to do the following:
   a. Avoid unnecessary sun exposure, especially when the rays are most intense (10 a.m. to 2 p.m.).
   b. Wear appropriate protective clothing (long-sleeved shirts, wide-brimmed hats, sun umbrella).
   c. Apply a sun-blocking agent when sun exposure is extended or unavoidable.
   d. Continue with follow-up medical supervision.

Evaluation criteria. *See* Overview. Patient verbalizes warning signs of recurrence.

MELANOMA

Malignant melanoma is a malignant neoplasm of the melanocytes that has the potential for invasion, widespread metastasis, and eventual death. It accounts for 1% of all skin cancers and 67% of the deaths due to skin cancer in the USA. Predisposing factors include pigmented hairy nevi, xeroderma pigmentosum, heredity, fair skin, and ultraviolet exposure.

Malignant melanoma is classified into three types: **Lentigo maligna melanoma** (type I) is a slowly evolving, hyperpigmented lesion, occurring on exposed skin surfaces. It usually affects the elderly and is related to chronic sun exposure. It first appears as a tan, flat lesion. **Superficial spreading melanoma** (type II) can occur anywhere on the epidermis, eventually penetrates the basement membrane, and metastasizes. It is most common in middle age. It tends to be circular with an irregular border, and it may have a varied combination of colors such as tan, brown, and black mixed with gray, bluish black, or white. **Nodular melanoma** (type III) affects patients ≤30 to 40 yr old. It tends to spring up suddenly from a mole or clear skin and tends to grow down to invade the dermis and subcutaneous tissue. It is a spherical blueberry-like nodule with a smooth surface and uniform blue-black color that may present as an elevated irregular plaque or may be polypoidal. Metastasis is the major *complication* of all three melanoma classifications. *Diagnosis* is made by the health history, physical exam, and lab tests.

Common interventions

Chemotherapy, regional isolation perfusion, radiation therapy, and immunotherapy are the main **medical** interventions. Wide excisional surgery with regional node dissection followed by skin grafting is the major **surgical** treatment. **Nursing** interventions are the same as for basal cell epithelioma (*see above*).

ULCERS

Ulcers are superficial losses of surface tissue due to cell death. Predisposing factors include compromised mobility, blood supply, and nutrition. Causes include infection and interference with blood supply (venous or aterial). The *symptoms* of **venous stasis ulcers** are slight edema and brownish discoloration of the skin, which eventually progress to a large patch of red, weeping, scaling, eczematous dermatitis that frequently ulcerates. The ulcers are usually located on the medial lower leg, near and above the ankle, and they may be painful and tender. **Arterial leg ulcers** begin as arterial insufficiency, with hair loss, nail dystrophy, and dry, cool, pale, atrophic skin of an extremity. They appear on heels, toes, or trauma sites and are pale or white with slightly elevated rolled edges that are rimmed in purple-red. They have a grey or yellow ulcer base and are painful. **Decubitus ulcers** are discussed in Chapter 7. The major *complication* of ulcers is infection. *Diagnosis* is made by the health history, physical exam, arteriography, skin temperature determination, oscillometry, blood studies, x-ray exams, phlebography, or ultrasonography.

Common interventions

For venous stasis ulcers, **medical** treatment consists of bed rest, elevation of feet, warm, moist compresses, antibiotics, bandages, and debriding agents. Skin grafting is the most common **surgical** intervention.

For arterial leg ulcers, medical and surgical treatment consists of topical corticosteroids; antibiotics; keeping the ulcer clean, dry, and pressure-free; and skin grafts.

Nursing interventions (venous ulcers)

Physical 1. Administer medications as ordered.
2. Cleanse the ulcer as ordered.
3. Apply dressings.
4. Apply elastic bandages.
5. Elevate leg(s).
6. Expose the ulcer to air at night when the patient is in bed.
7. Attend to skin grafts as needed.
Psychosocial 8. Explain all procedures, medications, and treatments.
9. Prepare the patient for surgery as needed.
Educational 10. Instruct the patient to do the following:
    a. Wear elastic support hose.
    b. Avoid prolonged standing or sitting with legs dependent.

    c. Elevate feet and legs a certain part of each day.
    d. Avoid crossing knees and ankles.
    e. Avoid extremes of temperature.
    f. Avoid wearing tight-fitting clothing (e.g., girdles), shoes, and stockings.
    g. Avoid trauma to the area.
    h. Wear a foam rubber pad around the ankle region to protect against trauma.

Evaluation criteria. *See* Overview.

Nursing interventions (arterial ulcers)

Physical 1. Administer medications as prescribed.
    2. Administer topical preparations.
    3. Keep the ulcer clean, dry, and pressure-free.
    4. Promote bed rest.
    5. Administer analgesia.
    6. Provide pre- and postoperative care as indicated.
Psychosocial 7. Explain all treatments, medications, and procedures.
    8. Explain the disease process and provide support.
    9. Prepare the patient for surgery.
Educational 10. Instruct the patient about preventing infection, reducing inflammation, enouraging healing, applying medications, and the need for bed rest.
Prevention 11. Instruct the patient to stop smoking.
    12. Instruct the patient to keep the affected areas warm and dry.
    13. Advise the patient to wear soft, woolen socks and well-fitting shoes, etc.
    14. Advise the patient to avoid injury and/or trauma to the affected limb.

Evaluation criteria. *See* Overview. Patient stops smoking.

LUPUS (SLE)

SLE is a chronic, inflammatory, multisystem disease that affects the connective tissue of the skin, vascular system, and the serous and synovial membranes. Lupus was originally described as a skin disorder and given the name lupus erythematosus because of the characteristic "butterfly rash" usually seen across the bridge of the nose. The rash may be macular to papular, mildly to severely inflamed, faint pink to red. Discoid lupus is the name now given to the disorder when involvement is limited to the skin. SLE affects >200,000 Americans, women more frequently than men, and blacks more than whites. The average age of onset is 30 yr. Heredity is the major predisposing factor, and it is believed to be caused by an autoimmune disorder. The disease is characterized by remissions and exacerbations.

Skin *symptoms* include an erythematous rash that may appear on the face ("butterfly rash"), the extremities, or the trunk. The cutaneous lesions that occur in sun-exposed areas may lead to hypopigmentation (vitiligo), hyperpigmentation, and alopecia, which may be patchy or circumscribed and is usually temporary. SLE may affect the skin, vascular system, lungs, heart, kidneys, joints, and CNS. *Complications* include infection and death from vital organ involvement.

Diagnosis is made by the health history, physical exam, and lab tests. Blood tests are performed to determine the erythrocyte sedimentation rate, albumin:globulin ratio, lupus erythematosus cell preparation, antinuclear antibody test, serologic test for syphilis (a biologic false-positive test is frequently seen in SLE), and serum complement levels. Urine tests check for profuse proteinuria, and immunoglobulins should be checked with a skin biopsy.

Common interventions

1. Rule out SLE.
2. Administer steroids, systemically or topically, as indicated.
3. Avoid sun exposure.
4. Use sunscreens when sun exposure is unavoidable.

Nursing interventions

Physical 1. Administer medications as prescribed.
2. Assist with treatments as needed.
Psychosocial 3. Explain all procedures and treatments.
4. Explain the disease process.
5. Provide reassurance and support.
Educational 6. Instruct the patient to do the following:
  a. Avoid sun exposure and reflected sun.
  b. Use sun-blocking agents.
  c. Wear protective clothing.
  d. Avoid sunbathing.
  e. Avoid the sun when it is most intense.
  f. Avoid fluorescent lighting.
  g. Keep his skin clean and moisturized.
  h. Use hypoallergenic cosmetics.
  i. Use gentle shampoos and avoid hair colorings and permanents (they may be harsh).
  j. Use a wig if needed.

Evaluation criteria. *See* Overview. Disease is controlled, and patient adjusts to changes in condition.

SCLERODERMA

Scleroderma is an insidious, multisystem disease characterized by proliferation of connective tissue in the skin and internal structures. It is an uncommon condition that occurs more frequently in women than in men. The cause is speculated to be of autoimmune origin.

Characteristically, the disease begins insidiously on the face and hands, but later involves the arms, neck, chest, abdomen, and back. Skin becomes tense, wrinkle-free, and bound to adjacent structures (or hard, thick, and unflexible). The face is immobile, expressionless, rigid, and masklike. The mouth and lips become small and taut. Increased skin involvement may also lead to areas of pigmentation and vitiligo, subcutaneous calcification, and telangiectasia. Sweat secretion is suppressed, and the skin becomes dry. The epidermis, appendages, and subcutaneous fat undergo progressive atrophy. Eventually, complete loss of appendages (hair, nails) results. Often, the fingers become fixed in a semiflexed position in advanced stages, and they may become atrophied, pointed, and ulcerated. *Complications* include immobility and multisystem organ involvement. *Diagnosis* is based on the health history, physical exam, erythrocyte sedimentation rate, and histologic examination.

Common interventions
1. Administer steroids for antiflammatory effect.
2. Administer salicylates.
3. Prescribe physical therapy.
4. Keep the patient's skin well-lubricated.
5. Treat additional organ involvement symptomatically.
6. Perform surgery for deformities.

Nursing interventions
Physical 1. Administer medications as prescribed.
2. Provide physical therapy.
3. Protect the skin from cold, trauma, and infection.
4. Keep the skin well-lubricated.
5. Provide symptomatic interventions for other organ involvement.
Psychosocial 6. Explain the disease process to the patient.
7. Provide emotional support.
Educational 8. Advise the patient to keep warm, take warm baths, etc.
9. Instruct the patient to administer medications and carry out treatments and procedures as prescribed.
Prevention 10. Advise mobility as prescribed.

Evaluation criteria.   *See* Overview.

POLYARTERITIS NODOSA

Polyarteritis nodosa is an acute multisystem disease characterized by diffuse inflammation of small and medium-sized arteries. Its cause is unknown. The cutaneous *symptoms* include linear subcutaneous nodules that are a result of aneurysms of small superficial blood vessels, a purplish rash with a meshed pattern (livedo reticularis), and/or superficial ulceration of the fingers and toes. Constitutional symptoms may also be present (e.g., fever, malaise, weakness, and pain). Infection, renal failure, and cardiac failure are associated *complications.*

Diagnosis is made by the health history, physical exam, and the following laboratory tests: blood (CBC, erythrocyte sedimentation rate, serum globulin level), urinalysis, and biopsy (histologic evaluation).

Common interventions
1. Treat symptoms and provide support.
2. Administer corticosteroids and immunosuppressants.
3. Avoid offending drugs that may precipitate disease.
4. Prevent and treat infections.

Nursing interventions
Physical 1. Provide symptomatic nursing care.
  2. Administer medications as prescribed.
  3. Protect the patient from infections.
  4. Monitor the patient's vital signs.
Psychosocial 5. Provide emotional support.
  6. Explain all treatments, medications, and procedures.
Educational 7. Explain the disease process.
  8. Instruct the patient to take medications as prescribed.
  9. Instruct the patient to be alert for signs of infection.
Prevention 10. Advise the patient to avoid drugs that may exacerbate his symptoms.
  11. Advise the patient to avoid exposure to infection.

Evaluation criteria.   *See* Overview. Symptoms are controlled.

BREAST COMPLICATIONS
The breasts involve a great deal of emotion for both men and women. Approximately 25% of women who see a physician do so because of concern related to abnormal findings or a lump in the breast. The majority of abnormal findings are either related to benign conditions or merely physiologic changes.

Anatomy and physiology review
The breast is a modified sebaceous gland located between the 2nd and 6th ribs between the sternal edge and midaxillary line (Fig. 12-2). The mammary glands (breasts) are paired organs that lie on the pectoral fascia and muscles of the anterior chest wall. The nipple is centrally located on each breast and is surrounded by the areola. Small elevations on the areola are sebaceous glands. Breast tissue has three major components: glandular tissue, fibrous tissue, and fat. The glandular tissue is organized into 15 to 20

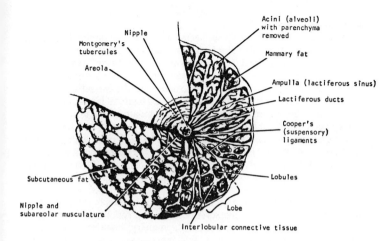

Acini (alveoli)
with parenchyma
removed

Nipple

Montgomery's
tubercules

Areola

Mammary fat

Ampulla (lactiferous sinus)

Lactiferous ducts

Cooper's
(suspensory)
ligaments

Subcutaneous fat

Lobules

Nipple and
subareolar musculature

Lobe

Interlobular connective tissue

Figure 12-2. Anatomy of the breast.

lobes, which further subdivide into lobules and acini. The acini branch into a ductal system that extends through the lobe and finally converges at the nipple. The glandular tissue is supported by the fibrous tissue and suspensory ligaments (Cooper's ligaments), which originate at the subcutaneous tissue layer, run through the breast tissue, and attach to the muscle fascia. Along with supporting the breast, the fibrous tissue allows for mobility of the breast. Fat surrounds the breast superficially and peripherally and provides support to the glandular tissue. The male breast consists mainly of a small nipple and areola. There are rudimentary ducts without any well-developed acini. A small proportion of fat is present between the ducts and above the pectoral fascia.

A knowledge of the breast lymphatics is essential because spread of cancer is frequently through this system. The major channels of lymphatic drainage of the breast occur through the axillary, transpectoral, and internal mammary channels. The axillary and transpectoral channels also have drainage into the infraclavicular and supraclavicular lymphatics. The axillary lymphatics are the major channels of drainage for the breasts. Metastasis from breast cancer is frequently located in this group. Because of the importance and complexity of the lymphatics of the breast area it is essential to carefully examine the indicated nodes.

Physiologically the breast is an endocrine target organ that is influenced by hormonal variations during a female's life-span. The developmental milestones occur at puberty, during each menstrual cycle, during pregnancy, and at menopause. Hormonal variations affect the physical and microscopic characteristics of breast tissue.

General assessment

A complete **history** must be collected with attention directed to reason for contact, current health status (nutrition), past health history (menstrual, obstetric), concurrent health problems (medications taken), family health history (especially mother, sister), and occupational/environmental history. Much of this information can be used to determine the patient's risk status for breast cancer. Questions specifically related to breast history (review of system) include inquiries regarding pain, tenderness, lumps, dimples, discharges, changes in nipples and breasts, development, and lactation.

A complete **physical assessment** should be performed with attention directed to the breasts. Physical assessment of the breasts consists mainly of the techniques of observation, inspection, and palpation. Good lighting is necessary. The patient should be disrobed to the waist, in a sitting position with arms at sides.

The **breast examination** includes the following steps: **(1)** Inspection and comparison of (a) the breasts (in the above position), making note of size (some size difference is normal), symmetry, contour (evidence of masses, dimpling, and flattening), skin (appearance, color, texture, and venous pattern), and areolar area; (b) the nipples, making note of size, shape, (long-standing, simple inversion is usually normal), discharge, rashes or ulceration, and direction in which they point; and (c) breasts, with patient raising arms over head and pressing hands on hips (to tense the pectoralis muscles), making note of any dimpling, retraction, changes in contour, flattening, edema, or redness. (If the patient has large, pendulous breasts, leaning forward may be useful for the examiner to note dimpling, flattening, edema, or redness. The examiner should at all times be bilaterally comparing the breasts.) **(2)** Palpation of the axilla and supraclavicular area for lymph nodes while the patient is seated with hands on hips. **(3)** Palpation of the breast while the patient is seated with arms at sides. Each breast should be completely and systematically palpated, quadrant by quadrant or in increasing or decreasing concentric circles. Whatever pattern is used, it is essential that the entire breast (including the tail, periphery, and areola) is palpated, making note of consistency of the tissue (elastic, lobular, stringy), premenstrual fullness, nodularity, tenderness, and areas of hardness. If present, nodules should be described in terms of location (quadrant and centimeters from nipple), size, shape, consistency, delimitation, mobility, and tenderness. **(4)** Palpation of the nipple to note elasticity, and compression of the nipple to determine the presence of discharge. **(5)** Palpation of the entire breast with the patient lying down, with a small pillow under the shoulder to spread the breast tissue evenly.

For the male breast examination, the patient should be disrobed to the waist and seated. The examination includes inspection of the nipples and areola for nodules, swelling, ulceration, and general breast enlargement; palpation of the breasts and areolae for nodules; palpation of an enlarged breast to differentiate between glandular enlargement and fatty enlargement of obesity; and inspection of the axilla, noting rashes and infections.

Diagnostic tests

The following is a list of the various diagnostic tests that are used in breast examinations.

1. Mammography: A screening x-ray procedure used to evaluate suspicious areas of the breast before a mass is detectable.
2. Thermography: A noninvasive screening procedure used to measure areas of heat. "Hot spots" are suspicious.
3. Xerography: A breast x-ray using a selenium-coated plate.
4. Transillumination: A visual examination of the breast using a cold light in a dark room. It demonstrates cysts or neoplasms not detectable on palpation.
5. Ultrasound (holography): A noninvasive technique using high-frequency sound waves to evaluate the various breast lesions.
6. Biopsy: A minor surgical procedure involving removal of part of a lesion, which is then examined histologically for definitive diagnosis.
7. Cytology: A cell examination used to identify suspicious or abnormal cells.

Common interventions

Specific **general** interventions are listed under each problem in the following sections. One of the most important **nursing** activities is to teach the patient breast self-examination (BSE). Through BSE, malignancies may be discovered early and receive early treatment. The importance of teaching BSE is emphasized even more so when one considers that 90% of breast cancers are initially discovered by the patient. The patient can be taught BSE while being examined. The American Cancer Society's suggestions for BSE are included in Table 12-2.

Evaluation criteria. Vital signs are within normal limits. Patient verbalizes an understanding of disease process. Patient knowledgeably participates in therapeutic care plan. Patient correctly demonstrates BSE.

MASTITIS

Mastitis, an inflammation of the breast, is most common in lactating women, but may occur at other times. Predisposing factors include lactation, poor hand-washing techniques, infected infant, and systemic infection. It is usually caused by *Staphylococcus aureus.* Infection usually begins in one lobule and extends to other areas.

Signs and symptoms include chills, fever, rapid pulse, pain in the affected area, a doughy and tough-feeling breast, stagnation of milk (if duct is infected), and discharge from the nipple. *Complications* include breast

TABLE 12-2

How to Perform BSE

Factor	Explanation
In shower	Hands glide more easily over wet skin. With fingers flat, move gently over every part of each breast. Use right hand to examine left breast, and left hand for right breast. Check for any lump, hard knot, or thickening.
Before a mirror	Inspect breasts with arms at sides. Next, raise arms high overhead. Look for any changes in contour of each breast, a swelling, dimpling of skin, or changes in the nipple. Then, rest palms on hips and press down firmly to flex chest muscles. Left and right breast will not exactly match (few women's breasts do). Regular inspection shows what is normal for each individual.
Lying down	To examine right breast, put a pillow or folded towel under right shoulder. Place right hand behind head to distribute breast tissue more evenly on the chest. With left hand, fingers flat, press gently in small circular motions around an imaginary clock face. Begin at outermost top of right breast for 12 o'clock, then move to 1 o'clock, and so on around the circle back to 12. A ridge of firm tissue in the lower curve of each breast is normal. Then move in an inch, toward the nipple, keep circling to examine every part of breast, including nipple. This requires at least 3 more circles. Now slowly repeat procedure on left breast with a pillow under left shoulder and left hand behind head. Notice how breast structure feels. Finally, squeeze the nipple of each breast gently between thumb and index finger. Any discharge, clear or bloody, should be reported immediately to a physician.
Rationale	Most breast cancers are first discovered by women themselves. Since breast cancers found early and treated promptly have excellent chances for cure, learning how to examine breasts properly can help save life. Use the simple 3-step BSE procedure shown above.
Timing	Follow the same procedure once a month about a week after menstruation, when breasts are usually not tender or swollen. After menopause, check breasts on first day of each month. After hysterectomy, check with a physician or clinic for an appropriate time of the month.
Findings	If a lump, dimple, or discharge is discovered during BSE, it is important to see a physician as soon as possible. Don't be frightened. Most breast lumps or changes are not cancerous, but only the physician can make the diagnosis.

Reprinted with permission from the American Cancer Society. How to Examine Your Breasts. American Cancer Society, Inc., New York. 1977.

abscesses. *Diagnosis* is made by the health history, physical exam, and culture and sensitivity of the mother's milk.

Common interventions
1. Stop breast-feeding (if indicated).
2. Administer antibiotics and analgesics.
3. Apply a firm breast support.
4. Apply heat locally.

Nursing interventions

Physical 1. Administer medications as prescribed.
2. Apply breast support and heat.
3. Assess for changes in condition.
Psychosocial 4. Provide emotional support if breast-feeding has been cancelled.
5. Explain the disease process, all treatments, and their rationales.
Educational 6. Teach the patient to practice meticulous personal hygiene with emphasis on hand washing.
7. Foster maximum participation in the care plan.

Evaluation criteria. See Overview. Pain diminishes and breast reverts to its normal consistency. Milk is expressed from breast. Discharge clears up.

BREAST ABSCESS

Mastitis often leads to the formation of an abscess, which is a localized collection of pus in the breast. The incidence, etiology, and predisposing factors to an abscess are the same as for mastitis (*see above*). The *signs and symptoms* include a very sensitive, dusky red area, a palpable mass, and pus expressed from the nipples. *Diagnosis* is made by the health history, physical exam, and culture and sensitivity of breast discharge. **General** treatment is similar to mastitis. In addition, **surgical** incision and drainage may be performed and dressings applied. **Nursing** care is similar to that for a patient with mastitis. Meticulous hand care and aseptic technique must be employed.

FIBROCYSTIC DISEASE

Fibrocystic disease is a benign neoplastic breast disorder characterized by increased formation of fibrous tissue, hyperplasia of epithelial cells of the ducts and breast glands, and dilation of the ducts. A major concern is that fibrocystic disease may mask underlying cancer. Although the cause is unknown, it is the most common lesion of the female breast, occurring most often in younger women (30 to 50 yr of age). Hormonal imbalance is the major predisposing factor.

Fibrocystic disease is *characterized* by a firm, mobile, smooth, round, well-delineated mass in the upper and outer quadrant of the breast. There is bilateral, but not necessarily equal, involvement. Single or multiple cysts are accompanied by dull, aching pain and a feeling of fullness, heaviness, and tenderness. Premenstrual accentuation of symptoms is not uncommon, with premenstrual fluctuation of mass size. Malignancy is the major related *complication. Diagnosis* is made by the health history, physical exam, and aspiration biopsy. Needle aspiration is the most frequent intervention, with surgical excision if the cyst recurs.

Nursing interventions

  Physical 1. Assist with surgical procedures as indicated.
  Psychosocial 2. Explain all procedures and the nature of the disorder.
  Educational 3. Emphasize the need for a breast examination.
  Prevention 4. Stress the importance of frequent reexamination.

  Evaluation criteria. *See* Overview.

ADENOFIBROMA

Adenofibroma is a benign neoplastic tumor of the fibrous and glandular tissue. It is a common lesion of the female breast, most frequently affecting women in their late teens and early twenties. *Characteristically,* the adenofibroma lesion is firm, smooth, rubbery, round, well-delineated, and freely movable. In addition, it is usually painless, occurring usually singly. It is not associated with nipple changes or discharges, and it is not characterized by malignant potential. *Complications* include infection and scarring. *Diagnosis* is made by the health history, physical exam, biopsy, and histologic evaluation. Common **interventions** include simple, local excision. **Nursing** interventions are similar to those of fibrocystic disease (*see above*).

HYPERTROPHY (FEMALE)

Female hypertrophy is an increase in the breast size that does not involve tumor formation. It usually occurs in adolescence through adulthood, with *symptoms* being moderate to massive breast hyperplasia and ptosis of hyperplastic breasts. *Complications* include limitation of physical activity, back and shoulder pain, excoriation of the inframammary area, and severe psychologic problems. *Diagnosis* is made by the health history and physical exam.

Common interventions

The treatment of choice is reduction or removal of breast tissue and transposition of the nipple to a suitable position on the chest (reduction mammoplasty). The goal is to construct normal-appearing, smaller breasts.

Nursing interventions

Physical 1. Provide pre- and postoperative care.

2. Observe for failure of the areolar graft, infection, effectiveness of healing, loss of sensation in the nipple, and venous thrombosis in the breast tissue.

Psychosocial 3. Provide emotional support in the immediate postoperative period.

4. Tell the patient about the inability to nurse after the surgical procedure.

Evaluation criteria. *See* Overview. Wound heals and patient verbalizes long-term aftereffects of surgery.

HYPERTROPHY (MALE)

Enlargement of the male breast (**gynecomastia**) may be produced by lobule formation or stromal proliferation (foundation tissue of the breast). Lobule formation is usually associated with an excess of estrogen or androgen. Stromal proliferation is usually associated with normal levels of testosterone and estrogen. Transient gynecomastia occurs in 50% of normal males at puberty. Predisposing factors include a familial trait. Causes include rapid changes and/or imbalances in hormone levels in adolescents, gonadal dysfunction, and systemic disorders (cirrhosis, ulcerative colitis, high spinal cord lesions, etc.), obesity, and renal failure with long-term hemodialysis. In addition, gynecomastia may be drug-induced (estrogen, testosterone, reserpine, spironolactone, digitalis, etc.). *Symptoms* include unilateral or bilateral breast enlargement, usually without symptoms but occasionally accompanied by tenderness. Psychologic disturbance is a related *complication. Diagnosis* is based on the health history, physical exam, and gonadotrophin and sex steroid levels.

Common interventions

If the individual appears to have an otherwise normal development, no treament is needed. Reduction mammoplasty is a surgical alternative available to the patient.

Nursing interventions

Physical 1. Refer to female reduction mammoplasty (*see above*).

Psychosocial 2. Provide emotional support to the patient.

3. Advise the patient regarding alternative treatments.

Evaluation criteria. Refer to female reduction mammoplasty (*see above*). In addition, patient chooses treatment that is most acceptable to him.

MALIGNANT NEOPLASMS

There is a rapid increase in the occurrence of malignant neoplasms after 40 yr of age, which is then followed by a gradual rise in occurrence with older women at high-risk. Malignant neoplasms are rare in men, accounting for 0.2% of all male cancers. In contrast, they are a major cause of cancer death in women, accounting for 18% of cancer deaths in the female population in the USA.

Predisposing factors include advanced age, a history of breast cancer or of breast cancer in the mother or a sister, early menarche and late menopause, birth of the first child after 30 yr of age, never having given birth to a child, exposure to ionizing radiation, estrogen replacement therapy, a history of cystic disease, and North American, European, or Jewish descent. The cause is unknown.

The numerous histologic types of breast cancer are classified for the specific tissue or origin and type of cancer cell. **Carcinoma of the ducts** is the most commonly affected site, originates from the epithelial cells that line the mammary ducts, may invade the breast tissue in irregular patterns, and may be infiltrating or noninfiltrating. **Lobular carcinoma** arises from the lobular tissue and may be infiltrating or noninfiltrating. **Mammary sarcoma** (rare) arises from the ligaments, tendons, and muscles of the breast. **Inflammatory carcinoma** (rare) is a lethal and aggressive form of cancer that involves the subdural lymphatics. **Paget's disease** is a carcinoma arising from the minute ducts of the nipple that affects the nipple, areola, and surrounding skin.

Characteristically, in breast cancer, the **mass** is usually singular and of irregular or stellate shape. It has a firm to hard consistency and is not clearly delineated. It is usually nontender, nonmobile, and fixed to the skin or tissues. The **skin** has dimpling, edema, a prominent vascular pattern, and abnormal contours. In the **nipple** there is inversion, flattening or retraction, deviation or pointing, edema of the nipple and areola, and discharge. In Paget's disease, redness, erosion, and ulceration or dermatitis of the nipple and areola may exist. *Complications* include metastases.

Diagnosis is made with the health history, physical exam, biopsy, and histologic exam. Early diagnosis and treatment of breast cancer improves the survival rate. Education of health professionals and the public is a critical element in early diagnosis. Public education must be informative without arousing anxiety. Individuals must regularly perform BSE to detect abnormalities early. Health professionals must view health education as one of their more important functions. Education is especially important for those considered to be at greater risk for developing breast cancer.

Common interventions

Treatment will depend on the extent and type of cancer, and on the patient. The objective is to remove or destroy the entire neoplasm. Much controversy exists as to the surgical procedures used.

Medical

Radiation is used as primary treatment, adjunct to surgery, for tumor reduction, and as a palliative measure. Chemotherapy (drug treatment) involves anticancer drugs, endocrine manipulation, and immunotherapy.

Surgical

1. Halsted radical mastectomy: Removal of the entire breast, skin, pectorales major and minor, axillary lymph nodes, and fat.
2. Extended radical mastectomy: Removal of all of the tissue involved in the Halsted procedure plus the internal mammary lymph nodes.
3. Modified radical mastectomy: removal of the breast, some fat, and most axillary nodes.
4. Simple mastectomy: Removal of the breast.
5. Simple mastectomy plus radiation or partial mastectomy plus radiation: Removal of the tumor and 2 to 3 cm of the surrounding tissue.
6. Tylectomy (lumpectomy, wedge excision, quadrant excision) plus radiation: Removal of the tumor mass and a small amount of the surrounding breast tissue.
7. Subcutaneous mastectomy: Removal of the internal breast tissue, leaving the skin.

Nursing interventions

Physical 1. Provide general pre- and postoperative care.
   2. Prevent postoperative arm edema on the operated side by correct positioning of the arm and by encouraging arm exercises as early as indicated.
   3. Prevent postoperative infection.

Psychosocial 4. Provide planned emotional support for the patient and her family pre- and postoperatively.
   5. Refer the patient to community resources (e.g., Reach to Recovery, other self-help groups).

Educational 6. Teach the patient how to perform wound care.
   7. Promote the use of a prosthesis.
   8. Advise the patient to continue follow-up examinations.
   9. Teach the patient the various arm exercises.
  10. Teach the patient and her family BSE.
  11. Involve the family and significant others in the care plan.
  12. Advise the patient about available community resources.

Prevention 13. Teach the patient and her family special arm and hand care.
   a. Apply lubrication to the hand several times daily.
   b. Wear rubber gloves when washing dishes, etc.
   c. Wear a thimble when sewing.
   d. Notify the physician if the arm gets red, hard, swollen, or hot.
   e. Wear a medical alert tag.

f. Return for follow-up care as ordered.
g. Avoid carrying a purse or heavy items or wearing jewelry or a wristwatch on the affected arm.
h. Avoid hangnails, cuts, scratches, burns, insect bites, and the use of strong detergents on the affected arm.
i. Avoid having blood drawn, injections, or BP measurements on the affected arm.
j. Avoid sunburn, tight-fitting sleeves, and the use of hormone or beauty creams before consulting with the physician.

Evaluation criteria. *See* Overview. Patient knowledgeably participates in therapeutic care plan. Patient demonstrates ability to cope with disease and returns to predisease socialization behaviors. Patient makes use of available community resources. Patient is able to discuss all measures to protect affected arm and hand.

CHAPTER 13

ALTERED FUNCTIONING OF THE HEAD AND NECK

Caroline Camuñas

Problems with the head and neck constitute approximately one third of the complaints for which care is sought. All of these problems have an enormous impact on the individual and society, ranging from days lost from work due to the common cold to the long-term and life-threatening results of neoplasm.

Because disorders of the head and neck are highly visible, deformities in these areas are often apparent to others. Body image and self-esteem may be severely compromised. Initiating and maintaining relationships may be very difficult, and a pattern of social isolation, reactive depression, and general helplessness may develop. A person undergoing radical facial surgery, for example, may be as sexually compromised as an individual who has had genital surgery.

Altered functioning of the head and neck involves the senses as well as body processes: sight, hearing, speech, smell, taste, equilibrium, eating, and breathing may all be affected. Sensory disturbance may cause serious social and communication problems because the senses provide information about the environment and one's spatial and interactive relationships with it.

EYE

OVERVIEW

Because ~90% of the information that people receive about their surroundings is obtained through the eyes, blindness is the most dreaded sensory loss, and any altered functioning of the eyes causes a high degree of anxiety.

Anatomy and physiology review

Components of the eye include external structures (Table 13-1 and Fig. 13-1), extraocular muscles (Table 13-2), internal structures (Table 13-3), refractory structures (Table 13-4), and an anterior chamber (Table 13-5). **Binocular vision,** the normal simultaneous use of both eyes, results in depth perception and enlarges the visual field. Visual images, which must be focused on identical points on the retinas, are received from slightly different angles, resulting in perspective and, consequently, depth perception. The necessary processes for binocular vision are convergence of visual axes, or the coordinated movement of both eyes (*See* Table 13-2); regulation of pupil size; refraction of light rays on the retinas; and accommodation or change of lens strength, depending on the distance of objects.

The **innervation** of the eye is presented in Table 13-6. In brief, the neural photosensitive receptors of the retina initiate the nerve impulse messages that travel through the optic nerves. The optic nerves join to form the optic chiasm, the crossing point for the fibers from the medial halves of the retinas. From the optic chiasm, the optic nerves continue to the cerebrum, where visual impulses are interpreted as sight. (Critical areas are nearby for visual interpretation and memory.)

General assessment

The **health hisory** includes the past health history, the family history, and a review of systems. The *past health history* should focus on endocrine

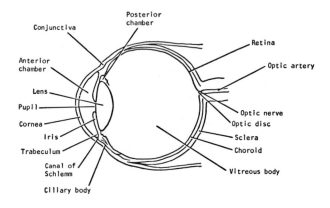

Figure 13-1. Cross section of the eye.

TABLE 13-1

External Structures and Functions of the Eye

Structure and components	Function
Orbit Frontal, sphenoid, zygomatic, maxillary, palatine, ethmoid, and lacrimal bones	Provides protective recess for the eye.
Extrinsic (extraocular) muscles	Hold eye in place and coordinate movement. Exert effect by contraction.
Eyelid (dense connective tissue around orbital septum)	Covers and protects eye.
Glands of eyelid Meibomian (sebaceous)	Produce an oil secretion that prevents overflow of tears, maceration of the lids by tears, and rapid evaporation of the normal tear layer.
Zeis's (sebaceous)	Produce an oil secretion and connect with follicles of eyelashes.
Moll's	Produce sweat.
Conjunctiva	Provides continuous covering of the inner surface of the lid. Becomes continuous with the epithelium of the cornea.
Lacrimal apparatus Lacrimal gland	Secretes tears, which keep cornea and conjunctiva moist and lubricated, protect against bacterial invasion, and wash off foreign particles.
Lacrimal canaliculus, lacrimal sac, and nasolacrimal duct	Carry excess tears to nose.

disorders (especially diabetes mellitus, thyroid disease, and pituitary adenomas), cardiovascular or hypertensive disease, and connective tissue disease. In addition to general, systemic disease, the *family history* should focus on eye disease (especially degenerative disorders, strabismus, myopia, and tumors). The *review of systems* should focus on the occurrence of previous disorders, injury, and the nature of visual symptoms (e.g., change in visual acuity, pain, and loss of vision).

TABLE 13-2

Extraocular Muscles

Muscle	Primary action	Secondary action
Lateral rectus	Abduction	None
Medial rectus	Adduction	None
Superior rectus	Elevation	Adduction and intorsion
Inferior rectus	Depression	Adduction and extorsion
Superior oblique	Depression	Intorsion and abduction
Inferior oblique	Elevation	Extorsion and abduction

The **physical examination** begins with an external examination. The *eyelids* are assessed for protection of the eyes by effective closure, indication of systemic disease (e.g., lid edema caused by CHF, kidney disease, allergy, or thyroid disease), malposition of the lids, and presence of local disease (e.g., tumor or infection). After the *eyelashes* and *lacrimal glands* are assessed, the *conjunctiva* should be examined for color, secretions, foreign bodies, smoothness, and thickness.

The *cornea* and corneal reflex are checked next. Fluorescein is used to test for corneal abrasions. The *pupil* should be assessed for size, shape, reaction to light, accommodation, and consensual pupil reaction. The *placement of the eyeball in the orbit* should be checked (note whether the eye is pushed forward or sunken), as well as the *extraocular muscles* (note if both eyes move together and if visual lines meet at the object of fixation). The normal *visual field* of each eye should extend ~60 degrees medially, 50 degrees upward, 90 degrees temporally, and 70 degrees downward. Visual fields may be altered by a CNS or ocular disorder. *Intraocular pressure* is measured by means of indentation (Schiötz) tonometry or applantation tonometry. *Visual acuity* and *refraction* should be tested. The *ophthalmoscopic examination* may be direct, indirect, or by means of biomicroscope (slit lamp).

Laboratory tests include retinal photography with fluorescein angiography, ultrasonography, electroretinography, radioisotope scanning, x-rays, and gonioscopy (visualization of the angle of the anterior chamber of the eye).

Common interventions

Medical interventions involve the use of drugs. Parasympathomimetic drugs cause miosis. Some examples are the cholinergic drugs (pilocarpine, carbachol, and acetylcholine chloride) and the cholinesterase inhibitors (e.g., echothiophate iodide). The parasympatholytic drugs cause mydriasis (pupil dilation) and cycloplegia (ciliary muscle paralysis). Some examples are the mydriatics (e.g., eucatropine hydrochloride) and the cycloplegics (atropine sulfate, homatropine hydrobromide, cyclopentolate hydrochloride, and tropicamide). The sympathomimetic drugs cause mydriasis and

TABLE 13-3

Internal Structures and Functions of the Eye

Structure and components	Function
Globe	
Sclera (posterior five-sixths of eye; tough, fibrous, white, opaque layer)	Provides rigid structure and protects internal components.
Cornea (anterior; transparent and colorless)	Provides rigid structure and allows passage of images to retina.
Uveal tract	
Choroid	Supplies nutrients to the retinal rod-and-cone layer and prevents internal reflection of light.
Ciliary body	Changes shape of lens and allows changes in focus.
Iris	Controls the amount of light reaching the retina.
Retina	
Macula	Contains photosensitive receptive end organs; contains cones, which provide color vision, respond to bright light, and differentiate fine details.
Retinal periphery	Contains rods, which respond to low levels of light and detect moving objects.
Optic disc	Constitutes anterior surface of the optic nerve; carries impulses to the brain.

vasoconstriction (e.g., phenylephrine hydrochloride). Other drugs that may be used are topical and systemic antibiotics, the sulfonamides (e.g., sulfisoxazole), adrenal corticosteroids, and carbonic anhydrase inhibitors (e.g., acetazolamide). **Surgical** interventions include extraocular muscle surgery, corneal transplantation, retinal surgery (cryotherapy, photocoagulation, laser surgery, scleral buckling, and circling procedures), peripheral iridectomy, and cataract extraction.

Nursing interventions

Physical 1. Assess for changes in signs and symptoms (changes in visual acuity, presence of floaters and light flashes, and changes in the nature of the pain).

TABLE 13-4

Structures for Refraction

Structure	Function
Cornea	Allows passage of images to retina.
Aqueous humor	Refracts light; supplies nutrients to the cornea, lens, and vitreous humor; maintains internal pressure; fills anterior chamber; and helps maintain slight forward curve of cornea.
Lens	Changes focus of the eye and performs function of accommodation.
Vitreous humor	Refracts light, fills posterior chamber, and maintains spherical shape of eyeball.

TABLE 13-5

Structures and Functions of the Anterior Chamber

Structure	Function
Anterior chamber angle	Formed at the site of the origin of the iris from the ciliary body; regulates aqueous outflow and maintains intraocular pressure.
Ciliary processes	Produce aqueous fluid.
Trabeculae	Allow aqueous humor to flow out of anterior chamber into canal of Schlemm.
Canal of Schlemm	Empties aqueous humor into veins within sclera and episclera for absorption into general circulation.

2. Report changes to the physician.
3. Administer eye medications. (Know correct eye for instillation; administer at specific time ordered.)
4. Administer local treatment (warm or cold compresses; clean prosthesis; remove contact lenses).

Psychosocial 5. Provide emotional support for the patient and significant others. Consider especially (a) any threat to vision and possibility of blindness, (b) any changes that necessitate a permanent modification of life-style and activities, and (c) the stresses that accompany major surgery.

TABLE 13-6

Innervation of the Eye

Nerve	Function
Optic nerve (2nd cranial nerve)	Carries visual impulses to the brain; spreads out over posterior two-thirds of the globe's inner surface, forming the retina.
Occulomotor (3rd cranial nerve)	Controls all movements of the eye except those listed below.
Trochlear nerve (4th cranial nerve)	Controls the superior oblique muscle (downward nasal movement).
Ophthalmic nerve (a branch of the 5th cranial nerve)	Carries sensory impulses (pain, touch, and temperature) from the eye and surrounding structures.
Abducens nerve (6th cranial nerve)	Controls the lateral rectus muscle (lateral deviation).

6. Use available resources to assist the patient and family to deal with the situation.

Educational 7. Teach protection of vision: (a) do not rub eyes; (b) wear shatterproof or unbreakable protectors (e.g., goggles when participating in sports such as tennis or swimming, sunglasses in bright sunlight); (c) use clean, well-fitted glasses; (d) do not use eyewashes or eye drops unless prescribed by a physician; (e) use a clean washcloth to wash around the eyes; (f) exercise caution when using sprays or chemicals (e.g., be certain the nozzle is pointing away from the eyes, and avoid splashing liquids); (g) use common sense when applying eye cosmetics (e.g., follow package directions, never apply them in a moving car, avoid hurried application, replace supplies of eye makeup [especially mascara] every 3 to 6 mo, avoid adding water to eye cosmetics, avoid sharing cosmetics with others, apply eyeliners outside the lashes, and apply makeup to skin that is clean); (h) comply with safety regulations; (i) supervise and instruct children with regard to eye care and protection; and (j) keep in mind the need for early consultation and treatment.

8. Teach self-care (which may be lifelong): administration of drugs, personal hygiene, indications of recurrence, need for follow-up care, importance of early recognition and reporting of symptoms, with immediate treatment, application of warm or cold compresses, insertion and removal of contact lenses, and when to call the physician.

Evaluation criteria

Symptoms are diminished or absent. The patient is assessed for changes in status, receives medication/treatments on time, verbalizes signs, symptoms, and importance of treatment, demonstrates proper care of eyes and good personal hygiene, keeps appointments, calls physician when problems occur, and participates in appropriate self-help groups. Visually handicapped patients familiarize themselves to new environments, achieve independence in self-care and other activities as appropriate, and learn to live with their disability. Complications are avoided.

REHABILITATION OF THE VISUALLY HANDICAPPED

Nursing interventions

   Physical 1. Orient the patient to the environment: (a) describe room, (b) walk around room, (c) describe bed as focal point of room and describe rest of room, (d) leave patient near a piece of furniture, never in middle of room, and (e) allow patient to unpack and place belongings.
   2. Keep the phone, water, call light, and TV and radio controls in the same position.
   3. Place food in the same position to allow eating without assistance: (a) cut food, butter bread, and pour coffee, and (b) do not force patient to perform these tasks until he or she is emotionally ready.
   4. Assist the patient with ambulation: (a) have the patient take your arm by using a three-point hold (thumb, index, and middle finger) at your elbow, (b) keep your arm close to your body to allow the patient to feel your direction, (c) usually, have the patient stay one step behind, (d) warn the patient of crowds, narrow doors, etc., by dropping your arm behind (which alerts the patient to walk behind you), and (e) inform the patient of obstacles.
   5. Encourage self-care (e.g., hygiene, dressing, etc.).
   Psychosocial 6. Visit the patient frequently: (a) knock before entering the room, and (b) identify yourself.
   7. Keep the patient oriented with regard to time: (a) encourage listening to radio or TV, (b) remind of time and day each shift, and (c) remove the face from an inexpensive clock so that the patient can tell time by touch.
   8. Allow the patient to plan his or her day.
   9. Assist the patient and family through the grief process over loss of vision. (The resolution of grief is necessary for patients to learn to live with disability, realize limitations, become involved with the outside world, and achieve life goals.)
   10. Initially, do not challenge the patient's use of denial. (Denial can be a healthy defense mechanism.)
   11. Allow the expression of anger and depression: (a) demonstrate

empathy and acceptance, and (b) recognize that the expression of grief is the first step in rehabilitation.
12. Discuss fears: (a) ask open-ended questions, and (b) allow the patient to talk about how blindness will affect relationships and the ability to earn a living.
13. Allow for value changes during adjustment to disability (e.g., from a refusal to use a cane to using one, and from a refusal to learn Braille to learning it).
14. Assist the patient in resolving independence/dependence conflict.
15. Assist the patient in developing ways to cope with unfamiliar situations (e.g., social communication or prejudice).
16. Understand your own feelings toward blindness in order to help provide positive feedback for the patient's self-esteem, body image, and adjustment.
17. Encourage the patient to participate in group discussions or therapy.
18. Make appropriate referrals.
    a. State blindness agency. Use the Directory of Agencies Serving the Visually Handicapped in the United States, available from:
       American Foundation for the Blind
       15 W. 16th St.
       New York, NY 10011
    b. Guide dog school.
       Seeing Eye
       Morristown, NJ 07960
    c. Textbooks and professional books.
       Recording for the Blind
       212 E. 58th St.
       New York, NY 10022
    d. Library in each state for books and magazines.
    e. Rehabilitation centers.

Evaluation criteria.   *See* Overview.

FOREIGN BODIES

Foreign bodies in the eyes may be superficial, embedded, or impaled. Eye injuries from foreign bodies are common, although safety programs have significantly reduced their incidence. Examples of these foreign bodies are dust, insects, metal fragments, plaster chips, and toys (e.g., darts). *Signs and symptoms* include a statement by the patient that something has hit his eye (foreign body sensation), normal or blurred vision, pain or no discomfort, and tearing. *Complications* include degeneration of the retina or destruction of the entire eye.

Diagnosis includes a health history (especially of how the trauma was caused) and a physical exam (with the eye adequately anesthetized) for amount of pain, visual acuity/deficit, and associated injuries to other structures. Fluorescein dye may be used because it concentrates in the area of irritated corneal tissue. (Fluorescein should never be applied to an eye with a soft contact lens in place because it may permanently stain the lens; the dye should always be rinsed out after the exam because it may cause chemical conjunctivitis.)

Common interventions

The eye should be patched and the patient sent to the ophthalmologist. (Removal of a nonmagnetic foreign body is much more hazardous than removal of a magnetic one.) Superficial injuries of the conjunctiva are not serious and may be safely cared for by first-aiders. Embedded foreign bodies should be removed by a physician, and objects that have impaled the eye should be removed by an ophthalmologist.

1. For superficial trauma to the conjunctiva:
   a. Remove the foreign bodies with a moist cotton applicator or with a spindle of clean cotton or facial tissue.
   b. Use saline and an irrigating syringe to wash out small particles.
   c. Use topical antibiotics only if the cornea is injured.
2. For superficial trauma to the cornea:
   a. Use saline and an irrigating syringe to wash particles off the surface.
   b. Use a moistened cotton-tip applicator.
   c. Do not push the foreign body along the epithelium.
   d. Do not roll the applicator on itself (may cause the foreign body to become embedded).
   e. Apply a topical antibiotic.
3. For embedded foreign bodies (which should be removed by a physician):
   a. Instill a topical anesthetic.
   b. Administer antibiotic eye drops.
   c. Patch the eye (for hours or days).
4. For impaled foreign objects (which should be removed and treated by an ophthalmologist):
   a. Leave the object intact.
   b. Stabilize the object by applying a wet saline dressing, securing the object (by means of a dressing) to the patient's head, immobilizing the patient's head, and avoiding pressure on the globe.

Evaluation criteria.   *See* Overview.

LACERATIONS

These common injuries may be caused by sharp objects such as knives, scissors, or projections on the dashboard of a car. (Blunt trauma can cause posterior lacerations without a penetrating eye wound.)

The *signs and symptoms* of lacerations without prolapse of tissue are bleeding, tearing, pain, foreign body sensation, open wound, hyphema, clear or blood-filled vitreous, and possible change in visual acuity. The *signs and symptoms* of lacerations with prolapse of tissue include (in addition to those listed above) prolapse of the iris through the wound. The presence of blood in the vitreous and a soft eye with no recordable intraocular pressure may indicate the posterior rupture of the globe. If uveal tissue is injured, sympathetic ophthalmia is a possible consequence. The *sign* of avulsion (tissue loss in the eye) is gross deformity, with extrusion of the eye from the orbit. (A change in visual acuity may or may not be present.) *Complications* include retinal detachment and rupture of the globe. There is a guarded prognosis for sight. *Diagnosis* is based on the health history and physical exam.

Common interventions

1. When administering first aid:
   a. Do *not* apply pressure to the lids of a severely injured eye to stop bleeding. (*Never* apply pressure to the globe.)
   b. Gently bandage the eye.
   c. Refer the patient to an ophthalmologist as soon as possible.
2. For avulsion of the eye:
   a. Treat as above.
   b. Shield the eye with a metal or plastic shield (or paper cup) before bandaging. (It is not necessary to shield the unaffected eye or to immobilize the head.)
   c. Avoid exerting the patient. (Transportation by automobile is advised. It is not necessary to immobilize the head.)
3. For superficial laceration of the conjunctiva:
   a. Irrigate the eye with saline.
   b. Suture the wound, if necessary. (The wound usually heals within 24 hr if the margins of the wound are in apposition.)
   c. Administer antibiotic eye drops.
   d. Patch the eye only for comfort.
4. For laceration without prolapse of tissue:
   a. Irrigate the blood clots from the anterior chamber.
   b. Reform the anterior chamber by the injection of normal saline or air.
   c. Suture the wound.
   d. Administer mydriatic eye drops.
   e. Administer systemic or local antibiotics.
   f. Apply bilateral eye bandages.
   g. Place the patient on bed rest.
5. For laceration with prolapse of tissue:
   a. Remove tissue at the level of the wound lip.
   b. Treat as for a laceration without prolapse of tissue.

c. Eviscerate or enucleate the eye if the wound is extensive, there is a great loss of intraocular contents, and there is no hope of useful functioning.

Evaluation criteria.   *See* Overview.

CHEMICAL BURNS

Chemical burns have a fairly common incidence and are caused by strong alkalis, acids, solvents, poisons, and similar substances that are used in the home (in the form of cleaning agents) as well as in industry and laboratories. These substances are extremely hazardous to delicate eye tissues. The *signs and symptoms* of chemical burns include severe pain, reddened conjunctiva, copious tearing (unless deep structures are involved), demarcation of the area (if a chemical acid is the cause), and opacification of the cornea. *Complications* may involve permanent ocular damage or blindness. *Diagnosis* is based on the health history (especially exposure to physical agents) and the physical exam.

Common interventions
First aid

1. Provide immediate first aid. (Chemicals burn for as long as they are in contact with tissue.)
2. Hold eyelids open and flush the conjunctiva of both lids, the sclera, and the cornea with water for 15 to 20 min. (Do *not* waste time looking for antidotes: seconds are precious.)
3. Get the patient to an ophthalmologist as soon as possible.

Medical

1. Maintain cycloplegia and prevent iritis by administering atropine 1% bid.
2. Prevent infection by administering topical antibiotics q 2 hr.
3. Limit degree of corneal damage with very cautious use of local corticosteroid.
4. Control pain with sedatives and narcotics.
5. Do not administer local anesthetics repeatedly because they inhibit healing.

Surgical intervention may involve a corneal transplant.

Evaluation criteria.   *See* Overview.

FLASH BURNS

Flash burns are fairly common and are caused by ultraviolet radiation from a variety of sources (e.g., sunlamps, welding torches, germicidal lights, and sunshine). Flash burns are asymptomatic for several hours after exposure; then severe eye pain occurs. (Often, the patient is awakened from sleep.) Other *signs and symptoms* are photophobia, blepharospasm, tearing, reddened conjunctiva, dull corneal surface, and diffuse punctate fluorescein staining. *Diagnosis* is based on the health history and physical exam.

Common interventions

1. Patch eyes.
2. Apply cold compresses.
3. Administer aspirin or codeine.
4. Administer cycloplegics (homatropine 2% or cyclopentolate 1%) for relief of pain associated with iritis.
5. Apply topical antibiotic qid.
6. Do *not* use topical anesthetic except for the initial examination; it delays corneal healing.
7. Reassure the patient that the corneal epithelium will heal without scarring or visual loss.

Evaluation criteria.   *See* Overview.

THERMAL BURNS

Thermal burns are fairly common and are caused by explosions, molten metal, fire, or steam. *Signs and symptoms* include edema of the face and eyelids, edema and hyperemia of the conjunctiva, charring of the lids, and pain. Possible *complications* include perforation of the cornea, loss of the eye, and the spread of infection to the brain. *Diagnosis* is based on the health history and physical exam.

Common interventions
First aid

1. Apply cold compresses over burned areas.
2. Wash off the lids with surgical soap before applying compresses if the tissue is contaminated.
3. Continue cold compresses for ≥20 min.
4. Refer the patient to a physician.
5. Transfer the patient to a burn center if necessary.

First- and second-degree burns

1. Apply antibiotic ointment to broken blisters.
2. Use cycloplegics if the cornea or conjunctiva is burned.

Third-degree burns

1. Keep the cornea covered to prevent permanent scarring (apply ointment, cover the eye area with plastic wrap, and apply the dressing).

2. Treat corneal burns with antibiotics and cycloplegics.
3. Remove crusting and discharge by using gentle swabbing and by applying warm, moist compresses.

Surgical interventions may include skin grafting (if lid retraction occurs), suturing the lids together (to prevent corneal perforation), corneal transplant (if peripheral tissues are strong enough), and blepharoplasty (at a later date).

Nursing interventions

Physical 1. Administer medications as ordered.
2. Provide burn care as necessary. (Care is the same as for burns elsewhere on the body.)
Psychosocial 3. Prepare the family and significant others for the gross change in the patient's appearance due to lid and facial edema. (Talk with them *before* they see the patient.)
4. Reassure the patient realistically about future vision.
5. Explain all procedures to the patient.
6. Refer the patient and family for counseling as appropriate.
Educational 7. Teach correct application of medications.
8. Teach need for follow-up care.
9. Teach prevention as appropriate.

Evaluation criteria. *See* Overview.

HYPHEMA

Hyphema is hemorrhage into the anterior chamber of the eye. It occurs frequently and results from rupturing of the vessels of the iris due to blunt or penetrating trauma or to surgical complication. *Signs* include blood that may be fairly obvious in the anterior chamber, either filling the entire chamber in severe cases, or settling and forming a visible level. Other signs are vision loss (degree depends on the extent of hyphema) and elevated intraocular pressure. *Complications* include glaucoma and permanent vision loss. *Diagnosis* is based on the health history and physical exam.

Common interventions

Medical treatment includes bed rest with both eyes patched, miotic drops to increase the absorption of blood, and cycloplegics to decrease the incidence of recurrent hemorrhage in the vessels of the iris. **Surgical** interventions include paracentesis of the anterior chamber and irrigation of the anterior chamber with fibrinolysin. (In general, the need for surgical intervention is a poor prognostic sign.)

Nursing interventions

Physical 1. Administer medications as ordered (eye medications, sedation to minimize movement and prevent further hemorrhage, and systemic medication to decrease intraocular pressure).

2. Elevate the head of the bed 30 degrees. This encourages blood to settle in the anterior chamber and may prevent the formation of synechiae (adhesions between the iris and adjacent structures).
3. Assess for elevated intraocular pressure (*see* section on acute glaucoma *below*).
4. Assess for recurrence of hemorrhage, evidenced by sudden pain, lethargy, or pain secondary to increased intraocular pressure.
5. Restrict activities for 4 to 5 days.
Psychosocial 6. Explain the need for rest and quiet.
7. Reassure realistically about future vision.
8. Explain all procedures to the patient.
9. Teach about prevention.
10. Explain the need for frequent evaluation by the physician.

Evaluation criteria. *See* Overview.

BLOW-OUT FRACTURE OF THE ORBIT

Fracture of the floor of the orbit is a fairly common result of blunt trauma to the eye. *Signs and symptoms* include (1) pain and nausea at the time of injury, (2) contusion and ecchymosis of the eye area, (3) diplopia on looking up or down, which may occur immediately or within a few days, (4) enophthalmos (backward displacement of the eye), (5) the affected eye's appearing lower than the normal eye, (6) limited movement of the eye, (7) crepitation (indicating fracture into a sinus), and (8) reduced sensation in the distribution of the maxillary branch of the trigeminal nerve on the cheek. A *complication* is loss of vision due to damage of the optic nerve. In addition to the history and physical exam, x-rays are used to make the *diagnosis*. **Surgical** reduction is required promptly.

Nursing interventions

Physical 1. Administer medications.
2. Assess for bleeding.
3. Allow diet and activity as tolerated.
Psychosocial 4. Reassure the patient about future vision and cosmetic effect.
5. Allow the patient to verbalize feelings about the accident.
6. Teach about appropriate preventions (e.g., use of seat belts).
7. Teach need for follow-up care.

Evaluation criteria. *See* Overview.

RETINAL DETACHMENT

Retinal detachment is separation of the sensory portion of the retina from the pigment epithelium of the choroid. This rare condition causes 1 in 10,000 persons/yr to develop a blind eye. It affects more men than women, most often after the age of 40. Usually occurring spontaneously, retinal detachment develops bilaterally in 10 to 25% of the spontaneous cases.

The primary cause is degenerative change resulting from aging. The mechanism of this change is as follows: the vitreous framework shrinks, the shrinkage pulls on the retina, forming a hole, and the fluid in front of the retina moves behind the retina. Some predisposing secondary factors are myopia (nearsightedness), aphakia (absence of the lens), and perforating or blunt trauma. Retinal detachment can also be the result of retinopathy from systemic disease (e.g., hypertension, diabetes mellitus, eclampsia, periarteritis nodosa, and chronic glomerulonephritis) or of vascular disturbances in the retina and choroid (e.g., retinal vein occlusion or choroidal carcinoma).

Retinal detachment may develop slowly or suddenly. The patient may complain of floaters (thickened particles that float within the vitreous cavity, caused by vitreous hemorrhage or thickened vitreous clumps and often described as spots, clumps, or a web). The patient may also complain of flashes, especially in the morning and when entering a darkened area. Flashes are caused by vitreous traction on the retina. (The traction stimulates the retina and is interpreted as light.) Retinal detachment causes a gradual, painless loss of vision. In areas where the retina is still attached, vision is normal. When the entire retina is detached, vision is poor, often allowing the patient only to count fingers; vision may often be worse. *Diagnosis* is based on the health history and physical exam, including a thorough examination of the eye with an ophthalmoscope after full pupil dilation.

Common interventions

The goal of preoperative **medical** treatment is to restrict eye movement by means of bed rest, sedation, patching of both eyes, and positioning in bed. To cause scar formation around the hole between the retina and choroid, the following **surgical** procedures may be used: photocoagulation (argon, ruby, krypton, or carbon dioxide lasers), diathermy, or cryothermy. To reattach the retina, scleral buckling may be used (which mechanically indents the globe, opposing the retina and choroid, and reduces vitreous traction on the retina). Circling procedures may also be used to reattach the retina. These procedures, which encircle the entire globe and indent it over the detachment, are often used to overlie and support the scleral implant.

Nursing interventions (preoperative)

Physical 1. Restrict eye movement by maintaining bed rest with bathroom privileges (decreases possibility of falling and enlarging detachment, in addition to decreasing stress on retina resulting from movement).

2. Administer eye medications (dilation by mydriatics and cycloplegics allows for examination of retina at any time and prevents iritis).

3. Apply bilateral eye patches if ordered (unilateral patches are not

useful because the eyes move simultaneously). The head of the bed can be raised for meals if the patches are in place.

4. Administer sedation, antibiotic eye drops, and preoperative medication as ordered.

Psychosocial 5. Allay anxiety and apprehension. (The patient has undergone an emergency admission on the day of diagnosis and has usually had some rapid loss of vision.)

6. Allow the patient to verbalize fears about loss of sight or blindness.

7. Reinforce the possibility of a favorable outcome. (Uncomplicated retinal detachment has a 70 to 90% chance of reattachment by a single operation; further procedures reattach another 6%; ~10% are cured; and ~5 to 10% develop new holes and problems.) If the prognosis is poor, however, do not instill false hope.

8. Orient the patient to hospital routines and procedures.

Educational 9. Inform the patient about what to expect on the day of surgery and in the postoperative period.

10. Teach deep-breathing exercises to prevent pulmonary complications.

11. Teach leg exercises to prevent thrombophlebitis and emboli.

Nursing interventions (postoperative)

Physical 1. Restrict eye movement by applying eye patches. (The operated eye is always patched for cleanliness and comfort. Bilateral patches, usually worn for 2 or 3 days, may be used to decrease eye movement and encourage the settlement of the retina against the choroid. They are not used if the retina is flat at the end of the procedure.)

2. Assist with activities of daily living.

3. Allow activity as ordered (bed rest with bathroom privileges beginning from day of surgery, if tolerated; provide assistance as needed.)

4. Provide a pillow under the head.

5. Elevate head of bed for meals as ordered (30 to 90 degrees).

6. Assist with ambulation, usually by 3rd postoperative day.

7. Administer analgesics as ordered: meperidine, 50 to 100 mg IM; acetaminophen with codeine No. 3, PO; or acetaminophen PO. The pain is often described as a frontal or temporal headache.

8. Administer antiemetics for nausea and vomiting.

9. Administer eye drops (cycloplegic, antibiotic, and anti-inflammatory).

10. Maintain the patient's head position if ordered (required for 4 to 5 days). This is done if air or solution was injected into the vitreous cavity to inflate a collapsed globe. The area needing flattening is positioned uppermost; a change of position is allowed as long as the head is parallel to the floor.

11. Assist with deep breathing and leg exercises.
12. Observe for complications (hemorrhagic choroidal detachment or retinal detachment).

Psychosocial 13. Reassure the patient that the presence of floaters is not a cause for alarm. (Preoperatively, poor vision prevented the patient from seeing them. Floaters usually disappear rapidly but may persist for years.)

14. Reassure the patient that the continuation of light flashes does not indicate that surgery was not successful. (It indicates that vitreous traction was not completely relieved by surgery. This condition requires close follow-up.)

Educational 15. Teach the need for and administration of eye medications.

16. Explain the need for and extent of activity limitations. The patient should avoid crowds (because of jostling), unfamiliar places (because of the possibility of falling), and reading (because it requires jerky, rapid eye movements).

17. Allow activities for self-care, watching TV (which requires straight-ahead vision), light housework, a return to sedentary work in 2 wk, and a return to normal physical activity in 6 wk.

18. Explain when to call the physician for emergency evaluation (sudden onset of many new floaters or progression of a visual field defect).

19. Stress the need for periodic examination of both retinas. The interval is determined by the condition of the vitreous and retina (usually q 6 to 12 mo).

Evaluation criteria.   *See* Overview.

INFLAMMATION/INFECTION

Blepharitis is a chronic infection of the glands and the lash follicles along the eyelid margins. A **sty** is an infected swelling near the eyelid margin. (A *chalazion* is an infection of a Meibomian gland; a *hordeolum* is an infection of the glands of Moll or Zeis.) **Conjunctivitis** is hyperemia of the conjunctiva. **Keratitis** is an inflammation of the cornea. **Uveitis** is an inflammation of the uveal tract.

These infections and inflammations are common and may be caused by local infection (viruses, bacteria, granulomatous inflammation, parasites, fungi, rickettsiae, allergy, or pediculosis), granulomatous infections (such as TB, leprosy, syphilis, allergy, and collagen diseases, especially rheumatoid arthritis), trauma (foreign bodies, chemicals, or other irritants), poor nutrition, or poor hygiene. Some causes remain unknown.

The local *signs and symptms* may be bilateral or unilateral and include pruritus, pain, burning, "tired" eyes, lid edema, and conjunctivitis. **Blepharitis** is *characterized* by scales (hard, tenacious, and difficult to remove if staphylococcal; greasy and easy to remove if seborrheic; nits on lashes if due to pediculosis), sensitivity to light, sticky, crusty eyelids on awakening, and occasional ulcers along the eyelid margin. Mixed types of blepharitis are common. **Conjunctivitis** is *characterized* by a purulent discharge that becomes worse at night and by preauricular lymph node involvement. The vision is generally not affected. A **sty** is *characterized* by a reddened, swollen eyelid, astigmatism, if the sty is very large, a hard, nonpainful lump pointing toward the conjunctival side of the eyelid, and an elevated red or red-yellow area on the conjunctival surface. **Keratitis** causes mild to severe pain. The vision is unaffected if the visual axis is not involved, and is markedly reduced if the central cornea is involved. Photophobia may be present if the inflammation is severe. **Uveitis** is *characterized* by blurred vision, floaters, visual defects, light flashes, a nonreactive pupil, an infected conjunctiva, moderate to severe eye pain, and sensitivity to light.

The *diagnosis* of these conditions is based on the health history, physical exam, and laboratory findings (culture and sensitivity, as well as microscopic examination of scrapings).

Common interventions
Medical
Blepharitis

1. If staphylococcal, treat with sulfonamide or antibiotic eye drops tid or qid, and topical or systemic antibiotics for skin infection.
2. If seborrheic, treat with an antifungal shampoo (scalp and eyebrows).
3. If a mixed type, treat the seborrhea first.
4. If due to pediculosis, remove nits and treat with ophthalmic physostigmine.

Sty and conjunctivitis

1. Treat with warm compresses and antibiotics or sulfonamide eye drops.
2. Systemic antibiotics may occasionally be necessary.
3. Remember that gonococcal conjunctivitis is an emergency; a delay in treatment may result in corneal ulceration or perforation.

Keratitis and corneal ulcers

1. Treat with specific topical antibiotics. (Therapy is begun as soon as cultures and smears are taken. Eye drops are administered hourly around the clock until the infection is under control.)
2. Treat with topical steroids. (Do not use if the causative agent is herpes, unless an antiviral agent is administered concomitantly.)

Uveitis

1. Treat with mydriatics to rest the eye and prevent the formation of posterior synechiae.

2. Treat with corticosteroids to reduce inflammation (eye drops, systemic corticosteroids, and subconjunctival or retrobulbar injections).
3. Prescribe analgesics (aspirin, acetaminophen, or propoxyphene).
4. Treat associated systemic disease.

Surgical
Sty

1. Incision and curettage.
2. Excision of cyst.

Corneal ulcer with fungal infection

1. Debridement.

Nursing interventions

Physical 1. Apply warm compresses and administer medications as ordered.
2. If blepharitis is present, use olive oil or hydrogen peroxide to soften and free crusts.
3. If pediculosis is found, assess the family and contacts.
4. If pediculosis or gonorrhea is found, notify local health authorities.
5. Bathe the eye as needed.
6. Assess the condition of the eyes.
Psychosocial 7. Encourage completion of the course of medication (to prevent recurrence and complications).
8. If conjunctivitis is present, encourage the patient to avoid contact with others. (The discharge is contagious.)
9. Inform the patient that early treatment prevents recurrence or complications.
10. Reassure the patient that if the treatment is followed, the condition should resolve without complications.
Educational 11. Teach the patient the signs and symptoms.
12. Teach the patient how to remove scales and crusts.
13. Teach the patient how to administer medication and apply warm compresses.
14. Stress the importance of personal hygiene (e.g., hand washing and not rubbing the eyes) and of a well-balanced diet.

Evaluation criteria. *See* Overview.

DIABETIC RETINOPATHY

Diabetic retinopathy refers to retinal abnormalities resulting from impaired carbohydrate metabolism. It may be proliferative or nonproliferative. Diabetic retinopathy, the second largest cause of blindness in the

USA, occurs ~20 yr after the onset of diabetes, despite the apparent control of the disease. It is related to the duration of the disease rather than to its severity: its incidence is increasing because of the lengthened life-span of diabetics. Its etiology, which is not well understood, involves vascular impairment due to abnormal carbohydrate metabolism.

The *signs* of diabetic retinopathy are (1) changes in vision (loss of vision ranging from mild reduction to perception of light only to blindness, reduced visual field, and sudden change in refractive error); (2) extraocular muscle palsy; (3) unexplained cataract or retinopathy; and (4) local changes. Nonproliferative local changes include neovascularization or fibrosis that is elevated or on the surface of the retina. Proliferative local changes include neovascularization and/or fibrosis, microaneurysms, blot hemorrhages, retinal edema, vitreous hemorrhage, and traction retinal detachment. The *diagnosis* includes the health history, physical exam, and laboratory tests. The absence of glycosuria and a normal fasting blood glucose level do not exclude diabetes. A further work-up may be necessary in the presence of local findings.

Common interventions

There is no need for **medical** treatment, except by control of diabetes. **Surgical** treatment may involve argon laser photocoagulation if changes in vision are present. This procedure, which can be performed on an outpatient basis, results in a 50% reduction in the rate at which blindness occurs, but it also compromises the visual field to some degree.

Nursing interventions

    Physical 1. Refer to nursing interventions for diabetes mellitus (*see* Chapter 22) and rehabilitation of the visually handicapped (*see above*).

    2. Administer medications and assist the patient with activities of daily living as needed.

    Psychosocial 3. Do not confront the patient with regard to denial. This state of shock and denial will usually persist until the patient is legally blind or close to it.

    4. Allow for the expression of anger and depression. Grieving over blindness involves coming to terms with future complications and death because 22% of diabetics die within 5 yr of being declared legally blind, and 62% die within 7 to 9 yr.

    5. Allow the patient to verbalize guilt about causing his or her own blindness. (There is no correlation between compliance and the progression of retinopathy.)

    6. During adjustment to disability, allow for value changes (e.g., from suicidal thoughts to hopefulness and realistic determination).

7. Provide support if the patient leaves the hospital with less vision than on admission.
8. For other psychosocial and educational interventions, *see* section on rehabilitation of the visually handicapped, *above*.

Educational 9. Assess the patient's knowledge of diabetes mellitus.

10. Teach care related to diabetics with a visual handicap: modify technique for drawing up and injecting insulin, obtain syringes that can be set to a prescribed dosage or make a template, provide the opportunity for practice.

Evaluation criteria.   *See* Overview.

GLAUCOMA

Glaucoma is a condition in which intraocular pressure becomes high enough to cause structural or functional damage. The three main types of glaucoma are adult primary, secondary, and congenital. (Congenital glaucoma, which is rare, will not be discussed.)

Adult primary glaucoma may be *open-angle* (chronic, wide-angle, or simple) or *closed-angle* (narrow-angle, acute, or congestive). Adult open-angle glaucoma causes 15% of the cases of blindness in the USA. It affects 1 to 2% of persons over age 40, and accounts for at least 90% of the cases of primary glaucoma. It also affects more women than men. Adult closed-angle (acute) glaucoma is relatively rare.

Open-angle glaucoma has a hereditary basis (multifactorial and autosomal recessive trait) and results from a loss of trabecular permeability. *Closed-angle glaucoma* results from the bundling up of the iris in the periphery of the anterior chamber, preventing aqueous access to angle structures. It is precipitated by dilation of the pupil, emotional upsets, and darkness.

Open-angle glaucoma causes no *symptoms* until vision is lost because of optic atrophy. The loss of vision is gradual, irreversible, and usually painless, although there may be occasional slight aching around the eyes. *Closed-angle glaucoma* is an emergency condition. Its *symptoms* are severe pain (localized to the eye initially, radiating to any part of the head later), nausea and vomiting, blurred vision and rainbow-colored halos around lights (both caused by corneal edema), extreme hardness of the eye, red eye, and a moderately dilated pupil that is nonreactive to light. Closed-angle glaucoma is usually unilateral and may result in permanent blindness within a few days if left untreated.

The *diagnosis* is based on (1) a health history, especially a family history of glaucoma, blindness, or serious visual loss and a past history of frequent, unsatisfactory changes in glasses, and (2) the physical exam, which reveals increased intraocular pressure as measured by tonometry. (Finger tension is not reliable in simple glaucoma, even when performed by an expert.) The ophthalmoscopic examination reveals cupping and atrophy of the disc when damage has occurred.

Common interventions

Medical (open-angle glaucoma)

1. Medical interventions are the treatment of choice. They involve the use of miotics (pilocarpine 1 to 4%), carbonic anhydrase inhibitors (acetazolamide [Diamox]), epinephrine eye drops, and timolol (Timotic) eye drops.

Surgical (open-angle glaucoma)

1. Surgical procedures, performed when optic and visual field changes progress even with maximum medical therapy, include trabeculectomy, cyclodialysis (separation of the ciliary body from the sclera to form an exit for the aqueous humor), and cyclodiathermy or cyclocryothermy.

Medical (closed-angle glaucoma)

1. Miotics (pilocarpine 4% may be instilled q 5 to 10 min until the pupil is constricted).
2. Osmotic drugs (mannitol or urea IV and glycerol PO).
3. Carbonic anhydrase inhibitors (administered in two to four times the usual dose).
4. Meperidine to control pain.
5. Although the reduction of intraocular pressure usually occurs within 4 to 6 hr, emergency surgery is indicated if the pressure remains high.

Surgical (closed-angle glaucoma)

1. Peripheral iridectomy is required for effective treatment. (Surgery may be deferred for a day until the eye is less inflamed if the medical regimen is successful in reducing pressure.)
2. Prophylactic peripheral iridectomy is recommended for the other eye because of a high incidence of an attack occurring in the other eye within a few years.
3. An argon laser may be used to make a small hole in the iris through the intact cornea. This procedure requires no anesthesia or hospitalization.

Nursing interventions (preoperative)

Physical 1. Administer glaucoma medication as ordered. (Use the medication that the patient has if there is a delay in obtaining a new supply from the pharmacy.)
2. Administer preoperative medication.

Nursing interventions (postoperative)

Physical 1. Administer eye drops as ordered. Miotic eye drops are used to maintain control of glaucoma in the unoperated eye. They are used in the operated eye for ~4 days postoperatively. (Miosis in the operated eye may not always be done.) After this time, mydriatic eye drops are used to prevent the formation of posterior synechiae.

2. Administer carbonic anhydrase inhibitors, if needed for the unoperated eye (not needed for the operated eye).
3. Administer codeine with aspirin or acetaminophen for the control of pain.
4. Administer an antiemetic for the control of nausea and vomiting.
5. Allow activity as tolerated (e.g., bathroom privileges on the day of surgery).
6. Tell the patient not to lie on the operated side.
7. Allow diet as tolerated.

Psychosocial 8. Discuss the fear of blindness with the patient. (Sight that is lost will not be regained because of damage to the optic nerve. Further loss of sight can be avoided by faithfully following the prescribed regimen.)

9. Discuss the impact of having a chronic condition. (Group sessions may be helpful.)
10. Include significant others in these discussions.

Educational 11. Teach the need for and administration of medications (eye drops and carbonic anhydrase inhibitors).

12. Teach about living with pupillary constriction (e.g., the increased difficulty of seeing at dusk or dawn, and the planning of activities, such as reading or traveling in unfamiliar areas, for when appropriate light will be available).
13. Stress the need for periodic examinations, and emphasize when to call the physician.
14. Teach the need for yearly tonometric examinations for family members over age 30 in order to ensure early detection.

Evaluation criteria. See Overview.

Secondary glaucoma, which accounts for 30% of all glaucoma, results from ocular disease other than a developmental abnormality: (1) inflammation, such as active iritis or cyclitis, (2) mechanical blockage, such as swelling of the lens or cataracts, (3) dislocation of the lens into the anterior chamber, (4) dislocation of the lens into the pupil, (5) trauma causing hemorrhage in the anterior chamber (glaucoma may develop immediately or years later), and (6) intraocular tumors. (For *signs and symptoms* and *diagnosis, see* adult primary glaucoma.)

Common interventions

Medical interventions are aimed at correction of the underlying cause. Secondary glaucoma is treated as simple glaucoma if the angle is open and as narrow-angle glaucoma if the angle is closed. **Surgical** interventions are the same as for open- or closed-angle glaucoma. **Nursing** interventions are the same as for adult primary glaucoma.

CATARACT

A cataract is an opacity of the lens caused by a degenerative process. **Senile** cataracts are common. **Traumatic** cataracts are the second most common kind. Cataracts due to **intraocular disease** are fairly common. **Congenital, developmental,** and **endocrine** cataracts are rare. Although cataracts occur frequently at all ages past 40, some degree of cataract is expected in all people >70 yr. It rarely occurs, however, in persons aged 20 to 30 yr.

The etiology of senile cataract is unknown, but changes in metabolism within the lens may be responsible. A congenital cataract is a hereditary condition whose enzymatic cause is unknown. It is associated with galactosemia, rubella, Down's syndrome, Werner's syndrome, and Lowe's syndrome. A developmental cataract is due to the failure of the lens fibers to remain transparent. A traumatic cataract is usually due to a metallic foreign body in the eye, but may also be caused by other foreign objects, heat (glassblower's cataract), or radiation. An endocrine cataract results from diabetes mellitus or hypoparathyroidism. Cataracts due to intraocular disease result from chronic or recurrent uveitis, glaucoma, retinitis pigmentosa, or retinal detachment.

Symptoms include a slow loss of vision that generally affects both eyes (often, one eye is worse than the other) and a change in vision: (1) an unpleasant glare in bright light due to the scattering of light within the eye; (2) progressive nearsightedness; and (3) distortions of sight or double vision due to an irregular clouding of the vision.

In addition to the health history and physical exam, the *diagnosis* of cataract is made by examination of the eye with an ophthalmoscope, loupe, or slit lamp, which reveals lens edema, protein alteration, necrosis, and disruption of the normal continuity of lens fibers.

Common interventions

There is no **medical** treatment at present. The most common **surgical** procedure and the treatment of choice is intracapsular cataract extraction, which involves removing the entire lens with the intact capsule. Another procedure is extracapsular extraction, which is used for some types of congenital and traumatic cataract. The anterior portion of the capsule is ruptured and removed, and the lens cortex and nucleus are expressed. The posterior capsule of the lens is left in the eye. The phacoemulsification procedure uses ultrasound waves the break up the lens and suction to remove the fragments. A fourth procedure, intraocular lens implant, may be performed after all of the above procedures. The implant may be an anterior chamber lens or an iris plane lens. Implants are performed with almost half of the cataract removal procedures in the USA. Most cataract surgery is performed under local anesthesia.

Nursing interventions (preoperative)

Physical 1. Administer eye medications as ordered: antibiotic eye drops instilled on morning of surgery, and "dilating series" as ordered (cycloplegic and mydriatic).

2. Administer preoperative sedation IM ~1½ hr before surgery: 100 mg secobarbital, 25 mg promethazine hydrochloride, and 50 mg meperidine.

Psychosocial 3. Orient the patient to surroundings and hospital routine.

4. Reassure the patient that surgery will improve vision.

Educational 5. Teach activity restrictions and eye care (*see below*).

Nursing interventions

Physical 1. Administer eye medications: mydriatic drops to dilate the pupil and keep it at rest, antibiotic ointment or drops to prevent infection, and steroid drops to reduce inflammation.

2. Administer analgesics: meperidine IM during initial postoperative period, then codeine with aspirin or acetaminophen.

3. Cleanse the eyelids.

4. Protect the eye from trauma: provide glasses or a shield during the day, and provide a shield at night.

5. Allow activity as tolerated (assist the patient to bathroom after recovery from anesthesia, allow the patient to lie on back or on unoperated side, elevate head or provide pillows as desired, and ambulate on 1st postoperative day).

6. Provide diet as tolerated (usually, regular diet by dinner if surgery takes place in the morning).

7. Observe for intraocular complications and report them immediately: increased intraocular pressure (assess for vomiting and for change in discomfort/pain); hyphema (assess for sudden sharp pain and for visible blood in a dependent position of the anterior chamber); prolapse of the iris or wound rupture (assess for bulging of the wound and for a pear-shaped iris); endophthalmitis; and vitreous loss.

Psychosocial 8. Reassure the patient that it will take several weeks to adjust to the new glasses (usually, 2 mo).

9. Teach the patient to begin using glasses only when sitting, to look through the center of the glasses (turning the head when looking to the side), and to practice activities with assistance until familiar with the perception of spatial relationships.

10. Inform the patient that plastic cataract eyeglass lenses are available and are lighter and more comfortable than glass lenses.

Educational 11. Teach the need for and administration of eye drops.

12. Advise the patient with regard to limitations of activity (avoiding heavy lifting and straining at stool, bending the knees to pick up objects from the floor , discussing with a physician the resumption of sexual activity, moving slowly and carefully for 3 to 4 wk, and avoiding falls).

Evaluation criteria. *See* Overview.

BLINDNESS

Blindness is the inability to perceive even light. (Legal blindness is vision with corrected eyeglasses of <20/200, or a visual field of <20 degrees in the better eye.) There are 28 million blind people in the world, 500,000 of them in the USA. Each year, ~50,000 Americans become blind.

Blindness may be congenital or acquired. It may develop suddenly or slowly at any time during life. Outside the USA, common causes of blindness are trachoma (chronic infection of the conjunctiva and cornea), onchocerciasis (roundworm infection of the eyes), and xerophthalmia (dryness and thickening of the conjunctiva and cornea caused by vitamin A deficiency). In the USA, common causes are glaucoma, diabetic retinopathy, and senile macular degeneration. Rarer causes in the USA are herpes simplex keratitis, cataracts, and retinal detachment. *Diagnosis* is based on the health history and physical exam. At present, there is no treatment for blindness. The development of artificial vision with the use of computers is being researched. For nursing interventions, refer to the section on rehabilitation of the visually handicapped (*see above*).

EXOPHTHALMOS (PROPTOSIS)

Exophthalmos is a displacement of the eyeball that makes it appear to bulge forward. It may be bi- or unilateral; it most commonly occurs with Graves' disease.

Exophthalmos may result from systemic disorders such as (1) hyperthyroidism (Graves' disease), which may result in thyrotoxic or thyrotrophic ("malignant") exophthalmos, (2) Paget's disease of the bone, and (3) leukemia or lymphoma. Other causes include inflammatory disorders (e.g., cellulitis, lacrimal gland inflammation, and cavernous sinus thrombosis); vascular disorders (e.g., spontaneous hemorrhage, aneurysms, and varicosities); various forms of trauma (e.g., fractures, emphysema [air from the sinus enters the orbit due to a rupture in the medial orbital wall], and hemorrhage); primary tumors of the eye or orbit (e.g., rhabdomyosarcoma, hemangioma, or dermoid tumors); metastatic tumors or those from surrounding structures (e.g., neuroblastoma, sinus carcinoma, or intra-cranial meningioma); and cysts (e.g., congenital dermoid cyst, parasitic cyst, or a mucocele from the sinuses).

Exophthalmos is *characterized* by the bulging of one or both eyeballs. If the condition is bilateral, the bulging may be more marked on one side. The change in position of the eyeball causes (1) dissociation of ocular movement, (2) diplopia, (3) infrequent blinking, and (4) pain as a result of extreme ocular swelling and irritation of the cornea due to inadequate protection by the eyelids. Lid lag is also a *sign* of exophthalmos: (1) lid closure lags behind, or does not follow, the descent of the eye when the patient is looking down; (2) lid closure occurs in jerky, stepwise movements. Lid retraction is almost pathognomonic of thyroid disease. The upper lid is elevated, and the sclera above the cornea is conspicuously exposed. (The presence of lid retraction excludes tumor as the etiology.) The *symptoms* of exophthalmos depend on the etiology: pain (when due to trauma), fever (when due to infection), paresis of the muscles supplied by the 3rd, 4th, and 6th cranial nerves (when due to cavernous sinus thrombosis), and con-junctival redness and edema (when due to cellulitis).

In addition to the health history and physical exam, the *diagnosis* is based on exophthalmometer readings, which demonstrate the antero-posterior distance between the lateral orbital rim and the corneal apex, as well as the difference in this distance between the two eyes. (The normal distance is 12 to 20 mm, and the normal difference between the two eyes does not exceed 2.5 mm.) The identification of cause involves assessing for thyroid disorder, x-ray (for fracture or tumor), CAT scan, culture and sensitivity, and biopsy.

Common interventions

The goal of **medical** treatment is to correct the underlying cause. Local treatment is provided as appropriate. Thyrotoxic exophthalmos is greatly improved when thyroid disease is controlled. Thyrotrophic exophthalmos is treated with corticosteroids (systemic, retrobulbar [behind the eye], and subconjunctival). **Surgical** interventions include a lateral tarsorrhaphy (narrowing the width of the palpebral fissure) to correct lid retraction, and Krönlein's operation to decompress the orbit, if vision is threatened.

Nursing interventions

Physical 1. Administer systemic medications, eye drops, and oint-ments as ordered.

2. Apply warm or cold compresses as ordered.

Psychosocial 3. Reassure the patient that appearance will improve when the underlying cause is treated.

4. Reassure the patient that surgery, if required, will improve ap-pearance.

Evaluation criteria.   See Overview.

EAR

OVERVIEW

The ear participates in the senses of hearing and position. Hearing is the appreciation of sounds. The sense of position includes orientation in space and movement of the body through space, which requires balance and equilibrium. Two common problems of the ear are deafness and vertigo.

Deafness is not an obvious disability and often goes unrecognized. It may, however, cause more serious emotional disabilities than blindness. The deaf are often ridiculed and treated with impatience. The hard-of-hearing and the deaf often feel that people are talking about them and may be depressed and insecure. The inability to hear may cause disorientation and suicidal depression.

Vertigo, a severe whirling sensation in which the individual or the environment seems to spin, may be produced by disturbances of the CNS or of the ocular, proprioceptive (muscle reflex), and vestibular systems. A reasonable degree of steadiness is retained if two of the three mechanisms for maintenance of equilibrium (vision, proprioception from muscles, and labyrinth function) are retained. Vertigo is not fatal but can cause serious, if not fatal, accidents. It can be mild or incapacitating, and it requires great adjustment in daily life.

Anatomy and physiology review

See Table 13-7 for the structures and functions of the ear; *see* Figure 13-2 for the anatomy of the ear.

General assessment

The **health history** includes the *past health history* of general, systemic diseases and of ear disease, as well as a *review of systems* that focuses on problems associated with the ear (vertigo, dizziness, nausea, and vomiting). The **physical examination** includes the following procedures: (1) assess the external ear for lesions, lumps, and inflammation (do this carefully and gently to prevent pain and bleeding); (2) tip the patient's head sideways (toward the opposite shoulder) in order to look into the ear; (3) straighten the canal by pulling the auricle upward and backward and the tragus forward; (4) inspect the canal and tympanic membrane with an aural speculum, otoscope, or an operating microscope; (5) assess general hearing (whisper, spoken voice, etc.); and (6) assess for vertigo and dizziness. **Laboratory tests** include (1) audiometry for quantitative hearing, (2) specialized tests for specific hearing difficulties, (3) a glycerol test for Ménière's disease, (4) x-rays, and (5) CAT scans.

Common interventions

Medical interventions involve the use of drugs (e.g., antibiotics, analgesics, vasodilators, antiemetics, and antihistamines) and hearing aids.

TABLE 13-7

Structures and Functions of the Ear

Structure and components	Function
Auricle (external ear)	Receives sound waves and directs them to middle ear.
External auditory canal (cartilaginous tissue with sebaceous glands, ceruminous glands, and hair follicles)	Protects ear.
Tympanic membrane	Divides external and middle ear, vibrates when reached by sound waves, and initiates vibration of ossicles of inner ear.
Middle ear	

Ossicles
    Malleus ("hammer")
    Incus ("anvil")
    Stapes ("stirrup")
	Amplify sound waves and transmit sound to inner ear.

Oval window	Transmits sound to inner ear.
Eustachian tube	Equalizes pressure.
Mastoid air cells	Form part of temporal bone.
Inner ear	

Vestibule
    Utricle
    Saccule
	Receptors for position of head in relation to gravity.

Cochlea (contains organ of Corti)	Receptor end organ of hearing.
Semicircular canals (contain sensory organs for equilibrium)	Receptor end organs for equilibrium.
Acoustic (8th cranial) nerve	
Cochlear nerve	Connects cochlea to brain.
Vestibular nerve	Connects semicircular canals, saccule, and utricle with brain.

Surgical interventions include myringotomy, myringoplasty, and stapedectomy.

Nursing interventions

Physical 1. Administer local/systemic medications as ordered.
  2. Irrigate the ear as ordered.
  3. Clean the ear for surgery if ordered.
  4. Position the patient as ordered postoperatively (operated ear up to protect grafts or operated ear down to encourage drainage, and head of bed flat or gatched 30 degrees).
  5. Assist the patient with vertigo and nausea by helping the patient maintain the position ordered, keeping the side rails up, assisting the patient with moving, avoiding jarring the patient or bed, and administering medications such as dimenhydrinate (Dramamine).

Altered Functioning of the Head and Neck 275

6. Provide nourishment as ordered (liquid or light diet).
7. Observe for and report postoperative complications such as infection (elevated temperature, drainage, and headache), changes in hearing, tinnitus, vertigo, nystagmus, disturbance of gait, bleeding (reinforce dressing as needed, do not disturb inner ear dressing), and injury to the facial nerve.
8. Provide eye care if the facial nerve is injured. (Assess for the ability to frown, wrinkle the forehead, pucker the lips, and bare the teeth.)

Psychosocial 9. Assist the patient to cope with hearing loss. (Speak normally, but ascertain that the patient follows the conversation.)
10. Reassure the patient that postoperative nausea and vertigo are temporary effects of the trauma and edema caused by surgery.
11. Encourage the hearing impaired to obtain professional diagnosis and treatment.

Educational 12. As preventive measures, teach the patient to clean the ears only with a wet washcloth over a finger (articles smaller than a finger can cause puncture of the tympanic membrane or scratches on the skin, which can lead to infection), have a physician remove foreign bodies, protect the ears from contaminated water by plugging them with petrolatum-soaked cotton or by wearing a bathing cap (especially if there is a history of ear infections or perforated eardrum), blow the nose with both nostrils and the mouth open during acute respiratory infections, avoid flying during an acute respiratory infection (if flying is necessary, take drying agents, such as antihistamines, or equalize pressure by chewing gum or swallowing), take no medications during pregnancy except those specifically prescribed by a physician, report any noticeable

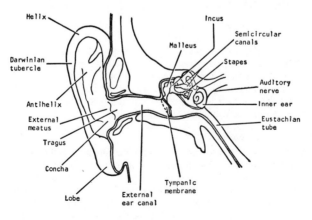

Figure 13-2. Cross section of the ear.

hearing loss to a physician, have ears pierced only under sterile conditions and follow directions in caring for newly pierced ears, and wear appropriate protective ear devices at work as needed.

13. As part of preoperative teaching, instruct the patient to reduce attacks of vertigo by slowing movements; to expect that hearing may not improve for several weeks postoperatively because of edema, dressings, and packings; to not blow the nose, sneeze, or cough postperatively; to learn deep-breathing exercises; to not touch the ear or the dressing; and to minimize vertigo and nausea by maintaining the ordered position, avoiding contraindicated activities and movements, moving slowly, and avoiding sudden movements.

14. As part of postoperative teaching, instruct the patient to avoid getting the ear wet from showering, shampooing the hair, or swimming; to avoid contact with persons with acute respiratory infections; to avoid bending, lifting heavy objects, and flying until permitted by the physician; to protect the external ear from burns, injury from hair dryers, shower, and elastic in caps if sensation is lost postoperatively; and to keep follow-up appointments with the physician.

Evaluation criteria

The patient is assessed for changes in status, receives medications and treatments on time, verbalizes signs and symptoms and importance of treatment, participates in self-care, and keeps follow-up appointments. Complications are avoided.

OBSTRUCTION OF THE EAR CANAL

Obstruction occurs when the ear canal is blocked by an object. It may be caused by (1) impacted cerumen (earwax), due to a narrow ear canal or excessive secretion of cerumen, or (2) a foreign body (insects, beans, peas, beads, toys, etc.). The *symptoms* of obstruction are pain (if the object is deep in the ear canal), conductive hearing loss, buzzing or a sensation of movement (if caused by an insect), and visualization of the foreign body. The *complications* are inflammation and/or infection. *Diagnosis* is based on the health history and physical exam.

Common interventions

Medical treatment for impacted cerumen involves softening the hard wax and removing it with irrigation or a cerumen spoon. For an insect caught in the ear, a few drops of mineral oil, olive oil, or 70% alcohol solution are instilled in the ear to kill the insect, which is then removed with forceps or a cerumen spoon. Before wet paper is removed, it should be allowed to dry. Vegetables should be irrigated with 70% alcohol solution to shrink them before removal. (Water should not be used because it makes vegetable matter expand.) Large, firmly embedded objects may require **surgical** removal under general anesthesia.

Nursing interventions

Physical 1. Instill ear drops and irrigate the ear canal as ordered.

Psychosocial 2. Reassure the patient that accumulated earwax is not a sign of uncleanliness.

Educational 3. Teach the patient not to put objects in the ears, how to clean ears, and how to instill softening agents as ordered.

4. Reinforce the need for follow-up visits to the physician for removal of cerumen.

Evaluation criteria. *See* Overview.

EXTERNAL OTITIS

External otitis is an inflammatory disorder of the auricle and external auditory canal. It is a common condition, especially in the summer (swimmer's ear), and it may be acute or chronic. Predisposing factors include moisture in the ear as a result of the climate or swimming; injury due to foreign objects, cleaning the ear with cotton swabs, or scratches as a result of itching; seborrheic and allergic dermatitis; and (in its severe, chronic form) diabetes mellitus, hypothyroidism, and nephritis. External otitis may be caused by bacteria (staphylococcal and gram-negative rods) or fungi (*Aspergillus* and *Mucor*).

Local *signs and symptoms* include moderate to severe pain, scales, crusts, pustules, erythema, edema, watery or purulent discharge (may be foul-smelling), and hearing loss. Systemic signs and symptoms include fever and adenopathy. *Diagnosis* is based on the health history, physical exam, and culture of drainage.

Common interventions

1. For acute otitis externa, relieve pain by applying heat and administering analgesics (aspirin, acetaminophen, or codeine).
2. Treat infection with antibiotics (given systemically and/or by ear drops with or without hydrocortisone).
3. For chronic otitis externa, remove debris and clean the ear.
4. Treat infection with antibiotic ear drops, antibiotic ointment or cream, or exfoliative, antipruritic ointment.
5. For mild chronic otitis externa, the patient should apply antibiotic ear drops once or twice a week and wear earplugs for showering, shampooing, and swimming.

Nursing interventions

Physical 1. Monitor vital signs.
2. Assess and record aural drainage.

3. Remove debris and clean the ear.
4. Apply heat (heat lamp; warm, moist compresses; or heating pad).
5. Administer medications.

Evaluation criteria.   *See* Overview.

OTITIS MEDIA

Otitis media is a common inflammation of the middle ear. Acute suppurative otitis media, occurs most frequently in children during the winter.

Serous otitis media may be acute or chronic. Causes include obstruction of the eustachian tube, prolonged accumulation of fluid in the middle ear, allergic reaction, or sudden pressure changes (e.g., rapid descent when flying if the person has an upper respiratory infection, or rapid underwater ascent when scuba diving). *Suppurative (purulent) otitis media* may also be acute or chronic. Pneumococci, beta-hemolytic streptococci, and *Haemophilus influenzae* are the most frequent causes. (Viruses and mycoplasmas have not been proven to cause it.) Other causes include infection that spreads from the nose and nasopharynx through the eustachian tube, perforated eardrum, infected material forced into the middle ear by improper blowing of the nose, and a condition that allows contaminated water to enter the middle ear while swimming. The chronic form may result from inadequate treatment of the acute form or from resistant strains of bacteria.

Serous otitis media is *characterized* by (1) a full, plugged feeling in the ear, (2) a conductive hearing loss that may be severe, (3) popping or clicking sounds when moving the jaw or swallowing, and (4) an echo when speaking. It may, however, also be asymptomatic. *Acute suppurative otitis media,* which may be asymptomatic, is usually *characterized* by the following local signs and symptoms: severe, deep, throbbing ear pain; a red, bulging tympanic membrane; purulent drainage, if the tympanic membrane ruptures; and a conductive hearing loss (usually mild). The systemic *signs and symptoms* include an upper respiratory infection and a mild to very high fever. *Chronic suppurative otitis media* is marked by a recurrent, painless discharge (foul-smelling or nearly odorless) from the ear and by hearing loss. (Pain or vertigo indicates impending complications.) The *complications* of otitis media include (1) a conductive hearing loss due to tympanic membrane destruction or ossicular destruction, (2) abscesses (intracranial, subperiosteal, or epidural), (3) cholesteatoma (a cystlike mass consisting of squamous epithelium), (4) meningitis, (5) suppurative labyrinthitis, (6) facial muscle paralysis, (7) sigmoid sinus or jugular vein thrombosis, and (8) mastoiditis.

In addition to the health history and physical exam, the following laboratory tests are used to make the *diagnosis:* for *acute suppurative otitis media,* an elevated WBC and, if drainage is present, culture and sensitivity;

for *chronic suppurative otitis media,* audiologic evaluation and mastoid x-rays.

Common interventions

For **serous otitis media, medical** treatment involves the use of nasal decongestants for at least 2 wk (sometimes indefinitely) and antihistamines if the cause is allergy. Other treatments include inflation of the eustachian tube and removal of fluid by needle aspiration. **Surgical** treatment involves myringotomy and aspiration of fluid with the insertion of a polyethylene tube.

For **suppurative otitis media, medical** treatment involves the use of systemic antibiotics; nasal decongestants (systemic and local); codeine, aspirin, and acetaminophen for pain; and aspirin and acetaminophen for fever. The patient is maintained on bed rest, local heat is used to speed up resolution, and local cold is used to decrease pain. **Surgical** treatment involves a myringotomy if purulent material is present and under pressure and if symptoms continue with the treatment (pain, fever, vertigo, and hearing loss).

For **chronic suppurative otitis media, medical** treatment involves the maintenance of a patent eustachian tube and ear canal by careful cleansing of the ear and removal of granulation tissue. Treatment may also involve the use of antibiotic and corticosteroid ear drops and systemic antibiotics (if the organism is known or if acute infection occurs). **Surgical** interventions may include mastoidectomy, excision of the cholesteatoma, myringoplasty, or tympanoplasty.

Nursing interventions

1. Same *physical* and *psychosocial* interventions as for external otitis.
Educational 2. Teach the importance of completing the course of antibiotics prescribed and of caring for upper respiratory infections.
3. Teach the correct use of decongestants.

Evaluation criteria.   *See* Overview.

MENIERE'S DISEASE

Ménière's disease is a disorder of the labyrinth. It is relatively common, affects slightly more men than women, and usually occurs between the ages of 40 and 50 yr. Its etiology is unknown, but it seems to be related to a dysfunction of the ANS, resulting in temporary vasoconstriction of the inner ear.

The *signs and symptoms* of an acute attack, which begins suddenly and lasts from 10 min to 3 hr, are (1) severe vertigo with loss of balance (usually, the patient must lie down or fall, and he or she staggers if there is an attempt to walk) and space disorientation (surroundings whirl wildly), (2) tinnitus, (3) hearing loss (sensorineural, usually unilateral, onset with first attack, progressive, rarely total, and usually permanent), and (4) the patient assumes a characteristic posture to help decrease the symptoms: lying on the unaffected ear and looking in the direction of the affected ear.

In addition to the health history and physical exam, the *diagnosis* is based on certain laboratory tests: (1) caloric testing for abnormal vestibular functioning, (2) electronystagmography (ENG), and (3) audiometric tests, which identify poor speech discrimination and sensorineural hearing loss.

Common interventions

For an acute attack, **medical** treatment involves bed rest and the following drugs: atropine sulfate SC, diazepam IV, Innovar IV or droperidol, and antiemetics. For long-term management, the following drugs are prescribed: antihistamines, drugs for motion sickness (dimenhydrinate, cyclizine, and meclizine), niacin, vasodilating agents, autonomic blocking agents, diuretics, and sedatives or hypnotics. The following interventions should be made with regard to diet: (1) low salt to prevent fluid retention (although the value of this has not been established), (2) diet therapy to control obesity and metabolic disorders, and (3) food allergies should be ascertained. The patient should be urged to discontinue smoking in order to avoid vasospasm and vasoconstriction. Ablation of the inner ear or labyrinth is a **surgical** procedure performed on patients who have incapacitating vertigo and have been unsuccessfully treated for 2 yr. This procedure, which is performed only if the disease is unilateral, leaves the patient with a deaf ear.

Nursing interventions

Physical 1. Provide a quiet, safe environment during an attack (keep the side rails up, provide assistance when the patient is out of bed, and keep the call bell within the patient's easy reach).
   2. Administer medications as ordered.
   3. Administer care in a calm manner (avoid bumping into or jarring the bed).
   4. Record intake and output if the patient is vomiting, and record the character of the emesis.
   5. Provide small amounts of fluids frequently.
Psychosocial 6. Provide emotional support (acute attacks are frustrating).
Educational 7. Teach the patient about the need for medication, the nature of the disease, and the rationale of treatment.
   8. Teach the patient that slow movement and position changes help to decrease the symptoms.
   9. Teach the patient about activity limitations (and the need for them) and about any modifications in the diet.
   10. Explain diagnostic tests.

Evaluation criteria.   *See* Overview.

OTOSCLEROSIS

Otosclerosis is a bony disorder of the otic capsule. It is the most common cause is conductive deafness. Its incidence is estimated at 1% in the white population (rarer among Asians and blacks), and 60% of patients have a family history. Bilateral involvement occurs in 75 to 85% of the cases. Otosclerosis is more common in women than in men. It may be transmitted by a monohybrid autosomal dominant gene with a 25 to 40% penetrance (genetic effect) or by an autosomal recessive gene. The early stage of otosclerosis is characterized by bone resorption and loose, spongy bone. The later stage is characterized by fewer vascular spaces and the re-deposition of bone. The *signs and symptoms* of otosclerosis are a gradual, progressive hearing loss, tinnitus, and a normal tympanic membrane. The *diagnosis* is based on the health history, physical exam, audiometric testing, and a tuning fork test (which demonstrates bone conduction lasting longer than air conduction). There is no **medical** treatment. The **surgical** treatment is stapedectomy.

Nursing interventions

Physical 1. Protect the graft: position the patient flat, with the operated ear up, and maintain bed rest as ordered.

2. Administer meperidine, 100 mg IM (usually only 1 or 2 injections required) and antibiotics to prevent infection.

3. Assess the ear canal for drainage (change the cotton in the canal as necessary, do not change the packing next to the eardrum, and avoid wetting the dressing).

Psychosocial 4. Explain that hearing will be decreased because of postoperative edema and packing.

Educational 5. Instruct the patient to avoid blowing the nose for 1 wk to prevent forcing air into the eustachian tubes, thereby loosening the eardrum and contaminating the operative site.

6. Instruct the patient to avoid loud noises and pressure changes until healing is complete (usually 6 mo).

7. Teach the patient how to change the dressing, which involves gently placing a piece of cotton in the meatus (*not* the ear canal). The cotton should be changed once or twice a day.

8. Teach the importance of completing the full course of prescribed antibiotics.

9. Teach the importance of keeping the follow-up appointment.

Evaluation criteria.   *See* Overview.

HEARING LOSS

Hearing loss refers to the inability to perceive sound. An estimated 13.2 million persons in the USA have impaired hearing in one or both ears, and 6.4 million of these have bilateral hearing loss, of whom >50% are age 65 yr or older. Hearing loss occurs more frequently in men than in women.

Congenital/neonatal hearing loss may be transmitted genetically or it may result from trauma, toxicity, or infection during pregnancy and delivery. **Sudden deafness** is a medical emergency that may be due to (1) *acute infections* (mumps, measles, influenza, and adenoviruses may cause viral endolymphatic labyrinthitis-type deafness; herpes zoster may cause viral neuronitis and ganglionitis; an active upper respiratory infection is present in 25% of patients), (2) *arteriosclerosis* secondary to aging, hypertension, diabetes, or hyperlipemia, (3) *blood dyscrasias* (accelerated coagulation, polycythemia vera, or macroglobulinemia), (4) *neurologic disorders* (multiple sclerosis or neurosyphilis), and (5) *lesions of the temporal bone* (acoustic neuroma, tumor, oval- or round-window fistula, or aneurysm of the anterior inferior cerebellar artery). **Noise-induced hearing loss** results from cochlear damage caused by exposure to noise levels of >85 to 90 decibels over a long period of time. (High-intensity music, such as rock music, will produce a temporary threshold shift.) **Presbycusis** may be due to sensory, neural, metabolic, or mechanical causes. The *sensory* form involves atrophy of the organ of Corti and of the auditory nerve in the basal end of the cochlea. This process begins in middle age and is slowly progressive. *Neural* presbycusis involves the loss of ganglion cells and the degeneration of nerve fibers. It occurs late in life. The *metabolic* form is due to atrophy of the stria, and the *mechanical* form may result from the stiffening of the basilar membrane.

Signs and symptms include loss of the perception of some or all sound frequencies, inability to understand the spoken word, and tinnitus. (Other symptoms depend on the etiology.)

The health history, physical exam, audiologic testing, x-rays, and scans are used in the *diagnosis* of hearing loss.

Common interventions

Medical treatment of sudden deafness must begin as soon as possible. It is ineffective when started 2 to 3 wk after onset. Treatment involves the use of steroids, vasodilators, IV histamine, anticoagulants, low molecular weight dextran, and urografin. A hearing aid is prescribed for patients with presbycusis. (Hearing aids are of no use for patients with noise-induced loss of hearing.) For the removal of tumors, the following **surgical** approaches may be used: middle cranial fossa, translabyrinthine, or posterior cranial fossa.

Nursing interventions

Physical 1. Refer to nursing interventions for otosclerosis (*see above*).
Psychosocial 2. Encourage the hearing impaired to obtain professional diagnosis and treatment.
3. Inform personnel of the patient's handicap.
4. Ascertain that the patient understands the tests and procedures.

5. Position the patient so that he or she gains as much information as possible from visual cues.
6. Speak slowly and distinctly, but do not shout.
7. If the patient can lip-read, stand directly in front of the patient and speak slowly and distinctly.
8. Gain the patient's attention by raising your hand or waving. (Touching may startle the patient.)
9. Refer the patient for rehabilitation as needed.

Educational 10. Teach the patient how the hearing aid works and how to maintain it.

Evaluation criteria.   *See* Overview.

NOSE

OVERVIEW

In addition to its important role in respiration, the nose is the organ of smell. It also participates in the production of speech and the sense of taste. Smell enhances the taste of foods and stimulates the appetite. The nose is an obvious organ and has an important influence on one's body image. Distortions of the nose, whether congenital or acquired, minor or major, can cause a great deal of unhappiness, psychic pain, or profound emotional disturbance.

Anatomy and physiology review

The nose consists of bones, the nasal processes of maxillary bones, a bony and cartilaginous septum, and cartilage. It opens posteriorly into the nasopharynx, and receives its size and shape from the nasal bones and cartilages. The **anterior nose** (1) is lined with skin that gives rise to vibrissae (nasal hairs), (2) extends posteriorly to meet the respiratory mucous membrane, (3) has ciliated mucosa, which moves mucus and other foreign materal, and (4) lies inferior to the olfactory epithelium (the end organ for the sense of smell). The nose has pH of 7.0, and it secretes nasal lysozyme, which is most active in a slightly acidic environment. (Alkaline or very acidic nose drops restrain lysozyme and ciliary action.) The nose functions best when the humidity is 45 to 55% and when the temperature is 21°C (70°F). It secretes 1,000 ml of fluid in 24 hr.

The nose has four major **functions**: (1) it serves as a passageway for air in respiration, (2) it warms, humidifies, and filters air during inspiration, (3) it serves as the organ of smell and aids in the sense of taste, and (4) it aids in phonation by amplifying sound and altering the timbre of the voice. The **paranasal sinuses** consist of cavities located in the frontal, sphenoid, ethmoid, and maxillary bones, and of mucous membrane lining. The **functions** of sinuses are to give resonance to the voice, to condition inspired air, and to lighten the weight of the skull.

General assessment

The **health history** includes current health status, the individual history, and a review of systems. The determination of *current health status* should include questions regarding the use of tobacco, alcohol, and drugs (prescribed, over-the-counter, or illegal, e.g., cocaine). The *past health history* should focus on acute or chronic infections and allergic reactions, trauma, and systemic disease (e.g., hypertension or pituitary tumors). The *review of systems* should focus on problems associated with the nose and ear: pain, discharges, changes in hearing, vertigo, and tinnitus. The **physical examination** should include an assessment of the external nose (symmetry, edema, erythema, tumors, and lumps). The nasal chambers are assessed anteriorly with a nasal speculum; a postnasal mirror is used for the nasopharynx. The mucous membrane is checked for pallor, redness, and edema. Mucous plugs and discharge are checked for color, consistency, amount, and odor. It may be necessary to shrink the nasal mucosa. Topical vasoconstrictors include ephedrine and cocaine. The paranasal sinuses are assessed by inspection and palpation of overlying tissues, location of purulent secretions in the nose, and transillumination of the maxillary and frontal sinuses. **Diagnostic tests** include nose and throat cultures, a WBC, and x-rays of the nose and sinus.

Common interventions

Medical interventions include the use of nasal packing, drugs (antibiotics, antihistamines, vasoconstrictor nose drops, analgesics, and antipyretics), forcing fluids, humidification, nasal irrigation, and bed rest in Fowler's position to facilitate drainage. **Surgical** interventions are usually performed under local anesthesia (aspiration, irrigation, correction of deformities, reconstruction, and removal of polyps and tumors).

Nursing interventions

Physical 1. Maintain a patent airway by suctioning as necessary and by positioning to facilitate drainage (e.g., Fowler's position).
2. Monitor vital signs (take rectal temperature, report temperature elevations, and assess for hypo- or hypertension).
3. Administer medications.
4. Perform nasal irrigation (not commonly ordered).
5. Provide adequate fluids and appropriate diet.
6. Provide oral hygiene and apply a lubricant/moisturizer to the lips.
7. Provide humidity.
8. Care for nasal packs.
9. Apply hot or cold packs.
Psychosocial 10. Explain all procedures and treatments.
11. Encourage diversions while the patient is on bed rest.
12. Encourage an adequate intake of fluids.
13. Explain the postoperative reactions that may be expected (dis-

coloration around the eyes, edema in the operative area, bleeding, and tarry stool due to the swallowing of blood).

14. Explain that time is needed for appearance to return to normal: 1 to 2 wk are needed for ecchymosis around the eyes to resolve; 4 to 6 wk are needed for edema to resolve after rhinoplasty.

Educational 15. Teach about the need to complete the course of antibiotics, use nose drops only as directed, and get adequate amounts of fluids, nutrition, rest, and humidity (use of humidifiers in winter and avoidance of air conditioning in summer).

16. Teach the patient preoperatively about the use of local anesthesia (pain not felt, but feeling of pressure), the necessity of breathing through the mouth postoperatively, the presence of nasal packs, and the necessity to expectorate secretions and to not blow the nose.

17. Instruct the patient about the need for follow-up care and about symptoms that require the attention of a physician.

Evaluation criteria

The patient is assessed for changes in status, has a patent airway, receives adequate nutrition, receives medications and treatments on time, verbalizes signs and symptoms and the importance of treatment, participates in self-care, and keeps follow-up appointments. Complications are avoided.

NASAL PACKING

Nasal packing is a procedure in which the nasal cavity is packed with gauze in order to control bleeding.

Nursing interventions

Physical 1. Assess the patient's condition during insertion of packs (make the patient comfortable in a seated position, which prevents gagging and choking on the blood in the pharynx; monitor vital signs as needed; lower the patient's head if the patient feels faint; and protect from injury if the patient faints).

2. Prevent packs from slipping and obstructing the airway (tape a string from the nasal pack to the patient's face; assess the position of the nasal pack frequently; keep scissors, a flashlight, and a hemostat at the bedside in case of emergency; and make sure that the call light is available and working and that the patient knows how to use it in case of emergency).

3. Assess the patient's status frequently.

4. Take rectal temperatures (the patient is unable to keep the mouth closed around an oral thermometer).

5. Report all temperature elevations to the physician (a slight temperature elevation is expected).

6. Assess for and report any ear symptoms (packing may obstruct the eustachian tube and cause otitis media).

7. Keep the patient comfortable by assessing position of the packing and reporting any displacement to the physician, administering sedation as ordered, and providing a liquid diet as long as the packing is in place (chewing and swallowing cause discomfort).
8. Change the gauze under the nose as needed.
9. Provide mouth care.
10. Use a moisturizer on the patient's lips to minimize dryness from mouth breathing.
11. Assist with removal of the packs by placing the patient in Fowler's position in bed, tying a towel around the neck, holding an emesis basis under the chin, and assessing condition (the patient may feel faint).

Psychosocial 12. Allay fear and anxiety by telling the patient to breathe through the mouth.
13. Reassure the patient that the difficulty in swallowing will be relieved as soon as the packing is removed.
14. Reassure the patient that the packing is lubricated and that removal will not be painful.
15. Explain that there may be minimal bleeding when the packing is removed.

Educational 16. Instruct the patient to expectorate the blood that accumulates in the nasopharnyx.
17. Instruct the patient to avoid blowing the nose or lifting for 1 to 2 wk.
18. Instruct about the need for follow-up care.

Evaluation criteria.   *See* Overview. Packing remains in place.

SUBMUCOUS RESECTION

Submucous resection (SMR) is the removal of cartilage or bone that lies between the mucous membrane and the perichondrium of the nasal septum. (It is usually performed under local anesthesia, and nasal packs are inserted.) Its purpose is to equalize the size of the right and left nasal cavities in order to prevent airway obstruction.

Nursing interventions

Physical 1. Refer to nursing interventions for nasal packing (*see above*).
2. Reduce pain by administering analgesics (meperidine 100 mg or morphine 10 mg IM for one or two doses) and by providing ice packs.
3. Prevent edema and encourage drainage (semi-Fowler's position, cool-mist vaporizer, and ice packs).
4. Change the dressing as needed (two to three times postoperatively).
5. Assess frequently for signs of hemorrhage: blood at the back of the

throat (examine with a flashlight), soaking blood on the nasal packing and mustache dressing, hemoptysis or hematemesis, frequent swallowing, belching, and systemic signs of hemorrhage (tachycardia, tachypnea, hypotension, etc.).

6. Provide a liquid diet on the day of surgery, regular diet afterward.

Psychosocial 7. Explain that edema and black eyes will resolve in 1 to 2 wk.

Educational 8. Instruct that blowing the nose must be avoided after the nasal packing is removed.

9. Instruct about limiting activity for 2 to 3 days postoperatively.

10. Instruct the patient to avoid smoking in the postoperative period.

Evaluation criteria. *See* nasal packing *above.*

RHINOPLASTY

Rhinoplasty is the reconstruction of the external nose. It involves sawing and/or chiseling the nasal bones, dividing and shortening cartilage, and possible implantation of silicon material. Rhinoplasty is usually performed under local anesthesia; bilateral nasal packs may or may not be used. It provides cosmetic repair of the nose for congenital or acquired deformity (disease or trauma) or for psychologic reasons.

Nursing interventions

Physical 1. Refer to nursing interventions for nasal packing and SMR (*see above*).

2. Provide IV fluids initially and PO fluids as tolerated.

3. Provide lubricant or moisturizer for the lips.

4. Administer medications: antiemetics (may be needed initially), analgesics, and antibiotics.

5. Do not alter dressings.

Psychosocial 6. Assess the patient's expectation of surgery and assist the patient in developing realistic expectations of surgery.

Educational 7. Instruct the patient to avoid removing or picking at the dressing.

8. Instruct the patient about the importance of keeping follow-up appointments.

9. Instruct the patient about the application of splints that may be used after discharge.

Evaluation criteria. *See* Overview. Patient verbalizes realistic expectations of surgery.

FRACTURE

A fracture of the nasal bones is the most common facial fracture and is often associated with other facial fractures. It may be caused by minor injuries such as falls or being struck by a ball, or it may result from severe trauma (car accidents or fights). With minor injuries, there is no displacement of the nose or nasal obstruction. With serious nasal fractures, there may be external deformity, nasal obstruction, other trauma to the face, copious bleeding (from the nostrils and back into the nasopharynx), and edema around the nose. Inadequate or delayed treatment may cause the *complications* of permanent nasal displacement, septal deviation, or obstruction. *Diagnosis* is based on the health history, physical exam, and x-ray. For minor injury, no treatment is necessary. (Often, the individual does not consult a physician.) For serious nasal fracture, the treatment consists of reduction of the fracture. (The use and choice of anesthesia depends on the kind of fracture.)

Nursing interventions (prereduction care)

Physical 1. Maintain a patent airway.
2. Apply ice packs to minimize edema.
3. Assess bleeding (control anterior bleeding with gentle, local pressure; posterior bleeding is rare and requires packs).
4. Assess for and report clear fluid drainage, which may be CSF.
Psychosocial 5. Encourage the patient to relax by breathing slowly through the mouth. (As edema increases, breathing becomes more difficult.)
6. Reassure the patient that ecchymosis will fade after ~1 wk.
7. Instruct the patient to avoid blowing the nose.
8. Instruct the patient that local anesthesia will prevent pain during the procedure, but that pressure will be felt.

Nursing interventions (postreduction care)

Physical 1. Refer to nursing interventions for nasal packing (*see above*).
2. Make sure that the external splint is applied correctly and that it does not cause undue pressure.
3. Administer analgesics and antibiotics as ordered.

Evaluation criteria. See nasal packing. Nasal splint applied correctly.

EPISTAXIS

Epistaxis (nosebleed) is of common incidence. Its most frequent cause is trauma (fractured nose, nose picking, fractured skull and middle third of the face, or foreign body), though it may also result from inflammatory processes (acute and chronic rhinitis and sinusitis), neoplastic disease, circulatory disease (hypertension or enlarged adenoids causing pressure to blood vessels), or septal deformity. In addition to nasal hemorrhage, the *symptoms* of epistaxis may include nausea and vomiting secondary to swallowing blood. Its *complications* may include hypotension and shock. *Diagnosis* is based on the health history, physical exam, and, if bleeding is severe, an Hct and Hb.

Common interventions
Medical

1. Treat the patient in a seated position (unless the patient is hypotensive).
2. Suction clots and blood from the nose.
3. Find the bleeding point and stop the bleeding by applying pressure, applying epinephrine or ephedrine packs, applying petrolatum gauze packs, or cauterizing with chemocautery (silver nitrate stick) or electrocautery.
4. Encourage bed rest (sedatives or morphine).
5. Transfuse the patient if necessary.
6. Severe epistaxis may require postnasal packing or surgery.

Surgical

1. Ligation of appropriate artery, SMR, or cryotherapy.

Nursing interventions

Physical 1. Refer to nursing interventions for nasal packing (*see above*).
2. Have the patient remain seated (unless the patient is hypotensive).
3. Apply pressure by pinching the nostrils.
4. Monitor vital signs.
5. Protect the patient's clothing.
Educational 6. Instruct the patient about techniques for stopping bleeding, indications of airway obstruction, and how to remove the packing if airway obstruction occurs. (Patients with postnasal packs are usually admitted to the hospital; those with anterior nosebleeds are seldom admitted.)
7. Teach the necessity of follow-up care.
8. Teach preventive measures: instruct the patient not to pick the nose or insert foreign objects into it, and provide information about the use of a humidifier and of water-soluble lubricants or nasal sprays in very dry environments.

Evaluation criteria.   *See* Overview and nasal packing.

RHINITIS

Rhinitis, a very common condition, is an acute or chronic inflammation of the mucous membrane of the nose. *Acute simple rhinitis* (coryza or the common cold) may be caused by rhino-, adeno-, or coxsackieviruses, or by ECHO or influenza viruses. *Allergic rhinitis* (frequently called hay fever) is caused by an allergen. The cause of *nonallergic vasomotor rhinitis* is unknown, although it may be due to (1) an unstable ANS, which allows the engorgement of the nasal mucosa and the overproduction of nasal mucus, (2) stress, or (3) some endocrine disturbances. *Rhinitis medicamentosa* is caused by the overuse of nose drops, resulting in a rebound swelling of the nasal mucosa. The *symptoms* of *acute simple rhinitis* are burning and irritation in the nasopharynx, sneezing, chills, malaise, muscle aches, mild fever, headache, copious nasal discharge (which may become purulent), and nasal obstruction. The *symptoms* of *allergic rhinitis* are sneezing; nasal obstruction; tearing of eyes; nasal discharge; frontal headache; itching of the eyes and nose; pale, edematous turbinates; and smooth, glistening nasal mucosa. The *symptoms* of *nonallergic vasomotor rhinitis* are chronic, intermittent nasal obstruction; nasal discharge; bluish, swollen nasal mucosa; and engorged turbinates. The *symptoms* of *rhinitis medicamentosa* are nasal obstruction and edematous nasal mucosa. *Diagnosis* is based on the health history, physical exam, and identification of the allergen.

Common interventions

Medical (acute rhinitis)

1. Symptomatic treatment: bed rest; avoid chilling; force fluids; take diet as tolerated; warm, salt-water gargles; nose drops; and antihistamines.

Medical (allergic rhinitis)

1. Removal of the allergen, if possible.
2. Desensitization of the patient.
3. Antihistamines.

Medical (nonallergic vasomotor rhinitis)

1. Antihistamines.

Medical (rhinitis medicamentosa)

1. Stop use of nose drops.
2. Medications for initial period: sedative to allow sleep at night; and PO nasal decongestants (chlorpheniramine maleate).

Surgical (allergic rhinitis)

1. SMR of the septum or inferior turbinates.
2. Polypectomy, if polyps are present.

Surgical (nonallergic vasomotor rhinitis)

1. SMR.

Nursing interventions

Physical 1. Administer medications as ordered.
2. Provide fluids.
3. Provide adequate rest.

Psychosocial 4. Urge those with acute rhinitis to avoid contact with others for the first 2 to 3 days, when the condition is contagious.
5. Reassure those with acute rhinitis that the condition is self-limiting and that the symptoms usually disappear in 6 to 7 days.
6. Reassure patients with rhinitis medicamentosa that the symptoms will disappear in 2 to 3 wk and that they will be able to breathe through the nose without medication.

Educational 7. Teach the correct use of medications; administration and side effects (drowsiness and dry mouth).
8. Teach individuals to call a physician if there are complications to acute rhinitis: pneumonia, bronchitis, sinusitis, otitis media, temperature elevation, or symptoms that last longer than 1 wk.

Evaluation criteria. *See* Overview.

SINUSITIS

Sinusitis is an inflammation and/or infection in one or more of the paranasal sinuses. It is of common incidence and may be an acute or chronic condition. The predisposing factors are chronic nasal infections (from a deviated nasal septum, nasal polyps, or edema of the turbinates) and excessive nose blowing during acute rhinitis. Causes include bacteria, viruses (less frequent), abscessed teeth, or tooth extraction.

Symptoms include pain (severe, constant headache and pressure over the region of the infected sinus), nasal obstruction and congestion, purulent discharge if the duct is open, cough and sore throat, postnasal drip, orbital edema or swelling over the sinuses, malaise, anorexia, nausea, fever (usually low-grade, but may reach 40°C [104°F] if the sinus is completely obstructed and the infection is severe), red and swollen mucosa, and pus in the nasal cavity or nasopharynx.

Diagnosis is based on the health history, physical exam, CBC (leukocytosis may be present), x-rays of the sinuses, and transillumination (the sinus will be opaque).

Common interventions

Medical (acute sinusitis)

1. Relieve pain by prescribing analgesics (aspirin, acetaminophen, codeine, meperidine, or morphine) and by the use of a heat lamp or hot, moist packs.
2. Drain the sinuses by ensuring an adequate fluid intake, the inhalation of warm, moist air, and the prescription of medications (nose drops to constrict the vessels and reduce hyperemia, and mucolytic agents).

3. Control infection by the use of broad-spectrum antibiotics.
4. Provide symptomatic relief with oral antihistamines early in the course of the treatment.

Medical (chronic sinusitis)

1. Repeated lavage of the sinuses.

Surgical (chronic sinusitis)

1. Correction of nasal deformities.
2. Removal of diseased mucous membrane.
3. Enlargement (or creation) of sinus openings to improve drainage.

Nursing interventions

Physical 1. Relieve pain by administering medications and applying heat as ordered, and by elevating the head of the bed no more than 30 degrees.
2. Encourage drainage of the sinuses (provide and encourage fluids, keep the windows closed if a room vaporizer is used, and administer nose drops if ordered).
3. Control infection by administering antibiotics as ordered and by monitoring vital signs.
4. Encourage bed rest, mental rest, and adequate dietary intake to increase resistance to infection.
5. For postoperative care, refer to nursing interventions for nasal packing and SMR (*see above*).

Evaluation criteria.   *See* Overview and nasal packing.

DEVIATED SEPTUM

A deviated septum is a shift from the midline of the nasal septum. It is of common incidence — most adults have a septum that deviates — and it may be due to normal growth or to the trauma of falls, blows, or surgery. *Symptoms* include a crooked nose, nasal obstruction, sinusitis, headache, or epistaxis. The patient, however, may be asymptomatic. *Diagnosis* is based on the health history and physical exam. SMR is the **surgical** treatment. Refer to **nursing** interventions for nasal packing and SMR (*see above*).

MOUTH AND THROAT

OVERVIEW

The mouth (oral cavity) and throat (pharynx) have important roles in nutrition, respiration, and phonation. The oral cavity, which is easily examined, connects with the pharynx.

During infancy, the mouth is associated with food, which in turn is associated with sucking, warmth, love, and security. This association of survival with the pleasurable sensations of love, acceptance, and belonging continues throughout life. As a result, severe emotional reactions may occur when the functioning of the mouth is altered.

Anatomy and physiology review

Table 13-8 lists the **structures** and **functions** of the mouth and throat. The **digestive process** begins with chewing, which involves the movement of the mandible, lips, tongue, and cheeks. The teeth divide solids into small pieces and mix them with saliva. (The tongue and cheeks pass food back and forth between the teeth, thus facilitating the grinding and dividing of food.) The bolus of food is then assembled for swallowing and voluntarily propelled back to the isthmus of the pharynx. Protective mechanisms occur at the pharynx, and the bolus is moved reflexively. The tongue remains elevated and the lumen of the pharyngeal isthmus is reduced, thus creating a negative pressure in the pharynx and nasopharynx. The nasopharynx is closed off by elevation of the soft palate. The pharynx is elevated by muscle contraction. The epiglottis covers the glottis to protect the larynx. Simultaneous closure of the glottis protects the airway. The cervical esophagus opens, and breathing stops. The negative intrathoracic pressure that is created helps to distend the esophagus. The bolus is then moved by peristalsis through the esophagus.

General assessment

The **health history** includes current health status, the past health history, and a review of systems. The *current health status* should include questions regarding the use of tobacco, alcohol, and prescribed and nonprescribed drugs. The *past health history* should focus on acute or chronic infections and allergic reactions, and trauma. The *review of systems* should focus on pain, soreness, lesions, changes in taste, chewing difficulties, dysphagia, bleeding, altered voice, hoarseness, and dental status. **Laboratory data** should include culture and sensitivity, and a WBC. Other tests include x-rays of the jaw and teeth and nasopharyngoscopy.

Common interventions

Medical interventions include the prescribing of drugs (antibiotics, antihistamines, analgesics, and antipyretics) and of a fluid or mechanically soft diet as well as irrigation, humidification, and bed rest with positioning to promote drainage. **Surgical** interventions include aspiration, drainage, the correction of deformities, reconstruction, the removal of polyps or tumors, and radical neck dissection.

Nursing interventions

Physical 1. Maintain a patent airway by suctioning as necessary and positioning to facilitate drainage.

TABLE 13-8

Structures and Functions of the Mouth and Throat

Structure and components	Function
Tongue	Propels food from teeth to pharynx and produces intelligible speech.
Intrinsic muscles	Control shape of tongue.
Extrinsic muscles	Move tongue.
Cranial nerves	
Lingual branch of 5th	Gives sensation to anterior two-thirds of tongue.
Chorda tympani branch of 7th	Gives taste to anterior two-thirds of tongue.
Lingual branch of 9th	Gives taste and sensation to posterior third of tongue.
Superior laryngeal branch of 10th	Gives sensation to area near epiglottis.
Hypoglossal nerve (12th)	Mediates all motor activity.
Salivary glands	Prepare food for digestion.
Parotid (located below and in front of ear)	
Submaxillary (located in posterior floor of mouth)	
Sublingual (located in anterior floor of mouth, under tongue)	
Teeth	Prepare food for digestion.
Palate	
Hard palate (part of maxillary bone; covered with mucous membrane)	Forms roof of mouth.
Soft palate (continuous with posterior margin of hard palate; contains muscles)	Closes off nasal cavity during phonation of certain sounds and during swallowing.
Pharynx	Passageway for respiratory and digestive tracts; forms vowel sounds.
Nasopharynx (adenoid or pharyngeal tonsil is a lobulated mass of lymphoid tissue)	Is active in immune system.
Oropharynx	
Tonsils (masses of lymphatic tissue)	Are active in immune system.
Laryngopharynx (hypopharynx)	
Larynx	Produces sound, assists in determination of quality of voice, and assists in coughing.
Epiglottis	Covers glottis during swallowing, prevents aspiration, and assists visceral musculature by helping to increase intra-abdominal pressure (e.g., in defecation or childbirth).

   2. Monitor vital signs. (Take rectal temperature and report elevations to the physician.)
   3. Administer medications.
   4. Provide mouth care (frequent oral hygiene, lubricants, moisturizers, and humidity).
   5. Provide and encourage the intake of adequate fluids and an appropriate diet.
Psychosocial 6. Explain all procedures and treatments.
   7. Provide support to cope with fear, anger, and grief.
Educational 8. Teach the need for and the essentials of good oral hygiene and dental care.
   9. Teach the need for a well-balanced diet.
   10. Teach about medications and their side effects.

Evaluation criteria

A patent airway and adequate nutrition are maintained, complications are avoided, and the patient verbalizes the components of self-care and the need for follow-up care.

FRACTURED JAW

A fractured jaw is a break in one or both of the maxillae or in the mandible. It is fairly common and results from accidents or fights. The *symptoms* of **maxillary fractures** (LeFort III) are the forcing of structures inward, elongation of the face, malocclusion of the teeth, large amounts of edema, soft tissue trauma, associated injuries (nasal and orbital fractures and CNS trauma), and a compromised airway. The *symptoms* of **mandibular fractures** are malocclusion of the teeth, pain, abnormal mobility of the jaw with irregularity of the dental arch, edema, and ecchymosis. *Diagnosis* is based on the health history, physical exam, and x-rays.

Common interventions
Medical

   1. Relieve airway obstruction.
   2. Start IV with Ringer's lactate solution.
   3. Control hemorrhage by suctioning and packing.
   4. Apply ice packs to control swelling.
   5. Assess neurologic status.
   6. Assess and treat other injuries. (More serious injuries may be present, which should take precedence once airway patency has been established and hemorrhage has been controlled.)

Surgical (maxillary fracture)

   1. Surgical repair by a team of specialized physicians.

Surgical (uncomplicated maxillary fracture and mandibular fracture)
1. Surgery with interdental wiring. If teeth are not present, Kirschner's wires or a metal plate are used for fixation.

Nursing interventions

Physical 1. Maintain a patent airway.
2. Keep a wire cutter and scissors at the bedside.
3. Suction the mouth with a soft catheter (insert behind molars and through the natural space between teeth).
4. Place the patient in Fowler's position to promote venous and lymphatic drainage.
5. Monitor vital signs.
6. Assess oxygenation, including color of fingers and toes. (A dusky face may be due to venous congestion; restlessness and apprehension may be due to air hunger.)
7. Minimize the possibility of vomiting by administering antiemetics and by maintaining the functioning of the nasogastric tube.
8. Provide liquids. (Administer IV fluids until PO liquids are tolerated; provide clear liquids initially, then progress to a high-calorie, blenderized diet; administer by straw or cup.)
9. Administer analgesics and antibiotics as ordered.
10. Provide frequent oral hygiene: brush the exterior surfaces of the teeth; rinse and irrigate the mouth frequently; use water under pressure, if possible; and lubricate or moisturize the lips frequently.

Psychosocial 11. Assist the patient to cope with fear, anger, and grief.
12. Assist the patient to communicate by providing paper, pencils, and a Magic Slate, by encouraging the patient to speak slowly in order to increase the intelligibility of speech, and by encouraging listeners to be attentive.
13. Provide realistic reassurance about appearance and the possibilities of plastic surgery.
14. Reassure the patient that immobilization is usually required for only 4 to 5 wk.

Educational 15. Teach oral suctioning as soon as the patient is capable of learning it.
16. Instruct the patient about the need for oral hygiene and a balanced diet, and instruct significant others in the care required (suctioning, oral hygiene, and diet).

Evaluation criteria. *See* Overview. Communication is facilitated.

ORAL INFECTIONS

Stomatitis is an inflammation of the mouth; **glossitis** is an inflammation of the tongue; and **gingivitis** is an inflammation of the gums. These conditions which are of common incidence, may be caused by local infection: viruses, bacteria, yeasts, molds, fungus ("thrush," or *Candida albicans* overgrowth, due to the depression of normal bacterial flora by antibiotics), and spirochete and fusiform bacillis in symbiosis (Vincent's angina, thought to be brought on by poor oral hygiene, nutritional deficiencies, or systemic debilitating disease). Other causes of oral infections are systemic disease, mechanical trauma (jagged teeth, biting cheeks, or mouth breathing), chemical trauma (mouthwashes or dentifrices), and chemotherapy. The *symptoms* of oral infections are a sore mouth, excessive salivation, malodorous breath, and inflammation of the mouth. Thrush and Vincent's angina also affect the pharynx. In thrush, white patches of exudate may be seen over the pharynx, tonsils, and base of the tongue. Vincent's angina (trench mouth) is *characterized* by infected gums, a fetid odor, bad taste, and circumscribed ulcers of the tonsil with bleeding bases. *Diagnosis* is based on the health history and physical exam.

Common interventions

Medical treatment involves removal of the cause, frequent oral hygiene, a bland, soft diet, and appropriate medication (antibiotics and local antiinfectives).

Nursing interventions

Physical 1. Provide frequent oral hygiene.
2. Administer medications as ordered.
3. Provide appropriate diet and fluids.
4. Assess the condition of the mouth.
Psychosocial 5. Encourage completion of the course of medication.
Educational 6. Teach the need for good oral hygiene and dental care.
7. Teach proper care of the mouth and teeth (brushing and flossing the teeth).
8. Teach the need for a well-balanced diet.
9. Teach about the administration and side effects of medication.

Evaluation criteria. *See* Overview.

CANKER SORES

Canker sores (aphthous stomatitis) are ulcers of the mouth and lips. Although they are of common incidence, their cause is unknown. They may, however, be related to emotional stress, trauma, vitamin deficiency, allergy to food or drugs, endocrine disorders, or viral infections (sometimes considered to be a manifestation of herpes). *Diagnosis* is based on the health history, physical exam, and x-rays.

Common interventions

Medical treatment includes correction of the underlying cause and topical or systemic steroids (which may suppress recurrence). Refer to **nursing** interventions for oral infections (*see above*).

CARIES

Dental caries, or tooth decay, is a common condition that depends on the resistance of tooth enamel and on the particular nature of the plaque formed (the most important factor in the development of caries). Tooth decay is caused by bacteria contained in plaque and by the diet. (Carbohydrates, especially sucrose, increase cavity production.) The *symptoms* of caries are dental cavities and pain, especially when the teeth come into contact with extremes in temperature. *Diagnosis* is based on the health history, physical exam, and x-rays.

Common interventions

Medical treatment involves cleaning of teeth by dental professionals and filling of cavities by a dentist.

Nursing interventions

Physical 1. Provide frequent mouth care to patients unable to do so.
2. Provide an appropriate diet.
Psychosocial 3. Explain the need for good oral hygiene as part of promoting general good health.
Educational 4. Teach the correct method of brushing and flossing teeth.
5. Teach about diet: decreasing the frequency of eating, and cutting down on between-meal sweets, especially soft, sticky, adherent ones.
6. Urge the use of toothpastes that contain fluoride.
7. Teach the use of pressurized irrigation devices as recommended by a dentist.

Evaluation criteria. See Overview.

PAROTITIS

Parotitis is an inflammation of the salivary glands. It is of common incidence and may be suppurative or nonsuppurative. *Infectious or epidemic parotitis (mumps)* is caused by a virus. *Obstructive parotitis* results from recurrent obstruction caused by mucous plugs and partial stricture. *Suppurative parotitis* is caused by bacteria, usually *Staphylococcus aureus.* The predisposing factors are dehydration (especially postoperative), dry mouth, poor oral hygiene, and decreased salivation.

The *symptoms* of *mumps* include (1) prodromal symptoms that last 24 hr (myalgia, anorexia, malaise, headache, and low-grade fever), (2) earache that is aggravated by chewing, (3) tenderness and swelling of the parotid glands, (4) elevated temperature (38.3 to 40.0°C [101 to 104°F]), (5) possible swelling of other salivary glands, and (6) clear secretion from the glands. The *complications* of mumps are orchitis (20 to 30% of males after puberty), meningitis, encephalitis, and pancreatitis. The *symptoms* of *obstructive parotitis* are swelling of the gland and ropy secretions from the gland. The *symptoms* of *suppurative parotitis* are swelling, pain, and redness of the gland, as well as a moderate or high fever.*Diagnosis* is based on the health history, physical exam, and, for mumps, serologic antibody testing.

Common interventions

Medical treatment for mumps includes analgesics for pain, antipyretics for fever, and fluids to prevent dehydration from fever and anorexia. (IV fluid may be administered if the patient is unable to swallow.) For obstructive parotitis, the treatment consists of correcting the cause. Suppurative parotitis is treated with antibiotics, although the **surgical** intervention of incision and drainage may be required.

Nursing interventions

Physical 1. Administer medications as ordered.
2. Provide adequate fluids and diet. (Avoid spicy, irritating foods.)
3. Monitor vital signs, especially temperature.
4. Provide for oral hygiene.
5. Apply warm or cool compresses to relieve pain.
6. For mumps, isolate the patient, observe for complications, and report the case to the local public health authorities.
7. For suppurative parotitis, provide frequent oral hygiene with an antiseptic mouthwash, maintain adequate hydration, record intake and output accurately, provide PO fluids as allowed, maintain IV fluids, and stimulate parotid secretions by giving the patient hard candy to suck.

Psychosocial 8. Encourage bed rest and explain the need for isolation.
Educational 9. Explain the treatment.
10. Teach oral hygiene.
11. Teach preventive measures for mumps: routine immunization at age 15 mo; immunization within 24 hr of exposure may prevent or attenuate the disease; immunity lasts 9½ yr.

Evaluation criteria. *See* Overview.

TONSILLITIS

Tonsillitis, inflammation of the tonsils, is a a common condition that may be acute or chronic and is caused by bacteria. The *symptoms* of acute tonsillitis are sore throat, swollen anterior cervical lymph glands, fever, chills, anorexia, malaise, muscle pain, headache, enlarged, brightly inflamed tonsils, and exudate on the tonsils (yellow follicles if *Streptococcus* is the cause). The local *complications* of acute tonsillitis include chronic tonsillitis, acute otitis media, acute sinusitis, and abscesses. The systemic complications are pneumonia, nephritis, osteomyelitis, and rheumatic fever. The symptoms of chronic tonsillitis are recurrent sore throat, enlarged tonsils, and purulent material that may be expressed from the tonsil crypts with a wooden tongue blade. The *diagnosis* is based on the health history, physical exam, and the following tests: elevated WBC and culture and sensitivity.

Common interventions

Medical treatment includes bed rest, fluids, antibiotics, aspirin or acetaminophen, and codeine, 32 mg q 3 hr. **Surgical** treatment is a tonsillectomy, which is performed ≥4 wk after all symptoms subside. (Surgery is not performed during the acute stage.)

Nursing interventions (general)

Physical 1. Provide fluids and appropriate diet.

2. Administer medications.

Psychosocial 3. Encourage bed rest for 48 hr after the patient's temperature returns to normal.

Educational 4. Teach the need to complete the course of antibiotic.

5. Teach the need for follow-up care.

Nursing interventions (preoperative)

Psychosocial 1. Reduce anxiety by discussing what to expect intra- and postoperatively.

2. Tell the patient that ~1 wk of work will be missed because of sore throat.

Educational 3. Explain that local anesthesia is used for adults. (It prevents pain but not the sensation of pressure.)

4. Tell the patient to expect considerable throat pain and that medication will be administered as needed.

5. Tell the patient to expect some bleeding postoperatively.

Nursing interventions (postoperative)

Physical 1. Maintain a patent airway.

2. Prevent aspiration by placing the patient on his or her side.

3. Monitor vital signs; assess for hemorrhage and report tachycardia or hypotension immediately.

4. Give the patient water to drink when the gag reflex returns.

5. Provide nonirritating fluids.

6. Administer analgesics as needed.

7. Encourage deep breathing.

8. Ambulate the patient when he or she is ready.

Educational 9. Instruct the patient to report bleeding, ear discomfort, or any fever lasting >3 days.

10 Instruct the patient to avoid analgesics that contain aspirin.
11 Instruct the patient to keep follow-up appointments.

Evaluation criteria.   *See* Overview.

CANCER

The following are the major types of cancer of the head and neck. (They are all more common in men than in women.) The 1983 estimated incidence of oral cancer is 4% in men and 2% in women (or ~3% of all cancer). The estimated new cases for 1983 is 27,100. The tongue is the most common site of oral cancer. More than 90% of oral cancers are of the squamous cell type. There is a 2:1 male:female prevalence with occurrence in all ethnic groups. Squamous cell carcinoma of the **lip** constitutes 15% of malignant tumors of the mouth (2.2% of all cancers). Basal cell carcinoma of the lip is much less frequent. Cancers of the **oral cavity** (95% of which are squamous cell carcinomas) constitute 8% of all malignant tumors. The tonsils are the most common site for malignant tumors of the **oropharynx**. Cancer of the **nasopharynx** constitutes only 0.5% of all cancers, but it is a common tumor among Filipinos, Malays, and Chinese. Cancer of the **hypopharynx** accounts for ~4% of all cancers in men. It is three to four times as common as cancer of larynx. Cancer of the **nasal cavity** and **paranasal sinuses** constitutes ~1% of all malignancies. Cancer of the **mandible** is uncommon. Cancer of the **salivary glands** accounts for ~0.33% of all malignant tumors. (Women with malignant salivary gland tumors have a higher incidence of breast cancer.) Most tumors of the **neck** (80%) are metastatic from another site. Primary cervical tumors are those of the major salivary glands and lymphomas of the cervical lymph nodes. (For cancer of the **larynx**, *see below.*) Although the predisposing factors of most of these cancers are unknown, this is not the case for cancers of the lip and the oral cavity. Predisposing factors in cancer of the lip are (1) exposure to sunlight (one third of all patients have a history of working outdoors, and the highest occurrence rates are in Florida and Texas), (2) complexion (fair-skinned, blond, and blue-eyed people are more susceptible), and (3) smoking (including pipe smoking). The predisposing factors in cancer of the oral cavity are smoking, heavy intake of alcohol, poor oral hygiene, and syphilis.

The *signs and symptoms* of these cancers depend on the location of the lesion. Among the signs are (1) leukoplakia, with underlying microscopic changes (hyperplasia, keratosis, which possibly precedes malignancy, and dyskeratosis, which is likely to precede malignancy), (2) ulceration, (3) masses or lumps, (4) tenderness or sore throat, (5) enlarged cervical lymph nodes, (6) malodorous breath, (7) pain, nasal obstruction, and persistent nasal secretion, if the nasal cavity and the sinuses are involved, (8) painless, slow-growing nodules in the mouth, (9) bulging, asymmetrical sinuses, (10) hoarseness and dyspnea, (11) interference with swallowing, and (12) choking or aspiration. *Diagnosis* is based on the health history, physical exam, and the following laboratory tests: nasopharyngoscopy, radiography (arteriography, laminography, and x-rays), biopsy, vital dyes, and oral cavity exfoliative cytology.

Common interventions

Medical treatment includes chemotherapy, immunotherapy, and radiotherapy. **Surgical** interventions include radical neck dissection (the most commonly performed major operation for cancer of the head and neck), superficial resection of the parotid gland, V excision of carcinoma of the lip, and resection of the maxillary antrum.

Nursing interventions (general)

Physical 1. Decrease discomfort of dry mouth by encouraging the use of lozenges and gum and by providing fluids and a humidifier.
2. Promote good oral hygiene by encouraging the use of a soft toothbrush, dental floss, and mouthwashes, and by providing mouth irrigation with diluted hydrogen peroxide or normal saline.
3. Provide a nonspicy diet without temperature extremes.
4. Assess drooling after mouth or facial surgery: encourage more frequent swallowing, provide tissues and a bag in which to dispose of them, and notify the physician if severe drooling continues. (The patient may need plastic reconstruction of the oral structure.)

Psychosocial 5. Explain the expected benefits of the treatment.
6. Explain that talking will be difficult or impossible with implants.
7. Explain that alcohol and tobacco should be avoided.

Educational 8. Instruct the patient about diagnostic tests and treatment.
9. Instruct the patient to avoid moving suddenly if implants are in place.

Nursing interventions (postoperative: head and neck dissection)

Physical 1. Maintain a patent airway.
2. Monitor intake and output.
3. Administer IV fluids and medications.
4. Assess for respiratory distress.
5. Assess for carotid artery rupture. (The physician should inform the nursing staff of the probability of this complication. Emergency equipment at the bedside should include packing, a cuffed tracheostomy tube, an endotracheal tube, and IV solutions.)
6. In the event of carotid artery rupture, apply pressure and call for assistance. (The patient will die without immediate surgery.)
7. Assess for infection.
8. Assess for chylous fistula (milky drainage, especially after meals).
9. Make sure that the Hemovac is functioning (to prevent hematoma formation) by frequently assessing its functioning, by attaching the

Hemovac to constant suction if needed and ordered, and by emptying the suction container as needed. (Expect ~70 to 120 ml of serosanguineous drainage the 1st day, 30 to 50 ml the 2nd day, and 0 to 30 ml the 3rd day.)

10. Place the patient in Fowler's position, which decreases pressure on the skin flap, promotes drainage, and eases breathing.

Psychosocial 11. Assist the patient in accepting his or her changed body image.

12. Explain that exercises will strengthen the remaining muscles and make up for those removed during surgery.

Educational 13. Teach measures to reduce pain and aching from missing muscles (the use of liniment and the application of heat).

14. Teach exercises to be done when the wound is well healed.

15. Teach the necessity of follow-up care.

16. Instruct the patient to report any new lesions as soon as possible.

Evaluation criteria. *See* Overview. Patient and family participate in rehabilitative measures.

NECK

OVERVIEW

The **larynx** provides an airway between the pharynx and the trachea, and it also produces speech. Altered functioning of the larynx has significant physiologic and psychologic consequences.

Anatomy and physiology review

Table 13-9 lists the **structures** and **functions** of the neck. **Phonation** is produced by the vibration of the vocal cords, which causes oscillations of pressure in expired air. These oscillations are accentuated or suppressed by changing the resonating qualities of the throat and mouth. **Speech** is produced by a delicate coordination of the intrinsic and extrinsic muscles of the larynx with those of the pharynx, soft palate, lips, and tongue.

General assessment

The **health history** includes current health status, the past health history, and a review of systems. The *current health status* should include questions regarding the use of tobacco and alcohol. The *past health history* focuses on acute or chronic infections and allergic reactions. The *review of systems* focuses on problems of the neck: (1) hoarseness, which may be caused by improper approximation of the vocal cords, inflammation of the larynx, or laryngeal paralysis, should be carefully investigated if it persists for >2 wk; (2) cough; (3) dyspnea (expiration is easy, inspiration is difficult, and it should be noted that slowly developing obstructions are tolerated better than sudden obstructions); (4) stridor (usually inspiratory);

TABLE 13-9

Structures and Functions of the Neck

Structure	Function
Larynx	Provides airway between trachea and pharynx; prevents aspiration into trachea; triggers cough reflex when foreign body touches mucosa; produces speech.
Thyroid cartilage ("Adam's apple")	Protects false cords (horizontal folds of mucous membrane), true cords, and ventricles.
Cricoid ("ringlike") cartilage	Protects larynx.
Arytenoid cartilage	Opens and closes glottis; relaxes or increases tension in cords.
Hyoid bone	Suspends cartilaginous larynx; provides attachment to many muscles.
Recurrent laryngeal nerves	Provide motor innervation.
Superior laryngeal nerve	Provides sensory innervation; provides motor innervation to cricothyroid muscle.
Glottis (space between true cords)	Closes and protects lungs if foreign body enters larynx; allows movement of cords.
True cords	Assist in production of speech.
Lymphatic drainage system	Drains to lymph nodes in middle and upper cervical chains along jugular vein.

and (5) pain, which occurs early in inflammatory disorders and late in neoplastic disorders.

The **physical examination** involves (1) checking for the symptoms described above; (2) assessing respiratory status by ensuring airway patency and checking for signs of respiratory distress (tachypnea, tachycardia, restlessness, and circumoral or nail bed cyanosis); (3) assessing the throat for the presence of inflammation, leukoplakia, and irregularities of size and shape; and (4) palpating the neck for signs of enlarged lymph nodes. **Laboratory data** include culture and sensitivity and a WBC. X-rays (tomography and barium esophagrams) and direct or indirect laryngoscopy are other assessment tools.

Common interventions
    Medical interventions involve endotracheal intubation, drugs (antibiotics, corticosteroids, antipyretics, analgesics, and cough suppressants), diet (fluids and mechanical soft), humidification, and bed rest. **Surgical** interventions include tracheotomy, laryngectomy, and arytenoidectomy (excision of arytenoid cartilage). Refer to **nursing** interventions for the mouth and throat (*see above*).

LARYNGEAL EDEMA

Edema of the larynx is an emergency condition that causes a reduction in airway size. It is fairly common and may be acute or chronic. Acute laryngeal edema may result from anaphylaxis, allergy, acute laryngitis, direct injury to the larynx during intubation or surgery, or inflammatory conditions such as erysipelas and scarlet fever. The chronic condition may result from radiotherapy or tumors of the neck and from obstruction of the laryngeal lymphatics secondary to infection. The *signs and symptoms* of airway obstruction are dyspnea, stridor, cyanosis, and retraction of the soft tissues around the thoracic cage on inspiration. *Diagnosis* is based on the health history and physical exam.

Common interventions
    For acute allergic laryngeal edema, **medical** treatment includes administration of a corticosteroid, administration of epinephrine 1:1,000 SC, local application of ice, and insertion of an endotracheal tube. Other acute forms of the condition require insertion of an endotracheal tube. For chronic conditions, treatment involves administration of a local vasoconstrictor, administration of a local corticosteroid, and insertion of an endotracheal tube. **Surgical** treatment (tracheotomy) may be necessary in both acute and chronic laryngeal edema.

Nursing interventions
    Physical 1. Assess airway status.
    2. Monitor vital signs.
    3. Provide appropriate care for an intubated patient by maintaining tubal patency, by avoiding injury to surrounding tissues (provide humidity, deflate cuff as necessary, and use sterile technique), and by providing respiratory support as needed.
    Psychosocial 4. Explain care to the patient and significant others.
    5. Reassure the patient and significant others that the patient will be able to speak by blocking the lumen of the tracheostomy tube.
    6. Provide an alternative means of communication (e.g., writing pad and pen).
    Educational 7. Teach the patient how to suction, clean, and change the tracheostomy tube, if appropriate.

8. Teach the patient to avoid allergens.
9. Teach about signs, symptoms, and care, as appropriate.

Evaluation criteria. Patient is assessed for changes in status, receives adequate nutrition and hydration, receives medications and treatments on time, verbalizes signs and symptoms and importance of treatment, participates in rehabilitation and self-care, demonstrates adjustment to altered body image, and keeps follow-up appointments. Complications are avoided.

LARYNGITIS

Laryngitis is an inflammation of the vocal cords. It is of common incidence and it may be acute or chronic. It may be caused by a bacterial or viral infection, excessive use of the voice, inhalation of smoke or noxious fumes, aspiration of chemicals, or coughing. The acute local *symptoms* are hoarseness (mild or involving loss of voice), pain, and laryngeal edema. The systemic symptoms are fear, cough, malaise, and the symptoms of an upper or lower respiratory tract infection. The symptoms of chronic laryngitis are persistent hoarseness, frequent cough, voice fatigue, and a tired, aching throat. *Diagnosis* is based on the health history, physical exam, and indirect laryngoscopy, which demonstrates reddened and inflamed vocal cords. Exudate may be present.

Common interventions

Medical interventions involve voice rest, antibiotics if the cause is bacterial, analgesics and throat lozenges for pain relief, elimination of the underlying cause, and hospitalization if warranted. **Surgical** interventions include a tracheotomy if airway obstruction occurs.

Nursing interventions

Physical 1. Encourage the patient to rest the voice: post a sign over the bed stating that the patient is to rest the voice and refrain from speaking; provide other means of communication (pad and pencil or Magic Slate); anticipate the patient's needs; and post a note stating that the patient cannot use the intercom.
2. Administer medications as ordered (antibiotics, analgesics, throat lozenges, and cough syrup with codeine if the cough is dry).
3. Alleviate throat discomfort by providing humidity and administering aerosol therapy.
Psychosocial 4. Explain the need for rest to the patient and significant others.
5. Encourage the patient to avoid smoking.
Educational 6. Teach the need for completion of the course of antibiotics.
7. Explain the importance of adequate humidification of air (use of a

vaporizer or humidifier in the winter, and avoidance of air conditioning in the summer).
8. Teach about the use of lozenges.

Evaluation criteria.   *See* Overview.

CANCER OF THE LARYNX

Malignant tumors of the larynx constitute <2% of all carcinomas. It is
the most common upper respiratory tract malignancy, and there are
~10,000 new cases every year. This cancer shows no racial predilection,
but the incidence is much greater in smokers than in nonsmokers (3:1).
Cancer of the larynx occurs most frequently at about age 60 yr. In 1982,
9,100 cases were predicted to occur in men, and 1,800 in women. The
cause is unknown. Predisposing factors are a familial history of cancer,
irritants such as alcohol, cigarette smoke, and noxious fumes, a history of
chronic laryngitis, and frequent abuse of the voice. The first *symptom* is
usually hoarseness, which may be slight and intermittent but gradually
becomes constant. Sounds become progressively more difficult to make.
Later signs include respiratory obstruction, which becomes progressively
worse. The patient uses accessory muscles to breathe, and an audible
stridor may be present. The late signs are malodorous breath, dysphagia,
weight loss, and hemoptysis. *Diagnosis* is based on the health history,
physical exam, direct or indirect laryngoscopy, x-ray, CAT scan, and
barium esophagram.

Common interventions

Medical interventions for cancers too advanced for surgical treatment
include chemotherapy and radiotherapy. Radiotherapy is used for cancers
confined to the true cords. **Surgical** interventions include partial or total
laryngectomy, the latter with or without radical neck dissection.

Nursing interventions (preoperative)

Physical 1. Administer antibiotics as ordered.
    2. Provide oral hygiene.
Psychosocial 3. Discuss concerns and fears about the forthcoming
    surgery and the changes it will bring (suffocation, choking, or death;
    mutilation; the inability to work or speak; and changes in relation-
    ships, especially rejection by significant others).
    4. Discuss fear of the recurrence of cancer.
    5. Reassure the patient that the total care required will be available.
    The patient will not be left alone until able to care for self.
    6. Refer to voice loss as temporary because the patient will learn to
    speak in a new way.
    7. Discuss esophageal speech in terms that are acceptable to the
    patient.

8. Arrange to have a person who has been successfully rehabilitated visit preoperatively (after discussing the visit with both the physician and the patient).
9. Arrange a consultation with the speech therapist to have rehabilitation begun preoperatively. (This may not be possible for all patients because of high anxiety.)
10. Establish a means for the patient to communicate with the staff and family, either by writing or hand signals.
11. Discuss postoperative care so that the patient knows what to expect and can ask questions.

Educational 12. Explain postoperative care (e.g., suctioning, care of the laryngectomy tube, tube feedings, and vital sign measurements).
13. Explain that the pain will not be severe and that medication will be administered as needed.

Nursing interventions (postoperative)

Physical 1. Maintain a patent airway.
2. Provide adequate humidification of air.
3. Suction through the tracheostomy as needed.
4. Suction the nose and mouth as ordered. (An order is needed because of the possible presence of the suture line. Use a new catheter to suction the tracheostomy.)
5. Provide constant attention during the early postoperative period.
6. Assess closely for complications (respiratory distress, hemorrhage from the wound or tracheostomy, shock, hemoptysis, and excessive coughing).
7. Monitor intake and output.
8. Administer IV fluids.
9. Administer analgesics. If opiates are ordered, observe closely for and report signs of respiratory depression. (The incisional pain is minimal, but headache and sore throat are common.)
10. Administer antibiotics and vitamins.
11. Administer tube feedings if ordered (started on 2nd postoperative day and provided q 2 to 3 hr to avoid gastric distension and nausea). Gastric suctioning may be ordered if nausea occurs.
12. Provide oral fluids/diet as ordered, which may be started on the 1st postoperative day. (A regular diet may be started on the 2nd postoperative day.)
13. Carefully supervise the patient's first attempts at taking water, which may cause coughing or choking. Provide only water until the patient can swallow well.
14. Report any return of feedings through the tracheotomy. (This indicates a fistula. It is confirmed by the appearance of methylene blue in the tracheal aspiration after the patient swallows fluid that contains the dye.)

15. Administer/provide frequent oral hygiene.
16. Assist the patient out of bed on the 1st postoperative day as ordered.
17. Refer the patient for speech therapy.

Psychosocial 18. Assist the patient to cope with the loss of (a) a means of verbal communication, (b) the personal qualities of the voice, (c) the ability to express emotions through tone of voice or laughter, (d) normal breathing, (e) the sense of smell, and (f) the ability to blow the nose, gargle, whistle, sip through a straw, and sip soup.
19. Assist the patient to cope with changes in sexual self-image. (Men may associate a laryngectomy with a loss of masculinity/castration. In addition, the voice is no longer available for sexual expression.)
20. Assist the patient with grief and depression over loss. (Depression is usually worse by the 3rd or 4th postoperative day.)
21. Because severe, prolonged depression is not normal, assess for and report indications of severe depression, refer the patient for psychiatric consultation if severe depression occurs, and place the patient on suicide precautions if necessary. (Women are often more depessed than men because of the change in appearance and the sound of esophageal speech.)
22. Provide support to the patient and family with regard to changing moods (anger, fear, apathy, depression, etc.).
23. Reduce the patient's anger by anticipating needs.
24. Inform the staff that the patient cannot speak; post a notice by the intercom.
25. Explain all procedures to the patient.

Educational 26. Begin teaching the patient for self-care early.
27. Teach the patient how to suction the tracheostomy on the 1st postoperative day.
28. Teach the patient to remove and clean the inner cannual, if present, by the 5th day.
29. Teach the patient how to remove and replace the entire laryngectomy tube by the time of discharge, if it is still being worn. (Most patients wear the tube for the first 3 to 8 wk. Some wear the tube at night after the initial period if the stoma tends to collapse or does not provide for adequate air exchange during sleep.)
30. Teach about the need for, and provision of, humidified air.
31. Teach the patient to prevent aspiration of water by wearing a protective covering when washing the hair, bathing, or showering, by using a mirror when washing the face, and by directing the water at chest height when showering.
32. Teach the patient to use special care to avoid aspiration of foreign objects: loose hair after haircuts, aftershave lotions, shaving lather, powder, and sprays such as deodorants or hair sprays.
33. Teach the patient to avoid contact with people who have upper respiratory tract infections.

34. Instruct a significant other in routine general care, as well as in mouth-to-neck resuscitation in case of respiratory depression or arrest.
35. Refer the patient to the Lost Chord Club, the New Voice Club, or other rehabilitation resources in the community (e.g., the local or regional branch of the American Cancer Society, the American Speech and Hearing Association, the State Office of Vocational Rehabilitation, and educational facilities with a speech and hearing department).
36. Instruct the patient to always carry an identification card that states that the patient has no vocal cords, gives information on how to do mouth-to-neck resuscitation, and provides the name of the person to be notified in an emergency. This card may be obtained by writing to

The International Association of Laryngectomies
American Cancer Society
219 E. 42nd St.
New York, NY 10017

37. Advise the patient to avoid smoking.

Evaluation criteria. *See* Overview. Airway is patent; communication is achieved and maintained.

CHAPTER 14

ALTERED RESPIRATORY FUNCTIONING

Sharon Brown and Marianne Taft Marcus

OVERVIEW

Definition

Respiration, the process of molecular exchange of oxygen and carbon dioxide within the pulmonary system, is basic to life. Respiration involves the exchange of gases (O_2 and CO_2) between atmospheric air and the tissues of the body. Alterations in respiratory functioning account for a wide range of acute and chronic illnesses from the "common cold" to obstructive lung disease and neoplasms. This chapter will provide the nurse with a review of the anatomy and physiology of respiration and a reference for identifying and intervening in specific alterations of respiratory functioning.

Anatomy and physiology review

The respiratory system can be divided into the conducting system, the lungs, pleurae, respiratory muscles, and the respiratory center (Fig. 14-1). The **conducting system** consists of the upper airway (nose, pharynx, larynx, and epiglottis) and the lower airway, or tracheobronchial tree (trachea, right and left main-stem bronchi, segmental bronchi, and bronchioles, which communicate directly with alveoli through alveolar ducts). The functions of the conducting system are to (1) conduct air, (2) filter inspired air by means of mucociliary clearance (entrapment of foreign

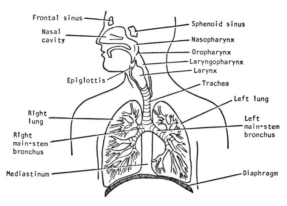

Frontal sinus
Nasal cavity
Epiglottis
Right lung
Right main-stem bronchus
Mediastinum
Sphenoid sinus
Nasopharynx
Oropharynx
Laryngopharynx
Larynx
Trachea
Left lung
Left main-stem bronchus
Diaphragm

Figure 14-1. The respiratory system.

bodies in mucus that is secreted by goblet cells of the tracheobronchial tree and movement of these foreign bodies by cilia to the pharynx, where they are expectorated or swallowed), and (3) warm and humidify air by means of the capillary blood supply in the submucosal layer of the airway.

The **lungs** (right and left) consist of the lobes and lung parenchyma. The right lung has three lobes (upper, middle, and lower) and the left lung has two lobes (upper and lower). The lung parenchyma consists of alveolar sacs (a healthy adult has >300 million) and pulmonary capillaries (blood supply from the right ventricle of the heart). The functions of the lungs are to exchange O_2 and CO_2 across the alveolar-capillary membrane (diffusion), to remove exogenous and endogenous wastes by the alveolar macrophages, and to secrete surfactant by the alveoli. (Surfactant is a detergentlike compound that prevents lung collapse by reducing surface tension of the lung.)

The **pleurae** are double-layered, serous membranes that line the thoracic cavity and encase the lungs. The outer layer — the parietal pleura — is adjacent to the chest. The inner layer — the visceral pleura — is adherent to the lung surface. A small amount of pleural fluid exists between membranes. Its functions are to lubricate the pleurae and to cause membranes to adhere to one another, thereby prohibiting separation between the lungs and thorax (potential space).

The **muscles of respiration** include the diaphragm and the external intercostals. The diaphragm separates the thoracic and abdominal cavities and flattens on inspiration to increase the longitudinal dimension of lungs. The external intercostals pull ribs up and out to increase the anteroposterior dimension of the lungs.

The **respiratory center** is located in the medulla oblongata in the brainstem, just above the spinal cord. The respiratory center responds to the

CO_2 and H^+ content of CSF in order to increase or decrease the respiratory rate (*see* Chapter 3). It also stimulates contraction of the diaphragm through nerve fibers that extend down the spinal cord to the phrenic nerves.

The **respiratory process** is a combined effort by the lungs and circulation to supply O_2 to body tissues and to remove CO_2 by means of ventilation and gas exchange. **Ventilation,** or air movement (inspiration and expiration), is modified by respiratory centers in the medulla and periphery (carotid and aortic bodies), PCO_2 (elevation increases respiration), PO_2 (elevation decreases respiration), the chemical content of CSF, pain, temperature, stress, alterations in physical activity, and the condition of the structures of the respiratory system. **Gas exchange** (the exchange of CO_2 and O_2) occurs at two levels: at the alveolar-capillary membrane (external respiration) and at the tissue-cellular level (internal respiration). Gas exchange requires adequate O_2 concentration in the alveoli, Hb concentration in the blood (combines with O_2 to transport), and rate of transport of oxyhemoglobin to the tissues in response to tissue needs. In addition, gas exchange also requires adequate O_2 diffusion from the alveoli and an adequate number of body cells that are capable of using O_2.

General assessment

The general assessment consists of a health history, physical exam, and various diagnostic tests. **Health history** data that are specific to the respiratory status are listed below. The *current health status* should include information about the chief complaint and personal behavior patterns, especially nutrition (diet, fluid intake, and change in appetite); cigarette smoking in pack-years (no. of packs/day $\times$ yr smoked); alterations in exercise tolerance and sleep due to breathing difficulties; and medications (antibiotics, cardiac medications, bronchodilators, antihistamines, diuretics, steroids, O_2, intermittent positive-pressure breathing [IPPB], nebulizer, or humidifier). The *past health history* should include relevant information regarding developmental data (scoliosis); frequency of examinations, immunizations, chest x-rays, and tuberculin skin tests; past illnesses (TB, respiratory infections); trauma or surgery involving the chest; allergies; and foreign travel (exposure to pathogens or toxins). The *family history* should include information about respiratory infections, TB, allergies, asthma, emphysema, and/or cancer. Relevant *social history* data include occupation (exposure to dust, fumes, chemicals, or asbestos), contact with animals, and living conditions (crowding increases the risk of respiratory infection). In the *review of systems* (including analysis of the symptom: onset, duration, characteristics, and aggravating and relieving factors), the patient is assessed for any recent weight changes, weakness, fatigue, malaise, fever, or chills. The nose and sinuses are assessed for pain, tenderness, discharge, obstruction, sneezing, and rhinitis. The mouth and throat are assessed for pain, soreness, lesions, dysphagia, and voice changes. The neck is assessed for pain, swelling, and limitation of movement. The respiratory system is assessed for pain, dyspnea, wheezing, coughing, sputum, and hemoptysis. The cardiovascular system is assessed for pain, edema, and syncope. The GI system is assessed for the presence of flatulence (which increases pressure on the diaphragm). The musculo-skeletal system (specifically related to the muscles of respiration) is assessed for pain, tenderness, weakness, deformities, and decreased range of motion. The hematopoietic system is assessed for anemia (Hb is required for O_2 transport). Finally, the patient's mental status should be assessed, because impaired emotional functioning may alter the respiratory rate.

During the **physical examination**, *inspection* is used to assess the patient's general appearance (restlessness, scars, posture) and skin color. (Pallor indicates anemia or hypotension; flushing indicates CO_2 retention; and cyanosis indicates hypoxia.) Inspection is also used to assess the patient's nail beds (cyanosis, clubbing), lips (pursed), nose (flaring), trachea (midline), chest symmetry and configuration, and the antero-posterior diameter of the chest (normal is 1:2). Finally, inspection can be used to assess the rate, rhythm, depth, and pattern of breathing; the use of accessory muscles; and the presence of intercostal bulging or retraction. *Palpation* is used to assess the patient's skin temperature, muscle tone or tenderness, respiratory excursion, and tactile fremitus. The patient's lung fields are *percussed* for resonance, hyperresonance, dullness, and flatness of all lung fields and diaphragmatic excursion. All of the patient's lung fields should be *auscultated* for normal breath sounds (vesicular, broncho-vesicular, and bronchial) and for adventitious breath sounds (rales, rhonchi, wheezes, and rubs).

The **diagnostic tests** used to assess the respiratory system include laboratory data, the chest x-ray, bronchography, bronchoscopy, and pulmonary function studies. *Blood tests* (specifically the RBC, Hb, and Hct) indicate the adequacy of Hb for O_2 transport. Blood tests are also used to determine the erythrocyte sedimentation rate (ESR), which indicates the presence of inflammation or infection; the WBC, which indicates inflam-mation, infection, or allergy; and the serum electrolyte levels, which reflect the fluid and electrolyte status of the patient. Finally, arterial blood gases are used to determine the following: (1) pH (normal: 7.35 to 7.45) indicates acid-base balance (*see* Chapter 3); (2) PCO_2 (normal: 35 to 40 mmHg) indicates adequacy of ventilation; (3) PO_2 (normal: 80 to 100 mmHg) reflects the ability of the lungs to diffuse O_2 across the alveolar capillary membrane; (4) O_2 saturation (normal: 95 to 98%) indicates the percentage of O_2 across the alveolar capillary membrane; and (5) serum bicarbonate (HCO_3^-) (normal: 22 to 26 mEq/liter) indicates compensatory metabolic response in acid-base variations. Other laboratory data include *sputum culture and sensitivity* (indicates the presence of bacteria and suggests approriate antimicrobial agents), *sputum for cytology* (indicates the presence of neoplastic cells), *biopsies* (lung, pleural, scalene, and medi-astinal nodes), and *skin test* for delayed hypersensitivity (PPD).

Chest x-rays are used for both screening and diagnostic purposes. *Bronchography* is x-ray visualization of the bronchial tree after the introduction of an iodized radiopaque liquid through a metal cannula and catheter. **Nursing** care of the patient undergoing bronchography is as follows:

1. Elicit any history of iodine sensitivity.
2. Provide scrupulous oral hygiene.
3. Keep the patient NPO for 8 hr before the examination.
4. Remove dentures.
5. Call the physician's attention to loose or capped teeth.
6. Provide postural drainage to remove secretions in the bronchioles.
7. Administer a short-acting barbiturate (secobarbital) 1 hr before the procedure.
8. Apply a local topical anesthetic spray (cocaine, tetracaine) before the introduction of radiopaque substances. (Observe for toxicity to the anesthetic, e.g., rapid pulse, excitation, headache. Notify the physician.)
9. After the procedure, provide postural drainage to remove any radiopaque material.

Bronchoscopy is visualization of the bronchial tree by means of a lighted hollow instrument (bronchoscope). During the procedure, a tissue biopsy may be obtained. The preparation is the same as for a bronchogram, although IV anesthesia may be indicated if a biopsy is performed or if the patient is very apprehensive. Follow-up **nursing** care is the same as for a bronchogram except for the following actions:

1. Position the patient as ordered (semi-Fowler's or flat).
2. Collect postbronchoscopy sputum for culture and cytology.
3. Observe for and report complications (e.g., hoarseness, laryngeal edema, and hemorrhage from biopsy site).

Pulmonary (ventilatory) function studies are performed to evaluate the bellows action of the lungs, chest wall, and diaphragm in order to determine the functional capacity/volume of the lungs by means of a spirometer. These studies are used for screening, classifying and determining the severity of respiratory impairment, evaluating the progression of pulmonary disease, determining the response to therapy, and predicting alterations in respiratory status following a pneumonectomy or lobectomy. Some examples of pulmonary function studies are listed below:

1. Tidal volume (TV or V_T): The amount of air inspired/expired during normal quiet respiration.
2. Vital capacity (VC): The maximal amount of air that can be expired after a maximal inspiration.
3. Inspiratory capacity (IC): The maximal amount of air that can be inspired after a normal expiration.

4. Forced expiratory volume (FEV_1) in 1 second: The amount of air expelled in the 1st sec of the forced VC maneuver.
5. Residual volume (RV): The volume of air left in the lung after maximal expiration.

Common interventions

O_2 therapy. O_2 is administered to treat hypoxemia resulting from pulmonary or nonpulmonary dysfunction (e.g., acute or chronic respiratory failure, pulmonary edema, airway obstruction, cardiac dysfunction, and shock). O_2 therapy increases alveolar O_2 tension, resulting in decreased respiratory and myocardial effort. O_2 therapy is administered via high- and low-flow systems.

Low-flow systems provide variable O_2 concentration (21 to 90%) and deliver less than the total inspiratory flow rate of required O_2. They balance the fraction of inspired O_2 (FIO_2) between room air and O_2 delivered. (Variation in the rate or depth of respiration alters the FIO_2; the larger the V_T, the lower the FIO_2.) Low-flow systems result in variable accuracy and dependability and are effective only in patients with an intact upper airway and stable ventilation. There are three kinds of low-flow systems. The *nasal cannula* (Fig. 14-2) is the most comfortable and supplies O_2 via nasal prongs. The flow rate of O_2 can be adjusted from 1 to 6 liters/min to deliver

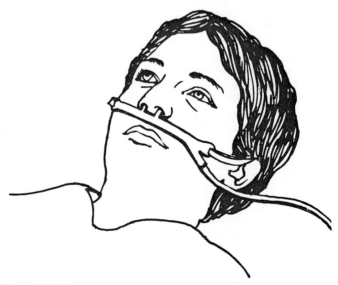

Figure 14-2. Nasal cannula.

from 24 to 45% FIO$_2$. However, the flow rate should not be adjusted >6 liters/min because it has no effect on FIO$_2$ and it results in drying of the nasal passages. The *face mask* (Fig. 14-3) provides an increased anatomic reservoir for O$_2$, but restricts eating and talking. The flow rate of O$_2$ can be adjusted from 5 to 8 liters/min to deliver 40 to 60% FIO$_2$. The face mask should never be used at <5 to 6 liters/min because the patient may rebreathe exhaled air. The *face mask with reservoir* comes in two types: the nonrebreather (one-way valve between the bag and mask) and the rebreather (no one-way valve between the bag and mask). For either type, the flow rate of O$_2$ can be adjusted from 6 to 15 liters/min to deliver 60 to 99% FIO$_2$. The face masks must fit securely, and the reservoir bag should never collapse more than halfway during inhalation.

High-flow systems deliver total inspiratory flow rate of required O$_2$. They provide a consistent and accurate FIO$_2$ (which may be measured directly with an O$_2$ analyzer), are capable of delivering high or low O$_2$ concentrations (30 to 100%), and allow for temperature and humidity control. The venti mask, the most common high-flow system, draws along room air at a specific ratio to liter flow of O$_2$. It does not change the FIO$_2$ if there are changes in the rate or depth of respirations (which is particularly important in the critically ill patient). The mask must fit securely, and the tubing must be free of kinks.

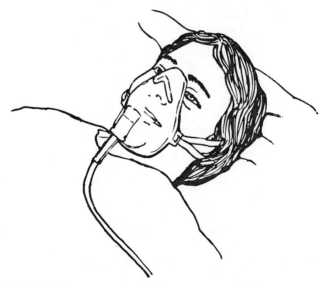

Figure 14-3. Face mask.

The main complications of O_2 therapy are atelectasis, due to the effect of O_2 on pulmonary surfactant (*see below*), and O_2 toxicity, which results from too high a concentration of O_2 over an extended period. Signs and symptoms include restlessness, paresthesias in extremities, nausea, vomiting, fatigue, lethargy, malaise, dyspnea progressing to severe respiratory distress, substernal pain, cyanosis, and asphyxia. The **nursing** interventions for O_2 therapy are as follows:

Physical 1. Position the patient for optimum comfort and chest expansion (semi-Fowler's or high Fowler's).
2. Maintain a patent airway.
3. Initiate and maintain O_2 flow rate/concentration and humidification as ordered. (Question high flow rate/concentration for extended period of time.)
4. Check O_2 devices frequently for patency and function.
5. Remove mask/cannula q 2 hr to observe skin and clean equipment.
6. Provide oral and nasal hygiene frequently.
7. Monitor vital signs q 15 min for 4 hr; then q 2 to 4 hr if stable.
8. Check level of consciousness q 15 min; then q 2 to 4 hr if unchanged.
9. Auscultate chest q 1 to 4 hr.
10. Monitor arterial blood gases.
11. Institute safety precautions to prevent fire.
    a. Ground all electrical plugs and equipment.
    b. Post and strictly enforce no smoking signs.
    c. Remove all smoking materials from the patient's room.
    d. Do not use combustible materials (such as oil, alcohol, or ether) when O_2 is being administered.
    e. Prevent static electricity. Remove wool, silk, and synthetic fabrics from the area.
12. Observe and report signs and symptoms of complications.
13. Assist the patient to cough, turn, and deep breathe q 2 hr.
Psychosocial 14. Remain with the patient during adjustment to O_2 therapy to reduce anxiety.
15. Reassure the patient concerning the safety of properly used equipment.
16. Assist the patient/family in acquiring O_2 devices for home use if indicated.
Educational 17. Explain the rationale for O_2 therapy.
18. Instruct the patient/family in the safe use of O_2 equipment.
19. Teach the patient/family to observe for and report signs and symptoms of complications.

The **evaluation criteria** are listed at the end of the Overview (*see below*).

Artificial airways. Artificial airways (Fig. 14-4) are used to establish and maintain a patent airway in any of the following situations: upper

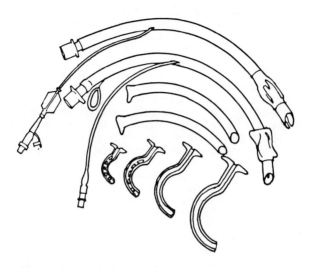

Figure 14-4.   Artificial airways. Top two, cuffed endotracheal tubes; middle two, nasopharyngeal tubes; bottom four, oropharyngeal tubes.

airway obstruction (mouth to larynx); respiratory insufficiency following surgery or trauma; and acute respiratory failure secondary to pulmonary, cardiovascular, or neuromuscular disease. In addition, they are used to prevent aspiration of oral and gastric secretions in the unconscious or paralyzed patient, facilitate suctioning when indicated, and provide for use of assistive mechanical ventilatory devices (IPPB, continuous mechanical ventilation). The two main kinds of artificial airways are pharyngeal tubes and endotracheal tubes.

Pharyngeal tubes provide an airway to the level of the larynx. One type of pharyngeal tube, the oropharyngeal tube, is inserted through the mouth. It keeps the tongue forward away from pharyngeal wall, acts as a bite block when used with an endotracheal tube (*see below*), and facilitates orotracheal suctioning. Complications of oropharyngeal tubes include gagging, vomiting, and laryngospasm in the conscious/semiconscious patient, and obstruction due to improper tube size. Another type of pharyngeal tube, the nasopharyngeal tube, is inserted through the naris. It lies in the posterior pharynx, is tolerated by the alert patient, and provides a means for pharyngeal suctioning. Complications of nasopharyngeal tubes include hemorrhage (particularly in the presence of bleeding disorders or anticoagulants), obstruction due to improper tube size, and infection (particularly in the presence of draining CSF or blood).

The **endotracheal tube,** which is reserved for situations in which simpler airways are unsuccessful, can be inserted through the nose or mouth. It provides an airway through the larynx to the trachea. The endotracheal tube may be inserted through an oropharyngeal tube (bite block) when required. The plain endotracheal tube is used for children. In order to ensure an airtight seal, a tube that fits the cricoid ring should be selected. The cuffed tube uses an inflatable sleeve near the distal tip to ensure a seal. A soft cuff is preferred over a rigid cuff. The cuffed tube maintains low pressure (maximum 15 to 20 mmHg measured on a manometer) during exhalation, prevents aspiration, and does not distort the tracheal wall (soft cuff). During intubation, complications of the cuffed tube include bruised lips or tongue, impaired vocal cords (hoarseness), dislodged adenoid tissue, ECG changes due to vagal stimulation (bradycardia, prolonged PR interval), vomiting, aspiration, and broken and displaced teeth. Once the tube is in place, complications include laryngeal edema (obstruction, stridorous respirations), respiratory fatigue due to resistance from the tube, and dyspnea due to improper placement, obstruction, or kinking of the tube. Postextubation complications vary from pharyngitis, laryngitis, and tracheitis, to vocal cord damage (ulceration, granuloma). The **nursing** interventions for artificial airways are as follows:

Physical 1. Monitor pulse and respirations for quality and rate hourly and prn.
2. Auscultate chest for breath sounds hourly.
3. Monitor BP and temperature q 4 hr.
4. Check level of consciousness hourly.
5. Provide oral/nasal hygiene frequently (water-soluble lubricants).
6. Suction hourly and prn (airway placement stimulates mucus secretion).
7. Maintain sterility during suctioning to reduce chance of infection.
8. Check placement and patency of airway q 30 min.
9. Change oral airway q 8 hr; nasal, q 72 hr and prn.
10. Administer O_2 when ordered (preoxygenate prior to airway insertion when possible).
11. Establish alternative means of communication when indicated (pad, pencil, call bell).
12. Provide humidification to prevent tenacious bronchial secretions.
13. Monitor intake and output.
14. Monitor for signs and symptoms of complications.
15. Assist the patient to cough, turn, and deep breathe.
16. Do not extubate until the patient is able to ventilate without assistance (gag and swallow reflexes intact).
17. Apply restraints (when ordered) to prevent accidental extubation.
18. Keep side rails in place if restlessness exists.
19. For endotracheal intubation, perform the following actions:
    a. Check the tube placement with a chest x-ray.
    b. Measure and adjust the cuff pressure q 4 to 8 hr.

c. Deflate the cuff for 5 to 10 min hourly if the patient can maintain respirations.

d. Suction the airway prior to deflation.

e. Observe the cuff for air leaks.

Psychosocial 20. Remain with the patient during intubation/extubation to decrease anxiety.

21. Reassure the patient about the temporary nature of artificial airways.

22. Respond promptly to the patient's call bell to reduce anxiety and establish trust.

Educational 23. Explain all procedures, despite the patient's level of consciousness.

24. Explain the rationale for the use of artificial airways.

25. Teach the patient alternative methods of communication.

The **evaluation criteria** are listed at the end of the Overview (*see below*).

Mechanical aids to ventilation. When disease, debility, or injury render the patient incapable of adequate pulmonary ventilation, mechanical assistance may be ordered. Positive-pressure ventilators are designed to provide short-term/intermittent assistance to ventilation, or continuous control of ventilation and O_2 administration. The two main kinds of mechanical aids are IPPB and continuous mechanical ventilation.

IPPB, the mechanical application of inspiratory positive pressure to the airway to facilitate a therapeutically slow inspiratory rate and phase, is used to provide optimal peripheral (alveolar) distribution of inspired air and to increase V_T, bronchodilation, and mean airway pressure. IPPB decreases respiratory effort and controls the inspiratory:expiratory ratio. It facilitates the removal of bronchial secretions and the delivery of aerosol medication and humidity (particularly in patients with decreased inspiratory capacity). While controversy exists regarding the advantages of IPPB over other methods of respiratory therapy, it may be ordered to treat atelectasis, pulmonary edema, respiratory acidosis, CO_2 narcosis, postoperative hypoventilation, and acute/chronic obstructive lung disease. IPPB should never be used in the presence of pulmonary hemorrhage, subcutaneous emphysema of unknown etiology, or a tracheoesophageal fistula. It should be used with extreme caution in the presence of pneumothorax, hemoptysis, active TB, hypovolemia, and severe cardiac diseases. IPPB complications include infection (aerosol or water left in tubing, mask, or nebulizer support bacterial growth); dizziness secondary to hyperventilation; gastric distension; tachycardia secondary to its effect on the cardiopulmonary circulation; ruptured alveoli resulting in mediastinal/subcutaneous emphysema; fatigue; and nausea and vomiting (if administered sooner than 1 hr after meals). **Nursing** interventions specific to IPPB use are as follows:

Physical 1. Monitor BP, apical pulse, skin color, breath sounds, and respiratory effort before and after treatment.

2. Position the patient in an upright sitting position.

3. Set the IPPB machine to the pressure limit (usually 15 to 20 cm H_2O pressure) and O_2 setting ordered.
4. Place aerosol medication, distilled water, or saline in the nebulizer as ordered.
5. Administer treatment (usually 15 min tid or qid) as ordered.
6. Monitor pulse 1 to 2 times during treatment.
7. Encourage effective coughing several times during, and at the end of, treatment to remove secretions.
8. Use individual tubing, mask/mouthpiece, and nebulizer for each patient. Clean and dry equipment thoroughly after use.
9. Assist with oral hygiene following treatment.

Psychosocial 10. Remain with the patient continuously during the first treatment to decrease anxiety.
11. Reassure the patient that treatments will become easier with practice.

Educational 12. Explain the procedure and its rationale to the patient.
13. Teach the patient to maintain a slow respiratory rate using diaphragmatic breathing.
14. Teach the patient to seal his lips tightly around the mouthpiece during inspiration.

The **evaluation criteria** are listed at the end of the Overview (*see below*).

Continuous mechanical ventilation (CMV) is indicated for continuous control of ventilation and O_2 administration, which may be necessary in the following situations: CNS disorders that compromise the respiratory center in the medulla, musculoskeletal diseases/injuries that limit chest expansion, neuromuscular disorders resulting in respiratory paralysis, left-sided heart failure/pulmonary edema, postoperative respiratory insufficiency, hypoxia secondary to respiratory infection in COPD, and upper airway obstruction due to laryngeal edema or trauma. CMVs, which are continually being modified, must include the capability to function dependably for long periods of time and to regulate the concentration of inspired O_2 from room air (20%) to 100%. They should provide warm humidification, be easily cleaned, and provide a means for measuring the volume of expired air. There are two main types of CMVs: pressure cycled and volume cycled. Pressure-cycled CMVs, which are relatively inexpensive and mobile, deliver a preset pressure (usually 15 to 25 cm H_2O) with each respiration. They do not necessarily provide for a constant volume of gas, they lack adequate alarm systems, and the inspired O_2 concentrations may vary and be unreliable. Volume-cycled CMVs, which are large, expensive and immobile, deliver a constant volume of air with each respiration. They deliver a more accurate O_2 concentration than pressure-cycled CMVs and have a built-in alarm system and a pressure cutoff valve to prevent delivery of pressures above a predetermined limit. The complications and side effects of CMVs include respiratory infection, O_2 toxicity (*see above*), fluid and electrolyte imbalance and positive water imbalance (*see* Chapter 3), gastric distension, stress response (gastric bleeding, ulcer), and dysrhythmias/cardiovascular impairment due to increased intrathoracic pressure (which decreases right-sided venous return), acid-base imbalances, or hypoxemia. Other complications include atelectasis, pneumothorax (subcutaneous/mediastinal emphysema due to excessive pressure and/or volume settings), and decreased urinary output due to an increase in vasopressin, reabsorption of water in renal tubular cells, an increase in ADH secretion, and/or sodium and water retention. CMVs are used almost exclusively in critical care areas. Before assuming responsibility for the care of a patient on a ventilator, the nurse must have an excellent understanding of the patient's pathophysiologic process, develop considerable skill and knowledge in the use of the machine, and be completely familiar with the manufacturer's instructions for the specific ventilator in use. **Nursing** interventions basic to all ventilator patients are as follows:

Physical 1. Establish a flow sheet on which to record arterial blood gas determinations at least twice a shift and more frequently on an unstable patient. Following any change in ventilator setting, indicate the setting at time blood is drawn.
2. Monitor the following factors and record them on the patient's flow sheet: serum electrolytes, intake and output, breath sounds, V_T, VC, pulse (cardiac monitor may be ordered), BP, level of consciousness, and temperature.
3. Monitor ventilator warning signals. (Alarms should be on at all times except during suctioning and weaning.)
4. Maintain O_2 level as ordered. (Check FIO_2 with O_2 analyzer.)
5. Continuously maintain patent airway; use strict aseptic technique for suctioning.
6. Observe for air leaks associated with cuffed endotracheal/tracheostomy tubes.
7. Never leave the patient unobserved.
8. Observe appropriate safety precautions with O_2 and electrical equipment (*see* O_2 therapy *above*).
9. Be prepared to ventilate the patient manually if the ventilator malfunctions or if power fails (Ambu bag, ~15 respirations/min).
10. Establish an alternative means of communication (pencil, paper).
11. Turn and position the patient at least q 2 hr to prevent atelectasis and pneumonia.
12. Maintain the patient in good body alignment.
13. Perform passive range-of-motion exercises at least q 4 hr to maintain muscle and skin tone.
14. Provide oral hygiene q 2 to 4 hr.
15. Provide for deep breaths ("sighs") several times an hour (mechanical or bag) to prevent atelectasis.
16. Test stools for blood (stress ulcers are a complication).

Psychosocial 17. Observe facial expressions/body language closely for indications of anxiety, fear, or pain.

18. Respond to the call bell promptly to reduce anxiety.
19. Anticipate the patient's needs.
20. Orient the patient to his surroundings frequently.

Educational 21. Explain all procedures, even when the patient is comatose.

22. Teach the patient/family the rationale for CMV, alternative means of communication, to avoid placing tension on the airway, and safety precautions associated with CMV.

Nursing interventions associated with weaning from CMV are as follows:

1. Establish rapport to reduce anxiety.
2. Anticipate fears associated with weaning.
3. Evaluate ventilatory parameters carefully before initiating weaning (blood gases, V_T, and clinical status).
4. Teach breathing exercises.
5. Begin with short periods of CMV.
6. Remain with the patient continuously during weaning.
7. Assess ventilation while the patient is off CMV. Check for cyanosis, tachycardia, diaphoresis, restlessness, and decreased V_T.

The **evaluation criteria** are listed at the end of the Overview (*see below*).

Drugs. The following major classifications of pharmacologic agents are used to treat patients with altered respiratory functioning.

Antitussives are used to depress the cough reflex. They are administered PO, and may be in lozenge or syrup form. Examples include codeine (narcotic) and dextromethorphan hydrobromide (Romilar), carbetapentane citrate (Toclase), and benzonatate (Tessalon) (nonnarcotic). **Nursing** interventions include the following:

1. Inform the patient/family not to take food or liquids PO for 15 min after taking antitussives in syrup form (reduces local soothing effect).
2. Warn women of childbearing age that antitussives are usually contraindicated during pregnancy.
3. Observe and record any effect and/or untoward reaction following drug administration.

Expectorants reduce the viscosity of secretions (mucolytics) and increase the flow of secretions. They are available as PO medications or as aerosols. Examples include acetylcysteine (Mucomyst), tyloxapol (Allevain), glyceryl guaiacolate (Robitussin), and terpin hydrate. **Nursing** interventions consist of the following:

1. Inform the patient/family not to take food or fluids PO for 15 min after taking PO preparations that produce local soothing effect.

2. Teach the patient/family to clean the nebulizer carefully following treatment.
3. Observe and record any effect and/or untoward reaction following drug administration.

Antihistamines antagonize histamine response in allergic conditions and prevent edema and bronchospasm in bronchial asthma. They are available as PO, parenteral, and per rectum medications. Examples include brompheniramine maleate (Dimetane) and chlorpheniramine maleate (Teldrin). **Nursing** interventions consist of the following:

1. Teach the patient/family that antihistamines may cause drowsiness. Warn against driving or working near machinery while medication is in effect.
2. Institute safety precautions (side rails) if the patient is sedated from antihistamine.
3. Caution the patient to avoid CNS depressants (alcohol, sedatives) while antihistamine response is present.

Antibiotics kill or inhibit growth of pathogenic organisms. They are available as PO, parenteral, and aerosol medications. Examples include penicillin, streptomycin sulfate, polymyxin B sulfate, and cephalosporins. **Nursing** interventions are as follows:

1. Elicit any previous history of allergic response to antibiotics.
2. Observe for allergic reactions.
3. Institute safety precautions for potential allergic response and have epinephrine readily available.
4. Teach the patient/family to take antibiotics only as ordered by the physician and to observe for any untoward response.
5. Monitor for superimposed fungal infections.
6. Observe and record any effect and/or untoward reaction following drug administration.

Bronchodilators relieve bronchospasm by direct action on the bronchial smooth muscle. They are available as PO, parenteral, per rectum, and aerosol medications. Examples include epinephrine hydrochloride (Adrenalin), ephedrine sulfate (Bofedrol), and pseudoephedrine hydrochloride (Sudafed) (sympathomimetics and adrenergics) and aminophylline and theophylline (theophylline derivatives). For the sympathomimetics/adrenergics, **nursing** interventions are as follows:

1. Monitor the cardiovascular response to adrenergics (BP, pulse, and chest pain).
2. Teach the patient/family not to take maintenance doses at bedtime (insomnia may result); to avoid overuse of adrenergics (reduced response or untoward cardiovascular response may occur); to report dizziness, chest pain, or lack of response; and to continue other

therapeutic measures for respiratory dysfunction even when symptoms appear improved by bronchodilators.

For theophylline derivatives, **nursing** interventions are as follows:

1. Monitor for clinical and toxic effects.
2. Teach the patient/family to notify the physician if nausea, vomiting, GI pain, or restlessness occurs.

Other drugs used in respiratory disorders include **adrenocorticosteroids** (prednisone) to reduce inflammation and the resultant thickening of bronchial walls and **narcotic antagonists** (nalorphine hydrochloride, naloxone hydrochloride) to reduce/prevent respiratory depression caused by narcotic analgesics, tranquilizers, and sedatives. Narcotic antagonists are particularly important in the presence of pulmonary insufficiency and chest trauma.

Diet.   The major dietary consideration for the patient with altered respiratory functioning is the provision of adequate nutrition and fluids. This goal is difficult to maintain because of anorexia due to fatigue from increased respiratory effort, foul odor and/or taste of sputum, and hypoxia secondary to decreased GI motility or fluid and electrolyte imbalance. Sodium restriction may be ordered if edema secondary to cardiovascular disease has compromised respiration. Elimination diets may be ordered when allergic response causes respiratory dysfunction. **Nursing** interventions are as follows:

1. Monitor daily weights.
2. Elicit a diet history.
3. Maintain an intake and output record.
4. Encourage adequate fluid intake (3 to 4 liters/day if not contraindicated by cardiovascular or renal insufficiency).
5. Assist with oral hygiene before meals to counteract taste of sputum.
6. Remove sputum containers before meals are served.
7. Provide small, frequent meals based on the patient's food preferences. Avoid gas-forming foods.
8. Teach the patient/family to maintain hydration (to prevent thick, tenacious secretions); to plan small, frequent, nutritious meals; and to perform oral hygiene before meals.

Surgical interventions

Tracheostomy.   A tracheostomy is a permanent or temporary surgical opening into trachea at second, third, or fourth tracheal ring that is used for placement of an indwelling tube. The opening is used to facilitate ventilation and aid in the removal of bronchial secretions. It is indicated in acute or chronic conditions that compromise the airway, including upper airway obstruction; laryngeal edema due to prolonged intubation; head, neck, or chest injuries; hemorrhage following a thyroidectomy or radical neck resection; neurologic disorders that impair respiration or swallowing;

severe respiratoy disorders (e.g., pulmonary edema, emphysema); and severe burns around the head and neck. A tracheostomy is best performed in the OR (if the situation allows). An endotracheal tube is put in place to maintain the airway during the procedure. A stoma is then created surgically, and the tracheostomy tube is inserted in the trachea. The flange of the tracheostomy tube is sutured in place, and the tube is secured with umbilical tape to prevent accidental extubation. Finally, a postoperative x-ray is used to check tube placement (center of trachea, distal end, not touching carina). Tracheostomy tubes vary in size and type. Diameters vary from 3.5 to 14.0 mm (external) and 2.5 to 10.5 mm (internal). Length varies from 44.45 mm (1.75 in.) outside curve to 101.60 mm (4.00 in.). Tracheostomy tubes may be metal or plastic (disposable), and plain or cuffed. They may have an outer cannula only or both an inner (removable for cleaning and suction) and an outer cannula. Complications during surgery include hemorrhage, airway obstruction, pneumothorax/pneumo-mediastinum due to laceration of pleural apices, air embolus, and sub-cutaneous emphysema. Complications with the tube in place include ulceration of tracheal mucosa, tracheal polyps, swallowing dysfunction or tracheoesophageal fistula (erosion of cartilaginous rings due to overinflated cuff), infection (stoma, lungs), hemorrhage due to erosion of blood vessels, and accidental expulsion of the tracheostomy tube. Postextubation complications consist of nonunion of the stoma with sinus formation, bleeding, and tracheal stricture. **Nursing** interventions for the patient with a tracheostomy are as follows:

Physical 1. Monitor vital signs q 4 hr for the first 48 hr (more often if indicated), then qid.
2. Auscultate the chest for breath sounds q 4 hr.
3. Monitor for signs and symptoms of complications.
4. Place the patient in a semi-Fowler's position, avoiding forward flexion of the neck.
5. Measure intake and output.
6. Maintain adequate hydration to help liquefy secretions. (Encourage fluids to 3,000 ml/day, unless contraindicated. Provide warm humidification to environment.)
7. Provide for removal of secretions. (Encourage the patient to cough. Suction when secretions are audible, rather than routinely, using a 14 to 16 Fr whistle-tip catheter.)
8. Provide frequent mouth care.
9. Deflate the cuff hourly for 5 min to reduce trauma to the tracheal mucosa.
10. Inflate the cuff prior to feeding to avoid aspiration.
11. Assist the patient to avoid constipation and straining at stool and possible accidental expulsion of tracheotomy tube. (Encourage proper diet and fluids. Administer stool softeners, suppositories, enemas, and laxatives as ordered.)
12. Assist the patient to turn, cough, and deep breathe q 2 hr.

13. Change the dressing frequently to prevent infection. (Maintain strict aseptic technique. Clean skin around stoma with hydrogen peroxide, rinse with saline, and dry. Clean inner cannula [when present] with hydrogen peroxide, then sterile water. Use a 4 × 4 in. gauze pad as a dressing, cut to fit. Change umbilical tape qd and prn.)

14. Provide for accidental expulsion of the tracheostomy tube. (Keep a matching obturator taped to the head of the bed. Keep extra tracheostomy tube [same size] available at the bedside. Keep a dilator/hemostat and tracheal hook at bedside.)

15. Observe correct procedure in the event of accidental expulsion of tracheostomy tube. (Remain calm and stay at the bedside. Do not attempt to replace the tube forcefully. Hold the incision open with the dilator/hemostat until help arrives.)

16. Culture bronchial secretions routinely, and culture the wound if signs and symptoms of infection occur.

17. Establish an alternative means of communication (pad, pencil, pictures, call light).

18. Keep side rails in place if restlessness exists.

19. Prepare for extubation when ordered. (Insert a tracheostomy button into the opening with the cuff deflated several hours qd to evaluate the patient's ability to ventilate. Administer O_2 via alternative route. Encourage the patient to expectorate secretions orally.)

Psychosocial 20. Remain with the patient during the surgical procedure and subsequent adjustment to the tracheostomy.

21. Maintain a calm environment, but respond promptly to the call bell to alleviate anxiety and establish trust.

22. Anticipate fear of suffocation and provide appropriate explanations and reassurance.

23. Encourage the patient to communicate his feelings.

24. Refer the patient/family to a social worker or visiting nurse for help with adjustment to a permanent tracheostomy, when indicated.

Educational 25. Preoperatively, explain the purpose of the tracheostomy, inform the patient/family of the need to establish an alternative means of communication, and explain the procedure.

26. Teach the patient and family care and cleaning of the tracheostomy tube, stoma care, suction technique, and the following hygiene modifications:
    a. Direct the shower spray below the neck.
    b. Cover the tracheostomy with waterproof material during showering.
    c. Avoid tub bathing.
    d. Exercise extreme caution with hair clippings, shaving lather, aerosols, sprays, powder, and lotions.

27. Teach the patient and family to report persistent cough/respiratory distress to the physician, to keep the stoma covered (scarves, etc.), to exercise to tolerance (swimming forbidden), and the importance of acquiring a medical alert band indicating that the patient is a neck breather.

The **evaluation criteria** are listed at the end of the Overview (*see below*).

Chest tube systems.   Chest tube systems involve one or more tubes (catheters) inserted into potential space between the pleura to evacuate air and/or fluid by means of gravity and/or suction. The distal ends of the tubes are connected to a water-seal system to prevent reentry of air into intrapleural space. With chest tube systems, air and fluid in the pleural space is forced out through the chest tube as the patient inspires. As the patient exhales, air is prevented from reentering the pleural space because of the pressure of the water seal. This results in reexpansion of the lung (suction enhances this process) and restoration of normal negative pressure between the pleura. It also prevents tension pneumothorax and mediastinal shift (*see below*) by equalizing pressure. Chest tube systems are indicated for any condition in which a disrupted pleural membrane permits atmospheric air (positive pressure) or fluid to enter the intrapleural space. Thoracic surgery, trauma, spontaneous pneumothorax, and rupture of emphysematous bleb are examples of such conditions. Complications consist of infection and tension pneumothorax or mediastinal shift secondary to kinked, clamped, or clogged tubing. There are two main kinds of chest tube systems: bottle systems and disposable unit systems.

Bottle systems (Fig. 14-5) employ large glass bottles, airtight stoppers, and glass rods in the stoppers. In a one-bottle system, a long glass rod placed 2 cm below the fluid level (sterile H_2O/saline) drains the pleural space by gravity and provides the water seal. A short glass rod vents air from the pleural space. The one-bottle system is used in emergencies and short-term situations. It requires constant monitoring because the rising fluid level creates resistane to further drainage. In a two-bottle system, the first bottle is used for drainage and as a water seal (as above), and the second bottle has a long glass rod with its tip under the fluid level at a depth to equal the desired amount of suction in centimeters (usually 10 to 20 cm H_2O) with the top open to vent air. It is connected to a suction source and requires constant monitoring (as above). In a three-bottle system, the first bottle is used for drainage collection only, the second bottle provides the water seal, and the third bottle, which is connected to a suction source, is used for suction control. A main advantage to this system is that a rising drainage level does not create resistance to further drainage.

Disposable unit systems (Pleurevac) (Fig. 14-6) consist of a single, disposable unit with three chambers corresponding to the bottle system, arranged from right to left. Valves are used to trap fluid and air in appropriate chambers. Disposable systems may be used with or without

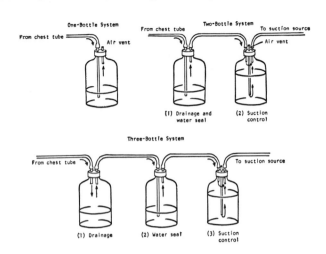

Figure 14-5. Chest drainage bottle systems.

suction. A collection chamber is calibrated to facilitate accurate measurement of drainage. Fluid levels in water-seal and suction chambers are monitored, and fluid lost by evaporation is replaced as indicated. The advantages of this system are that it is lightweight, unbreakable, and disposable.

Nursing interventions for the patient with chest tube systems are as follows:

Physical 1. Monitor amount, color, and consistency of drainage. (Mark level of drainage with adhesive strip, indicating date and hour when bottle system is used. Notify the physician of drainage in excess of 200 ml/hr, or 100 ml/hr if grossly bloody.)
2. Monitor bubbling in water-seal chamber. (Moderate bubbling is normal; indicates expulsion of air from the intrapleural space. Excessive continuous bubbling or absence of bubbling may indicate a leak in the system.)
3. Check site of tube insertion and surrounding area q 2 to 4 hr for crepitus and air leaks.
4. Monitor fluctuation (oscillation) of water in the tube (water-seal bottle). It should move up when the patient inhales/coughs and down when the patient exhales.
5. Monitor and record vital signs q 4 hr and prn.
6. Auscultate and record breath sounds q 2 to 4 hr and prn.
7. Check suction (when ordered) frequently.
8. Check tubing and connections frequently for leaks.

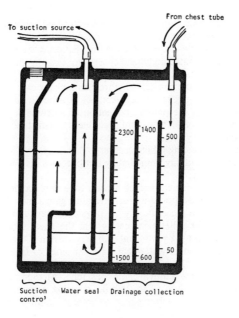

Figure 14-6. Disposable unit (Pleurevac).

9. Maintain the patency of the tubing by milking the tube hourly in the direction of the drainage apparatus to remove air, clots, and accumulated fluid, and by coiling and attaching excess tubing to the bed to prevent dependent loop formation.
10. Maintain bottles in an upright position, below chest level, at all times.
11. Keep glass bottles in a protective rack (cage) to prevent breakage, and avoid breaking bottles when side rails/bed are lowered.
12. Maintain an open air vent tube at all times, permitting the escape of intrapleural air from the bottle.
13. Administer pain medication as ordered.
14. Assist the patient to turn, cough, and deep breathe q 2 hr to facilitate drainage.
15. Splint the patient's chest when coughing to decrease pain.
16. Assist the patient to ambulate and sit in a chair with chest tubes in place.
17. Provide for emergency situations. (Keep two [6 to 8 in.] hemostats with rubber-covered ends at the bedside. Have a new water-seal system readily available.)

18. Clamp tubing immediately if glass water-seal bottle breaks. (Apply one hemostat ~10 in. from tube insertion site. Apply second hemostat 2 to 4 in. distal to the first hemostat to secure. Notify the physician immediately, and observe for tension pneumothorax and mediastinal shift.)

19. Check with the physician before clamping the chest tube for any of the following reasons: replacement of a bottle or the Pleurevac, transport of the patient, collection of a drainage specimen, and determination of the patient's readiness to withstand removal of the chest tube system.

20. Tape connecting tubing securely.

21. Reconnect tubing immediately if it becomes disconnected. Maintain sterility.

22. Do not attempt to replace a chest tube that accidently pulls out. Cover the insertion site with petrolatum gauze and a 4 ×4 in. gauze pad taped in place. Notify the physician immediately.

23. Monitor for criteria indicating that the chest tube is no longer needed. (Chest x-ray reveals full reexpansion of the lung. Absence of fluctuation in water-seal tube. Absence of drainage from the intrapleural space.)

24. Assist with the removal of the chest tube. (Medicate for pain 30 min before procedure. Tape sterile dressing securely to site [dry dressing or petrolatum gauze, as ordered] following removal of the tube.)

Psychosocial 25. Explain all procedures to the patient/family in order to decrease anxiety.

26. Encourage the patient/family to verbalize any concerns relative to chest tube insertion.

27. Reassure the patient/family that the need for the chest tube is temporary.

28. Reassure the patient/family concerning the safety of properly used equipment.

29. Anticipate the patient's needs and respond promptly to the call bell.

Educational 30. Explain the rationale for chest tube insertion to the patient/family.

31. Instruct the patient/family regarding the correct procedure for sitting in a chair and ambulating with the chest tube in place.

32. Inform the patient/family of safety precautions required with chest tubes (e.g., the need to clamp the tube immediately if water-seal bottle is broken; call for help).

The **evaluation criteria** are listed at the end of the Overview (*see below*).

Thoracentesis. Thoracentesis involves the insertion of a needle through the chest wall into the pleural space for aspiration of fluid from that area. It is used therapeutically to drain fluid in order to relieve lung compression and prevent or treat infection. It is used diagnostically to determine the cause and extent of a respiratory disorder. Laboratory tests on the fluid include specific gravity, WBC, RBC, protein concentration, glucose concentration, amylase content, cytology, and culture and sensitivities. Thoracentesis is indicated in the presence of empyema, hydrothorax, hemothorax, and pleurisy with effusion. During a thoracentesis, the patient should be placed in one of two appropriate positions: either (1) an upright, sitting position with neck and dorsal spine flexed, arms and shoulders raised, and head on pillow on over-the-bed table, or (2) turned on unaffected side, with arm over head (if unable to sit up). Local anesthetic is applied to the site of needle insertion, and the needle (17-gauge) is inserted into the pleural space under sterile conditions. Fluid is aspirated ($\leq$1,200 ml) slowly with a 50-ml syringe. Pressure and sterile dressings are applied to the aspiration site after the procedure. Complications include shock due to a fluid shift from the vascular to pleural space, infection, mediastinal shift or tension pneumothorax, pneumothorax, and inadvertent liver or spleen puncture.

Nursing interventions are as follows:

Physical 1. Administer sedation if ordered.
  2. Assist the patient to assume and maintain the proper position.
  3. Monitor the patient closely during the procedure for cardiovascular and respiratory changes (vital signs, dyspnea, cyanosis, and diaphoresis).
  4. Monitor vital signs q 15 min for 4 hr, then q 2 to 4 hr or prn.
  5. Auscultate the patient's chest q 4 hr, then prn.
  6. Check the dressing site for leakage.
  7. Position the patient on the unaffected side for 1 hr after the procedure.
  8. Administer pain medication if indicated.
  9. Assist with turning, deep breathing, and coughing as the condition improves.
  10. Record a description of the specimen and the patient's response to the procedure.
Psychosocial 11. Explain the procedure and rationale to the patient to allay fears.
  12. Remain with the patient during the procedure to reassure him.
Educational 13. Instruct the patient not to move or cough during the procedure.
  14. Tell the patient to report any pain or dyspnea during or after the procedure.

The **evaluation criteria** are listed at the end of the Overview (*see below*).

Pulmonary surgery. Surgical interventions for disorders in pulmonary functioning include exploratory thoracotomy, resectional surgery, decortication, and thoracoplasty.

Exploratory thoracotomy is used to locate bleeding and injury and to inspect the disease process and obtain a biopsy. A posterolateral parascapular or anterior incision is made through the intercostal space. The pleura is opened, and the ribs are spread to expose the lung. Closed chest drainage is usually required postoperatively.

Resectional surgery, surgical removal of lung tissue, is indicated in the presence of bronchiectasis, pulmonary TB (rare), chronic localized infections, cysts, lung abscesses, bronchial adenoma, and bronchogenic carcinoma. A posterolateral parascapular incision is made through the 4th, 5th, 6th, or 7th intercostal space, or an anterior approach is made through the 3rd, 4th, or 5th intercostal space. A pneumonectomy (removal of a lung) involves the crushing or severing of the phrenic nerve on the operative side in order to paralyze the diaphragm in an elevated position and reduce the size of the cavity. Closed chest drainage is not used. Serous exudate is allowed to consolidate in order to prevent mediastinal shift. A clamped chest tube may be placed to facilitate inspection of drainage for bleeding and regulation of intrathoracic pressure. A lobectomy (removal of a lobe) involves suturing of the associated bronchus. Overexpansion of the remaining lung tissue occurs in order to fill the thoracic space (compensatory emphysema). A lobectomy requires closed chest drainage postoperatively. Segmental resection is removal of one or more segments of a lobe of the lung. It requires closed chest drainage. Wedge resection, removal of a small wedge-shaped portion of a lung segment, also requires closed chest drainage.

Decortication is indicated in the presence of a thick, fibrous membrane over the visceral pleura secondary to empyema or to prolonged presence of blood or serous fluid in the pleural space. Decortication involves the dissection or peeling away of the restrictive membrane and the application of closed chest drainage with suction to facilitate rapid reexpansion of the lung.

Thoracoplasty is a procedure that is used to reduce the thoracic space before or after resectional surgery (when indicated by potential or actual failure of lung reexpansion). It is also indicated for closure of a chronic empyema space. The procedure involves the removal of ribs or portions of ribs, which permits weakening and collapse of a portion of the chest wall, and stripping of the periosteum (which is left in place in the chest wall to stimulate growth of bony substances for chest wall stabilization). Thoracoplasty requires closed chest drainage only if the pleura is entered inadvertently.

Postoperative complications specifically associated with pulmonary surgery include inadequate respiratory functioning (hypoxia, hyperventilation, CO_2 retention, hypercapnia, and respiratory arrest); tension pneumothrax; mediastinal shift; residual pleural space due to inadequate reexpansion of lung tissue; bronchopleural fistula; subcutaneous emphysema; acute pulmonary edema; atelectasis; pneumonia; and hemothorax. Other related complications include shock (hypovolemic, cardiogenic, and neurogenic); circulatory disorders (arrhythmias, MI, pulmonary embolism, thrombophlebitis, and cardiac arrest); and gastric distension (which causes an elevated diaphragm and, thus, decreased ventilation).

Preoperative **nursing** interventions are listed below:

Physical 1. Monitor parameters indicative of general health status (intake and output, sputum, pulmonary function tests, chest x-ray, bronchoscopy, ECG, CBC, serum electrolytes, urinalysis, arterial blood gases, history, and physical exam).
  2. Institute measures ordered to improve physical status, e.g., force fluids (unless contraindicated); allow no smoking; provide a high-protein, high-caloric diet, antibiotics, postural drainage, IPPB, breathing exercises, and oral hygiene; and medicate immediately preoperatively (atropine) to decrease secretions.
Psychosocial 3. Explain all diagnostic tests and activities associated with the perioperative period to decrease anxiety.
  4. Permit the patient/family to verbalize concerns relative to surgery.
  5. Encourage and support compliance with the smoking restriction.
  6. Reassure that medication will be used to decrease postoperative pain.
Educational 7. Explain the anatomy and physiology of the respiratory tract.
  8. Explain the rationale for surgery.
  9. Teach the patient/family about the routine and the equipment necessary in the postoperative period.
      a. Cough, deep breathe, and change position hourly for 24 hr.
      b. Ambulate, cough, deep breathe, exercise q 4 hr.
      c. Perform leg, arm, and shoulder exercises.
      d. Use respiratory therapy to drain secretions and help reexpand the lung as indicated.
      e. Use artificial airway, O_2 therapy, and CMV and chest tubes if indicated.
  10. Document teaching in chart.
  11. Evaluate the patient's understanding of the information presented.

Postoperative **nursing** care is as follows:

Physical 1. Monitor vital signs q 15 min for 4 hr, then q 30 to 60 min until stable.
  2. Monitor arterial blood gases, serum electrolytes, and central venous pressure (CVP) and arterial pressures.
  3. Have a cardiac monitor in place (when ordered).
  4. Auscultate the patient's chest for breath sounds q 2 hr.
  5. Record intake and output.
  6. Check the level of consciousness/sensorium frequently.
  7. Check chest tubes q 1 to 2 hr.
  8. Observe for crepitation (crackling noise).

9. Observe the dressing q 2 hr. (Bleeding on the dressing is unusual.)
10. Inspect, percuss, and auscultate the abdomen.
11. Monitor IV fluids (type, rate, amount, and site).
12. Observe and report signs and symptoms of complications (*see above*).
    a. Hemorrhage (bloody drainage, pallor, dyspnea, cyanosis, tachycardia, and tachypnea).
    b. Shock (hypotension with systolic BP <90 mmHg, oliguria/anuria).
    c. Absent/diminished breath sounds on unaffected side.
    d. Acute chest pain.
    e. Temperature elevation >37.2°C (99°F).
13. Frequently check the rate and functioning of the equipment in use.
14. Administer O_2 as ordered.
15. Maintain a patent airway.
16. Suction as ordered (usually nasopharyngeal q 2 hr, then prn). Deep tracheal suctioning should be performed only by the physician because of the delicate bronchial suture line.
17. Force fluids to liquefy bronchial secretions, unless contraindicated.
18. Administer pain medication as ordered with care (usually merperidine HCl). It is important to balance the pain relief necessary to accomplish breathing excercises against a depressed respiratory level.
19. Assist the patient with coughing and deep breathing as ordered (usually hourly for 24 hr).
    a. Medicate 20 to 30 min before the procedure.
    b. Take vital signs.
    c. Perform a respiratory assessment.
    d. Assist the patient to a sitting position.
    e. Splint the incision.
    f. Reassure the patient that the incision will not open.
    g. Encourage the patient to take several deep breaths and then cough.
    h. Assess vital signs and respiratory status after the procedure.
    i. Assist the patient with oral hygiene.
    j. Record the time of treatment, the amount and description of sputum produced, and vital signs and respiratory status before and after the procedure.
20. Assist with exercises as ordered (passive/active range of motion to arm of operative side is especially important to prevent "frozen" shoulder/arm contractures).
21. Assist the patient with turning as ordered (usually q 1 to 2 hr).
22. Follow any specific orders for positioning. General considerations: avoid Trendelenburg's; maintain dorsal recumbent until vital signs

stable; do not turn patient on unaffected side following pneumonectomy; usually can allow full lateral turning after lobectomy; avoid compressing or putting tension on chest tubes when positioning.

23. Assist with ambulation as ordered (usually by evening of operative day or following morning).

24. Ambulate the patient with O_2/chest tubes in place when ordered.

25. Provide for emergency situations. The following equipment should be within reach: Ambu bag, tracheostomy set, laryngoscope, bronchoscope, and crash cart.

26. Institute appropriate measures related to O_2 and electrical hazards.

Psychosocial 27. Explain all ongoing procedures to the patient/family to reduce anxiety.

28. Allow the patient to verbalize concerns and fears associated with altered respiratory status.

29. Reassure the patient/family concerning the safety of properly used equipment.

30. Maintain a calm environment and anticipate the patient's needs.

Educational 31. Reinforce the teaching provided to the patient/family in the preoperative period.

32. Teach the patient/family about any new equipment or procedures that may be required by the postoperative condition.

33. Teach about the need to practice scrupulous oral hygiene, avoid individuals with respiratory infections, provide for adequate rest periods, exercise to tolerance, continue range-of-motion exercises for the affected arm, and avoid irritants to the respiratory tract.

34. Teach about the need to take medications as prescribed.

35. Advise the patient to report any of the following to the physician: pain, swelling, redness, or drainage at the operative site; symptoms of an upper respiratory infection; shortness of breath; and side effects of medications.

36. Refer the patient to a social worker for counseling if modifications in life-style or occupation are necessitated by a diminished respiratory capacity.

37. Inform the patient/family about community resources available for support.

The **evaluation criteria** are listed at the end of the Overview (*see below*).

Nursing interventions

Nursing care for patients with altered respiratory status includes education and assistive measures to promote optimum ventilatory effort and ensure effective removal of secretions.

Turning and **positioning** the patient with altered respiratory status mobilizes secretions, provides for optimum chest expansion, reduces pressure of abdominal contents on the diaphragm, and facilitates deep breathing.

1. Encourage and assist the bed-bound patient to turn in a side-back-side rotation unless contraindicated.
2. Assist the patient to change position frequently.
3. Position the patient with dyspnea in a high Fowler's or semi-Fowler's position unless contraindicated. Keep side rails in place if confusion is present.

Activity aids in the mobilization of secretions, stimulates coughing (*see below*), and improves chest expansion.

1. Encourage and assist the patient to do as much activity as his condition permits (sitting in chair, ambulating, active/passive exercises).

Breathing exercises are used to reduce the patient's respiratory rate, produce more effective coughing, and help with controlled breathing. Instruct the patient in diaphragmatic breathing (augmented abdominal breathing):

1. Position the patient for comfort and optimum chest expansion.
2. Teach the patient to inhale deeply through the nose and exhale slowly through pursed lips.
3. Teach the patient to expand and contract his abdominal muscles during inhalation and exhalation.
4. Apply manual pressure on the upper abdomen to assist the patient during exhalation.

Coughing is a reflex or voluntary action that involves deep inspiration, closure of the glottis, muscular contraction (compression of chest wall and abdomen), opening of the glottis, and expulsive exhalation of alveolar air. Coughing removes irritants and secretions from the tracheobronchial tree and helps to prevent and treat respiratory disorders. Coughing is contraindicated in the presence of severe chronic lung disease (ruptured alveolar blebs may result), unstable cardiovascular conditions, and unstable cerebral conditions.

1. Institute measures to stimulate coughing (e.g., deep breathing, activity, position, slight manual pressure over the suprasternal notch, fluids, percussion, and vibration).
2. Provide for comfort. (Administer analgesics as ordered, and splint chest/abdominal incisions with hand, rolled blanket, or pillow.)
3. Instruct the patient in the most effective coughing technique: take deep breath, contract diaphragm/intercostal muscles, and exhale forcefully.

4. Teach the patient to expectorate (not swallow) sputum.
5. Provide encouragement and support.
6. Auscultate the patient's lung fields before and after the procedure to note effectiveness.
7. Observe and record results.

Suctioning involves the introduction of a sterile catheter and the application of intermittent suction to aspirate bronchial secretions from the trachea. It is indicated in the presence of conditions that render the patient unable to clear his own secretions, such as absent cough reflex, extreme debility, copious or tenacious secretions, and endotracheal intubation. Complications of suctioning include irritation or inflammation of tracheal mucosa due to improper technique and cardiac arrest secondary to hypoxia from prolonged suctioning.

1. Explain the procedure to the patient/family.
2. Position the patient appropriately: semi-Fowler's position if possible; head turned to side; pillow under shoulders to hyperextend neck.
3. Auscultate the chest to locate pooled secretions.
4. Preoxygenate and ventilate before the procedure and between aspirations if indicated.
5. Maintain sterile technique and dispose of equipment after use (catheter, glove, water-soluble lubricant, water).
6. Insert appropriate size, lubricated catheter into airway gently without applying suction.
7. Apply intermittent suction while withdrawing or rotating the catheter.
8. Aspirate 3 to 10 sec each time, as tolerated.
9. Monitor the pulse rate during the procedure.
10. Observe for signs and symptoms of hypoxia.
11. Auscultate the chest to determine the effectiveness of the procedure.
12. Record the patient's response to the treatment.

Humidification is the introduction of moisture to the environment in order to reduce bronchial irritation and liquefy secretions. Humidifiers are devices that electrically vaporize water with or without heat. Certain models also supply O_2. Nebulizers add aerosol water droplets to inspired air (medication maybe added). They may be hand-held or mechanical, intermittent or continuous.

Percussion/vibration and **postural drainage** are usually performed in combination to aid in the removal of secretions from the bronchopulmonary tree. Percussion (clapping) involves striking the chest wall rhythmically with cupped hands for 1 to 5 min over the affected lung field. It creates an air cushion between the hand and the chest wall that loosens secretions. Vibration involves compressing and vibrating the chest wall with the hands (fingers extended) as the patient exhales. Vibration, which follows percussion and is repeated for 3 to 5 exhalations, helps move secretions along the bronchial passages. Postural drainage uses positioning for maximal gravitational effect for the removal of secretions from the bronchopulmonary tree. Secretions are moved by gravity to the main-stem bronchi and trachea from which they may be suctioned or coughed up. Postural drainage follows chest physiotherapy when both procedures are ordered. These procedures are indicated in the presence of conditions that result in excessive or thick bronchial secretions (COPD, pneumonia, chronic bronchitis, cystic fibrosis) and the presence of diminished respiratory effort or secretion retention (obesity, immobility, postoperative status, debility, quadriplegia). These procedures are also used in the prevention of respiratory complications. Contraindications to these procedures include unstable cardiovascular disease (pulmonary edema, hypertension, CHF, pulmonary emboli) and trauma (spinal injury, head injury, fractured ribs, untreated tension pneumothorax). These procedures are also contraindicated in the presence of extreme age or debility, TB, resectable carcinoma, bony metastasis, lung abscesses/empyema, pulmonary effusion, extreme dyspnea, hemorrhage, and mastectomy with silicone implant. (Vibration alone may be indicated following thoracic surgery, chest trauma, or in severe debilitation.) Complications consist of dizziness, nausea (due to odor or taste of sputum), and vomiting/aspiration.

1. Monitor the patient before the procedure for signs and symptoms of contraindications (*see above*).
2. Determine which lung segments are to be drained. (Auscultate lung fields and monitor chest x-ray.)
3. Schedule therapy to avoid complications (before meals, at least 1 hr before tube feedings, tid or qid).
4. Administer medications/humidification (if ordered) 15 to 20 min before therapy (bronchodilators, liquefying agents).
5. Position the patient for maximum therapeutic effect and comfort (Table 14-1).
   a. Position the patient so that the segment to be drained is uppermost and in a vertical position.
   b. Use a tilt board, automatic bed, strong chair, and/or pillows to achieve the appropriate position.
   c. Position to drain the upper lobes first when several are to be drained.
   d. Modify the position as indicated by the patient's condition. (Debilitated and elderly patients may not be able to tolerate a head down position.)
6. Carry out drainage and percussion procedures according to accepted technique.
   a. Establish a rhythmic motion with cupped hands over the affected lung field.

TABLE 14-1

Positions for Postural Drainage and Chest Percussion

Lobe	Segments	Position	Percussion area
Upper	Right and left apical	Sitting upright (leaning forward for posterior; backward for anterior).	Upper back and scapulae.
	Right and left anterior	Supine, with pillow under knees.	Upper chest; below clavicles.
	Right and left posterior	Upright on unaffected side, at 45° tilt forward against pillow.	Scapula of affected side.
Middle	Right medial/ lateral	Trendelenburg's position (12-16 in); on back with 45° tilt toward left side; support with pillow under back.	Anterior chest; below clavicles. Anterior and lateral right chest between 4th and 6th ribs.
	Lingula	Trendelenburg's position (12-16 in); on back with 45° tilt toward right side; support with pillow under back.	Left chest; axillary fold to midanterior.
Lower	Right and left apical	Prone; pillow under hips and abdomen.	Posterior chest; both sides over lower portion of scapulae.
	Right and left anterior basal	Supine; Trendelenburg's position (14-18 in).	Anterior chest; both sides. Avoid sternum and stomach.
	Right and left lateral basal	Trendelenburg's position (14-18 in); turn on unaffected side; pillow under hips.	Affected side at level of 10th rib.
	Right and left posterior basal	Trendelenburg's position (14-18 in); prone; pillow under hips.	Posterior chest at level of 10th rib. Avoid kidneys.

b. Do not percuss over bare skin, spine, bony prominences, or soft tissue.
c. Instruct the patient to breathe deeply during percussion and vibration.
d. Follow percussion with vibration to the same area.
e. Apply compression and vibration only during exhalation.
f. Position the patient for postural drainage.

g. Encourage the patient to cough and deep breathe before changing positions.
h. Monitor cardiac and respiratory status during therapy.
i. Continue treatment for 10 min at first and progress to 30 min according to the patient's tolerance.
j. Encourage the patient to cough and deep breathe after the treatment.
k. Assist the patient to a comfortable position following therapy.
l. Assist with oral hygiene.
m. Observe the amount and characteristics of sputum.
n. Dispose of sputum carefully to prevent infection. Use appropriate hand washing techniques.
o. Assess respiratory status following therapy.
p. Record the time of therapy, tolerance to therapy, amount and characteristics of sputum, and respiratory status.
7. Remain with the patient continuously during postural drainage for the first few treatments, then prn, to allay fears.
8. Refer the patient to a social worker for aid in arranging respiratory care after discharge.
9. Explain the rationale for therapy to the patient/family.
10. Teach the patient/family each step of the procedure.
11. Teach the patient/family postural drainage before discharge.
12. Teach the patient/family how to dispose of sputum safely (wash hands after treatment).

Evaluation criteria

Risk factors/complications minimized or absent. Vital signs stable. Safety measures implemented. Patient and family demonstrate adequate knowledge base, e.g., list hazards and signs and symptoms of complications and recurrence, and participate in therapeutic regimen, medication regimen, therapies, and preventive practices.

DEVIATIONS

NEAR-DROWNING

Near-drowning is asphyxia secondary to accidental or intentional submersion. Each year in the USA, there are 7,000 fatalities and an estimated 8,000 near-drowning victims. Of the victims who live long enough to receive medical care, 90% survive. It occurs most often in children and young adults; 80% of the victims are males. Swimming and boating accidents are the most common causes of near-drowning. Suicide attempts are also frequent. "Dry-drowning," which accounts for 10 to 20% of all victims, is asphyxia secondary to reflex laryngospasm and closure of the glottis. No water is aspirated. "Wet-drowning" involves aspiration of water. The resultant laryngospasm, bronchospasm, and airway obstruction (particulate matter) cause hypoxia, which, when prolonged, results in pulmonary edema. If fresh water aspiration occurs, fluid shifts out of the lung into the circulation, pulmonary surfactant is destroyed, atelectasis occurs, and hypoxemia results. If salt water aspiration occurs, there is a rapid shift of plasma protein and water from the circulation to the alveoli, resulting in pulmonary edema and hypoxemia.

The severity of symptoms depends on whether or not water was aspirated, type and amount of water aspirated, length of submersion, temperature of the water, and promptness/effectiveness of treatment. *Symptoms* may include mild cough, tachypnea, pulmonary edema (frothy sputum, rales); altered mental status; coma; speech, motor, and visual abnormalities; seizures; arrhythmias and tachycardia secondary to acidosis and hypoxia; elevated temperature in the first 24 hr; vomiting associated with gastric distension; and cyanosis. *Complications* include neurologic disorders secondary to cerebral anoxia (5 to 20% of victims have permanent neurologic sequelae, hypothermia moderates the cerebral O_2 requirement) and renal failure secondary to hypoxia and hypotension. Pulmonary disorders may also occur, including atelectasis, bacterial pneumonia, lung abscess, empyema, and adult respiratory distress syndrome (ARDS). Finally, chest injuries (pneumothorax, mediastinal shift) secondary to resuscitation efforts may also occur.

Diagnosis is based on the health history, physical exam, and such laboratory tests as arterial blood gases (to identify the degree of hypoxia), chest x-ray, serum electrolytes (acidosis may occur), WBC (leukocytosis occurs in the first 1 to 2 days), and sputum culture and sensitivities.

Common interventions

Methods of treatment involve airway establishment, CPR, O_2 therapy (100%, then concentration adjusted according to arterial blood gases), observation in a medical facility (even if asymptomatic after resuscitation), and ventilatory support for respiratory failure. IV solutions are used to treat fluid and electrolyte imbalance (e.g., sodium bicarbonate for metabolic acidosis), aerosol bronchodilators are used for bronchospasm, and a cardiac monitor may be indicated. A nasogastric (NG) tube may be used to relieve gastric distension. Antibiotics are used if infection occurs (prophylactic antibiotic use is controversial).

Nursing interventions

Physical 1. Monitor and record vital signs on admission and as indicated by the condition. Notify the physician of any changes. (Cardiac monitor may be ordered.)

2. Monitor neurologic vital signs on admission and as indicated by the condition. Notify the physician of changes in level of consciousness or of seizure activity.

3. Monitor arterial blood gases and electrolytes.

4. Observe for signs and symptoms of complications.
5. Maintain a patent airway (artificial airway may be indicated). Suction if indicated.
6. Support ventilatory efforts (mechanical ventilator may be ordered).
7. Administer O_2 therapy as ordered.
8. Administer medications as ordered (bronchodilators, antibiotics).
9. Institute safety measures (side rails, seizure precautions, O_2 precautions, CMV precautions).
10. Observe the proper technique for NG tube insertion when ordered.
11. Monitor IV fluids.
12. Maintain an intake and output record.
13. Monitor and record resolving symptoms.
Psychosocial 14. Explain all procedures even when coma is present.
15. Support psychotherapy if the condition is a result of a suicide attempt.
Educational 16. Educate the public regarding water safety measures and CPR training.

Evaluation criteria.   *See* Overview.

ACUTE AIRWAY OBSTRUCTION

Acute airway obstruction is an emergency condition created by the presence of a foreign body (usually a bolus of food) in the larynx or trachea. Its incidence is not reliably documented. Predisposing factors include alcohol ingestion, extreme debility, and failure to chew food properly. Obstruction is often caused by accidental aspiration of a foreign body and by traumatic lesions (e.g., assaults, vehicular accidents, sports-related accidents). Airway occlusion by a foreign body results in death from asphyxia in 4 min. *Symptoms* include marked respiratory distress, inability to breathe, cyanosis, inability to speak, clutching of throat, and collapse. *Diagnosis* is based on the health history and physical exam.

Common interventions

Emergency methods of treatment include the delivery of four blows to the back between the shoulder blades, the Heimlich maneuver, and/or a tracheostomy. The **Heimlich maneuver** (abdominal thrust) elevates the diaphragm, compresses air in the lungs, increases tracheobronchial pressure, and forces the obstruction out of the airway. The procedure for the sitting or standing victim is to stand or kneel behind the victim, place a fist against the victim's abdomen between the umbilicus and xiphoid process, and grasp the fist with the other hand and apply a quick upward thrust. For the supine victim, the procedure is to kneel astride (facing) the victim, place one hand on top of the other, with the heel of the bottom hand on the victim's abdomen between the umbilicus and xiphoid process, and apply a quick upward thrust. The procedure may be repeated, if necessary. If rescue measures fail, a tracheostomy is indicated (*see above*).

PULMONARY EMBOLISM

Pulmonary embolism is a complete or partial obstruction of the pulmonary arterial flow to the distal lung. There are 50,000 deaths in the USA annually due to pulmonary embolism. The overall estimated annual incidence in the USA is over 500,000. Predisposing factors include venous stasis due to prolonged immobility, postpartum status, obesity, or burns; alterations in blood coagulability, as seen with neoplasms, anovulatory drug use (controversial), pregnancy, and sickle cell anemia; disease, e.g., chronic deep venous insufficiency, chronic pulmonary disease, CHF, diabetes mellitus, and infection; and venous injury due to surgery (particularly legs, pelvis, abdomen, and chest) or fractures or injuries to the lower extremities. The causative factor is foreign matter occluding the pulmonary artery, e.g., thrombi (most common), air, fat, amniotic fluid, and neoplasm. The affected area of lung cannot participate in gas exchange due to inadequate perfusion. Constriction of associated air spaces may result. Hypoxemia frequently occurs. Finally, increased resistance to pulmonary blood flow may result in pulmonary hypertension and acute right heart failure.

Symptoms vary from mild to severe. With a massive pulmonary embolism, the symptoms include sudden shock; respiratory distress (tachypnea, diminished breath sounds, rales); cyanosis; cerebral ischemia (restlessness, anxiety, syncope, convulsions); and crushing substernal pain. Pulmonary embolism may also be asymptomatic, with vague, nonspecific symptoms, including tachypnea; tachycardia; pleuritic chest pain, friction rub, fever hemoptysis (with infarction); anxiety and restlessness; dyspnea; and cough. *Complications* include pulmonary infarction, extension of emboli, acute MI, cerebrovascular occlusion, shock, ARDS (*see below*), bronchopneumonia, pulmonary abscess, cardiac dysrhythmias, and hepatic congestion or necrosis.

Diagnosis is based on the health history, physical exam, and the following laboratory tests: CBC (to identify elevated WBC, ESR), arterial blood gases ($PO_2 \leq 80$ mmHg; $PCO_2 < 35$ mmHg), serum electrolytes (respiratory alkalosis may occur), blood enzymes (to identify increased lactic dehydrogenase), ECG (normal unless acute pulmonary hypertension develops), chest x-ray (nonspecific or shows infarction), lung scan (demonstrates ventilation in excess of perfusion), and pulmonary angiogram (reveals clots and/or obstruction).

Common interventions

Medical treatment consists of the use of anticoagulation therapy (initially heparin IV or deep SC, then coumadin derivatives PO, and long-term maintenance with thrombolytics). Fibrinolytic drugs (streptokinase, urokinase) are also used, but may cause a severe allergic response. IV dextran is used to decrease blood viscosity and reduce aggregation of blood cells. Analgesics are used judiciously to reduce pain but not to depress respirations. O_2 therapy is used for respiratory distress, and vasoconstrictors may be used for shock, if indicated. **Surgical** treatment consists of interruption of the inferior vena cava by means of ligation, clipping, plication, or filter procedures performed in conjunction with the use of an intracaval umbrella. Surgical interruption is used in the presence of recurrent emboli or when anticoagulant therapy is unsuccessful. A rarely performed surgical procedure is the pulmonary embolectomy (surgical removal of emboli), which is used in the presence of massive embolism with cardiovascular collapse.

Nursing interventions

Physical 1. Monitor vital signs hourly, then prn. Notify the physician of adverse signs. (Cardiac monitor may be ordered.)
2. Auscultate chest for breath sounds q 2 to 4 hr.
3. Monitor sputum for amount, color, and character.
4. Monitor lab values (arterial blood gases, serum enzymes and electrolytes, WBC, clotting time, and prothrombin time).
5. Observe for signs and symptoms of complications.
6. Measure and record intake and output.
7. Administer medications as ordered: anticoagulants, thrombolytics, analgesics, vasoconstrictors (shock), cardiotonics.
8. Maintain parenteral fluids as ordered.
9. Observe for bleeding secondary to anticoagulants (stools, urine, sputum, injection sites, wounds).
10. Administer O_2 therapy as ordered.
11. Maintain activity levels as ordered (bed rest; semi-Fowler's position; no knee gatch during acute phase; increase activity as tolerated; turn q 2 hr; active and passive range-of-motion exercises q 2 to 4 hr when indicated).
12. Encourage the patient to deep breathe q 2 to 4 hr.
13. Encourage fluids (2,000 to 3,000 ml/day) unless contraindicated by cardiovascular status.
14. Administer oral hygiene after coughing.
15. Assist the patient to avoid constipation and straining. (Provide stool softeners and administer laxatives as ordered.)
16. Assess lower extremities frequently (calf measurement; warmth, tenderness in calf muscle; pedal pulses; proper placement of antiembolism stockings).
17. Assist with hygiene and avoid back rubs during the acute phase.
18. Use side rails if restlessness or confusion exists.
19. Have antidotes to anticoagulation readily available (protamine sulfate for heparin, vitamin K for coumadin, and aminocaproic acid for streptokinase).
Psychosocial 20. Remain with the patient during dyspneic episodes to decrease anxiety.

Educational 21. Teach the patient and family preventive measures to formation of emboli (avoid constricting clothing and crossing legs, wear antiembolism stockings, avoid sitting or standing longer than 1 hr, avoid rubbing the legs, particularly when calf tenderness is present, and maintain exercise).
22. Instruct the patient/family about follow-up visits to monitor anticoagulation.
23. Encourage the patient to obtain and wear a medical alert bracelet.
Prevention 24. Prevent stasis, particularly in postoperative, postpartum, and immobilized patients.

Evaluation criteria.   *See* Overview.

ADULT RESPIRATORY DISTRESS SYNDROME

ARDS is a form of pulmonary insufficiency, characterized by hypoxia and decreased pulmonary compliance, that develops after shock or shocklike states. The incidence of ARDS is undocumented but believed to be on the increase. Predisposing factors consist of many diverse conditions that produce stress, including trauma, hemorrhagic shock, fat embolism, multiple transfusions, drug ingestion, gram-negative sepsis, severe viral pneumonia, amniotic fluid embolism, major surgery, hemorrhagic pancreatitis, smoke inhalation, and thermal burns. Causation has not been precisely identified, but factors under study include ischemic pulmonary injury, increased circulating humoral agents in the blood during hemorrhagic or hypotensive shock (e.g., histamine, serotonin, complement), bacterial toxins that damage alveolar-capillary membranes, O_2 toxicity, microembolism secondary to trauma, and altered permeability of the alveolar-capillary membranes. During ARDS, increased capillary membrane permeability allows protein and water to shift into interstitial and alveolar spaces, resulting in edema and decreased functional VC. Also occurring are pulmonary hypoperfusion, hypoxemia, impaired surfactant production, decreased pulmonary compliance, atelectasis, hyperventilation, and hypocapnia.

Symptoms include dyspnea, tachypnea, cyanosis, confusion progressing to loss of consciousness, hypotension, and fine rales progressing to marked pulmonary edema. *Complications* include pneumonia, lung abscesses, pulmonary emboli, heart failure, septicemia, disseminated intravascular coagulation, irreversible lung damage, and death.

Diagnosis is based on the health history, physical exam, and the following laboratory tests: arterial blood gases (to identify hypoxemia, hypocapnia), chest x-ray (to identify alveolar infiltrates), and pulmonary function studies (revealing decreased compliance and functional residual capacity).

Common interventions

Medical treatment consists of ventilatory support (intubation, CMV with high pressure and flow capacity, PEEP), hemodynamic monitoring, and O_2 therapy. Other treatments include diuretics and fluid restriction in order to decrease circulating fluids; corticosteroids (use is controversial); antibiotics if the infection is identified; analgesics for pain (to reduce O_2 consumption associated with pain and hyperventilation); bed rest; bronchodilators, if indicated; and volume expanders (salt-poor albumin) to increase the serum colloidal osmotic pressure. Fever should be reduced to decrease O_2 consumption. **Surgically**, a tracheostomy may be indicated to establish and maintain an airway.

Nursing interventions

Physical 1. Monitor respiratory status closely (q 30 min or prn) for breath sounds, adventitious sounds, respiratory rate and depth, and arterial blood gases.
  2. Monitor cardiovascular status frequently for BP, apical pulse, neck vein distension, hepatojugular reflux, peripheral pulses, temperature, and color of extremities.
  3. Check level of consciousness hourly.
  4. Check temperature q 4 hr, then prn.
  5. Measure and record intake and output. Notify the physician if urinary output is <30 ml/hr.
  6. Monitor hemodynamic readings.
  7. Monitor weight daily.
  8. Monitor serum electrolytes. Monitor parenteral fluids closely; fluid overload is life threatening.
  9. Administer medications as ordered.
  10. Maintain O_2 at correct rate and concentration.
  11. Provide mechanical ventilation as ordered (*see* CMV *above*).
  12. Maintain a patent airway. (Encourage coughing and deep breathing if no airway is in place. Provide care for artificial airways or tracheostomy. Suction as indicated.)
  13. Institute safety precautions (side rails, O_2 precautions, CMV precautions).
  14. Position the patient for comfort and optimum ventilation (semi-Fowler's to high Fowler's).
  15. Maintain bed rest. Passive range-of-motion exercises may be indicated to promote venous return.
  16. Promote restful sleep at night; schedule blood work during the day.
  17. Assist with hygiene and provide back rubs to increase comfort and relaxation.
  18. Provide adequate nutrition to meet the demands of the critically ill patient.
  19. Encourage return to activity when indicated.

Psychosocial 20. Remain with the patient on CMV and/or during periods of dyspnea to decrease anxiety.

21. Permit family members to participate in the care, and provide support, when possible.

Educational 22. Instruct the patient/family in supportive pulmonary care when irreversible lung damage occurs.

Evaluation criteria. See Overview.

TRAUMA

Thoracic injuries are a leading cause of death and are frequently part of multisystem trauma. Of trauma deaths in the USA, 25% are due to chest injuries. Thoracic trauma includes **penetrating** or **perforating injuries** from bullets, knives, and shrapnel or other free-flying objects, and **blunt injuries** resulting from automobile accidents (steering wheel strikes chest, or victim is thrown from car), falls, blasts, explosives, and crushing accidents (machinery). Blunt injuries usually affect only the chest wall; the pleural cavity is not entered. Compression may rupture alveoli, damage the lungs and heart, and cause hemorrhage. Penetrating injuries cause communication with the pleural cavity, which permits the entrance of atmospheric air, thereby disrupting ventilation. Underlying organ damage may occur, depending on the course of the wound (i.e., the heart, lungs, and major thoracic vessels may be involved).

The *symptoms* and *complications* are listed with each specific injury below; however, complications are more likely to occur in the presence of massive multisystem trauma, obesity, advanced age, chronic pulmonary disease, and preexisting cardiovascular disease.

Diagnosis is based on the health history, physical exam, arterial blood gases, serum electrolytes, CBC, ECG (to identify cardiac damage), chest x-ray (to identify the nature and extent of injury to the chest), and other lab tests as indicated by the nature and extent of associated injuries (e.g., abdominal x-ray).

Medical and **surgical** treatments are directed toward (1) establishing and maintaining an airway via intubation, suctioning, and removal of secretions, bone fragments, blood, and vomitus; (2) restoring adequate ventilation with O_2 therapy, CMV, and positioning and ambulation when the condition permits; (3) preventing and treating shock with blood replacement and hemodynamic monitoring; and (4) relieving pain with analgesics (avoid depressing the cough reflex), nerve blocks, and splinting. Other important goals include (5) stabilizing the chest wall; (6) removing fluid and air from the pleural space; (7) recognizing associated injuries (visceral, head); (8) restoring fluid and electrolyte balance by administering IV fluids (avoid circulatory overload) and NG tube feedings (after danger of abdominal distension is past), and by resuming the diet as the condition permits; and (9) caring for external wounds (suturing, dressings).

There are four main kinds of the thoracic trauma: pneumothorax, hemothorax, flail chest, and rib fractures. These specific traumas are discussed below.

Pneumothorax is a collection of air in the pleural space due to (1) a puncture of the chest wall or diaphragm ("open"), or (2) a tear in the internal structures of respiration ("closed," "spontaneous," or "tension"). The *symptoms* of open pneumothorax include sudden, pleuritic chest pain, dyspnea, tachypnea, tachycardia, diminished or absent breath sounds on the affected side, hyperresonance on percussion, spontaneous emphysema, and positive x-ray findings. A *complication* is shock. The *symptoms* of closed (spontaneous or tension) pneumothorax include respiratory distress, progressive cyanosis, mediastinal shift and tracheal displacement (away from the affected side), hyperresonance on percussion of the affected side, displaced point of maximum impulse (away from the affected side), distended neck veins, and distant or absent breath sounds (on the affected side). A *complication* is shock. The treatment for open pneumothorax is as follows:

1. Do not remove the penetrating object (if it is still present) until medical support is available.
2. Apply an occlusive petrolatum gauze dressing.
3. Remove air and fluid (if in large amounts) with a large-bore needle or chest tubes.
4. Place the patient in the semi-Fowler's position.
5. Administer O_2 therapy to relieve hypoxia.

The treatment for closed pneumothorax is listed below:

1. Remove air and fluid with a large-bore needle or chest tubes.
2. Administer O_2 therapy with positive pressure.
3. Place the patient in the semi-Fowler's position.

Hemothorax, the collection of blood in the pleural cavity, is *characterized* by respiratory distress, tachycardia, hypotension, dullness on percussion (affected side), and absent or distant breath sounds (affected side). Hemothorax may lead to shock. Treatment involves the removal of blood from the chest cavity with a large-bore needle or chest tube, and the replacement of circulating blood volume.

Flail chest results from a crushing injury (fractured ribs) that causes loss of chest wall stability and paradoxical movement of the affected area of the lung. The chest wall over the flail area moves inward on inspiration and bulges outward with expiration. *Symptoms* include rapid and shallow respirations, cyanosis, pain at the site of injury, paradoxical chest motion, and bony crepitation at fracture sites. *Complications* include shock and pulmonary contusion. Treatment includes emergency stabilization of the chest wall with adhesive strips, sandbags, and manual pressure; keeping the patient off of the flailed side; tracheostomy; positive-pressure ventilation; and treatment of the underlying injuries (keeping the patient NPO until the extent of the underlying injuries is known).

Rib fractures, secondary to trauma, are common in the elderly, athletes, and patients with severe coughing. *Symptoms* of rib fractures include pain (which may be severe and aggravated by deep breathing or movement), splinting on movement, dyspnea, and an ecchymotic area on the chest wall. A chest x-ray should reveal the fracture. Underlying and associated injuries include (1) 1st rib: neck injury, brachial plexus injury, pneumothorax, aortic tear. clavicle and scapula fractures, and (2) 9th to 12th ribs: splenic rupture, and liver damage. Subcutaneous emphysema (*see below*) is a *complication*. Treatment includes intercostal nerve block, analgesics, and bronchial hygiene.

Subcutaneous emphysema is escaped air in subcutaneous tissues associated with chest injury, thoracic surgery, and CMV. *Symptoms* include distortion of areas of the body due to air in the tissues (face, neck, scrotum) and a characteristic crackling sound/sensation on palpation of skin. Respiratory distress may result from swollen neck. No treatment is necessary because subcutaneous emphysema usually resolves spontaneously.

Nursing interventions

Physical 1. Perform a careful initial assessment and an ongoing evaluation of the injury to include data regarding vital signs, color and temperature of skin, level of consciousness, respiratory pattern, use of accessory muscles, auscultation of chest for breath sounds and cardiac sounds, and peripheral circulation.
2. Institute emergency measures indicated by the specific injury.
3. Institute and maintain treatment as ordered. (*See* specific nursing interventions related to artificial airway, O_2 therapy, CMV, chest tubes, suctioning, positioning, pulmonary surgery, and drugs.)
4. Provide adequate nutrition to meet the demands of the critically ill patient.

Educational 5. Educate the public regarding prevention of accidents and first aid information.

Evaluation criteria. *See* Overview.

INFLUENZA

Influenza is an acute, highly contagious viral infection characterized by headache, fever, and malaise. Annual outbreaks are common and tend to spread very rapidly, particularly in urban populations. Epidemics generally occur every 3 to 5 yr. Pandemics (world-wide epidemics) occur approximately every 10 yr. Three causative viral agents have been identified: types A, B, and C. Although the three types have similar properties, infection by one type does not confer immunity to the other two types. **Type A**, the most common type, is usually responsible for epidemics, pandemics, and annual outbreaks. It can undergo certain antigenic variations from time to time, resulting in recurrent disease in susceptible persons. **Type B**, which is usually milder than influenza A, occurs frequently in localized outbreaks, such as in school children. It can result in Reye's syndrome, a condition causing cerebral edema and fatty infiltration of the liver. **Type C** is less frequently identified than types A and B, but seems very prevalent, as indicated by antibody studies.

Persons who are particularly vulnerable to influenza include school children (considered to be primary contributors to the spread of the disease) and the elderly debilitated population (particularly those with chronic illness). Persons with chronic respiratory and/or cardiac disease are considered to be at risk for developing the complications associated with influenza. Influenza viruses attack the pulmonary endothelial lining, resulting in inflammation, necrosis, and sloughing of the airways. The viral agent is spread in droplet form, probably most often via coughing and sneezing of infected secretions. The incubation period is usually 24 to 48 hr.

Symptoms include headache (most common initial symptom), fever of 37.8 to 40.0°C (100 to 104°F), generalized muscular aching with malaise and weakness, chills, sore throat, cough, watery nasal discharge, anorexia, nausea, and adventitious breath sounds, which are usually absent unless the lower pulmonary tract is involved as a result of secondary pneumonia. Occasionally, however, diffuse rhonchi, rales, and wheezes can be identified in uncomplicated influenza. The most common *complication* of influenza is pneumonia, which occurs most frequently in the aged, patients with mitral stenosis secondary to rheumatic heart disease, and chronic respiratory patients. Symptoms that might indicate secondary pneumonia are dyspnea and cyanosis (rare in uncomplicated influenza), sputum change from clear to purulent or bloody, and recurrence of fever after the initial episode of influenza. Other complications of influenza include otitis media, cervical lymphadenitis, sinusitis, tracheobronchitis, cardiovascular disease, and Reye's syndrome.

Diagnosis is based on the health history, physical exam, laboratory tests (throat culture, elevated or normal WBC [>15,000 suggests a secondary bacterial infection]), and a chest x-ray (usually normal; increased vascular markings and atelectasis sometimes seen).

Common interventions

Medical treatment is primarily symptomatic and may involve bed rest until after the fever subsides (premature return to activities is discouraged) and the administration of antipyretics and analgesics such as aspirin or acetaminophen. These drugs can cause discomfort by causing profuse sweating during the course of alleviating the fever. The patient's fluid intake should be increased, and he should be provided with cough medications and saline gargle. (Codeine is frequently prescribed to alleviate the cough associated with influenza.) Humidifiers are used for steam or cool vapor inhalation. Prophylactic antibiotics are sometimes prescribed; however, current studies demonstrate that antibiotic therapy is not effective against viral infections or in preventing secondary bacterial disease. Antiviral medications are currently under investigation. Some of these medications are claimed to be effective in shortening the course of influenza when inhaled by infected persons.

Nursing interventions

Most infected persons do not seek medical attention unless complications arise. The following nursing actions are helpful and can be recommended to patients and families.

Physical 1. Provide comfort measures such as back rubs and tepid sponge baths.
2. Encourage fluids and a light diet of foods that appeal to the patient.
3. Provide a restful environment.
4. Observe for signs of complications such as prolonged fever, productive cough, and dyspnea.
Educational 5. Encourage an adequate recovery period after the symptoms disappear in order to prevent secondary bacterial infections and relapse.
6. Teach the patient proper fever control (e.g., the use of antipyretics and tepid sponge baths).
7. If an antibiotic is ordered for prevention of a secondary bacterial infection, instruct the patient to take the prescription at regular intervals and to use all of the medication even though symptoms may subside in a few days.
8. Inform the patient of the signs and symptoms of complications that are usually bacterial in origin.
9. Teach the patient and family the following preventive measures: to avoid crowds and infected persons and to obtain vaccinations during epidemic periods if the individual is vulnerable (e.g., elderly, debilitated, chronically ill, health-care workers, and others providing needed public services). For adults, 0.5 ml of vaccine is given in September followed by 0.5 ml 2 to 3 mo later and a booster annually.

Evaluation criteria.   *See* Overview.

PNEUMONIA

Pneumonia is an acute inflammation of the parenchyma of the lung involving the respiratory bronchioles and alveolar sacs. It results in exudation, consolidation, and impairment of respiratory functioning. Although mortality rates have been lower since the advent of antibiotics, pneumonia is still very common. It is thought to affect 1% of all Americans annually. Persons who are predisposed to pneumonia include infants and young children (because of a poorly developed immune system), elderly and debilitated persons, and patients with decreased immune responses (which interfere with macrophage activity and are associated with certain types of cancer and cancer therapies). Also predisposed are patients with altered states of consciousness, which lead to an impaired ability to cough adequately, depress the reflexes responsible for glottic closure, and contribute to pooling of secretions or aspiration of gastric contents or feedings. Other predisposing factors include alcohol intake, head injury, drug overdose, seizures, general anesthesia, and cerebrovascular disease. Pneumonia may also develop in patients with inadequate coughing mechanisms and shallow breathing because the lung's ability to adequately clear pulmonary airways is impaired. Pneumonia can also occur in postoperative patients (particularly after abdominal or thoracic surgery), patients with artificial airways such as endotracheal and tracheostomy tubes, and chronic respiratory patients with obstructive and/or restrictive pulmonary disease (emphysema, bronchitis, tumor). Another group that is predisposed to the development of pneumonia includes patients with damaged cilia, which impairs mucociliary transport, causing retention of pulmonary secretions and foreign material. This condition is caused by smoking, alcohol ingestion, and bronchial epithelial damage resulting from previous respiratory infections.

There are five basic causative factors of pneumonia. **Bacterial** pathogens include the following: *Diplococcus pneumoniae* (pneumococcus), the most common cause of bacterial pneumonia (90%), usually follows a noncomplicated course; *Haemophilus influenzae* usually occurs in chronic respiratory patients; *Neisseria meningitidis* usually follows a viral respiratory infection; *Klebsiella pneumoniae* and *Staphylococcus aureus* are relatively uncommon, but may cause chronic respiratory difficulties; *Pseudomonas aeruginosa,* the most common nosocomial pneumonia, is acquired by patients with depressed immunity. **Viral** pneumonia, which usually occurs in immunosuppressed patients, may begin as influenza and result in a secondary bacterial pneumonia. **Fungal** pneumonia, which results in necrosis and cavitation of the lung (as does TB), is caused by inhalation of spores present in the soil. **Aspiration** pneumonia most frequently occurs in infants, anesthetized patients, or patients with depressed gag or swallowing reflexes. It is caused by aspiration of gastric contents and results in chemical irritation from gastric acids and infection from mixed bacterial flora. **Hypostatic** pneumonia is caused by shallow breathing or splinting of the chest and results in an accumulation of fluids in the lung bases.

Pneumonias can be classified as **lobar,** which causes large, sometimes massive areas of consolidation, and **bronchopneumonia,** which causes diffuse, patchy areas of consolidation. The effects of pneumonia vary, depending on the infecting organism and the individual host response. Lung tissue usually returns to normal once the lungs are cleared.

Symptoms include chills, fever of 40.0 to 41.1°C (104 to 106°F), pleuritic chest pain, cough (dry cough in viral pneumonia), rust-colored sputum progressing to yellow and purulent during the course of the disease (characteristic of bacterial pneumonias), dyspnea, tachypnea, tachycardia, hypoxemia, and adventitious breath sounds (rales, friction rub). *Com-*

plications include pleural effusion, bacteremia (associated with an increased mortality rate), lung abscess, emphysema, meningitis, bacterial endocarditis, respiratory failure, pulmonary edema, otitis media, sinusitis, and disseminated intravascular coagulation (DIC).

Diagnosis is based on the health history, physical exam, chest x-ray, and the following laboratory tests: CBC, including differential (leukocytosis [20,000 to 35,000 mm³] indicates bacterial pneumonia); sputum culture and sensitivity; and blood culture.

Common interventions

Viral pneumonias usually run an uneventful course without intervention beyond rest and fluids. The medical treatment of bacterial pneumonias includes the use of antibiotics (based on the results of sputum culture and sensitivity), O_2 therapy if the patient is hypoxemic, bed rest at least until after the fever subsides, antipyretics and analgesics, increased fluid intake (unless contraindicated), and humidifiers for steam or cool vapor inhalation.

Nursing interventions

Physical 1. Monitor vital signs q 4 hr. (Take more often during febrile episodes. Obtain rectal temperatures if the patient is dyspneic.)
2. Provide humidification to prevent mucous membrane dryness and to help loosen secretions.
3. Provide O_2 therapy if prescribed.
4. Perform respiratory assessment each shift and q 2 to 4 hr during the acute phase.
5. Assist the patient to turn, cough, and deep breathe q 2 hr unless contraindicated.
6. Observe sputum for color, amount, and consistency.
7. Discourage smoking.
8. Provide oral hygiene to combat the effects of sputum production and mouth breathing.
9. Maintain an accurate intake and output record to prevent potential dehydration.
10. Encourage 3,000 ml of fluids daily (unless contraindicated) to facilitate loosening of secretions and to prevent dehydration.
11. Assess skin turgor daily to determine fluid balance.
12. Monitor parenteral fluids if prescribed.
13. Encourage a diet high in calories and carbohydrates unless contraindicated.
14. Provide small, frequent meals if the patient is dyspneic or anorexic.
15. Isolate the patient as per the hospital policy manual.
16. Control visitors to provide rest and to decrease the spread of infection.
17. Maintain good hand washing techniques.
18. Dispose of sputum and contaminated tissues properly.

19. Suction the patient with pulmonary congestion unless contraindicated.
20. Prevent over-medication with respiratory depressants and drugs that depress the cough reflex.
21. Check NG tubes consistently for placement before instillation of fluids for feeding or irrigation.
Psychosocial 22. Allow the patient to express fears and concerns.
23. Prepare the patient for discharge by explaining reportable symptoms of elevated temperature, persistent cough, or dyspnea; importance of increased fluid intake; importance of two to three rest periods during the day; continuation of deep-breathing exercises for 6 to 8 wk after discharge; proper medication administration; and importance of keeping future appointments.
Educational 24. Instruct the patient on methods of preventing the spread of infection, such as turning head away from others when coughing, properly disposing of contaminated tissues, and using frequent hand washing.
25. Teach the procedure for effective coughing.
26. Encourage immunization against flu in predisposed persons (elderly, chronically ill).

Evaluation criteria. *See* Overview.

BRONCHITIS

Bronchitis is an acute or chronic condition characterized by hypertrophy of mucous glands and inflammation of the large bronchi, resulting in excessive mucous production and airway narrowing. Bronchitis is a frequent contributing factor in COPD along with emphysema and asthma. The overlapping criteria for the diagnosis of bronchitis, emphysema, and asthma make the incidence of each difficult to determine. The exact nature of heredity as a predisposing factor is unclear; however, there is a possible underlying genetic predisposition in affected individuals. Cigarette smokers have a 20 times greater chance than nonsmokers of acquiring bronchitis. Air pollution is another cause (incidence is higher in urban areas where industrial air pollution is greater). Patients with a history of chronic respiratory infections are predisposed to bronchitis.

Hypertrophied mucous glands and impaired respiratory defense mechanisms lead to pulmonary infection, bronchial edema, and bronchial inflammation. Airway narrowing results in increased airway resistance, impaired ventilation, and decreased alveolar gas exchange, causing hypoxia and hypercapnia.

Symptoms include chronic cough and sputum production, particularly on rising every morning. (This is a diagnostic criterion if present for a minimum of 3 mo/yr for at least 2 consecutive yr.) Other symptoms include increased temperature; dyspnea; cyanosis ("blue bloater" appearance); rales, rhonchi, and wheezes on auscultation; acidosis; and polycythemia (resulting from the compensatory mechanism to hypoxemia). *Complications* include recurrent infections during cold weather; pulmonary emphysema; right heart failure (cor pulmonale), resulting in dependent edema, jugular venous distension, hepatomegaly, and ascites; respiratory failure; and bronchopneumonia.

Diagnosis is based on the health history, physical exam, arterial blood gases (to identify decreased PO_2 and increased PCO_2 levels), and sputum collection for culture, sensitivity, and cytology. Also used in the diagnosis are a chest x-ray to identify heart enlargement and pulmonary congestion, and pulmonary function studies, which may indicate decreased FEV and increased RV.

Common interventions

Medical treatment includes counseling the patient to stop smoking and reduce weight (if the patient is obese) and the administration of bronchodilators, expectorants, steroids (must be strictly controlled and carefully monitored), and antibiotics (during infectious episodes). Low-flow O_2 is used to prevent CO_2 narcosis, and O_2 therapy is carefully titrated according to arterial blood gas readings.

Nursing interventions

Physical 1. Discourage smoking and exposure to pollution.
2. Provide humidification to prevent mucous membrane dryness and to help loosen secretions.
3. Assist the patient to perform postural drainage q 4 hr (if able to tolerate procedure).
4. Position the patient in semi-Fowler's to high Fowler's position (unless contraindicated) to facilitate chest expansion and effective coughing.
5. Provide small, frequent feedings to prevent dyspnea after meals.
6. Take vital signs q 4 hr and auscultate the chest q 4 hr and prn.
7. Observe sputum for amount, color, and consistency.
8. Monitor arterial blood gases.
9. Administer low-flow O_2 carefully titrated to arterial blood gas readings.
10. Monitor the patient's level of consciousness to identify changes signifying deterioration of arterial blood gases.
11. Provide adequate rest periods.
12. Assist the patient to turn, cough, and deep breathe q 2 hr.
13. Provide oral hygiene after coughing and before meals.
14. Administer the prescribed medications on time.
15. Increase hydration to an intake of 3,000 ml/day (unless contraindicated) to liquefy secretions.
16. Assess the effectiveness of IPPB treatments if prescribed.
Psychosocial 17. Remain with the patient during dyspneic episodes to alleviate anxiety.

18. Maintain a nonjudgmental attitude toward the patient's smoking.
19. Provide the names of community resources to aid the patient to stop smoking.
20. Accept the patient's behavior as a reflection of altered oxygenation and the chronic impact of the disease.
21. Refer the patient to social workers and therapists for help in maintaining an optimum level of activity and in coping with the considerable financial burden resulting from any decreased ability to work and the cost of medications and equipment.

Educational 22. Teach the patient diaphragmatic breathing and effective coughing.
23. Prepare the patient for discharge (*see* pneumonia). In addition, advise small, frequent meals that are high in protein and carbohydrate.

Prevention 24. Encourage cessation of smoking.
25. Encourage avoidance of occupational exposure to noxious fumes and dust.
26. Encourage persons with respiratory symptoms to seek early medical attention.
27. Encourage avoidance of weight gain because morbid obesity may contribute to respiratory dysfunction.
28. Encourage annual flu vaccine and avoidance of exposure to colds.

Evaluation criteria. *See* Overview. Ability to maintain maximal functioning and live with altered life-style despite chronic illness.

BRONCHIECTASIS

Bronchiectasis is a chronic, permanent dilation of bronchi due to weakened bronchial walls resulting from chronic inflammation. Its incidence is less common since the advent of antibiotics. It can occur following a cycle of persistent pulmonary infections after antibiotic treatment that has been administered for recurrent lung infections. Bronchiectasis usually occurs as a result of chronic inflammatory changes in bronchial mucosa and muscular coat from persistent infection seen particularly in immunodepressed patients. It is caused by bronchial obstruction resulting from mucus, neoplasm, or aspiration of a foreign body. It is also caused by infections resulting from TB, chronic bronchitis, aspiration of gastric contents, or as a complication of various childhood diseases (measles, whooping cough, influenza).

The chronic anatomic changes of the bronchi can appear as saccular dilations (more common in children) or as cylindrical or tubular dilations (more common in adults). Pathologic changes of bronchiectasis are irreversible. Conditions that may mimic bronchiectasis (atelectasis, tracheobronchitis) are reversible, making an accurate diagnosis imperative.

Symptoms include chronic cough (which produces large amounts of mucopurulent, foul-smelling sputum, sometimes as much as 200 ml/day), hemoptysis, cyanosis, fever, weight loss, dyspnea on exertion, weakness, fetid breath, and inspiratory rales. *Complications* include recurrent pneumonia, malnutrition, cor pulmonale associated with right heart failure, digital clubbing, and lung abscess.

Diagnosis is based on the health history, physical exam, an immune survey to detect immune-deficiency diseases, sputum stains and cultures, and a CBC, which may detect an anemia or a leukocytosis. Also used in the diagnosis are x-rays (bronchography, routine chest x-ray), bronchoscopy to identify sources of bleeding and/or secretion, and pulmonary function studies, which yield varying results depending on the extent of the disease.

Common interventions

Medical treatment involves vigorous bronchial hygiene, including postural drainage if tolerated, O_2 therapy, and the administration of bronchodilators and expectorants. Antibiotics may be used for 5 to 7 days or longer for well-established infections. Bronchoscopy is used to lavage and remove inspissated bronchial secretions. Resectional **surgery** is performed as a last resort.

Nursing interventions

Physical 1. Record vital signs q 4 hr.
2. Assist the patient to perform postural drainage q 4 hr (if able to tolerate procedure).
3. Position the patient with the head of the bed elevated.
4. Assist the patient with turning, coughing, and deep breathing q 2 hr.
5. Assess respirations and characteristics of sputum (color, amount, consistency).
6. Discourage smoking.
7. Administer prescribed antibiotics on time.
8. Provide humidification to prevent mucous membrane dryness and to help loosen secretions.
9. Provide O_2 therapy if prescribed.
10. Increase hydration to an intake of 3,000/day (unless contraindicated) to liquefy secretions.
11. Provide adequate rest periods.
12. Provide a well-balanced, high-protein, high-carbohydrate diet.
13. Provide frequent oral hygiene, particularly prior to meals.
Psychosocial 14. Remain with the patient during dyspneic periods.
Educational 15. Teach the patient diaphragmatic breathing and effective coughing techniques.
16. Advise the patient to eat small, frequent meals high in proteins and carbohydrates.

Prevention 17. Encourage vaccination against childhood diseases commonly complicated by pneumonia.

18. Encourage genetic counseling for patients with inheritable diseases that may predispose to bronchiectasis.

Evaluation criteria.   *See* Overview. Maintenance of normal body weight.

TUBERCULOSIS

TB is an acute or chronic, infectious, communicable disease caused by the tubercle bacillus (*Mycobacterium tuberculosis*). It results in lesions of the lungs but can disseminate to other organs. In 1981, 10 million people had TB. Of these, one quarter to one third died. In the USA, ~14.9/100,000 people have TB. There is a positive TB skin test in 30% of persons >50 yr of age. Race is a predisposing factor to TB, with Caucasian and Mongolian races seeming to have a natural resistance, and American Indians, Eskimos, and Africans having less resistance. Other predisposing factors include the virulence of the organism (some strains are more virulent than others), corticosteroid administration (known to reactivate dormant disease), and sociocultural factors such as crowded living conditions, poor nutrition, and inadequate medical care. TB is caused by the aerobic, gram-positive, acid-fast bacillus, *Mycobacterium tuberculosis* (pasturization destroys the bacillus). Of the two strains, the **human** strain is the most frequent cause in the USA, and the **bovine** strain is common in countries with inadequate sanitation practices. TB can be transmitted by inhalation of droplets dispersed by a contaminated person via coughing, sneezing, or talking or by ingestion of contaminated milk.

The incubation period is ~4 to 8 wk. Most lesions occur in the lower two-thirds of the lungs. The tissue reaction involves granuloma formation, caseation (a formation of a cheeselike substance), cavitation and scarring, and resolution with calcification (if the host's defenses are adequate). TB may lie dormant for years before becoming an active infection.

Symptoms include fever with night sweats, a cough producing purulent and/or bloody sputum (particularly heavy in early morning), pleuritic chest pain, anorexia with subsequent weight loss, malaise, fatigue, tachycardia, headache, amenorrhea (late in the disease), rales on auscultation, and a positive TB skin test (an indurated area measuring $\geq$10 mm indicates exposure, not necessarily active disease). *Complications* include cavitation, hemoptysis, effusion, bronchopleural fistula, empyema, pneumothorax, and dissemination to other organs via lymph or circulatory systems, including lymph nodes, bones, kidneys, genital tract, brain, and meninges.

Diagnosis is based on the health history, physical exam, and a culture of the organism (slow growing: takes $\geq$2 wk to grow) obtained from sputum, gastric washing, urine, or CSF. In addition, chest x-rays are used to identify area(s) of cavitation and pleural effusions. Bronchoscopy and lung biopsy (including biopsy of mediastinal nodes) are also used diagnostically.

Common interventions

Medical treatment involves the administration of two or three of the following medications for 18 to 24 mo: isoniazid (INH) (most effective antituberculosis drug), rifampin, ethambutol hydrochloride, streptomycin sulfate, and para-aminosalicylic acid (PAS). The patient should be told that the medications do not cure, only control, the disease. **Surgical** treatment, which was used more frequently as a treatment method before the advent of drug therapy, is used for exploration and resection to (1) diagnose when adequate cultures cannot be otherwise obtained, and (2) to treat hemorrhage.

Nursing interventions

Physical 1. Provide small, frequent feedings high in protein and carbohydrates.
2. Encourage fluids to an intake of 3,000 ml/day (unless contra-indicated).
3. Assist the patient to exercise to tolerance, encouraging adequate rest and avoidance of fatigue.
4. Provide respiratory isolation by placing the patient in a private room, peforming good hand washing techniques, avoiding contact with sputum, and wearing a face mask when in close contact with the patient or if the patient is unable to follow instructions regarding the disposal of sputum, etc.
5. Collect sputum specimens early in the morning and via gastric washings, if prescribed.
6. Take vital signs q 4 hr.
7. Assist the patient to turn, cough, and deep breathe q 4 hr.
8. Auscultate breath sounds q 4 hr.
9. Administer chemotherapy on time to maintain adequate blood levels.
Psychosocial 10. Encourage communication with family members and/or significant others.
11. Provide diversional therapy.
12. Assist the patient with stigma and discrimination that still exist for TB victims (e.g., in the job market).
Educational 13. Provide preoperative teaching if surgery is planned (*see* Chapter 9).
14. Prepare the patient and family for discharge (*see* pneumonia).
15. Stress the need for ongoing care because the disease is not cured, only controlled.
16. Stress the importance of moderate exercise with planned rest periods.
17. Advise the patient to report the following symptoms: hemoptysis, dyspnea, chest pain, and decreased hearing.
18. Stress the importance of a diet high in protein and carbohydrates.

19. Instruct the patient and family about methods to prevent transmission of the disease: proper disposal of sputum and contaminated
tissues, turning head away from others when coughing or sneezing,
and avoidance of over-the-counter medications without physician/
nurse approval.

Prevention 20. Encourage screening of family and close contacts of
persons with TB by chest x-ray or skin testing.

21. Encourage follow-up of the patient's family and contacts.

22. Administer isoniazid (if prescribed) to prevent dormant lesions
from becoming active in persons who convert from tuberculin
negative to positive with no evidence of clinical disease, who come
in close contact with the infected person, or who receive long-term
steroid therapy.

Evaluation criteria.   *See* Overview.

PLEURISY

Pleurisy (pleuritis) is a symptom of many respiratory conditions caused
by inflammation of the pleural membrane of the lungs, frequently resulting
in chest pain. Any predisposing factor that can contribute to respiratory
disease can be considered a contributing factor to pleurisy. In addition, any
condition resulting from or causing decreased resistance to any of the
following disease conditions is a predisposing factor to pleurisy: pneumonia,
viral respiratory infections, TB, pulmonary abscess, pulmonary infarction,
bronchial cancer, leukemias, lymphomas, breast cancer, trauma, pulmonary edema, cirrhosis, systemic infections, nephrosis, CHF, and
collagen diseases (such as disseminated lupus erythematosis).

Pleurisy may be either **fibrinous** ("dry" pleurisy without an increase in
pleural fluid) or **serofibrinous** ("wet" pleurisy with a pleural effusion).
Associated chest pain arises from inflammation of parietal pleura (visceral
pleura has no pain receptors).

Symptoms include severe chest pain, which may be sharp, stabbing,
localized to one side of the chest, and aggravated by deep inspiration,
coughing, or sneezing. Other symptoms include shallow breathing (as an
attempt to splint the chest and thereby decrease pain), dyspnea, fever,
malaise, weight loss, cough (purulent sputum may be associated), and
auscultatory findings of a friction rub (usually 24 to 48 hr after the onset of
chest pain) and/or decreased or absent breath sounds. *Complications*
include atelectasis, empyema, mediastinal shift, and chronic adhesive
pleuritis, a condition involving marked pleural thickening that interferes
with pulmonary functioning.

Diagnosis is based on the health history, physical exam, cytology
studies to identify an underlying malignancy, cultures of sputum and/or
aspirated pleural fluid, WBC, chest x-ray (300 to 500 ml of pleural fluid
must be present to be visible on x-ray), thoracentesis to aspirate pleural
fluid, and pleural biopsy.

Common interventions

Medical treatment is directed toward the primary disease and involves splinting of the involved area, bed rest, heat applications over the involved area, and the administration of analgesics, antitussives, SC injections of procaine and intercostal nerve blocks, and instillation of chemotherapy into the pleural space in cancer patients. **Surgical** treatment may involve decortication (removal of thickened pleura) in chronic conditions, thoracentesis to relieve respiratory distress, and chest tubes to closed chest drainage.

Nursing interventions

Physical 1. Position the patient on the affected side to splint the chest.
   2. Provide manual splinting of the chest during coughing.
   3. Observe and report respiratory distress.
   4. Assist the patient with turning, coughing, and deep breathing q 2 hr if the patient is on bed rest or breathes shallowly.
   5. Administer the prescribed medications on time.
   6. Position the patient in a semi-Fowler's to high Fowler's position (unless contraindicated) to facilitate chest expansion and effective coughing.
   7. Auscultate chest sounds q 8 hr.
   8. Take vital signs q 4 to 8 hr.
   9. Assess chest pain q 4 hr.
   10. Observe sputum for color, consistency, and amount.
   11. Monitor any chest tubes and drainage.
Psychosocial 12. Remain with the patient during dyspneic episodes to alleviate anxiety.
   13. Explain any diagnostic tests and the rationale for any procedures.
   14. Provide emotional support during invasive procedures by explaining procedures, explaining how the patient can assist during procedures, and remaining with the patient during procedures.
Educational 15. Teach the patient effective coughing techniques.

Evaluation criteria. *See* Overview.

FUNGAL INFECTIONS

Fungal infections consist of a group of lung diseases caused by inhalation of fungal spores found in soil and dust. Many of these infections are endemic to certain geographic areas around the world and in the USA. A high prevalence of positive skin tests (90 to 95%) in endemic areas in the USA suggests a high incidence. The most important fungal diseases in the USA are **histoplasmosis**, which is endemic in the Midwest and East and has a higher prevalence in adult males, **coccidioidomycosis**, which is endemic in the Southwest, and **blastomycosis**, which is endemic in the Southeast. Predisposing factors include a possible hypersensitivity to fungal disease in affected individuals and a decreased host resistance secondary to chronic illness, in infants, and in adults >50 yr old. Fungal infections are not communicable between humans. Histoplasmosis, which is caused by the fungus *Histoplasma capsulatum*, is found in the soil of areas inhabited by chickens, birds, and bats. Coccidioidomycosis, which is caused by the fungus *Coccidioides immitis*, occurs in the soil of arid regions where dust is blown by the wind and inhaled. Blastomycosis, which is caused by the fungus *Blastomyces dermatitidis*, does not appear to reside in soil. The portal of entry is not clear, but may possibly be the skin or lungs.

Fungal pulmonary infections can easily be confused with TB. After inhalation,the spores cause an allergic reaction resulting in inflammation, tubercle formation, caseation, scarring, calcification, and cavitation. The infections may be asymptomatic and self-limiting. *Symptoms* may include benign pneumonitis, fever, dyspnea, chest pain, weight loss, headache, nonproductive cough, hepatomegaly, and splenomegaly. *Complications* of fungal infections involve dissemination to various organs (more common in infants): liver, spleen, intestines, lymph nodes, brain, kidney, eye, skin, endocardium, oropharynx, larynx, and adrenal glands. Other complications include subacute bacterial endocarditis, meningitis, pneumonia, Addison's disease, and pleural effusion.

Diagnosis is based on the health history; physical exam; cultures of sputum, biopsied lesions, gastric washings, blood, urine, and bone marrow; chest x-rays to identify pulmonary infiltrates, cavitation, lymphadenopathy, and effusions; and skin testing, which becomes positive several weeks after exposure.

Common interventions

Medical treatment consists of the administration of medications (amphotericin B is the drug of choice). Medications must be administered carefully IV. Hospitalization is necessary. **Surgical** treatment involves excision of residual peripheral granulomas, particularly in the treatment of secondary infection or hemoptysis.

Nursing interventions

Physical 1. Administer IV medications. Monitor carefully and watch for the following symptoms of toxicity: venous thrombosis at the injection site; nausea, vomiting, and diarrhea; and impaired renal and/or liver functioning.
2. Assist with diagnostic testing.
3. Take vital signs q 4 hr.
4. Auscultate lungs q 8 hr.
5. Provide adequate rest periods.
Psychosocial 6. Explain all tests and procedures.
7. Provide emotional support during dyspnea and diagnostic procedures.

Educational 8. Teach the patient and family about the nature of the disease, methods of prevention, medications (names, purposes, dosages, times of administration, side effects), reportable symptoms (fever, chest pain, productive cough), and need for follow-up appointments.

9. Provide preoperative teaching for planned surgery (*see* Chapter 9).

Prevention 10. Teach farmers to keep farm buildings clean and dry.

11. Teach farmers to rinse floors of farm buildings before sweeping in order to decrease inhalation of contaminated dust.

Evaluation criteria.   *See* Overview.

MALIGNANT NEOPLASMS

Since only 3 to 10% of all pulmonary tumors are benign, this section will focus on malignant tumors only. Malignant neoplasms are a group of rapidly spreading pulmonary tumors that metastasize to other areas of the body and produce multiple systemic symptoms and effects. The neoplasm may be a primary tumor, originating in lung tissue, or a metastatic tumor, usually adenocarcinomas from GI, GU, and glandular tissues. Malignant lung tumors comprise 90 to 97% of all surgically resected pulmonary tumors. Lung cancer is the primary cause of cancer deaths in men. The average length of survival after diagnosis is 6 to 9 mo. Only 5% of diagnosed patients survive 5 yr. Scarred, chronically diseased lungs are a predisposing factor, and there is a possible hereditary predisposition. The incidence increases with age. The sex incidence is 5:1 male:female, although it is currently increasing in females. Urban dwellers are at higher risk than rural dwellers, and certain occupations increase exposure to carcinogens. A stressful life-style may be a predisposing factor, although this is not well supported by research at this point. There is a high correlation between cancer incidence and the number of cigarettes smoked. Exposure to coal tars, asbestos, and certain metals (e.g., arsenic, nickel) may cause malignant tumors, as may air pollution, exposure to ionizing radiation, and certain viruses.

Squamous cell (epidermoid) carcinoma, which is almost always associated with cigarettes, is usually centrally located and produces symptoms relatively early. **Adenocarcinoma** usually results from lung scarring, is usually peripherally located, and produces symptoms relatively late, resulting in a late diagnosis. **Oat cell** carcinoma usually occurs in males and metastasizes early. Lung cancers metastasize by direct extension, lymphatic spread, hematogenous spread, and transbronchial spread.

Lung cancer may be asymptomatic in early cases. *Symptoms* include cough (particularly a change in pattern), chest pain, rust-streaked or purulent sputum production, hemoptysis, dyspnea, wheezing on auscultation emphasized by forced expiration, anemia, coagulation disorders (bleeding, DIC), and symptoms of metastasis to other organs, such as the brain, bone, or liver. A major *complication* of lung cancer is the paraneoplastic syndrome, which is produced by a tumor that secretes hormones such as ADH, parathyroid hormone, and ACTH. This syndrome is most frequently associated with the oat cell type carcinoma. Other complications include superior vena caval obstruction, recurrent pleural effusions, pneumonitis, shoulder or arm pain from tumor compression of the brachial plexus, atelectasis, bronchial obstruction, and coagulation abnormalities.

Diagnosis is based on the health history, physical exam, sputum cytology, CBC, arterial blood gases, chest x-ray (fluoroscopy, tomography, angiography), bronchoscopy, percutaneous needle biopsy, scalene node biopsy, bronchial brush biopsy, mediastinoscopy, bone marrow biopsy, and pulmonary function tests.

Common interventions

Medical treatment consists of immunotherapy with BCG given intrapleurally. Radiotherapy is used in nonresectable, localized tumors; for palliation of metastatic disease; postoperatively for remaining pleural or nodal disease; and in patients whose physical condition makes surgery too great a risk. Chemotherapy is used for recurrent or metastatic disease and palliation in nonresectable tumors. **Surgical** intervention is the treatment of choice for localized, resectable tumors. The usual treatment is a lobectomy or pneumonectomy, depending on the extent of disease. Surgery is contraindicated in metastatic disease.

Nursing interventions

Physical 1. Assess nutritional status, daily weight, and intake and output.
   2. Monitor parenteral hyperalimentation, if prescribed.
      a. Follow strict aseptic technique during dressing and bottle changes.
      b. Follow hospital guidelines for care of the catheter insertion site.
      c. Use a pump to regulate flow. Never speed up rate to "catch up."
      d. Observe for signs of electrolyte imbalance or overload.
      e. Measure intake and output.
      f. Weigh daily.
      g. Monitor vital signs q 4 hr.
      h. Test urine for glucose and acetone q 6 hr.
   3. Assist with pain control (*see* Chapter 4).
      a. Assess pain frequently.
      b. Administer prescribed analgesics on time.
      c. Decrease stress in the environment.
      d. Prevent sensory deprivation or sensory overload, which may decrease the patient's resistance to or tolerance for pain.
      e. Consider group therapy (sometimes helpful).
      f. Utilize distractions.

4. Maintain activity level.
   a. Keep the patient mobile as long as possible to prevent disuse and circulatory impairment.
   b. Assist with planning activities and rest periods.
   c. Use a variety of methods to induce sleep and rest. (Avoid the use of medications, if possible.)
   d. Refer the patient to community groups to provide assistance at home.
5. Provide postoperative care (*see* Chapter 11).
   a. Observe for postoperative complications (pulmonary embolism, pulmonary edema, bronchopleural fistulas, cor pulmonale, cardiac arrythmias).
   b. Assess respiratory status hourly.
   c. Assist with turning, coughing, and deep breathing hourly.
   d. Position the patient in semi-Fowler's or high Fowler's position to facilitate expansion of the affected lung.
   e. Splint the patient's chest with a pillow or towel to facilitate deep breathing and coughing.
   f. Perform range-of-motion exercises of the arm and shoulder on the affected side to maintain muscle tone, prevent ankylosis of the shoulder, and increase circulation.
   g. Monitor chest tubes, if inserted postoperatively, or for treatment of effusion: position the patient on his affected side after tube insertion to facilitate drainage; record the amount, color, and consistency of drainage q 2 to 4 hr; and assess the chest tube site q 2 to 4 hr for drainage and air leaks.
   h. Auscultate breath sounds q 2 to 4 hr.
6. Provide specific care for patients undergoing chemotherapy (*see* Chapter 8).
   a. Assess the patient for nausea.
   b. Administer antiemetics, if prescribed, either prophylactically or to alleviate nausea.
   c. Provide frequent mouth care.
   d. Provide reverse isolation for marrow-depressed patients.
   e. Observe laboratory work to monitor the patient's status/progress.
   f. Encourage fluids of high nutritive value.
   g. Assess vital signs q 4 hr.
   h. Provide support if the patient experiences alopecia (hair loss). Tell the patient that the hair will regrow after the treatment, and encourage the use of scarves, wigs, and hairpieces in the interim.
7. Provide specific care for patient's undergoing external radiation.
   a. Provide good skin care.
   b. Avoid application of ointments and lotions to the radiation site.
   c. Expose the skin to air.
   d. Employ gentle washing techniques to the area of skin receiving radiation.

     e. Encourage avoidance of exposure to sunlight.

     f. Encourage the patient to not eat immediately before treatments.

     g. Encourage the patient to avoid foods that aggravate nausea (such as milk products).

     h. Observe for bleeding from mucous membranes (such as hematuria and nosebleeds).

8. Provide specific care for patients undergoing sealed internal radiation.

     a. Follow hospital policy regarding the treatment of the specific type of radiation sources and sites.

     b. Watch for dislodgment of implants.

     c. Check all linens, dressings, etc., for radioactivity before discarding.

     d. Maintain distance from sources of radiation; use a lead shield during patient care when possible.

     e. Organize care to minimize the time spent in close contact with the patient.

9. Provide specific care for patients undergoing unsealed internal radiation.

     a. Follow hospital guidelines for disposal of dressings and linens and radiation precautions for specific types of therapy.

     b. *See* Chapter 8.

Psychosocial 10. Provide emotional support for the patient and family during the diagnostic phase.

11. Assess the patient and family coping abilities/capabilities.

12. Encourage patient and family contact with community resources, such as the American Cancer Society and Visiting Nurses' Association.

13. Assist the patient with altered body image: provide instructions on how the patient can participate in care, encourage routine hygiene practices and the use of attractive clothing and scarves, wigs, or hairpieces (for alopecia).

14. Allow patient and family input into care to avoid feelings of loss of control.

15. Assist with the solving of unique patient concerns, e.g., transportation for frequent medical treatments, child care, and cost of treatments.

16. Encourage family and patient participation in support groups.

17. Provide opportunities for the patient and family to verbalize feelings about death/loss.

18. Recommend referral for religious counseling and/or psychologic evaluation and intervention, if indicated.

19. Provide continuity of care.

Educational 20. Instruct the patient and family about the condition, procedures, and treatments (especially side effects of medications).

21. Advise the patient about pain control techniques, including group and individual counseling, distraction, behavior modification, medications, and control of anxiety.

Prevention 22. Encourage public participation in education programs that stress annual physical exams, awareness of cancer warning signs, awareness of harmful effects of smoking and air pollution, and awareness of symptoms of lung cancer and need for early detection.

23. Encourage people with a chronic cough or a change in the nature of cough to seek medical attention.

24. Encourage frequent screening of habitual smokers and persons with chronic respiratory infections.

Evaluation criteria.   *See* Overview. Patient and family demonstrate acceptance of altered body image and diagnosis of cancer. Effective use of pain control techniques.

PULMONARY EMPHYSEMA

Emphysema is a chronic condition involving distension of alveoli with destruction of alveolar walls resulting in airway narrowing and decreased lung elasticity. Emphysema is the most common chronic lung condition; however, its incidence is difficult to determine due to varying diagnostic criteria. Possibly 5% of the population in the USA carry the hereditary factor sometimes associated with the disease, and possibly 10 million people in the USA have the disease. Heredity is a predisposing factor: a deficiency of alpha 1-antitrypsin has been identified in many emphysema patients. In addition, during the normal aging process, there is a normal loss of lung elasticity. Of all emphysema patients, 90% smoke heavily. Its incidence is increased in urban areas (air pollution). The relationship of occupational hazards with emphysema is unclear.

Loss of alveolar surface area and decreased elasticity of supportive tissues result in expiratory airway narrowing, increased lung compliance (particularly RV) and decreased gas exchange. There are two types of emphysema, and they usually occur together. **Panlobar** emphysema is hereditary, the least common form, and usually seen in primary emphysema without bronchitis. It involves peripheral destruction, affects all portions of the lungs, and has an equal incidence in both sexes. **Centrilobar** emphysema is associated with chronic bronchitis and involves destruction of respiratory bronchioles. It affects the lung apices, is more common in males than females, and is seldom found in nonsmokers.

Symptoms of emphysema include shortness of breath, decreased tolerance to exercise, usually no cough or slight cough with minimal sputum production (unless bronchitis is superimposed), orthopnea, tachypnea, anorexia, cyanosis (rare), weight loss, hyperresonance to percussion, decreased breath sounds, occasional expiratory wheezes, barrel-shaped chest, increased width of costal angle, and the use of the accessory muscles of respiration (intercostals, sternomastoids, abdominal). Cor pulmonale is a rare *complication* except late in the disease process. It is evidenced by hepatomegaly, jugular venous distension, peripheral edema, ascites, and chest pain. Other complications include emphysematous bullae and blebs (which can rupture, causing a spontaneous pneumothorax), respiratory failure, pulmonary thromboembolism, and chronic bronchitis.

Diagnosis is based on the health history, physical exam, CBC, arterial blood gases (may be normal until late in the disease), chest x-ray (may show low, flattened diaphragm and narrowing of pulmonary vessels), fluoroscopy, pulmonary angiography, ECG, and pulmonary function studies, which may show airway obstruction, increased RV, and decreased elastic recoil.

Common interventions

Cessation of smoking and the avoidance of air pollution can help alleviate the symptoms of emphysema. **Medical** treatment consists of the administration of antibiotics (if complicated by infection), bronchodilators for bronchospasm, cough depressants, steroids, and prophylactic influenza vaccine. Treatment includes low-flow O_2 therapy (usually 2 to 3 liters/min nasally) and the administration of IPPB therapy with bronchodilators and mucolytics. **Surgical** treatment includes resection of large bullae or removal of nonfunctioning lung tissue.

Nursing interventions

Physical 1. Discourage smoking and exposure to pollution.
2. Administer O_2 therapy with humidity (≤ 2 liters/min, unless prescribed or carefully titrated to arterial blood gases).
3. Administer IPPB treatments with medication and/or nebulization, if prescribed.
4. Administer prescribed medications on time.
5. Assess vital signs q 2 to 4 hr and prn. Take rectal temperatures during periods of dyspnea.
6. Auscultate lung sounds q 2 to 4 hr and prn, depending on the patient's condition.
7. Provide oral hygiene q 4 hr.
8. Position the patient in a high Fowler's or semi-Fowler's position to facilitate ventilation.
9. Assist the patient to turn, cough, and deep breathe q 2 to 4 hr.
10. Monitor the results of arterial blood gases.
11. Encourage 2,000 to 3,000 ml of fluids q 24 hr (unless contraindicated) to liquefy secretions.
12. Provide skin care q 2 to 4 hr for patients on bed rest.
13. Assist the patient to maintain or increase his level of activity according to his tolerance.

14. Provide adequate rest periods.
15. Provide a diet high in protein and carbohydrates.
16. Provide small, frequent feedings to decrease postprandial dyspnea.
17. Assess the patient's level of consciousness q 2 hr.
18. Monitor intake and output.

Psychosocial 19. Remain with the patient during dyspneic or anxious episodes.
20. Encourage the patient to participate in self-care as much as physically possible.
21. Provide referrals to resource people to assist the patient in coping with role reversal due to disability, altered body image, and the financial burden of the disability and the cost of medications and equipment.

Educational 22. Provide preoperative instructions if surgery is anticipated.
23. Teach the patient and family about the need for increased fluid intake, the need for any dietary alterations, energy-conserving skills for activities of daily living, breathing exercises (pursed lips, diaphragmatic breathing), methods of preventing infection (avoiding crowds, avoiding people with upper respiratory infection), the use of oxygen and other equipment (if prescribed), limiting outdoor activities during days of high air pollution, reportable symptoms (fever, increased dyspnea, increased cough, increase or change in sputum production or characteristics), the need for ongoing care, and the need for a medical alert band.

Prevention 24. Encourage participation in public education regarding the hazards of smoking and air pollution.
25. Encourage persons with respiratory symptoms to seek early medical attention.

Evaluation criteria. *See* Overview. Patient acceptance of altered life-style.

CHRONIC OBSTRUCTIVE PULMONARY DISEASE

COPD is a functional category alluding to a syndrome that results in airway narrowing of a chronic, progressive nature. COPD usually involves one or more of the following diseases: chronic bronchitis, bronchial asthma, and pulmonary emphysema. There has been an increased incidence in COPD during the last few years, particularly in women. In the USA, ~13 million people may be affected by one or a combination of the above conditions. Infection is a possible predisposing factor, although no specific etiologic agent has been identified. Heredity may also be a factor: a deficiency of alpha 1-antitrypsin has been identified in many emphysema patients. The normal loss of lung elasticity during the aging process can cause COPD. Allergies (only clearly related to asthma) may also cause

COPD. Major causes of COPD are cigarette smoking (the disease is uncommon in nonsmokers), air pollution (the incidence is higher in urban areas), and occupational hazards (inhalation of certain chemicals and dusts).

An increased difference between the ventilation:perfusion ratio occurs as a result of the underlying pathology. An irreversible change of decreased elasticity of the lungs results in obstruction, particularly during expiration. There are reversible changes of bronchospasm, increased mucous production, and bronchial edema, causing narrowing of airways.

Symptoms include hypoxemia, dyspnea (particularly on exertion), productive cough (increased in the morning, after eating a large meal, or during periods of high humidity), weight loss, anorexia, headaches, insomnia, polycythemia (resulting from hypoxemia), CO_2 narcosis (increased PCO_2, decreased pH, confusion, and loss of memory), use of accessory muscles of respiration (particularly on expiration), decreased breath sounds, hyperresonance to percussion, rales, rhonchi, and expiratory wheezes. *Complications* may include peptic ulcer, respiratory failure, recurrent respiratory infections, and cor pulmonale caused by pulmonary hypertension (evidenced by peripheral edema, hepatomegaly, ascites, jugular venous distension, orthopnea, and chest pain).

Diagnosis is based on the health history, physical exam, CBC, arterial blood gases, sputum culture and sensitivity, lung scans, pulmonary function studies, ECG, and the chest x-ray, which, although a poor tool for screening purposes, may be used to diagnose other associated diseases and is helpful when compared with previous chest films.

Common interventions

Medical treatment is similar to that for pulmonary emphysema (*see above*). It also involves assistance with chest physiotherapy (postural drainage, vibration, clapping), if needed. IV fluids are administered to maintain fluid and electrolyte balance, provide a route for administering medications, and provide adequate hydration. Respiratory functioning may be maintained by intubation with mechanical ventilation (if arterial blood gases do not adequately respond to other methods or are in the critical range). **Surgical** treatment may consist of resection of large bullae in emphysematous lungs or removal of nonfunctioning lung tissue. **Nursing** interventions are the same as for bronchitis and emphysema (*see above*).

Evaluation criteria. See Overview.

ASTHMA

Asthma is a condition characterized by spontaneous attacks of dyspnea and wheezing, lasting from several minutes to several hours. Of all cases, 50% occur before age 10. Asthma occurs in boys two times more frequently than girls. In adults, there is an equal incidence in men and women. Predisposing factors include inadequate bronchodilator tone and an inherited tendency of hypersensitive response to bronchoconstrictive stimuli of a minor nature (such as cold air, dust, psychic stimuli, and exercise). In some cases, asthma is idiopathic (no demonstrable allergen or other cause). More frequently, however, asthma is caused by an allergy to external allergens (usually inhaled pollens, molds, drugs, dusts, food); viral or bacterial respiratory infections; or psychologic stress (rarely the single causative agent).

Between attacks, there are no noted abnormalities: pulmonary functioning is near normal, and there are no symptoms. During attacks, pulmonary changes include bronchial edema, airway narrowing, altered ventilation:perfusion ratio as a result of uneven aeration, and increased bronchial secretions. Chronic pulmonary changes consist of hypertrophy of bronchial smooth muscle and hyperinflation of alveoli *without* destruction of alveolar walls (as in emphysema).

Symptoms include sudden onset of audible inspiratory and expiratory wheezes, air hunger, short inspiratory period, dyspnea on exertion, retraction of intercostal and sternal muscles, cyanosis, tachycardia, dry cough (usually after the attack subsides), decreased or absent breath sounds, rales, decreased level of consciousness, hypotension, dehydration, and anxiety from fear of suffocation and death. *Complications* include pulmonary edema, pulmonary infection (with symptoms of fever, purulent sputum, increased sputum culture and sensitivity), status asthmaticus (a severe attack lasting for 24 hr with minimal improvement from treatment), chronic bronchitis or bronchiectasis, emphysema, respiratory failure, atelectasis, cardiac failure (cor pulmonale), drug toxicity as a result of treatment, and (rarely) pneumothorax.

Diagnosis is based on the health history, physical exam, sputum culture and sensitivity, arterial blood gases, serum immunoglobins (may show increased levels of IgE), chest x-ray to distinguish asthma from other respiratory diseases (such as emphysema), lung scan, pulmonary function studies, and skin testing to identify possible allergens.

Common interventions

Medical

1. Encourage decreased exposure to allergens and such respiratory irritants as smoke, perfumes, paint fumes, cold air, and strong odors.
2. Provide immunotherapy or desensitization for identified allergens.
3. Encourage the avoidance of obesity, excessive exertion, fatigue, and smoking.
4. Encourage prompt treatment of respiratory infections.
5. Encourage indoor humidity levels of ≥30%.
6. Provide chest physiotherapy.
7. Prescribe medications (e.g., epinephrine, aminophylline, antihistamines, antibiotics, expectorants, steroids).

8. Provide IV fluids to replace fluid losses, maintain electrolyte balance, and adminster medications.
9. Prescribe O_2 during an acute attack (mechanical ventilation may be required).
10. Monitor theophylline levels to maintain a therapeutic level and avoid toxicity.
11. Prescribe IPPB with nebulization (sometimes contraindicated).
12. Recommend a change in climate in some cases.

Surgical

1. Perform bronchoscopy to aspirate secretions.
2. Perform endotracheal intubation to provide mechanical ventilation.

Nursing interventions

Physical 1. Assist the patient to a high Fowler's position in order to facilitate chest expansion.
2. Take vital signs q 2 to 4 hr. Take rectal temperatures during periods of dyspnea.
3. Auscultate lung sounds hourly to qid, depending on the patient's condition.
4. Assess the patient's level of consciousness q 2 hr.
5. Monitor arterial blood gases to detect hypoxemia.
6. Monitor intake and output.
7. Encourage increased fluid intake to 2,500 to 3,000 ml/day (unless contraindicated).
8. Observe and record color, amount, and consistency of sputum.
9. Administer and carefully monitor prescribed IV fluids.
10. Collect sputum specimens for cultures, if requested.
11. Provide oral hygiene q 2 to 4 hr and prn.
12. Provide adequate rest for the patient by limiting visitors and organizing nursing care to decrease frequent interruptions of rest periods.
13. Encourage the patient to maintain as much activity as possible. (The patient may feel well between episodes of respiratory distress.)
14. Provide a diet high in calories and protein.
15. Administer prescribed medications on time.
16. Suction the patient prn.
17. Provide humidity through bedside humidifiers in order to loosen secretions and prevent mucous membrane dryness.
18. Administer low-flow O_2 therapy, if prescribed. (Oxygen masks may increase feelings of suffocation.)
19. Administer and/or assess the effectiveness of IPPB treatments, if prescribed.
20. Decrease environmental respiratory irritants, such as smoke, flowers, and dust.

21. Discourage smoking and exposure to pollution.
Psychosocial 22. Remain with the patient during periods of anxiety or dyspnea.
23. Decrease the patient's anxiety by explaining procedures and treatments and anticipate the patient's needs and questions.
24. Recommend psychotherapy for patients with asthma of psychic origin (rare).
Educational 25. Teach the patient breathing exercises.
26. Teach the patient the reportable symptoms suggesting an upper respiratory infection or influenza, or an attack not relieved by usual measures.
27. Teach the patient the appropriate care during attacks (correct use of medications, provision of adequate rest).
28. Teach the need for a medical alert band.
Prevention 29. Encourage early treatment of respiratory infections.
30. Teach the patient and family to prevent future attacks by maintaining a balanced diet, adequate rest, and moderate exercise; avoiding fatigue and environmental irritants; and using air conditioners, humidifiers, and air filters.

Evaluation criteria. *See* Overview.

SARCOIDOSIS

Sarcoidosis is a systemic, granulomatous disease of unknown etiology in which tubercles arise in many organ systems, causing a variety of symptoms and effects. Sarcoidosis is a very widespread disease found in every country. It is twice as common in blacks as in whites, and twice as prevalent in females as in males. It occurs most frequently in the 20- to 40-yr-old age group. Of all cases, only 5 to 10% result in death (usually from pulmonary disease). A genetic susceptibility may be inherited because there seems to be a familial tendency. A possible genetic predisposition is inherited involving some unknown factors of hypersensitivity. Although the etiology is unknown, sarcoidosis is possibly a special form of TB.

Most frequently, sarcoidosis is a benign disease in which remission occurs during the first 2 yr. Hard, clearly demarcated tubercles occur associated with minimal inflammation and no necrosis or caseation (as in TB). Granulomas occur in the lungs (most common site), lymph nodes, skin, liver, spleen, heart, skeletal muscle, and bones.

Symptoms are variable, depending on the organ system(s) involved. The most common symptoms include persistent fever, spiking to 38.3°C (101°F), weight loss, fatigue, enlarged lymph nodes (most frequently mediastinal and hilar), dyspnea, cough with minimal sputum production, wheezing, rales, visual impairment, facial lesions of varying description, alopecia, pruritus (in liver involvement), renal calculi, and arthralgia. *Complications* include pulmonary insufficiency, cor pulmonale, hemoptysis (can be severe and fatal), spontaneous pneumothorax, blindness, and pulmonary infections, including TB (sarcoidosis seems to increase a person's risk to TB) and fungal infections (may be a result of long-term steroid and/or antibiotic therapy).

Diagnosis is based on the health history, physical exam, CBC (may indicate anemia and decreased WBC), arterial blood gases (usually show decreased PO_2 and PCO_2; CO_2 retention very late in disease), serum globulins (usually elevated), and serum calcium (sometimes elevated). A chest x-ray may show enlarged nodes and fibrosis, and a skull x-ray may be used to detect bony changes. Pulmonary function studies may show a decreased VC with a progressive deterioration of pulmonary functioning over time. A TB skin test may be negative or less reactive in persons who previously had a positive reaction. Finally, tissue biopsy of nodes, lesions, and affected organs can be diagnostic.

Common interventions

Most cases are benign and require no treatment. The most common **medical** treatment is the use of adrenal corticosteroids (tapered to lowest effective dosage, may be required for long-term therapy), chloroquine (not as effective as steroids), and antituberculosis therapy (not effective against sarcoidosis, preventive therapy due to increased risk to TB). Except for diagnostic purposes, **surgical** intervention is usually not indicated.

Nursing interventions

Most patients have a benign course with spontaneous remission. The nursing care of patients with a progressive disease is highly variable, depending on the nature of involvement.

Physical 1. Assist the patient to a high Fowler's position during dyspneic periods in order to facilitate lung expansion.
2. Take vital signs q 4 hr.
3. Provide adequate rest periods.
4. Auscultate lung sounds hourly to qid, depending on the patient's condition and the extent of lung involvement.
5. Monitor arterial blood gas results.
6. Encourage increased fluid intake to 2,500 to 3,000 ml/day to prevent urinary stasis and formation of calculi (unless contraindicated).
7. Administer prescribed medications on time, particularly observing for side effects of steroid therapy.
8. Observe any sputum for blood or other change.
Psychosocial 9. Remain with the patient during periods of anxiety or dyspnea.
10. Decrease the patient's anxiety by explaining procedures and treatments.

Educational 11. Teach the patient and family about the nature of the disease and its treatment, continuance of increased fluid intake, and information regarding the correct use of steroids.
12. Encourage avoidance of exposure to upper respiratory infections.
13. Encourage the patient to avoid strenuous exercise.
14. Encourage ongoing medical care.

Evaluation criteria. *See* Overview.

ATELECTASIS

Atelectasis is a generally preventable condition characterized by collapse of alveoli as a result of compression or bronchial obstruction. It is common postoperatively, particularly after abdominal or thoracic surgery, and in critically ill patients, who are prone to retention and/or aspiration of pulmonary secretions. Predisposing factors include prolonged bed rest and depressed lung defense mechanisms secondary to smoking, surgical anesthesia, chronic lung disease, or decreased levels of consciousness with potential aspiration of gastric contents. Shallow respirations as a result of pain, weakness, or abdominal distension also predispose to atelectasis. Bronchial obstruction, the most common cause, is a result of retained secretions or mucus. Compression, less common than obstruction, is usually a result of cancer, enlarged lymph nodes, aneurysm, scar tissue, abdominal distension, pneumothorax, or pleural effusion.

Absorption of alveolar gas into the circulation without the ability to replenish alveolar air results in alveolar collapse. The resultant hypoventilation of the involved areas causes pathologic shunting of unoxygenated blood from the right to left heart. Fibrosis and decreased lung functioning occur in chronic persistent conditions.

Symptoms include dyspnea on exertion, tachypnea, fever (often first sign), pleuritic chest pain, tachycardia, weakness, dullness to percussion over involved area, asymmetric chest movements on inspiration, rales (if retention of secretions occurs), and decreased or absent breath sounds over the affected area (frequently lung bases). Other symptoms are mild hypertension, anxiety, restlessness, confusion, cyanosis in severe cases, and signs of shock if the large bronchus is involved. *Complications* include more extensive atelectasis, pneumonia, and fibrotic lung disease.

Diagnosis is based on the health history, physical exam, arterial blood gases (to determine the level of hypoxemia), and chest x-rays (to detect the area involved, possible elevation of diaphragm on the affected side, and possible mediastinal shift toward the affected side in severe cases).

Common interventions

Medical treatment is based on the etiology. General methods include O_2 therapy, pulmonary hygiene techniques, early mobilization of patients, IPPB, incentive spirometry (Fig. 14-7), antibiotics for treatment of any

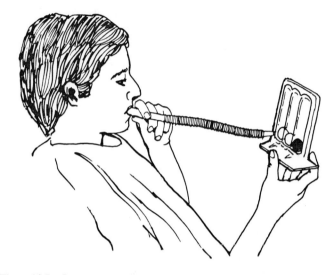

Figure 14-7. Incentive spirometer.

resultant infection, bronchoscopy for aspiration or removal of obstructions, and thoracentesis to remove any fluid or air from the pleural space. **Surgical** treatment involves the removal of the cause of lung compression and/or the affected lung segment in chronic cases.

Nursing interventions

Physical 1. Auscultate breath sounds q 2 to 4 hr as well as before and after ventilation exercises.
2. Take vital signs q 2 to 4 hr and prn.
3. Assist the patient to deep breathe and cough q 1 to 2 hr and prn.
4. Position the patient on his unaffected side or in high Fowler's, if tolerated. Alternate height of head of bed periodically.
5. Encourage use of incentive spirometry devices or blow bottles.
6. Suction the patient prn.
7. Relieve pain and splint surgical incisions to facilitate the patient's ability to perform deep breathing and coughing.
8. Administer O_2 and IPPB as prescribed.
9. Assist the patient with postural drainage and perform clapping qid and prn.
10. Observe sputum and collect specimens.
11. Increase hydration to 2,000 to 3,000 ml of fluid intake q 24 hr, unless contraindicated.

12. Provide humidification through the use of humidifiers.
13. Administer medications (antibiotics, antipyretics, analgesics) on time.
14. Avoid the administration of large doses of sedatives and narcotics, which inhibit cough.

Psychosocial 15. Explain tests and procedures to allay anxiety.

Educational 16. Provide preoperative teaching for planned surgery.

17. Teach the patient and family about pulmonary hygiene techniques and the need to avoid respiratory infection, smoking, and fatigue.

Atelectasis is a condition that can usually be prevented by good nursing care:

1. Assess the depth and rate of respirations q 1 to 2 hr in predisposed individuals.
2. Provide adequate hydration.
3. Encourage mobility and early ambulation.
4. Prevent and detect abdominal distension.
5. Avoid large dosages of respiratory depressants.
6. Encourage coughing and deep breathing exercises in predisposed individuals.
7. Position unconscious patients on their side with their head elevated in order to prevent aspiration.
8. Turn and position the patient hourly.

Evaluation criteria. *See* Overview.

CYSTIC FIBROSIS

Cystic fibrosis is a multisystem disease characterized by thick mucous secretions, pancreatic insufficiency, and an increase in the concentration of sodium and chloride in sweat. Cystic fibrosis occurs in 1 in 1,600 births. It primarily affects infants and young children; however, more adult cases have been seen due to advances in management. Heredity (autosomal recessive trait) is a predisposing factor. Its cause is not known.

During the course of the disease, thick mucous secretions block the intestines, lungs, and biliary ducts. These blockages result in ileus, fecal impaction, rectal prolapse, pulmonary disease, cirrhosis, and portal hypertension. Normal pancreatic tissue becomes replaced by cysts, fibrotic tissue, mucus, and fat. Electrolyte transport is abnormal: there is excessive salt in the sweat and resultant salt depletion.

Symptoms are diverse and dependent on the degree of clinical involvement, e.g., chronic bronchitis, bronchopneumonia, respiratory failure, diabetes mellitus, malnutrition (vitamin deficiencies), cirrhosis, portal hypertension, and hypersplenism. Specific pulmonary manifestations include wheezing; dry, nonproductive, paroxysmal cough; dyspnea; tachypnea; atelectasis; emphysema; recurring bronchitis and pneumonia; nasal polyps; and sinusitis. Specific GI manifestations include meconium ileus, intestinal obstruction, and rectal prolapse from wasting of the perirectal supporting tissues. Obstruction of the pancreatic ducts and deficiency of trypsin, amylase, and lipase may result in frequent, bulky, foul-smelling, pale stools that have a high fat content; poor weight gain; ravenous appetite; a distended abdomen; and sallow skin with poor skin turgor. Deficiency of fat-soluble vitamins (A, D, E, K) may cause clotting abnormalities and poor bone growth and development. Symptoms of pancreatic insufficiency include insufficient insulin production, abnormal glucose tolerance, and glycosuria. *Complications* consist of cor pulmonale, intestinal obstruction, esophageal varices, demineralization of bones, sterility (males), decreased fertility (females), and heat stroke.

Diagnosis is based on the health history, physical exam, sweat test (sodium concentration >60 mEq/liter), the absence of pancreatic enzymes from duodenal contents, and the absence of trypsin in the stools. Other diagnostic tests used to determine the extent of organ involvement include sputum culture, chest x-ray, arterial blood gases, liver function studies, and ECG.

Common interventions

Medical treatment consists of pancreatic enzyme replacement, sodium replacement, and the administration of fat-soluble vitamins and diet therapy (high protein, high calorie, low fat, high sodium). Other methods of treatment involve pulmonary support (postural drainage, percussion/vibration, and exercise), bronchodilators when indicated for bronchospasm, antibiotics for infection, and appropriate therapeutic measures for complications.

Nursing interventions

Physical 1. Assist the patient/family with therapeutic pulmonary measures: positioning, suctioning, percussion/vibration, postural drainage, humidification, and coughing and deep breathing.
2. Administer medications as ordered.
3. Encourage adequate nutrition. Small, frequent feedings may be indicated when dyspnea or digestive disturbances are present.
4. Provide adequate hydration: 3,000 ml/day (unless contraindicated) to liquefy secretions and prevent impaction.
5. Provide oral hygiene after meals and postural drainage procedures.
6. Encourage activity and rest periods as the condition permits.
7. Institute and maintain ventilatory support when indicated: CMV with positive pressure, O_2 therapy.
8. Monitor respiratory status q 4 hr and prn.
   a. Determine rate and rhythm of respirations.
   b. Observe for use of accessory muscles.
   c. Auscultate the chest for breath sounds.

    d. Palpate for tactile fremitus.
    e. Percuss the chest for dullness.
    f. Monitor blood gases.
  9. Observe sputum for amount, color, and consistency.
10. Monitor for signs and symptoms of complications.

Psychosocial 11. Provide constant encouragement and support to the patient/family. The social and emotional aspects of cystic fibrosis are considerable.

12. Refer to social workers, therapists, and community agencies for assistance with equipment in the home, the financial burden of the chronic disease, and any altered life-style.

Educational 13. Teach the patient/family to observe/report signs of respiratory infection (sputum changes, fever, dyspnea, increased cough), avoid crowds and respiratory pollutants, maintain appropriate diet and hydration, take medications as ordered and observe for side effects, maintain a regular schedule for postural drainage and breathing exercises, and keep follow-up appointments for care.

14. Encourage the patient to seek genetic counseling.
15. Stress the need for lifelong care.

Evaluation criteria. *See* Overview.

CHAPTER 15

ALTERED CARDIOVASCULAR FUNCTIONING

Mary Alice Higgins Donius

THE HEART

OVERVIEW

The heart is one of the most vital organs in the body. Heart disease affects more than 30 million Americans and is the leading cause of death in the USA. Cardiac disease has physical as well as psychologic, social, and economic sequelae. Nursing interventions are directed toward prevention and control of symptoms and complications and patient and community education to decrease risk factors.

Anatomy and physiology review

The normal heart lies within the pericardial sac in the thoracic cavity, just slightly left of the midline. The anterior portion of the heart consists of the right atrium and ventricle, and the posterior portion includes the left atrium and ventricle. (The major components of the heart are illustrated in Figure 15-1.)

The circulation of blood through the right heart (**pulmonary circulation**) begins with blood from the entire venous system returning to the right atrium by way of the superior and inferior venae cavae. The blood then passes to the right ventricle, from where it is pumped, via the pulmonary artery, to the lungs. In the lungs, CO_2 is removed and oxygenated blood

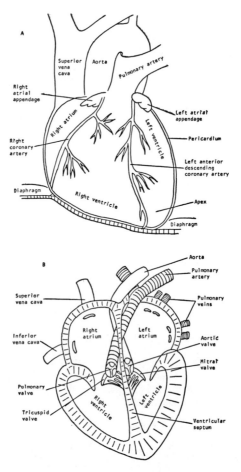

Figure 15-1. Major components of the heart. (A) Exterior view; (B) interior view.

returns to the left heart via the pulmonary veins. The circulation of blood through the left heart (**systemic circulation**) begins with oxygenated blood returning to the heart via the left atrium and passing into the left ventricle. When the left ventricle contracts, it propels blood through the aorta and into the systemic circulation.

The **coronary circulation** occurs via two main coronary arteries (the right and left), which supply the normal heart and the proximal portions of the great vessels with blood (Fig. 15-2). The left coronary artery divides into the anterior descending branch and the circumflex branch. The coronary veins drain directly into the coronary sinus (Fig. 15-3).

Conduction of the cardiac impulse is illustrated in Figure 15-4. The cardiac impulse originates in the sinoatrial (SA) node, spreads through the atrial muscle, and passes across the atrioventricular (AV) node. It then passes down the bundle of His, descends through the right and left bundle branches, and reaches the Purkinje fibers. These fibers spread the impulse to the ventricular myocardium and ventricular contraction occurs. The cardiac cycle refers to the sequence of events that occur and cause the heart to beat. The electric impulses can be followed on an **ECG tracing** of the normal conduction of an impulse through the heart. The ECG represents the sequential de- and repolarization of the atria and ventricles with corresponding contraction and relaxation of the cardiac muscle.

The heart is innervated by cholinergic fibers from the vagus nerve and adrenergic fibers from the sympathetic nervous system. **Cholinergic fibers**

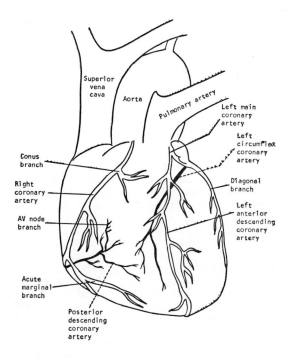

Figure 15-2.   Coronary circulation — arteries.

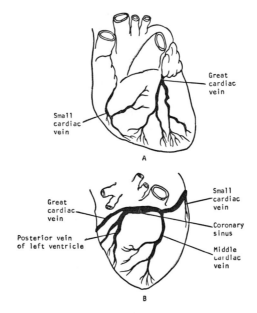

Figure 15-3.   Coronary veins and coronary sinus. (A) Anterior view; (B) posterior view.

are confined to the atria. The right vagus nerve supplies the SA node and controls heart rate and the force of atrial contractions. The left vagus nerve supplies the AV node. **Adrenergic fibers**, which are confined to the ventricles, increase the force of contraction. Reflexes are sensitive to pressure and chemical changes within the heart and great vessels. They exert control over the heart rate and peripheral vessels. **Baroreceptor reflexes** respond to changes in pressure within the vessels. **Chemoreceptor reflexes** respond to chemical changes in the blood and heart.

The main **function of the heart** is to supply the body with adequate amounts of blood for its metabolic needs during rest, normal activity, and periods of stress. Certain regulatory control mechanisms (factors affecting the cardiac cycle) (1) assist the circulatory system to adapt to the varying needs of the body and (2) support and reinforce one another. Factors affecting the **cardiac cycle** include (1) the movement of Ca^{++} in and out of the muscle cell, resulting in contraction and relaxation of the muscle, (2) the length-tension relationships in cardiac muscle (stretched muscle permits the release of Ca^{++}, an increased Ca^{++} level increases the force of contraction [Frank-Starling law], and increased contraction causes increased cardiac volume), and (3) the excitation-contraction coupling,

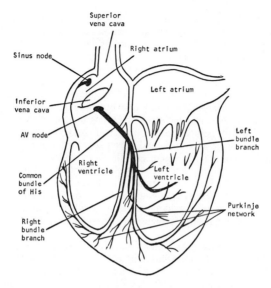

Figure 15-4. Conduction system of the heart.

which changes the rate of cardiac contractions and increases the force of contractions and the emptying rate of the heart.

CO, the amount of blood ejected by the ventricles each minute, is determined by the stroke volume (i.e., the amount of blood ejected with each beat) and the heart rate. CO can vary if the stroke volume or the heart rate changes.

General assessment

Components of the **health history** that are particularly relevant for the cardiac patient are current health status (specific complaint, present symptoms, duration, and personal behavior patterns), past health history of illnesses, family history (e.g., hypertension, heart disease, or jaundice) to identify risk factors, social history (relationships and occupation/school) to identify risk factors, and review of systems, with emphasis on the cardiovascular system.

In the **physical examination**, the initial observation and assessment should focus on the adequate functioning of the cardiovascular and peripheral vascular systems and include base-line vital signs as diagnostic, prognostic, and evaluative measures. The examination of the anterior and posterior chest begins with assessment of the lungs. The rate and rhythm of respirations is monitored, and the shape of the chest and the slope of the ribs is inspected. The chest is inspected for impaired respiratory movement (i.e., abnormal retraction on inspiration or abnormal bulging on expiration), and it is palpated to identify areas of tenderness, assess abnormalities noted on inspection, assess respiratory excursion, and elicit vocal fremitus. The chest is then percussed to assess (1) any abnormalities noted on inspection and palpation, (2) the symmetry of vibrations, and (3) diaphragmatic excursion. The chest is auscultated to assess and compare (1) the symmetry of breath sounds, and (2) any abnormal breath sounds (e.g., rales, rhonchi, wheezing, friction rubs, and stridor). During the cardiac assessment, the apical pulse at the point of maximal impulse (PMI) is inspected at the end of normal and forced expiration and is palpated for thrills or murmurs; the cardiac borders are percussed; and the heart sounds (Table 15-1) are auscultated at all valves and at Erb's point (3rd intercostal space, to the left of the sternum). Heart murmurs are a prolonged series of vibrations that vary in intensity, frequency, quality, and duration. They are characterized as systolic, diastolic, or continuous, and as either organic or functional. They develop as a result of structural or hemodynamic changes in the heart or blood vessels.

Diagnostic tests include chest x-ray (posterior, lateral, and right and left oblique) and the following laboratory tests: CBC with erythrocyte sedimentation rate, C-reactive protein, antistreptolytic O (ASO) titer, cardiac enzymes, serum electrolytes, BUN, serum creatinine, serum lipids, arterial blood gases (ABGs), and urinalysis. Diagnostic studies of the cardiovascular system are performed either for functional or structural evaluations of the heart. They are either invasive or noninvasive.

Noninvasive studies include the ECG, which is the graphic representation of the electric activity of the heart as the impulse initiated at the SA node travels through the conduction pathway of the heart (Table 15-2). Echocardiography is an ultrasonic examination of the heart that provides a graphic visualization of the cardiac structures, including chamber size, anatomy, and mobility. (A transducer placed on the chest and angled in various directions reflects the "echoes" on an oscilloscope.) The Doppler examination is an ultrasonic examination of the blood vessels of the body. (A transducer placed on the skin records a graphic representation of the blood flow through various vessels.) Halter monitoring is achieved via a small, portable, battery-operated ECG that permits ambulatory readings. The monitor is worn for 10 to 24 hr, thus providing a continuous ECG recording during unrestricted activity. The ECG is recorded on magnetic tape and marked with time intervals. A stress test involves ECG monitoring during physical stress in a laboratory setting under supervised conditions. The test stresses cardiovascular capacity and is terminated when the patient reaches the maximum level, experiences signs of ischemia on the ECG, or exhibits physical manifestations.

Invasive diagnostic procedures include cardiac catheterization, which is a cardiographic visualization of the heart that permits functional assessment of cardiac structures and that facilitates the diagnosis of cardiac

TABLE 15-1
Heart Sounds

Sound	Implication
Normal	
S_1	Is a loud, long, high-pitched sound heard at the mitral valve (PMI) and tricuspid valve; coincides with ventricular contraction; indicates closure of the mitral and tricuspid valves at the beginning of ventricular systole.
S_2	Is a higher pitched sound than S_1 heard at the pulmonic and aortic valves; indicates closure of the semilunar valve and the onset of diastole.
Abnormal	
S_3	May be heard as a gallop rhythm; is a faint, dull, low-pitched sound heard after S_2; is related to ventricular filling and may indicate mitral or tricuspid dysfunction.
S_4	Is heard just prior to S_1; is related to ventricular filling due to contraction of an enlarged atrium and may indicate aortic incompetency and pulmonary or systemic hypertension.
Systolic ejection click	Occurs in early systole; related to opening of the aortic or pulmonic valve or rapid distension of the proximal aorta or pulmonary artery.
Systolic nonejection click	Occurs in mid-to-late systole; related to mitral or tricuspid valve dysfunction.
Diastolic click	May be related to the opening snap of the mitral or tricuspid valve, to the precordial knock of pericarditis, or to a prosthetic valve; may be extracardiogenic.

PMI, point of maximal impulse.

disease related to anatomic malfunctioning. A catheter is inserted into the chambers of the heart, and contrast material is injected through it to provide opacification of the heart chambers and valves during fluoroscopy (angiography). Another invasive procedure is coronary arteriography, which allows visualization of the coronary arteries. (Contrast material is injected under fluoroscopy.)

Nursing care includes preparing the patient physically for the specific diagnostic exam, and providing the health teaching necessary for patient preparation. This is based on the specific exam, the patient's previous experiences with the same or a similar procedure, the effects of the actual or

TABLE 15-2

ECG Tracing

Tracing	Implication
P wave	Is the 1st wave of the cardiac cycle; represents the initiation of the impulse at the SA node; is the origin of atrial activity.
P-R interval	Is measured from the beginning of the P wave to the appearance of the next wave; represents the length of time the electric impulse takes to spread from the SA node though the AV node and the conduction system of the ventricles.
QRS complex	Represents ventricular depolarization and systole.
T wave	Represents ventricular repolarization, the end of systole, and the period of relaxation.
ST segment	Is measured from the QRS complex to the T wave; represents the time that the ventricles remain contracted.
U wave	Follows the T wave; may or may not be present in normal sinus rhythm; represents ventricular relaxation.

AV, atrioventricular; SA, sinoatrial.

potential illness, and the expectation of this procedure. In addition, the nurse provides postprocedure assessment and care related to the specific test.

Common interventions

Medical interventions may involve the following drugs: digitalis preparations, diuretics, vasodilators (nitrates), antiarrhythmic agents, beta blockers, calcium antagonists, anticoagulants, antihypertensive agents, analgesics, sedatives, and stool softeners. Various diets that may be prescribed are sodium restricted, polyunsaturated fatty acid, low cholesterol, and weight reduction, in addition to a reduced consumption of alcohol and caffeine. A planned exercise program is also initiated.

(The discussion of each **surgical** intervention will be followed by a listing of the **nursing** interventions that are specific to it.)

Coronary artery bypass graft (CABG) is the anastomosis of a saphenous vein autograft to an area proximal and distal to the coronary occlusion. Immediate preoperative care for open heart surgery is the same as for any thoracic surgery (*see* Chapters 9 and 14). Immediate postoperative care takes place in an intensive care setting for ~24 to 48 hr. The general guidelines for postoperative management apply (*see* Chapter 11). Guidelines specific for nursing management after cardiac surgery include the following:

1. Check and record central venous pressure (CVP) q 15 min.
2. Monitor the ECG for arrhythmias, especially forerunners of lethal arrhythmias.
3. Milk the chest tubes hourly and record the amount and color of the drainage from them hourly.
4. Measure and record intake and output hourly.
5. Weigh the patient daily and record the weight.
6. Assess the patient for signs of cerebral ischemia, hemorrhage, cardiac tamponade, cardiac shock, arrhythmia, renal shutdown, MI, and electrolyte imbalance.

Percutaneous transluminal coronary angioplasty (PTCA), an alternative to CABG surgery, involves dilation of the stenosed coronary artery by compression of the atherosclerotic material against the arterial lining. The vessel wall is dilated using a specially developed catheter. The double-lumen, balloon-tipped catheter is directed under fluoroscopy to the lesion. The balloon is placed within the lesion and is inflated for 4 to 5 sec with saline and contrast media. (The procedure may be repeated.) After the balloon is deflated and pulled back, contrast media is injected to evaluate the compression. Nursing interventions before PTCA are as follows:

1. Explain the purpose and rationale of this procedure to the patient and family.
2. Prepare the patient for the usual preoperative tests (see Chapter 9), coagulation survey, electrolyte survey, and myocardial radionuclide.
3. Administer preoperative medications (aspirin to decrease platelet adhesiveness, beta blockers to decrease ischemic symptoms, and a calcium antagonist to decrease the potential for coronary spasm).
4. Shave the patient's chest, groin, and upper thighs, and scrub the patient's chest and legs with Betadine three times.
5. Prepare the patient for the possibility of emergency bypass surgery.

Nursing interventions after PTCA are as follows:

1. Administer the usual postoperative care (See Chapter 11).
2. Assess, prevent, and treat complications, including hemorrhage, thrombus formation in the femoral artery, coronary spasm or thrombosis, hypovolemia, and hypokalemia.

Pacemaker insertion involves the introduction of an electrode into the right atrium or ventricle in order to help maintain normal cardiac rhythm. (The insertion may be temporary or permanent.) The procedure includes the following steps: (1) a bi- or unipolar electrode is inserted through the subclavian vein into the right atrium or ventricle (accomplished under fluoroscopy and ECG monitoring); (2) the electrode is tested for proper placement; (3) the electrode is connected to a pacer. If the pacer is temporary, the electrodes are sutured to the site and the pacer is secured to the upper arm. If permanent, the pacer is inserted into a small pocket made in the subcutaneous tissue of the chest.

There are two pacemaker models: fixed and demand. A fixed pacemaker delivers the electric impulse at a predetermined rate. It is continuous and does not respond to the patient's heart rate. With demand pacemakers, the electrode senses ventricular contraction and fires only when no contraction occurs. The electrode also senses atrial contraction and fires only if sequenced ventricular contraction does not occur. If no atrial contraction occurs, the electrode stimulates the atrium and ventricle.

Nursing care is as follows:

1. Provide general pre- and postoperative care (see Chapters 9 and 11).
2. Monitor heart rate and rhythm for pacing function.
3. Monitor for complications such as lethal arrhythmias, myocardial hemorrhage, and rapid hiccuping.
4. Provide emotional support to the patient and family.
5. Explain the function and use of the pacemaker.
6. Teach the patient related discharge management (to check the rate and rhythm of the pulse for 1 full min/day, to follow periods of activity with periods of rest, to be careful using electric tools, devices, and microwave ovens, and to use a safety razor rather than an electric shaver).
7. Report prolonged spells of hiccuping to the physician.
8. Schedule periodic checkups to evaluate the pacer's functioning and battery.

Evaluation criteria

Reduction/reversal of symptoms. Maintenance of normal cardiac rhythm. Reduction of fear and anxiety. Absence of complications. Patient and family verbalize medical regimen and necessary adaptations in lifestyle, as appropriate. Adherence to medical regimen.

CARDIAC ARREST

Cardiac arrest, a frequent cause of death, is the sudden cessation of CO that results from underlying cardiovascular pathology or hemorrhage. *Symptoms* include absence of pulses and respirations, cyanosis, unconsciousness, and dilated pupils. *Complications* include acidosis, hypoxia, hyperkalemia, and sudden and unexpected death. *Diagnosis* is based on the health history, physical exam, and an ECG tracing that shows a lethal arrhythmia or ventricular asystole.

Common interventions

Medical interventions for patients being monitored include identification of the underlying arrhythmias and appropriate treatment, defibrillation, CPR, and the treatment of acidosis, hypoxia, and hyperkalemia. For patients not being monitored, the treatment consists of CPR and defibrillation.

Nursing interventions

Physical 1. Identify the emergency, call for help, and administer CPR.
2. Prepare and/or administer medications as ordered, IV fluids, O_2 therapy, defibrillation, intubation, and ventilation.
3. After the emergency, carefully monitor the ECG, vital signs, CVP, ABGs, and intake and output.
4. Maintain IV fluids, O_2 therapy, and bed rest.
5. Assess and treat the underlying pathology.
Psychosocial 6. Provide emotional support for the patient and family during and after the cardiac arrest.

Evaluation criteria. *See* Overview.

MYOCARDIAL INFARCTION

An MI is the ischemic necrosis of myocardial tissue as a result of an abrupt decrease in blood flow to the myocardium. The most common site of an MI is the anterior wall of the left ventricle. The etiology of an MI may be any of the following: atherosclerotic plaque formation and hemorrhage within the wall of one or more of the main coronary arteries; hypertrophy of the heart muscle, leading to increased blood need; occlusion of a main coronary artery by embolism; gradual sclerotic occlusion; temporary decreased blood flow due to postoperative or traumatic shock; myocardial aneurysm. The severity of an MI depends on the location and extent of ischemia, the presence of previously infarcted myocardial tissue, and the adequacy of collateral circulation.

Symptoms include severe and prolonged substernal pain, with or without radiation; anxiety and apprehension; nausea and/or vomiting; signs of shock; signs of left-sided heart failure; and a low-grade fever. *Complications* include hypoxia, arrhythmias (including ventricular fibrillation), thromboembolism, mitral insufficiency, pericarditis, cardiac shock, ventricular aneurysm, CHF, acute renal failure, cerebral infarction, and cardiac arrest.

Diagnosis is based on the health history, physical exam, and elevated levels of the following lab studies: WBC, erythrocyte sedimentation rate, glucose (initially), creatine phosphokinase-myocardial band (CPK-MB) (increases within 4 to 8 hr, peaks within 24 hr, and returns to normal 6 to 8 days after MI), SGOT (increases within 6 to 8 hr, peaks within 18 to 36 hr, and returns to normal 6 to 8 days after MI), and lactic dehydrogenase (LDH) (increases within 24 to 48 hr, peaks within 3 to 6 days, and returns to normal 8 to 14 days after MI).

Common interventions

The goals of therapy are to reduce myocardial ischemia and necrosis by increasing myocardial perfusion and decreasing potential cellular damage. **Medical** interventions are designed to prevent and treat tachyarrhythmias by the use of medications and a temporary pacemaker, to treat left ventricular failure by the use of medications, O_2 therapy, and defibrillation, to maintain BP, to prevent cellular damage by the use of medications, and to relieve pain by the use of analgesics and sedatives. **Surgical** interventions include intra-aortic balloon pulsation, CABG, and PTCA.

Nursing interventions

The goals of nursing intervention include treatment of the acute attack and prompt alleviation of symptoms, prevention of complications and further attacks, rehabilitation of the patient, and teaching of the patient and family.

Physical 1. Administer medications as ordered.
2. Maintain the patient on complete bed rest in semi-Fowler's position.
3. Administer O_2 therapy.
4. Monitor the ECG for signs of arrhythmias, especially ventricular arrhythmias.
5. Monitor vital signs and intracardiac pressures.
6. Observe for signs of cardiogenic shock and left ventricular failure.
7. Maintain fluid and electrolyte balance (administer IV fluids and monitor intake and output).
8. Gradually increase the patient's activity and self-care.
9. Provide care that will continue to assess, treat, and prevent complications and associated diseases.

Psychosocial 10. Provide a calm, quiet atmosphere.
11. Provide reassurance to the patient and family during and after the attack.
12. Provide emotional support with regard to hospitalization and rehabilitation.
13. Prepare the patient for diagnostic tests and surgery, if necessary.
14. Help the patient to identify risk factors and precipitating conditions that may be modified and the resultant changes in life-style.
15. Support the patient and family with necessary life-style changes.

Educational 16. Teach the pathophysiology of the disease process and the rationale for treatment.
17. Teach the medical regimen for discharge (diet therapy, medication therapy, and exercise regimen as prescribed).
18. Teach the importance of weight control, smoking cessation, stress reduction, the exercise and medication regimens, diet therapy, relaxation techniques, and individual responsibility for management.

19. Teach ways of controlling associated disease such as diabetes and gout.

Evaluation criteria.   *See* Overview.

PULMONARY EDEMA

Pulmonary edema is a medical emergency in which fluid from the circulating blood floods the alveoli, bronchi, and bronchioles because of cardiac decompensation. The phases of pulmonary edema are presented in Table 15-3.

CARDIOGENIC SHOCK

Cardiogenic shock is reduced tissue perfusion as a result of severe cardiac dysfunction, such as acute MI or severe left ventricular dysfunction from any source. *Symptoms* include (1) signs of decreased CO (right- and left-sided heart failure), (2) signs of poor tissue perfusion of the brain, kidneys, liver, lungs, and heart, (3) signs of decreased peripheral vascular circulation, and (4) increasing signs of shock (hypotension, unresponsiveness, oliguria, diaphoresis, and metabolic acidosis). *Complications* include hypovolemia, ventricular arrhythmias (especially fibrillation), and death. *Diagnosis* is based on the health history, physical exam, ABGs, direct measurement of intravascular pressure, ECG, and left-sided cardiac catheterization.

Common interventions

Medical treatment includes intra-aortic balloon pulsation, vasodilation therapy, treatment of the underlying pathology, prevention and treatment of complications, and O_2 therapy.

Nursing interventions

Physical 1. Administer medications as ordered and assess for side effects.
2. Reduce pain.
3. Assess vital signs and monitor intake and output.
4. Monitor the ECG.
5. Assess the patient for signs of increasing shock.
6. Maintain the patient on bed rest.
7. Maintain IV fluids at the prescribed rate.
8. Administer O_2 therapy.
Psychosocial 9. Provide emotional support to the patient and family during and after cardiogenic shock.

Evaluation criteria.   *See* Overview.

TABLE 15-3

Phases of Pulmonary Edema

Parameter	Initial phase (I)	Advanced phase (II)	Acute phase (III)
Etiology	The interstitial space fills with fluid because of left-sided failure.	Fluid in the pulmonary circulation increases and fills the interstitial tissue. The lymphatic system is unable to handle the overload. The peripheral alveoli and small bronchi are filled with fluid.	The bronchial tree fills with fluid.
Symptoms	Dry cough, exercise intolerance, restlessness, anxiety and feeling of dread, dyspnea, orthopnea, increased BP, rales, and S_3 or diastolic gallop.	Acute SOB, productive cough (frothy hemoptysis), shallow and rapid respirations, cyanosis, diaphoresis, hypotension, tachycardia, moist rales, rhonchi ("cardiac asthma"), and anxiety.	Progressive symptoms of phases I and II, severe hypoxia (decreased level of consciousness, ventricular arrhythmias, metabolic/respiratory acidosis, and shock), diminishing breath sounds, and a rapid and irregular heart rate.
Complications	Advanced and acute phases.	Acute phase.	Ventricular fibrillation, acidosis, shock, and death.
Diagnosis	Health history and physical exam. Laboratory data: decreased $PaCO_2$ and mild decrease in PaO_2.	Health history and physical exam. Laboratory data: $PaCO_2$ begins to fall considerably below normal.	Health history and physical exam. Laboratory data: marked rise in $PaCO_2$.
Medical interventions	Oxygen therapy, semi-Fowler's position, and sedation.	Same as for phase I, plus digitalization, diuresis, bronchodilators, phlebotomy, and rotating tourniquets.	Same as for phases I and II, plus cardioversion, respiratory resuscitation, and cardiac resuscitation.

| Nursing interventions | 1. Assess respiratory distress: auscultate the heart and lungs, assess the apical and radial pulses, monitor ABGs, monitor respiratory rate and rhythm, and monitor systemic signs of decreased oxygenation.
2. Administer O_2 therapy and medications.
3. Position the patient (semi-Fowler's).
4. Provide physical and mental rest.
5. Provide emotional support for the patient and family.
6. After the emergency, maintain the patient on complete bed rest, a low-sodium diet, fluid restriction, and diuretic therapy, and teach the patient to prevent recurrence. | 1. Continue respiratory assessment to determine progression.
2. Monitor intake and output.
3. Monitor the ECG tracing.
4. Assess respiratory alkalosis.
5. Assess metabolic acidosis.
6. Administer medications.
7. Prepare for specific treatments: tourniquets and phlebotomy.
8. *See* 2–6 of phase I | 1. Continue as per phases I and II.
2. Prepare for and assist with specific treatments: cardioversion, respiratory resuscitation, and cardiac resuscitation. |
| Evaluation criteria | *See* Overview, | | |

ABG, arterial blood gas; SOB, shortness of breath.

CARDIAC TAMPONADE

Cardiac tamponade is a collection of fluid in the pericardial sac that results in compression of the heart. Causes include injury (blunt or penetrating chest trauma or cardiac surgery) and infection (related to pericardial effusion, pericarditis, pericardial constriction, or hemodialysis). Pericardial effusion may occur with acute rheumatic fever, SLE, and after MI or cardiac surgery. Pericarditis may result from viral, fungal, or bacterial (including tubercular) infection; uremia; malignant diseases (e.g., leukemia, lymphoma, and malignant melanoma); pericardial tumor metastasis; and as a side effect of medication. Pericardial constriction may be related to radiation therapy.

Cardiac tamponade occurs when fluid or blood collects in the pericardial sac and the pressure in the cavity rises to a level equal to the diastolic pressure. This equal pressure results in inadequate filling of the ventricles and a reduced CO. *Symptoms* include extreme anxiety, mental changes (e.g., confusion and combativeness), shortness of breath, dyspnea, orthopnea, increased rate and depth of respirations, clear and normal breath sounds, diaphoresis, pulsus paradoxus (a fall of systolic pressure on inspiration), Kussmaul's sign (a rise of venous pressure on inspiration), the inability of the apical pulse to be palpated, tachycardia, increased CVP, muffled or distant heart sounds, and friction rub. *Complications* include right-sided heart failure, progressive shock, and cardiac arrest.

Diagnosis is based on the health history, physical exam, and chest x-ray. Other tests include the ECG (in which there may be no specific changes), the echocardiogram (which determines the amount and location of the fluid), the taking of intracardiac pressure via CVP, and pericardiocentesis.

Common interventions

Medical interventions include pericardiocentesis and antibiotic therapy to treat the underlying pathology. **Surgical** treatment involves repair of the injury or trauma.

Nursing interventions

Physical 1. Assess the predisposing conditions that lead to cardiac tamponade.
2. Assess the symptoms of cardiac tamponade.
3. Administer medications as ordered.
4. Assess for the side or toxic effects of medications.
5. Monitor all vital signs, including CVP, BP, pulse, respirations, pulsus paradoxus, and pulse pressure.
6. Maintain the patient on bed rest in semi-Fowler's position.
Psychosocial 7. Allay the fear and anxiety of the patient and family.
8. Provide support during and after cardiac tamponade.

Evaluation criteria.   *See* Overview.

RHEUMATIC FEVER

Rheumatic fever is an infection of connective and endothelial tissue. It is caused by group A beta-hemolytic streptococci, but a possible genetic aberration of the immune system may also be involved. Phase 1 of rheumatic fever is marked by the presence of an acute streptococcal infection. The symptoms include fever, chills, enlarged lymph nodes, tonsillitis, nasopharyngitis, and otitis media. Phase 2, the latent period of sensitization, may last 1 to 5 wk and is asymptomatic after recovery from phase 1 occurs. Phase 3, the acute phase, involves systemic disease and inflammatory lesions of connective and endothelial tissue. The major *symptoms* of rheumatic fever are a low-grade and intermittent fever, polyarthritis (inflammation of the synovial joint linings), and carditis that involves the myo-, endo-, and pericardium. Other symptoms are malaise, anorexia, weight loss, and epistaxis. *Complications* include myo-, endo-, and pericarditis.

Diagnosis is based on the health history, physical exam, blood tests (increased erythrocyte sedimentation rate, WBC, and ASO titer) and on a positive culture for group A beta-hemolytic streptococcal infection.

Common interventions

Medical treatment includes bed rest with early ambulation as dictated by progress, analgesics, antipyretics, corticosteroids (especially with carditis), antibiotic therapy for 10 days to 2 wk, a bland diet with increased calories and protein, the treatment of specific complications, and prophylactic antibiotics for up to 5 yr.

Nursing interventions

Physical 1. Maintain the patient on bed rest and follow periods of activity with rest.
2. Prevent the complications of prolonged bed rest.
3. Offer the patient small, frequent feedings.
4. Administer medications as ordered and assess for side effects.
5. Encourage fluid intake.
6. Monitor vital signs.

Psychosocial 7. Provide a relaxing, quiet atmosphere and emotional support.

Educational 8. Teach the patient about medications (rationale, proper dosage and administration, potential annoying and harmful side effects, adaptation of medical regimen into life-style, and increased dose, per a physician's orders, when undergoing tooth extraction or a surgical procedure).
9. Instruct the patient as to the proper care of teeth and gums.
10. Advise the patient to avoid people with upper respiratory or streptococcal infections.
11. Instruct the patient to identify and report the symptoms of streptococcal infection.

Prevention 12. Teach the patient to obtain a culture for the symptoms of streptococcal infection and to maintain proper medical management of streptococcal infection, including taking medication for the prescribed time period despite the remission of acute symptoms.

Evaluation criteria.   *See* Overview.

ENDOCARDITIS

Infectious endocarditis refers to an inflammation of the valvicular surface, endocardium, and arterial wall of the heart. The most common causes are *Streptococcus viridans* or *Staphylococcus aureus.* A characteristic lesion in the endocardium consists of an irregular nodule of blood elements, deposited as vegetation, with resultant ulceration and destruction of tissue. *Symptoms* include fever, malaise, fatigue, the general symptoms of CHF, symptoms due to emboli, recent infection, a recent history of possible contact with an infective agent (e.g., dental work or a gynecologic or urologic procedure), a previous heart murmur, and the heart sounds of specific valvular heart disease and associated complications. *Complications* include emboli and cardiac valve involvement.

Diagnosis is based on the health history, physical exam, positive blood cultures, and an echocardiogram (to identify vegetation with the extent and location of heart damage).

Common interventions

Medical treatment consists of antibiotic therapy and bed rest. **Surgical** treatment involves valvular replacement.

Nursing interventions

Physical 1. Administer antibiotic therapy and assess the side effects of medication.
2. Assess and prevent infection.
3. Maintain the patient on bed rest and assess and prevent the complications of bed rest.
Psychosocial 4. Provide a quiet, relaxing atmosphere and emotional support.
Educational 5. Teach the patient to avoid infection.
6. Teach the patient to recognize and report the symptoms of infection (especially streptococcal).
7. Teach the patient to obtain a culture for the symptoms of infection and to maintain proper management of infection.

Evaluation criteria.   *See* Overview. Patient adherence to antibiotic therapy and verbalization of importance of detection, prevention, and treatment of infection.

CHRONIC VALVULAR DISEASE

Chronic valvular disease is the permanent damage to the structure of the cardiac valves that occurs after a single or multiple untreated episodes of acute rheumatic fever (ARF). The mitral and aortic valves are most commonly affected. Chronic changes in the valves may occur within months or years of ARF. Valvular dysfunction is of two types: **stenosis,** which restricts the valve opening and obstructs normal blood flow, and **regurgitation,** in which the valve fails to close and seal properly, thus allowing the blood to flow backward. The etiology, symptoms, complications, diagnosis, and medical and surgical interventions for chronic valvular disease are included in Tables 15-4 to 15-6. (*See also* Table 15-1.)

Nursing interventions

Physical 1. Administer anticoagulant and antibiotic therapy as ordered.
2. Assess for the side effects of medications.
3. Prevent infectious endocarditis and ARF.
4. Determine the patient's necessary life-style adaptations to prevent complications.
5. Provide general preoperative care (*see* Chapter 9).
6. Prepare the patient for preoperative procedures, including cardiac catheterization.
7. Prepare the patient and family for the surgery with regard to the surgical procedure, type of valve, and cardiopulmonary perfusion machine.
8. Provide general postoperative care for thoracic surgery (*see* Chapter 11).
9. Splint the thoracic incision when moving the patient or doing exercises with him.
10. Administer antibiotic and anticoagulant therapy and assess for the side effects of medications.
11. Prevent the complications of hemolytic anemia.
Psychosocial 12. Provide the patient with emotional support for coping with chronic illness and the life-style adaptations related to the illness and its complications.
Educational 13. Instruct the patient to take the anticoagulant as ordered.
14. Instruct the patient about the side effects of anticoagulant therapy (hematuria, hematemesis, dark and tarry stools, bleeding gums or oral mucosa, ecchymosis, purpura, petechiae, epistaxis, abdominal or lumbar pain, increased menstrual flow, and prolonged oozing from a minor injury).
15. Instruct the patient about factors that increase bleeding (fever, alcoholism, hot weather, renal insufficiency, x-ray, and medications such as aspirin and mineral oil).
16. Instruct the patient about factors that decrease bleeding (diarrhea, a diet high in fat and vitamin K, dichloro-diphenyl-trichloro-ethane [DDT], and medications such as oral contraceptives and vitamins K and C).

TABLE 15-4

Comparison of Mitral Valve Diseases

Stenosis	Regurgitation
Etiology	
Progressive narrowing of the orifice between the left atrium and left ventricle results in inhibition of normal blood flow in the left side of the heart, left ventricular hypertrophy, pulmonary hypertension due to overload of blood in the right atrium, decreased CO, right ventricular hypertrophy, tricuspid regurgitation, and systemic venous congestion.	Causes include ARF, congenital anomaly, bacterial endocarditis, and aortic valve disease. Atrophy of the valve results in increased blood volume in the left atrium and right ventricle, dilation and hypertrophy of the left atrium and right ventricle, increased pulmonary congestion, decreased CO, and increased systemic venous congestion.
Symptoms	
Gradual or sudden onset, fatigue, dyspnea, SOB, DOE, PND, orthopnea, abdominal discomfort, pain, and anorexia.	Weakness, fatigue, dyspnea, DOE, palpitations, symptoms of left-sided failure, and eventually, symptoms of right-sided failure.
Complications	
Atrial fibrillation and/or flutter, pulmonary edema and acute dyspnea precipitated by atrial fibrillation or flutter, systemic emboli, and CHF.	CHF, atrial arrhythmias, and emboli.
Diagnosis	
Health history and physical exam: S_1 greater in intensity (snapping sound); presystolic rumbling murmur near the apex. Chest x-ray (depending on the extent of stenosis and associated complications) may show enlarged left atrium and right ventricle, increased pulmonary artery prominence, increased pulmonary venous markings, and mitral valve calcification. ECG may show bifid P waves, right axis deviation, and right ventricular hypertrophy. Echocardiogram will show mobility of the mitral valve and will be specific for stenosis. Cardiac catheterization denotes size of the orifice and evaluates the heart for associated and other pathology.	Health history and physical exam: S_1 may be diminished; S_3 gallop sound; blowing, high-pitched systolic murmur; displaced apical pulse (because of enlarged left ventricle). Chest x-ray may show an enlarged left atrium and ventricle, pulmonary vascular engorgement, and an enlarged right ventricle. ECG may be nonspecific, or show left ventricular or biventricular hypertrophy. Echocardiogram may be nonspecific. Cardiac catheterization denotes mitral valve disease or incompetency and evaluates the heart for associated and other pathology.
Medical interventions	
Treatment and prevention of atrial arrhythmias, CHF, and emboli; anticoagulant and antibiotic therapy; prevention of endocarditis and ARF.	Treatment and prevention of atrial arrhythmias, CHF, and emboli; antibiotic therapy; prevention of endocarditis and ARF.
Surgical interventions	
Mitral valve commissurotomy; mitral valve replacement.	Mitral valve replacement.

ARF, acute rheumatic fever; DOE, dyspnea on exertion; PND, paroxysmal nocturnal dyspnea; SOB, shortness of breath.

TABLE 15-5
Comparison of Aortic Valve Diseases

Stenosis	Regurgitation
Etiology Causes include ARF and atherosclerosis. Progressive narrowing of the orifice between the left ventricle and aorta results in increased pressure and blood volume in the left ventricle, hypertrophy of the left ventricle without dilation, corresponding left atrial hypertrophy, decreased CO, and increased pulmonary congestion.	Causes include ARF, bacterial endocarditis, and congenital anomaly. Results include increased blood volume in the left ventricle, decreased CO, hypertrophy and dilation of the left ventricle, pulmonary congestion, and left-sided heart failure.
Symptoms Progressive symptoms of left-sided failure. Initial stage: fatigue, angina, and DOE. Later stage: orthopnea, PND, pulmonary edema, and increased diastolic pressure.	Heart murmur, sinus tachycardia with emotional stress or exertion, DOE, angina with rest and exertion, nocturnal angina, orthopnea, PND, excessive diaphoresis, and Marfan's syndrome.
Complications Acute pulmonary edema, atrial arrhythmias, myocardial ischemia, angina, left- and right-sided CHF, and infectious endocarditis.	Pulmonary edema and left- and right-sided CHF.
Diagnosis Health history and physical exam: systolic thrill over the aortic valve and harsh systolic murmur. Chest x-ray is normal. ECG may show increased amplitude of QRS complex. Echocardiogram will denote restrictive movement of the aortic valve. Cardiac catheterization denotes valve dysfunction and evaluates the heart for associated and other pathology.	Health history and physical exam: visible, forceful pulsation at the aortic valve; high-pitched, blowing diastolic murmur; Austin Flint murmur; S_3 and S_4 sounds with CHF; premature systole. Chest x-ray shows cardiomegaly. ECG may show increased amplitude of QRS complex and ST and T wave aberrations. Echocardiogram may show a deformed valve and a dilated left ventricle. Cardiac catheterization denotes valve disease and incompetence and evaluates the heart for associated and other pathology.
Medical interventions Treatment and prevention of complications associated with left-sided failure and pulmonary edema.	Treatment and prevention of complications associated with CHF and pulmonary edema.
Surgical intervention Aortic valve replacement.	Aortic valve replacement.

ARF, acute rheumatic fever; DOE, dyspnea on exertion; PND, paroxysmal nocturnal dyspnea.

TABLE 15-6
Comparison of Tricuspid Valve Diseases

Stenosis	Regurgitation
Etiology	
Caused most commonly by ARF.	May be associated with right ventricular failure or mitral valve disease.
Symptoms	
Increased right-sided volume and pressure, and general signs of right-sided heart failure.	Same as for stenosis.
Complications	
Right-sided heart failure, infectious endocarditis, and arrhythmias.	Same as for stenosis.
Diagnosis	
Health history and physical exam: auscultation of heart sounds (rumbling diastolic murmur associated with opening snap that is increased on inspiration). Chest x-ray shows enlarged right atrium and ventricle. ECG may have P wave aberrations. Cardiac catheterization shows valve dysfunction or disease, and helps to evaluate heart and associated disorders.	Health history and physical exam: auscultation of heart sounds (pansystolic murmur that is increased on inspiration, and S_3 gallop sound). Chest x-ray, ECG, and cardiac catheterization are the same as for stenosis.
Medical interventions	
Treatment and prevention of mitral stenosis, the underlying cause of right ventricular failure, and complications associated with right-sided failure.	Same as for stenosis.
Surgical intervention	
Tricuspid valve replacement.	Same as for stenosis.

ARF, acute rheumatic fever.

17. Instruct the patient to return to the clinic to have blood tests.
18. Instruct the patient to discontinue the anticoagulant and consult a physician if excessive bleeding occurs.
19. Instruct the patient to terminate anticoagulant therapy gradually in order to prevent thromboembolitis.
20. Instruct the patient to apply ice and pressure to the bleeding site.
Prevention 21. Advise the patient to use a soft toothbrush and an electric razor.
22. Advise the patient to wear gloves when gardening or doing similar work.
23. Advise the patient to carry vitamin K in case of blood loss and to wear medical alert identification.

Evaluation criteria. *See* Overview.

MYOCARDITIS

Myocarditis, an inflammation of the myocardium, is most commonly seen as a result of a systemic illness or infection. Because its clinical manifestations may be associated with the primary illness, myocarditis may go unnoticed unless it is a serious sequela. *Symptoms* include vague complaints of fever, fatigue, anorexia, and nausea; chest pain; dyspnea; palpitations; and tachycardia. *Complications* include arrhythmias, systemic and pulmonary emboli, CHF, pulmonary edema, and cardiac failure.

Diagnosis is based on the health history, significant findings of the physical exam (CHF, gallop rhythm, and friction rub associated with pericarditis), and chest x-ray that reveals cardiomegaly (especially ventricular enlargement) and pulmonary edema.

Common interventions

Medical interventions include treatment of the underlying illness or infection, antibiotic therapy, and treatment and prevention of cardiac failure (including digitalis therapy).

Nursing interventions

Physical 1. Maintain the patient on bed rest.
2. Administer antibiotic and digitalis therapy.
3. Prevent infection, cardiac failure, and the complications related to myocarditis and to prolonged bed rest.
Psychosocial 4. Provide the emotional support related to bed rest.
5. Provide a quiet, relaxed atmosphere.
Educational 6. Instruct the patient on the necessity of maintaining bed rest.
7. Teach the patient to avoid infection and to identify and report any signs of infection.

Evaluation criteria. *See* Overview.

PERICARDITIS

Pericarditis is an inflammation of the pericardium. Acute pericarditis is an acute inflammation, with or without fluid accumulation in the pericardial sac. It may result from a viral infection, TB, bacteremia, or septicemia of the pericardium or a contiguous organ. *Symptoms* include serous, purulent, or hemorrhagic fluid in the pericardial sac; chest pains (sharp and of sudden onset, they are aggravated by inspiration, coughing, or swallowing, and are relieved by sitting up); dyspnea; tachycardia; elevated temperature; pallor; anxiety; and restlessness. *Complications* include pericardial effusion and cardiac tamponade.

Diagnosis is based on the health history; physical exam (especially a friction rub that may be accentuated on inspiration); chest x-ray (which may be normal or reveal increasing heart size); an elevated ST segment on ECG; an elevated WBC; and culture of fluid from the pericardial sac.

Common interventions

Medical treatment includes antibiotic therapy, bed rest, analgesics, the prevention of complications, pericardial paracentesis, and treatment of the underlying cause.

Nursing interventions

Physical 1. Maintain the patient on bed rest.
2. Administer antibiotic therapy and analgesics as ordered.
3. Assess, treat, and prevent complications.
4. Prevent complications related to bed rest.
Psychosocial 5. Provide the emotional support related to bed rest.
6. Provide a quiet, relaxed atmosphere.
Educational 7. Instruct the patient on the necessity of maintaining bed rest.
8. Teach the patient to identify and report signs of infection and to avoid infections that may result in pericarditis.

Evaluation criteria. *See* Overview.

PERICARDIAL EFFUSION

Pericardial effusion is the accumulation of a small or large amount of fluid in the pericardial sac. When the volume is large, normal ventricular functioning is impaired and tamponade may occur. Table 15-7 compares and contrasts two forms of pericardial effusion, with and without cardiac tamponade.

CONSTRICTIVE PERICARDITIS

Constrictive pericarditis is a chronic inflammation of the pericardium, resulting in the thickening and fibrosis of the pericardial membrane. It is often a sequela of TB. *Symptoms,* which result from the inability of the ventricles to fill, may include right-sided heart failure, or the patient may be asymptomatic. The *complications* include atrial arrhythmias and CHF. *Diagnosis* is based on the health history; significant findings of the physical exam (e.g., loud and sharp third heart sound ["pericardial knock"]); chest x-ray (e.g., prominent pulmonary vascular system); ECG (atrial arrhythmias and T wave inversion); and cardiac catheterization that reveals a noncompliant pericardial sac.

Common interventions

Medical interventions aim at treating the underlying cause and the symptoms of CHF and other complications. **Surgical** treatment includes pericardiectomy (excision of the damaged, constricting pericardium). **Nursing** interventions are the same as for CHF and for TB (if it is the underlying cause). Refer also to nursing interventions for thoracic surgery (*see* Chapters 9, 11, and 14).

Evaluation criteria. *See* Overview.

TABLE 15-7

Pericardial Effusion, with and without Cardiac Tamponade

Without tamponade	With tamponade
Etiology	
Complication of acute pericarditis.	Complication of acute pericarditis and pericardial effusion.
Symptoms	
Nonspecific; symptoms of acute pericarditis and of systemic illness; quiet heart sounds; cardiac dullness on percussion.	Symptoms of pericardial effusion and cardiac tamponade.
Complications	
Cardiac tamponade.	Venous congestion, shock, and death.
Diagnosis	
Health history and physical exam. Chest x-ray shows cardiomegaly. Echocardiogram is highly specific for diagnosing and measuring pericardial fluid. Needle aspiration shows the presence of fluid.	Health history and physical exam. Needle aspiration shows the presence of fluid.
Treatment	
Pericardial paracentesis; the same as for acute pericarditis.	Emergency treatment (pericardial paracentesis and the prevention of shock); the same as for cardiac tamponade and acute pericarditis.
Nursing interventions	
The same as for acute pericarditis; pre- and postpericardial paracentesis care.	The same as for cardiac tamponade, pericardial effusion without tamponade, and acute pericarditis.

CONGESTIVE HEART FAILURE

CHF is a syndrome that results from the inability of the heart to pump sufficient blood to meet the metabolic demands of the body. It occurs in 50 to 60% of those with organic heart disease. There are three physiologic aspects of CHF: (1) pathologic cardiac overloading, (2) compensatory responses of the cardiovascular system to this overloading, and (3) cardiac decompensation as a result of the failure of cardiac compensation. These phenomena happen sequentially and may last for varying lengths of time. Pathologic cardiac overloading can result from three causative factors that can work singularly or in combination (Table 15-8). As a result of cardiac overloading, the heart attempts to maintain normal CO by a variety of compensatory mechanisms (Table 15-9). Cardiac decompensation occurs (1) if the compensatory mechanisms are unable to mediate the cardiac overloading, or (2) if these mechanisms fail. The *symptoms* produced because of decompensation are varied and depend on a number of factors, including the patient profile, the type and degree of underlying cardiac and

TABLE 15-8

Factors That Cause Cardiac Overloading

Factor	Cause	Effect/demand
Pressure overloading	Aortic stenosis, pulmonary hypertension, systemic hypertension, coronary artery disease	Increased force of cardiac contraction.
Volume overloading	Mitral regurgitation, aortic regurgitation, excessive venous return, and intracardiac shunt anomalies	Excessive filling of the ventricles during diastole, and increased force of cardiac contraction.
Loss of functional tissue	MI	Inability to maintain normal cardiac functioning.

TABLE 15-9

Compensatory Mechanisms for Cardiac Overloading

Mechanism	Effect
Frank-Starling law	Increased ventricular dilation, stroke volume, and CO.
Sympathetic nervous system	Cardiac level: increased pulse rate and myocardial contractility. Peripheral vascular level: increased vasocontractility to increase venous return and volume expansion.
Ventricular hypertrophy	Increased ventricular contractility.
Oxygen extraction	Increased oxygen extractions from circulating blood.

systemic disease, the functioning or failure of compensatory mechanisms, and the development of right- or left-sided failure. Left-sided heart failure is the more common form of decompensation in patients who have an MI. Right-sided heart failure almost always results from left-sided heart failure; it seldom exists independently. The differences in right- and left-sided failure are listed in Table 15-10.

Nursing interventions

  Physical 1. Increase cardiac contractility by administering a digitalis preparation.
   2. Assess the clinical effects of digitalization (reduced heart rate and decrease in presenting symptoms).
   3. Assess for and prevent digitalis toxicity.

TABLE 15-10
Comparison of Right- and Left-Sided Failure

Left-sided failure	Right-sided failure
Definition	
Failure of the left side of the heart to pump effectively.	Failure of the right side of the heart to pump effectively.
Etiology	
Hypertension, myocardial ischemia, MI, aortic valve disease and mitral valve disease (rarely).	Left-sided failure, pulmonary diseases (chronic emphysema and COPD), constrictive pericarditis, tricuspid stenosis (rarely), and congenital pulmonic stenosis (rarely).
Symptoms	
Cardiovascular/respiratory	*Cardiovascular/respiratory*
Dyspnea, DOE, PND, SOB, orthopnea, fluid at the base of the lungs, rales, rhonchi, friction rub, diminished breath sounds, muffled heart sounds, murmur (if valve disease), and a dry cough.	Increased venous pressure, hypertension, rales, and rhonchi.
Hepatorenal	*Hepatorenal*
Daytime oliguria, nocturia, and increased weight.	Hepatomegaly and pain.
Cerebrovascular	*Cerebrovascular*
Irritability, restlessness, mental confusion, syncope, hypertension, and cerebral anoxia.	Restlessness.
Abdominal	*Abdominal*
Anorexia and constipation.	Ascites, distension, pain or discomfort in the upper right quadrant, anorexia, bloating, nausea, and constipation.
Peripheral vascular	*Peripheral vascular*
Cold and pale extremities; cyanotic lips, nail beds, and extremities; fatigue and muscle weakness.	Cold extremities and cyanotic nail beds; dependent, pitting edema; distended neck veins and increased venous pressure.
Mental	*Mental*
Anxiety and depression related to chronic illness.	Apprehension, anxiety, and depression related to chronic illness.
Complications	
Pulmonary edema, pleural effusion, right-sided failure, cachexia, and shock syndrome.	Hypertension, acute pulmonary edema, cachexia, and shock syndrome.
Diagnosis	
Health history and physical exam. Laboratory data: increased BUN, Na^+, uric acid, and creatinine; mild proteinuria; decreased $PaCO_2$, increased pH. Chest x-ray shows hazy lung fields and distended pulmonary veins.	Health history and physical exam. Laboratory data: same a for left-sided failure. Chest x-ray is nonspecific.
Treatment	
Digitalization, diuresis, and increased tissue oxygenation.	Same as for left-sided failure.

DOE, dyspnea on exertion; PND, paroxysmal nocturnal dyspnea; SOB, shortness of breath.

4. Reduce fluid and Na^+ retention by administering diuretic agents, providing a low-sodium diet, and limiting fluid intake.
5. Assess for diuresis and prevent complications.
   a. Monitor intake and output accurately.
   b. Obtain daily weights.
   c. Check for decreasing pulmonary, abdominal, and peripheral edema.
   d. Monitor serum electrolytes and renal function blood studies.
   e. Monitor signs of dehydration.
   f. Assess for the reduction of presenting symptoms.
6. Increase tissue oxygenation and decrease O_2 need.
   a. Administer O_2 therapy, which should result in decreased respiratory symptoms, an increase in peripheral vascular and systemic perfusion, decreased arterial BP and heart rate, and an increased PO_2 level.
   b. Administer vasodilators as prescribed.
   c. Assess the clinical effects and potential side effects of specific vasodilation.
   d. Maintain the patient on bed rest.
   e. Prevent the complications related to prolonged bed rest.
   f. Monitor vital signs and auscultate heart and lung sounds.
   g. Provide for progressive periods of activity followed by rest.
   h. Provide relaxation measures.

Psychosocial 7. Provide a quiet, restful environment and reduce emotional stress.
8. Identify the necessary adaptations in life-style to decrease the symptoms and maintain the medical regimen.
9. Provide emotional support for coping with a chronic illness.

Educational 10. Teach the patient and family about digitalis therapy.
   a. Rationale for taking the drug.
   b. Potential side and toxic effects.
   c. Medication regimen (check the pulse before taking the drug, noting the rate and rhythm; take the drug according to the prescribed dose and time; and have routine blood studies, e.g., electrolytes and digitalis levels).
11. Teach the patient and family about diuresis.
   a. Rationale for Na^+ and fluid restriction.
   b. Need for low-sodium diet.
   c. Actual effects and potential side effects of the specific diuretic.
   d. Need for routine blood studies.
   e. Rationale for procedures that monitor Na^+ and fluid retention.
   f. Need for keeping accurate intake and output records.
12. Teach the patient and family about activity and rest (the rationale for mental and physical rest, a planned program for increasing activity, relaxation techniques, and stress-reduction techniques).

Evaluation criteria.   *See* Overview.

SINUS BRADYCARDIA

Sinus bradycardia, a benign arrhythmia, is *characterized* by a heart rate of <60 bpm. It is common among young adults, trained athletes, and the elderly. It may occur in the early stage of acute MI, or it may be the result of an increase in vagal tone due to carotid massage, digitalis or morphine sulfate, or vomiting. *Complications* include hypotension, syncope, ischemic chest pain, and heart failure. *Diagnosis* is based on the health history, physical exam, and a normal but prolonged ECG.

Common interventions

No treatment is necessary unless there are complications. In the event of complications, medical treatment includes IV atropine and the insertion of a pacemaker.

Nursing interventions

Physical 1. Monitor vital signs, especially pulse rate.
2. Assess, treat, and prevent complications.
3. Administer prescribed medication.
Psychosocial 4. Provide support during an episode.
Educational 5. Prepare the patient and family for pacemaker insertion.
6. Teach the patient to avoid complications.
7. Teach the patient safety measures with regard to complications.

Evaluation criteria. *See* Overview. Accurate pulse checking daily.

SINUS TACHYCARDIA

Sinus tachycardia, one of the two most common arrhythmias, is *characterized* by a heart rate of >100 bpm. It may result from pathologic conditions such as fever, anemia, hyperthyroidism, shock, CHF, pulmonary embolus, acute MI, and pericarditis. Sinus tachycardia may also result from physiologic conditions such as exercise, anxiety, and excitement, or from the use of cardioacceleration drugs. *Complications* include severe left ventricular failure. *Diagnosis* is based on the health history, physical exam, and a normal but rapid ECG.

Common interventions

Medical interventions include treating the underlying pathology, sedating the patient, and administering propranolol.

Nursing interventions

Physical 1. Monitor vital signs, especially the pulse rate.
2. Administer prescribed medications.
Psychosocial 3. Provide emotional support during an episode.
Educational 4. Instruct the patient with regard to the regimen for the underlying pathology.

Evaluation criteria. *See* Overview.

HEART BLOCK

Heart block, which may be permanent or transient, is the anatomic or functional disturbance of an impulse through the conduction system. Heart blocks are classified as first, second, or third degree (Table 15-11).

Nursing interventions

Physical 1. Administer prescribed medications.
2. Monitor vital signs and the ECG.
3. Assess the underlying pathology and prevent complications.
Psychosocial 4. Provide emotional support related to medical and surgical management.
Educational 5. Teach the proper administration and side effects of medications.

Evaluation criteria. See Overview.

VENTRICULAR TACHYCARDIA

Ventricular tachycardia, *characterized* by a heart rate of 130 to 250 bpm, is most frequently associated with coronary atherosclerotic heart disease, but may also be caused by any form of heart disease or by digitalis toxicity. An impulse originating from an ectopic focus in either ventricle gives rise to this condition. *Symptoms* include a series of three or more rapid heart beats that occur in a predominantly regular rhythm or that occur as the dominant rhythm. *Complications* include ventricular fibrillation, MI, cerebral ischemia, CHF, and shock. The *diagnosis* is based on the health history, physical exam, and the ECG: the QRS complex will be wide and bizarre, and the P wave may be present but exhibit no relationship to the QRS complex, or it may be indistinguishable because of the rapid heart rate.

Common interventions

Medical treatment includes the administration of lidocaine or procainamide (Pronestyl). Defibrillation is used when there are complications.

Nursing interventions

Physical 1. Administer prescribed medications.
2. Monitor vital signs, especially the pulse rate.
3. Assess for, treat, and prevent complications.
4. Prepare the patient for defibrillation.
Psychosocial 5. Provide emotional support during the episode and treatment for the patient and family.
Educational 6. Instruct the patient to rest as quietly as possible.
7. Instruct the patient to notify a physician or seek treatment if tachycardia occurs or persists.

8. Teach proper management of the underlying disease or condition.
9. Teach the patient the proper administration of digitalis.
10. Teach the patient to monitor his own pulse.

Evaluation criteria. *See* Overview.

VENTRICULAR FIBRILLATION

Ventricular fibrillation is an uncoordinated, chaotic rhythm with no effective ventricular contractions. It may result from severe myocardial damage, drug toxicity (digitalis, quinidine, or epinephrine), or from ventricular tachycardia and other arrhythmias. Impulses originate at multiple ventricular ectopic foci and spread simultaneously within the ventricular conduction system. *Symptoms* include generalized signs of ineffective CO. *Complications* include shock and death. *Diagnosis* is based on the health history, physical exam, and abnormal ECG findings that include a completely irregular pattern with no well-defined waves (which may range from coarse to very fine).

Common interventions

Medical interventions include treatment of the preceding arrhythmia, defibrillation, administration of lidocaine or procainamide, epinephrine or isoproterenol, and CPR.

Nursing interventions

Physical 1. Administer CPR.
2. Assist with emergency care.
   a. Set the defibrillator at 400 watts.
   b. Maintain the IV.
   c. Administer sodium bicarbonate and lidocaine as ordered.
   d. Hyperventilate the patient with O_2 before and after defibrillation.
   e. Assist with defibrillation.
   f. Monitor the patient after defibrillation (ECG, pulse, respiration, and level of consciousness).
Psychosocial 3. Provide emotional support for the patient and family.
Educational 4. Teach the patient the proper administration of medication.
5. Teach the patient to monitor his pulse.

Evaluation criteria. *See* Overview. Patient demonstrates pulse monitoring.

ATRIAL FIBRILLATION

Atrial fibrillation is marked by an extremely rapid and irregular atrial rate, the loss of synchronized atrial contractions, and an irregular ventricular rate. It is associated with mitral valve disease, coronary athero-

TABLE 15-11

Types of Heart Block

| Parameter | First degree | Second degree | | Third degree |
		Type I	Type II	
Definition	Impulse originates in the SA node and follows the normal conduction pathway through the AV node, but with a delay in conduction time. (Most common form of heart block.)	Conduction delay, usually within the AV node, which produces a partial and progressive AV block until no longer conducted ("dropped beat").	Periodic blocked impulse in the bundle of His or right and left bundle branches. (Less common than type I.)	Inability of any impulse from the SA node to be conducted to the AV node and into the ventricles (RBBB and LBBB).
Etiology	Result of coronary heart disease, digitalis toxicity, or ARF.	Associated with CHF, ventricular ectopic beats and syncope.	May result from MI.	Causes include congenital heart disease, cardiac valve disease, connective tissue disorders, MI, myocardial ischemia, cardiac tumor, hypokalemia, and drug toxicity.
Symptoms	Asymptomatic; recognized on ECG.	Transient; recognized on ECG.	Recognized on ECG.	Recognized on ECG; underlying pathology.
Complications	CHF, ventricular ectopic beats, and syncope.	Complete heart block.		Periods of asystole; Adams-Stokes syncope (loss of consciousness due to slow heart beat).

Diagnosis	Health history and physical exam. ECG: the P-R interval is prolonged but constant, and the P wave is followed by a normal QRS.	Health history and physical exam. ECG: the P-R interval progressively increases with each beat until a blocked P wave occurs. The next P wave is conducted, and the sequence begins again.	Health history and physical exam. ECG: blocked P wave without change in the P-R interval, which may be either prolonged or normal, but will remain constant. The QRS complex will widen if the block is below the AV node. Conduction is noted as 2:1 or 3:1, indicating the number of impulses blocked for every impulse conducted.	Health history and physical exam. ECG: presence of P waves without relation to the QRS complex. If the block occurs within the AV node, the QRS will be normal. If the block occurs below the AV node, the QRS complex will be wide and bizarre.
Medical intervention	No specific treatment.	No specific treatment unless complications occur, atropine.	Atropine.	Treatment of underlying pathology.
Surgical intervention	None.	Pacemaker.	Pacemaker.	Pacemaker (temporary or permanent).

ARF, acute rheumatic fever; AV, atrioventricular; LBBB, left bundle-branch block; RBBB, right bundle-branch block; SA, sinoatrial.

sclerotic heart disease, hypertensive heart disease, thyroid toxicosis, and acute MI. Less common causes include COPD and pulmonary embolism. Impulses originate from multiple ectopic foci in the atrium. *Symptoms* include a rapid and irregular heart rate. *Complications* include a decreased CO, thrombus formation, and embolization. *Diagnosis* is based on the health history, physical exam, and a characteristic ECG: an indistinguishable P wave, a base line that is wavy and irregular or flat and straight, an irregular PR interval, and a normal QRS complex.

Common interventions

Medical interventions include treatment of the underlying cause of the arrhythmia, digitalization, and defibrillation (in an emergency situation).

Nursing interventions

Physical 1. Treat the underlying cause of the arrhythmia.

2. Administer a digitalis preparation.

3. Observe for the side and toxic effects of digitalis.

4. Assist with defibrillation.

5. Maintain the patient on bed rest.

6. Monitor vital signs and the ECG.

7. Assess for and prevent associated complications.

Psychosocial 8. Provide the patient and family with emotional support during and after the episode.

Educational 9. Teach the patient about digitalis therapy.

Evaluation criteria. *See* Overview.

PREMATURE ATRIAL CONTRACTION (PAC)

PAC is an ectopic atrial impulse that occurs prematurely in normal sinus rhythm. Once the impulse reaches the AV node, it follows the normal conduction path into the ventricles. It is frequently associated with organic heart disease or enlargement of the atria, and may be precipitated by fatigue, anxiety, tobacco, and caffeine. The major *symptom* is an irregular heart rate. Its *complications* include atrial tachyarrhythmias. *Diagnosis* is based on the health history, physical exam, and a characteristic ECG: a normal QRS complex and a P wave that appears close to the preceding beat or that may be hidden by the T wave. The ectopic P wave is not of normal configuration and may be followed by a pause before the sinus beat.

Common interventions

Medical interventions include digitalization (if the PACs are symptomatic) and treatment of the underlying cause of the arrhythmia.

Nursing interventions

Physical 1. Treat the underlying cause of the arrhythmia.

2. Administer a digitalis preparation.

3. Observe for the side and toxic effects of digitalis.
4. Maintain the patient on bed rest.
5. Monitor vital signs and the ECG.
6. Assess for and prevent associated complications.

Psychosocial 7. Provide the patient and family with emotional support during and after the episode.

Educational 8. Teach the patient about digitalis therapy.

Evaluation criteria. *See* Overview.

PREMATURE VENTRICULAR CONTRACTION (PVC)

A PVC is an ectopic beat that occurs when one or more impulses originate in the ventricles. A single or multiple focus (origin) may be involved. This is the most common arrhythmia and is benign in healthy adults, but can be a dangerous sign in association with heart disease. It can be caused by anxiety, exercise, an acute MI, open heart surgery, any form of heart disease or other serious illness, and digitalis toxicity. *Symptoms* include occasional or recurrent irregular heart rate, ventricular bigeminy (PVCs alternating with a normal QRS complex), and ventricular trigeminy (PVCs occurring with every third beat). *Complications* include ventricular tachycardia and fibrillation. *Diagnosis* is based on the health history, physical exam, and an ECG that shows no P wave preceding the QRS complex, which is wide and bizarre. A compensatory pause may follow a PVC or a PVC may be interpolated between two normal beats with no change in rhythm.

Common interventions

Medical treatment may not be necessary in healthy adults. Digitalization is used in the presence of heart disease; lidocaine or procainamide in the presence of an acute MI.

Nursing interventions

Physical 1. Treat the underlying pathology.
2. Administer a digitalis preparation as prescribed.
3. Observe for the side and toxic effects of digitalis.
4. Administer medications as prescribed.
5. Monitor vital signs and the ECG.
6. Assess for and prevent associated complications.
7. Reduce the precipitating factors.

Psychosocial 8. Provide emotional support for the patient and family during and after the episode.
9. Reassure the healthy adult that PVC is benign.

Educational 10. Teach the healthy adult about precipitating factors and ways to reduce them.
11. Teach the patient about digitalis therapy.

Evaluation criteria. *See* Overview.

CORONARY HEART DISEASE

Coronary arteriosclerosis is a generic term that refers to the sclerotic changes occurring in the coronary arteries. It does not indicate the underlying disease process. **Coronary atherosclerosis** refers to the immediate pathology of the coronary artery(ies). It is a localized lesion of the arterial intima and media characterized by lipid and fibrous tissue collection in the vessel wall, affecting the structure and functioning of the vessel and the ability of blood to flow to the myocardium. Susceptibility to the disease increases with the number of risk factors present. Major risk factors include age, sex (males until age 50 yr), family history of coronary atherosclerosis, hypercholesterolemia, hyperlipidemia, hypertension, smoking, obesity, diabetes mellitus, gout, prostaglandin production, oral contraceptives and hormonal factors, stress, sedentary life-style, and physical inactivity. Coronary atherosclerosis may be caused by phospholipid production in the arterial wall as a response to local injury or by an obstructive lesion that develops as a result of a narrowing lumen, intramural hemorrhage, or thrombus formation. *Symptoms* and *complications* include angina, acute MI, metabolic acidosis, arrhythmias, hypertension, CHF, decreased ventricular functioning, and sudden death. *Diagnosis* is based on the health history, physical exam, chest x-ray (e.g., cardiomegaly), and myocardial ischemic response to stress tests. Cardiac catheterization helps to visualize lesions in the coronary arteries, identify the areas and effects of collateral circulation, and evaluate associated and other conditions of the heart.

Common interventions

Medical treatment includes decreasing the risk factors and prescribing medications to decrease the cardiac work load and increase O_2 delivery to the myocardium (digitalis preparations, nitrates, beta blockers, and calcium antagonists), treating the resulting pathology, prescribing a diet low in calories, cholesterol, and saturated fats, and treating related pathology (i.e., diabetes mellitus, gout, and increased BP). **Surgical** treatment includes CABG and PTCA (*see* Overview).

Nursing interventions

Physical 1. Administer medications as ordered.
2. Assess for the side and toxic effects of medications.
3. Administer O_2 therapy.
4. Assess for risk factors.
Psychosocial 5. Help the patient to identify personal risk factors and ways to change or modify them.
6. Assess the patient's responsibility for medical management.
Educational 7. Teach the patient and family ways to reduce risk factors.

a. Appropriate diet, drug therapy, and exercise regimen.
b. Association of the disease process, risk factors, and sequelae.
c. Rationale for and the effects of change.
d. Medical regimen with related diseases or complications.
e. Hereditary aspects.
f. CPR.
8. Discuss with the patient and family the psychosocial aspects of the disease (need to identify and reduce risk factors, need to change or modify life-style and ways to do it, responsibility of the individual to maintain health, and aspects of chronic illness).

Evaluation criteria.   *See* Overview. Identification and reduction of risk factors.

ANGINA PECTORIS

Angina pectoris is chest pain associated with myocardial ischemia. It is frequently the initial sign of cardiac ischemia. Precipitating conditions include severe aortic stenosis or insufficiency, severe mitral stenosis or regurgitation, hypotension, hyperthyroidism, marked anemia, polycythemia, and ventricular arrhythmias. Precipitating factors include physical and emotional stress, heavy exercise, cold weather, large meals, obesity, smoking, caffeine, extreme excitement, anger, and sexual activity. Any conditions or factors that decrease the O_2 delivered by the coronary arteries, increase the cardiac work load, and/or increase the myocardial need for O_2 may result in angina. The diagnostic *symptom* of angina is chest pain: squeezing, strangling, vicelike; burning sensation; retrosternal; radiating to the neck, mandible, arms, and teeth; lasting 3 to 5 min; and relieved by nitroglycerin. There is also a sense of impending doom. Stable angina is usually predictable and is controlled by rest or cessation of the predisposing activity and/or by nitroglycerin. Unstable (crescendo) angina follows a history of stable angina or exertion, but occurs with less exertion, at rest, and during sleep. It increases in duration, changes character, is not relieved by nitroglycerin as promptly, and gradually worsens. Prinzmetal (variant) angina results from coronary artery spasm, occurs at rest, and is induced by cold, coronary angiogram, and drug toxicity. *Complications* include MI and sudden death. *Diagnosis* is based on the health history, physical exam, and an ECG, which may show ST or T wave changes during an attack. The stress test may induce angina and produce changes in the ECG. Cardiac catheterization may show changes from coronary artery disease or changes in the cardiac valves. Tests for underlying causes other than cardiac-related ones may also be part of the diagnosis.

Common interventions

Medical treatment includes the prescription of medications (nitrates, beta-adrenergic blocking agents, calcium antagonists, digitalis preparations, sedatives, tranquilizers, antidepressants, and anticoagulants); reduction of all possible risk factors; a diet low in calories, cholesterol, and saturated fat; a planned program of exercise; and the reduction of physical and emotional stress. **Surgical** treatment includes CABG and PTCA.

Nursing interventions

Physical 1. Relieve pain by having the patient stop all activity, maintain bed rest, and eliminate precipitating factors.
2. Administer medication as prescribed.
3. Assess pain accurately and record the findings with regard to sensation, location, duration, and how relieved.
4. Prevent attacks by controlling precipitating conditions and high-risk factors.
Psychosocial 5. Provide a calm, quiet atmosphere.
6. Reassure the patient and family during an attack.
7. Assess the patient's emotional response to the attack and illness.
8. Assess the patient's responsibility for medical management.
9. Help the patient to identify personal risk factors and precipitating conditions that can be modified.
Educational 10. Teach the patient and family about the pathophysiology of angina, daily and prn medications to be taken and their side effects, carrying nitroglycerin at all times, preventing and treating pain, diet therapy, relaxation exercises, calling a physician or going to the ER if an attack does not subside with treatment, and CPR.
11. Discuss with the patient and family the psychosocial aspects of angina (need to identify and reduce risk factors, need to change or modify life-style to prevent angina, responsibility of the individual to maintain his own health, and aspects of chronic illness).

Evaluation criteria. See Overview.

THE VASCULAR SYSTEM

OVERVIEW

The vascular system is composed of arteries and veins that provide systemic circulation. Diseases of the vascular system are common, chronic, frequently incurable, and often necessitate changes in life-style. They occur as the result of the aging process or acquired disease (e.g., thromboangiitis obliterans). Interventions are directed toward prevention and control of symptoms and complications. Patient education is a major component of nursing care.

Anatomy and physiology review

In the systemic circulation, blood travels from the aorta to all parts of the body via the arteries and arterioles and returns to the heart via the venules and veins. **Arteries** are characterized by a thick vascular wall. They transport blood rapidly and under high pressure. **Arterioles**, the smallest branches of the arteries, are characterized by a strong muscular wall. They control blood flow into the capillaries. **Capillaries** are characterized by a semipermeable membrane. They transport oxygen and nutrients from the arterioles to interstitial tissue, and they transport carbon dioxide and waste products from interstitial tissue to the venules. **Venules**, the smallest branches of veins, collect blood from the capillaries and transport it to the veins. **Veins**, characterized by thin, muscular walls, transport blood to the heart. Veins in the extremities may contain valves, which prevent the backflow of blood. (The usual quantity of blood and pressure within components of the circulatory system are listed in Table 15-12.)

Normal arterial pressure in a young adult is 120 mmHg (systolic) and 80 mmHg (diastolic). The difference between these two pressures is known as the pulse pressure. Two factors influencing the amount of blood flow are (1) the differences in arterial and venous pressures within the vessels that supply an organ, and (2) the vascular resistance of the organ, which is influenced by the caliber of the vessels and the presence of new vascular channels. **Blood flow** is regulated locally and centrally. Acute local regulation involves the following responses: active hyperemia responds to metabolic changes; reactive hyperemia responds to short-term ischemia; and autoregulation responds to arterial pressure changes. Long-term local regulation responds to the same changes as the acute regulation mechanisms, but over a longer period of time (i.e., hours to weeks), and provides for a more complete regulation. Thus, the tissue needs and the flow of blood to these tissues control CO.

TABLE 15-12

Characteristics of Systemic Circulation

Vessel	Quantity of blood	BP
	%	*mmHg*
Heart	9	0
Pulmonary vessels	12	100
Aorta	} 8	100
Large arteries		95-97
Small arteries	5	85
Arterioles	2	55
Capillaries	5	30
Venules	} 25	25
Small veins		20
Large veins	} 34	10
Vena cava		5

Central regulatory mechanisms for maintaining blood flow include neural, hormonal, and chemical controls. Neural control involves ANS (sympathetic [norepinephrine] and parasympathetic [acetylcholine]) circulatory effects. The CNS is responsible for vasomotor-center response to stimulation. In addition, baro- or pressoreceptors respond to pressure changes in the walls of the large arteries. Hormonal control makes use of aldosterone, epinephrine, norepinephrine, kinins, angiotensin II, vasopressin, serotonin, histamines, and prostaglandins. Chemical control makes use of calcium, potassium, magnesium, sodium, acetate, citrate, hydrogen, and carbon dioxide. All of these control mechanisms work together to provide adequate tissue perfusion.

General assessment

The **health history** includes an assessment of current health status (chief complaint, e.g., symptoms, duration, treatment, relief, and use of tobacco and medications), the individual and family history of cardiovascular problems, and a review of systems. The respiratory system is assessed for dyspnea, shortness of breath, orthopnea, and rhonchi. The cardiovascular system is assessed for chest pain, palpitations, increased BP, and medications to improve cardiac functioning and decrease BP. The peripheral vascular system is assessed for varicose veins, edema, tingling, claudication, leg cramps, and color and temperature of the lower extremities. The **physical examination** involves observing the patient's color, respirations, and emotional state; monitoring BP in both arms (supine position and standing); and auscultating and palpating the peripheral pulses. **Diagnostic tests** include laboratory data (CBC and ABGs), x-rays (arteriography, phlebography, and retrograte filling tests), and Doppler studies.

Common interventions

Amputation, the severing and removal of a limb, may be of two types: open or closed. Open amputations are performed if infection is present. They permit drainage of purulent material. In open amputations, the stump is not closed with a skin flap until the infection is cleared. A second procedure then closes the wound. Closed or flap amputations are performed if no infection is present. A small drain is left in the incision site to prevent the accumulation of blood and fluids, or pressure dressings may be applied during surgery to help evaluate drainage. The stump is then covered with a skin flap. The location of amputation depends on the level of involvement of the extremity and on the adequacy of the circulation necessary for healing. Leg locations include above the knee (AKA) and below the knee (BKA). **Nursing** interventions include the following (*see* Chapters 9 and 11):

1. Assess circulation preoperatively to assist in determining the level of the amputation.

2. Prepare the patient for tests and procedures (e.g., angiography, oscillometry, and Doppler study).
3. Initial postoperative care is dictated by the type of surgical procedure. For an open amputation, elevate the stump and change the wound dressing using sterile technique; administer antibiotics; observe for bleeding, hemorrhage, hematoma, and edema; and prevent contractures by proper positioning of the extremity.
4. For a closed-flap amputation, check the dressing and reinforce it as necessary; assess for signs of bleeding, hemorrhage, hematoma, infection, and edema; prevent contractures by proper positioning; wrap and shape the stump; and assist with early ambulation.
5. Maintain skin integrity.
6. Manage phantom limb pain. (Reposition the stump and massage the extremity.)
7. Help the patient identify the restorative purpose of the amputation.
8. Help the patient achieve physical and psychologic readiness for rehabilitation.
9. Promote rehabilitation for the amputee.
   a. Prepare the patient emotionally.
   b. Assist the patient to function independently with the prosthesis.
   c. Assist the patient to be independent with a wheelchair if a prosthesis is contraindicated.
   d. Consult with the physician and physical therapist with regard to fitting the patient for a prosthesis (e.g., delayed fit with peripheral vascular disease, until healing of, and increased circulation to, the stump; immediate fit with traumatic amputation and unimpaired vascular supply).
   e. Teach the patient exercises to prevent contractures and promote muscle strengthening for ambulation.

In **femoral-popliteal bypass**, an autogenous saphenous vein is grafted from above to below the occluded portion of the artery to provide continuous blood flow. The nursing interventions are the same as for atherosclerosis (*see below*). **Endarterectomy** is the surgical removal of a thrombus. The nursing interventions are the same as for atherosclerosis (*see below*). **Saphenous vein ligation** involves ligation of the saphenous vein at the saphenofemoral junction. The nursing interventions are the same as for varicose veins (*see below*). **Embolectomy** is the surgical removal of an embolus in order to reestablish peripheral circulation after medical treatment has been unsuccessful. The nursing interventions are the same as for acute arterial occlusion (*see below*).

Evaluation criteria

Reduction/reversal of symptoms. Absence of infection and other complications, and/or recurrence of problem. Adequate circulation to extremities. Patient/family verbalization of medical regimen, preventive factors, and necessary adaptations in life-style, as appropriate. Evidence of adherence to medical regimen (including control of risk factors).

ACUTE ARTERIAL OCCLUSION

The blockage of a large or small peripheral artery as a result of embolism, a thrombus, or trauma is referred to as acute arterial occlusion. It is caused by the embolization of a central thrombus in the left side of the heart, occlusion due to atheromatous plaque formation or embolization, or thrombi from aneurysms, and is associated with atrial fibrillation, MI, mitral valve disease, valvular replacement, endocarditis, and CHF. *Symptoms* distal to the site include pain (sudden or preceded by numbness and paresthesias) that is increased with movement, decreased peripheral vascular circulation, and ischemia of the extremities. *Complications* occur as a result of decreased blood flow to the extremities. *Diagnosis* is based on the health history, physical exam, and arteriography.

Common interventions

Medical treatment includes anticoagulant therapy, bed rest, the application of heat to promote vasodilation, and the intra-arterial administration of vasodilators. **Surgical** treatment includes embolectomy, vascular bypass, and amputation, if gangrene develops.

Nursing interventions

Physical 1. Administer anticoagulant medication.
   2. Implement measures to reduce and relieve pain, including the administration of prescribed medication.
   3. Implement measures to promote vasodilation.
   4. Maintain the patient on bed rest.
   5. Prevent trauma to the affected extremity.
   6. Prevent complications related to anticoagulant therapy, immobility, and decreased peripheral vascular circulation.
   7. Prevent further complications from the underlying pathology.
   8. Preoperatively, assess the extremity distal to the occlusion, evaluate the return of peripheral circulation due to medical management, and prepare the patient for the specific surgical procedure (*see* Chapter 9).
   9. Postoperatively, assess the area distal to the embolectomy for adequate circulation, promote adequate circulation to the extremities, maintain the patient on bed rest, prevent complications related to decreased circulation, immobility, and anticoagulant therapy, and prevent trauma (with injury to the extremity) (*see* Chapter 11).
Psychosocial 10. Provide emotional support related to the disease process and treatment.
Educational 11. Teach the patient health practices related to the

prevention of conditions that may result in embolus formation, the prevention of complications related to anticoagulant therapy, the promotion of adequate arterial circulation, and the prevention of complications related to ischemia.

Evaluation criteria.   *See* Overview. Prevention of subsequent emboli.

CELLULITIS

Cellulitis is an inflammatory process that occurs in the dermis and subcutaneous tissues. It may be caused by a localized infection as a result of the skin on the face, neck, and extremities being burned, injured, or wounded; a hemolytic streptococcal infection, which results in a widespread infection; a *Staphylococcus aureus* infection, producing a limited area of infection; or a sterile infection in the lower extremities as a result of chronic venous insufficiency. Local *symptoms* include diffuse edema and hot, tender skin. There are also systemic signs of infection. *Complications* include (1) the spread of the streptococcal infection to the heart valves, if the condition is left untreated, (2) streptococcal gangrene from the spread of the infection into subcutaneous tissue, and (3) lymphangitis with symptoms of fever, chills, malaise, and headache. The *diagnosis* is based on the health history, physical exam, and culture of the affected area.

Common interventions

Treatment includes antibiotic therapy, bed rest, warm soaks, and heat applications.

Nursing interventions

Nursing interventions will be dictated by the site of the infection as well as the particular causative organism.

Physical 1. Administer antibiotic therapy.

2. Apply warm soaks and dressings as prescribed.

3. Maintain the patient on bed rest.

4. Prevent the further spread of infection and resultant complications.

5. Prevent trauma to the affected area and complications related to bed rest.

6. Promote increased circulation to the lower extremities, if they are affected.

Psychosocial 7. Provide emotional support related to the disease process and its effects on the body, especially on appearance.

8. Provide emotional support related to the effects of immobility and other treatments.

Educational 9. Teach the patient health practices related to the prevention of infection and of trauma or injury to the skin, the promotion of increased circulation to the lower extremities, and the care of the feet and legs.

Evaluation criteria.   *See* Overview.

THROMBOPHLEBITIS

Thrombophlebitis is an inflamed vein wall with clot formation. The causes include venous stasis as a result of a variety of physiologic, pathologic, or environmental conditions; injury to the vein wall from trauma, chemicals, or bacteria; and changes in the blood that increase coagulation. Previous history is a predisposing factor. Thrombophlebitis has a sudden occurrence, and its severity is related to the size and location of the involved vein. *Symptoms* include pain and tenderness, redness, warmth, edema, and a positive Homans' sign. A *complication* is the possibility of pulmonary emboli occurring. The *diagnosis* is based on the health history, physical exam, isotope studies, phlebography, and ultrasound (Doppler studies for measuring palpitations).

Common interventions

Treatment includes anticoagulant therapy, bed rest, elastic stockings or Ace bandages, the application of heat, relief of pain, and antibiotic therapy (if the injury is due to bacteria).

Nursing interventions

Nursing interventions focus on preventing complications, reducing the thrombus, and promoting venous circulation.

Physical 1. Administer anticoagulant therapy.

2. Apply heat to the site.
3. Implement measures to reduce and relieve pain, including administering prescribed medication.
4. Maintain the patient on bed rest.
5. Apply elastic stockings or Ace bandages.
6. Prevent complications related to anticoagulant therapy and immobility.
7. Prevent trauma and injury to the site.

Psychosocial 8. Provide emotional support related to the disease process and treatment.

Educational 9. Teach the patient health practices related to the prevention of conditions that can result in thrombophlebitis, the prevention of complications related to anticoagulant therapy, the promotion of venous circulation by exercise and elevation of the extremities, and the proper application and use of elastic stockings.

Evaluation criteria. *See* Overview.

PRIMARY (ESSENTIAL) HYPERTENSION

Essential hypertension is a sustained or intermittent increase in both the systolic and diastolic BP (>140/90 mmHg) with no well-defined etiology. Two types of essential hypertension have been identified: benign (gradual onset and prolonged course) and malignant (abrupt occurrence, short and dramatic course, and fatal if untreated). Essential hypertension is the leading cause of morbidity in the USA, and its incidence increases with age. In general, premenopausal women have a lower BP than men. Blacks have a higher incidence than whites. The etiology is unknown. Theories being investigated include (1) the correlation between a defect in renal hormonal regulation and hypertension, and (2) the antihypertensive effects of prostaglandins. Contributing factors include age, sex, familial history, race, increased sodium intake, obesity, stress, inactivity, smoking, atherosclerosis, and diabetes. Underlying changes include an increase in CO with normal peripheral vascular resistance, or a normal CO with increased peripheral vascular resistance. *Symptoms* include gradual or abrupt rise in BP. *Complications* are caused by an acceleration in the development of atherosclerosis in the major arteries, increased peripheral vascular resistance by the fibrotic narrowing of the smaller arteries in the systemic circulation, and hypertrophy of the left ventricle with a cyclical consequence of higher systemic pressures. Complications, which can range from minor disabilities to death, include CHF, arteriosclerosis, MI, cerebrovascular accident, renal failure, and ophthalmic damage. *Diagnosis* is based on the health history, physical exam, CBC, serum electrolytes, urinalysis, and chest x-ray. Other tests include an ECG (specific for left ventricular functioning) and specific tests to rule out secondary hypertension, including tests for renal and adrenal functioning, tests for increased intracranial pressure, and cardiac angiography.

Common interventions

Medical treatment focuses on control. (The disease cannot be cured.) Medications include diuretics, sympathetic blocking agents, and vasodilators. In addition, a low-sodium diet, relaxation techniques, and the reduction of stressors are prescribed.

Nursing interventions

Physical 1. Assess BP q 2 to 4 hr as ordered. (Measurements are taken in both arms while the patient is resting and standing.)
2. Assess the potential and actual complications related to increased BP.
3. Assess the risk factors associated with increased BP.
4. Administer prescribed medications, including antihypertensive agents and sedatives.
5. Assess the side effects of medications.
6. Provide a restful, quiet hospital atmosphere.
7. Provide a low-sodium diet.
Psychosocial 8. Provide emotional support to the patient and family related to the disease process, prognosis, and treatment (chronic illness, reduction of risk factors, and change in life-style).
9. Listen to the patient's fears, worries, and concerns and offer reassurance.

10. Help the patient identify specific stressors.

Educational 11. Teach the patient and family the pathophysiology of hypertension and its complications.

12. Teach the patient and family the risk factors related to hypertension.
13. Teach the patient and family how to reduce risk factors (low-sodium diet, reducing diet, relaxation techniques, stopping smoking, and exercise program).
14. Teach the patient management of related diseases, especially diabetes (if appropriate).
15. Teach the patient to report the signs and symptoms of related complications and the side effects of medications.

Evaluation criteria.   See Overview. BP ≤140/90 mmHg.

SECONDARY HYPERTENSION

Secondary hypertension is a consequence of another primary disease process occurring in the body. Its incidence increases with age. Secondary hypertension is classified according to the organ system that is affected. Causes related to body systems include renal (parenchymal hypertension and renovascular damage), adrenal cortex (Cushing's disease and primary aldosteronism), adrenal medulla (pheochromocytoma), neurologic (polyneuritis and increased intracranial pressure from brain tumors and hematomas), mechanical (coarctation of the aorta), and pregnancy-related. The *symptoms* include those associated with the primary disease and those of primary hypertension and its complications. Refer to Primary Hypertension for the diagnosis and common interventions (*see above*).

ANEURYSMS

An aneurysm is a localized or diffuse enlargement of an artery. A **saccular** aneruysm involves only one side of the artery and has a pouchlike appearance. A **fusiform** aneurysm involves the dilation of the entire circumference of the artery. A **dissecting** aneurysm refers to a cavity formed as a result of blood being forced between the layers of the artery wall. Aneurysms are most often the result of arteriosclerosis. (Dissecting aneurysms occur most frequently.) A number of pathologic processes can result in the formation of aneurysms: trauma of the artery, congenital weakness, arteriosclerosis, and previous infections such as subacute bacterial endocarditis and syphilis. Aneurysms usually occur either in the thoracic or abdominal aorta (Table 15-13).

ATHEROSCLEROSIS

Atherosclerosis is the formation of an atheroma (lipoid deposit) in the intima and media of the arterial wall. It primarily affects the aorta and its large branches. The etiologic factors for coronary artery atherosclerosis (*see above*) are also applicable to the atherosclerotic conditions of the

TABLE 15-13

Comparison of Thoracic and Abdominal Aneurysm

Parameter	Thoracic aneurysm	Abdominal aneurysm
Symptoms	Usually asymptomatic; dictated by size and location; compression or obstruction of adjacent structures (pain and aortic insufficiency).	Asymptomatic; or pulsating abdominal mass that may be palpated on physical exam, continuous or intermittent pain in the abdomen and back, decreased renal circulation, and decreased peripheral vascular circulation.
Complications	CHF as a result of aortic insufficiency, expansion and rupture of the aneurysm, hemorrhage, and death.	Expansion and rupture of the aneurysm, hemorrhage, and death.
Diagnosis	Health history, physical exam, chest x-ray, angiography, and CAT scan. The ECG is either normal or shows nonspecific changes.	Health history, physical exam, abdominal x-ray, and IVP.
Surgical intervention	Surgical resection of the aneurysm, with replacement graft of the aorta.	Same as for thoracic aneurysm.
Nursing interventions (*See also* Chapter 11.)	Preoperatively, prepare the patient for diagnostic tests and the specific operative procedure; postoperatively, provide care for thoracic surgery (*see* Chapter 14).	Same as for thoracic aneurysm.

IVP, IV pyelogram.

mesenteric, renal, cerebral, and iliac-femoral arteries. The symptoms depend on the location and extent of the vascular occlusion, the rapidity of its onset, and the presence and extent of collateral circulation. The primary *symptom*, claudication from ischemic muscle, occurs proximal to the site of arterial obstruction. General symptoms include intermittent claudication, which may progress to pain at rest; diminished or absent peripheral pulses below the site of obstruction; cool, dry, shiny skin, which may appear cyanotic or show signs of pallor when elevated and of rubor when dependent; atrophy of the skin, with loss of hair and hard, thickened nails; delayed healing of minor lesions; diminished or absent sensory or motor functioning; possible edema; and ulcerations or superficial gangrene. *Diagnosis* is based on the health history, physical exam, x-ray (angiography), oscillometric readings indicating arterial flow, skin temperature studies, and ultrasound or Doppler studies.

Common interventions

Treatment focuses on reducing the risk factors. **Medical** treatment includes anticoagulant therapy, vasodilators, and fibrinolytics. **Surgical** treatment includes vascular bypass, endarterectomy (removal of the thrombus), and amputation.

Nursing interventions

Interventions focus on minimizing the effects of decreased blood flow to the extremities and reducing or eliminating the risk factors involved in further development of atherosclerosis.

Physical 1. Maintain adequate circulation to the extremities.

2. Maintain skin integrity (especially foot care).

3. Maintain the patient on a program of moderate exercise.

4. Protect the extremities from trauma, pressure, and infection.

5. Preoperatively, teach the patient pre- and postarteriogram care (*see* Chapter 20).

6. Postoperatively, assess the limb distal to the operative site for signs of adequate circulation, maintain the patient on bed rest for 3 to 5 days, and prevent complications related to bed rest (*see* Chapter 7).

Psychosocial 7. Provide emotional support related to chronic illness, change in life-style, maintenance of the therapeutic regimen, and pain.

Educational 8. Teach the patient health practices to prevent progression of the disease process and its complications.

9. Promote patient responsibility for maintaining a regimen of treatment and prevention.

Evaluation criteria.   *See* Overview.

ARTERIOSCLEROSIS

Arteriosclerosis is the gradual loss of vessel elasticity with thickening and induration of the medial layers of the vessel wall. Arteriosclerosis obliterans is a degenerative and obstructive disorder of an artery. It affects the intimal and medial layers of the vessel wall, and often represents the late stage of atherosclerosis. Arteriosclerosis usually occurs in older age-groups and is thought to be part of the normal aging process. Its causes include (1) the occlusion of a peripheral vascular artery as a result of an atheroma formation on the intima of the vessel, and (2) loss of elasticity of the media of the vessel wall. The arteries become elongated and tortuous, and thus weak and susceptible to hemorrhage and dilation. *Symptoms* may occur both distal and proximal to the obstructed segment of the artery, and they reflect the progressive nature of the disease. Initial symptoms include changes in skin temperature, a difference in the color and size of the extremities, altered peripheral pulses, bruits, and intermittent claudication. Later symptoms include pain at rest, pain at night that subsides with exercise, tingling and numbness in the toes, and delayed healing. *Diagnosis* is based on the health history and physical exam. Diagnostic studies as well as the common interventions are the same as for atherosclerosis (*see above*), with the addition of measures to provide warmth to the extremities and general exercises to maintain circulation.

BUERGER'S DISEASE

Buerger's disease is an inflammatory type of obstructive vascular disease that affects the peripheral arteries and veins in the upper and lower extremities. It occurs most frequently in young adult males, is rare in women and blacks, and is prevalent among Jews. There is no generally accepted cause. Potential factors include smoking, infections, toxic agents, and hypercoagulability of the blood. *Symptoms,* which depend on the vessel involved, the extent of involvement, and the degree of collateral circulation, usually begin in the feet and move up the legs to the upper extremities. These symptoms include persistent coldness in the extremities; diminished or absent peripheral pulses; numbness and tingling; aching pain in the digits, instep, ankle, calf, wrist, and forearm; the aggravation of symptoms with exposure to cold; red, hardened, painful areas over the affected vessels; cutaneous color changes, including cyanosis and rubor; a constant burning or boring pain that is increased by chilling, smoking, and tension; and dependent cyanosis and elevated pallor. *Complications* result from tissue ischemia and necrosis. *Diagnosis* is based on the health history and physical exam.

Common interventions

Medical treatment involves prescribing the cessation of smoking or the use of tobacco in any form, using methods to increase circulation (such as warmth), effecting vasodilation, and prescribing moderate exercise. **Surgical** treatment includes a paravertebral injection of alcohol, which may be used to block sympathetic impulses and promote vasodilation, or a bilateral preganglionic sympathectomy, which may be performed to provide permanent vasodilation of the blood vessels in the lower extremities. **Nursing** interventions are the same as for athero- and arteriosclerosis (*see above*), but also include teaching the patient about preventing vasoconstriction by stopping smoking and by keeping the hands and feet protected from the cold.

Evaluation criteria.   *See* Overview.

RAYNAUD'S DISEASE

Raynaud's disease involves a reduction of blood supply in the extremities (most commonly the hands) as a result of arterial spasm. It occurs almost exclusively in women; the symptoms are usually evident before age

40. The etiology of Raynaud's disease is unknown. (It is not to be confused with Raynaud's phenomenon, which refers to localized changes in the peripheral circulation as a result of vasospasms produced by underlying pathology.) *Symptoms* are a direct result of the arterial spasms, which may be precipitated by cold and emotional stress. They include pallor and cyanosis during spasm, rubor as a result of vasodilation, and signs of adequate circulation when spasms are not occurring. *Complications* include recurrent infections and gangrene that necessitates amputation. *Diagnosis* is based on the health history and physical exam.

Common interventions

Medical treatment involves the use of sedatives or tranquilizers, vasodilators, and sympathetic blockers (experimental).

Nursing interventions

Physical 1. Make sure that the patient avoids cold and tobacco.
2. Administer medications as ordered.
Psychosocial 3. Reduce emotional stress.
4. Reassure the patient that Raynaud's disease is a benign condition.
Educational 5. Teach the patient the importance of reducing stress.
6. Teach the patient relaxation techniques.
7. Advise the patient to avoid cold and tobacco.

Evaluation criteria. *See* Overview.

VARICOSE VEINS

Varicose veins are superficial veins that are dilated, elongated, and tortuous as a result of incompetent valves in the surface veins of the lower extremities. The condition occurs in the greater and lesser saphenous veins and their tributaries. Primary causes include congenital weakness of the veins, pregnancy, obesity, standing for long periods over the course of years, and extreme tallness. Secondary causes include thrombophlebitis, arteriovenous fistula, and pressure on the inferior vena cava or iliofemoral vein. The changes resulting from the primary or secondary disease include the following: the veins of the legs become weak and distended; the leaflets of the valves within the veins are prevented from closing properly; these changes cause the backflow of blood, venous stasis, and increased venous pressure. *Symptoms* resulting from increased venous pressure (which interferes with the compression of the deep veins by the skeletal muscles) include edema, brownish pigment on the skin (resulting from RBCs in the surrounding tissue), and muscle cramps and fatigability in the lower extremities. *Complications* include inflammation, cellulitis, stasis dermatitis, ulcerations, and atrophy. *Diagnosis* is based on the health history, physical exam, phlebography, and a retrograde filling test.

Common interventions

Medical treatment includes the prevention of venous stasis by elevating the extremities and wearing elastic stockings. It may also involve the injection of a sclerosing solution to produce obliteration of the varicosity and communicating vein. **Surgical** treatment includes saphenous vein ligation.

Nursing interventions

Physical 1. Improve venous return by elevating the patient's legs frequently, elevating the foot of bed for sleeping, and applying elastic stockings before the patient rises.

2. Prevent venous stasis by having the patient avoid standing or sitting for long periods of time, crossing the legs at the knees or using the knee gatch of the bed, and wearing restrictive clothing (such as garters and girdles) around the lower extremities.

3. Provide general preoperative care (*see* Chapter 9).

4. Postoperatively, provide general care (*see* Chapter 11), keep the patient's legs tightly wrapped in elastic bandages or stockings, keep the patient's legs straight, and elevate the foot of the bed to a level above the heart.

Educational 5. Teach the patient to wear specially prescribed stockings, to avoid sitting for long periods of time, to elevate the legs when not standing, to rest with the body straight and the legs elevated, and to resume normal activities gradually.

Evaluation criteria.   *See* Overview.

CHAPTER 16

ALTERED GASTROINTESTINAL FUNCTIONING

Mary D. Smith

OVERVIEW

Concepts

Numerous signs, symptoms, and complaints related to GI functioning are associated with varying degrees of health or disease. Dyspepsia, for example, is a common cause of absenteeism from work or disruption of role fulfillment. Absenteeism and interference with role functioning are standard criteria used by the public to evaluate wellness.

Signs and symptoms

Indigestion, nausea, vomiting, constipation, diarrhea, and malabsorption are related to altered GI functioning. Indigestion, nausea, and vomiting may appear singly or in some combination, briefly or for prolonged periods.

Indigestion is a subjective observation; may be confirmed with objective signs such as belching; may be experienced as heartburn or overacid stomach; may be called dyspepsia; and produces a burning sensation in the upper abdomen for 1 hr or more after eating. Indigestion is aggravated by caffeine, alcohol, and spicy foods. When long-standing, it may lead to gastritis (inflammation of the stomach) and, eventually, to peptic ulcer. Prolonged indigestion may also be associated with the development of gastric or esophageal cancers or of hiatus hernia (protrusion of the stomach into the thoracic cavity). Indigestion is relieved by ingesting milk, antacids (such as Gelusil, Maalox, and Mylanta), and bland foods; by avoiding spicy and irritating foods; by getting adequate rest; and by avoiding stress. Gastritis and long-standing dyspepsia often require the use of anticholinergic drugs, such as Pro-Banthine and Valpin. Chronic gastritis is treated with such drugs as Pro-Banthine and Bentyl. Belching is treated by avoiding air-swallowing (aerophagia) and gas-forming foods (such as those in the cabbage family), by taking small bites and chewing food well, and by using such drugs as Mylicon after meals. Belching that is related to gallbladder disease is treated with Pro-Banthine and Bentyl.

Nausea and **vomiting** serve to rid the body of an irritating substance. The most common cause is gastroenteritis (inflammation of the stomach and intestines), but nausea and vomiting are also related to the use of drugs, both oral (such as aspirin, codeine, and digitalis) and parenteral (such as meperidine HCl and morphine). Many illnesses and conditions involve nausea and vomiting, including acute abdominal illness (e.g., gallbladder disease, obstruction of the GI tract); infectious hepatitis (usually accompanied by nausea); chronic ear, nose, and throat disorders (e.g., postnasal discharge resulting in persistent, early morning vomiting; pregnancy; and psychologic distress. The *effects* and *complications* of nausea and vomiting include decreased appetite, diminished nutritional status, and fluid and electrolyte imbalance. *Treatment* is effected by providing small, frequent meals; a diet high in protein and calories; cold foods, especially if nausea is induced by odors; home-cooked foods, when possible; an emesis basin, tissues, and frequent mouth care and mouthwashing; a quiet environment and/or distractors of the patient's own choosing; and antiemetics as ordered.

Constipation and **diarrhea** may be chronic or sporadic problems of altered GI functioning. The various signs and symptoms identified for differential diagnosis are as follows.

Belching: Air-swallowing, stomach distension, ingestion of ethyl alcohol, chronic gallbladder disease, cancer of the stomach, and hiatus hernia are related to belching.

Constipation: Sluggish bowel, inactivity, medication, cancer of the bowel, rectal fissure, cryptitis, and psychic depression are associated with constipation.

Malabsorption: Malabsorption is related to sprue, celiac disease, and diarrhea (cause unknown).

Dyspepsia: Gastritis, peptic ulcer, cancer of the stomach, hiatus hernia, gallbladder disease, and abdominal epilepsy are related to dyspepsia.

Diarrhea: Diarrhea is associated with viral gastroenteritis, food poisoning, ulcerative colitis, cancer of the large intestine, vitamin deficiency, regional enteritis, pancreatitis, and overactive thyroid.

Nausea and vomiting: Viral gastroenteritis; ingestion of medications, ethyl alcohol, and narcotic drugs; infectious hepatitis; acute appendicitis; gallbladder disease; peptic ulcer with obstruction; a chronic ear, nose, or throat infection; emotional distress; and pregnancy are related to nausea and vomiting.

Constipation, a common complaint that results from slowed functioning of the GI tract, accompanies the aging process or a decrease in activity. Signs and symptoms of a sluggish bowel include hard, dry feces; a feeling of fullness; a vague urge to defecate; and dull, aching rectal discomfort. Streaks of blood may be seen on the outside of the stool if a hemorrhoidal vessel ruptures or the rectal lining is torn. However, no hidden (occult) blood is mixed with the stool in such instances, as would be seen with conditions involving more serious lower intestinal tract bleeding. Factors that cause, aggravate, or contribute to constipation include inadequate fluid intake, sedentary habits, failure to respond promptly to the urge to defecate, use of such medications as belladonna derivatives and opiates, bed rest, depression, and the presence of rectal disorders, diverticulitis (inflammation of pockets in the lower rectum), or mechanical obstruction due to cancer. The *effects* and *complications* of constipation are decreased appetite, abdominal discomfort (a feeling of fullness), headache, discomfort on defecation, and fecal impaction. *Treatment* includes increased fluid intake, increased roughage and bulk in the diet, the development of good bowel habits, and the use of stool softeners (such as Colace) or added bulk medications (such as Metamucil).

Diarrhea is a condition characterized by the frequent passage of watery stools. Viral gastroenteritis is the most common cause; it is characterized by profuse, watery, greenish, blood-streaked stools and is associated with malaise, fever, vomiting, and loss of appetite. Food poisoning is another cause usually involving ingestion of poisonous mushrooms or of *Salmonella* (in leftover fish and poultry) or staphylococcus (in warm, creamy mixtures) organisms. Food poisoning also produces abdominal cramps and vomiting. Food allergies may result in cramps, diarrhea, nausea, and vomiting. Ulcerative colitis results in diarrhea with blood in the feces; when severe, it may be accompanied by fever, rectal pain, and mucus in the feces. Cancer or partial obstruction may cause diarrhea and abdominal cramps as a result of excessive mucous secretion by intestinal cells; cancer of the large intestine may be accompanied by blood in the feces, and advanced cancer may produce diarrhea, nausea, anorexia, and weight loss. Other causes of diarrhea include vitamin deficiencies, regional enteritis, deficiency of pancreatic enzymes, and hyperthyroidism.

The *effects* and *complications* of diarrhea include decreased appetite, fluid and electrolyte imbalance, an irritated or excoriated anal area, and changes in life-style and/or self-image. *Treatment* may include the use of Lomotil and Kaopectate, rest, restriction of irritating foods, and ingestion of fluids and bland foods. Toilet facilities or a bedpan and room deodorants should be readily available; skin care requires special attention.

Malabsorption is evidenced by the following symptoms: malnutrition; multiple, foul, bulky, foamy, greasy stools; abdominal distension due to accumulated undigested foods and gas; and secondary vitamin and mineral deficiencies. A partial listing of causes can be remembered with the aid of the mnemonic WAISTED:

W   Whipple's disease, intestinal lipodystrophy (very rare), and other causes of steatorrhea
A   Anorexia nervosa and depression
I   Inflammations: tuberculosis, Crohn's disease, ulcerative colitis, and subacute bacterial endocarditis
S   Surgical causes: gut resections and stomach and bowel internal fistulas
T   Tumors
E   Endocrine-related causes: thyrotoxicosis, Addison's disease, Conn's syndrome, and pituitary abnormalities (Sheehan's syndrome)
D   Diabetes mellitus

This adaptation of Shipman's mnemonic for assessment of the causes of severe weight loss indicates conditions that may contribute to malabsorption of essential nutrients.

Adult nontropical sprue is sometimes associated with malabsorption. This disorder may follow its childhood version, celiac disease, and is characterized by diarrhea, with stools of high fat content (malabsorption of fat); anemia (malabsorption of iron); hemorrhagic tendencies (malabsorption of vitamin K); and tetany (malabsorption of calcium).

Malabsorption is *treated* with either hyperalimentation or specific dietary adjustments, such as providing diets that are gluten-free, low in fat, or high in caloric value (*see* Chapter 2).

UPPER GI TRACT OVERVIEW

Anatomy and physiology review

Figure 16-1 illustrates major and accessory organs and structures of the GI tract. Chapter 2 describes the specific functions of digestion and absorption.

General assessment

A **health history** should be obtained, including a detailed nutrition status and review of the head, the nose and paranasal sinuses, the mouth and throat, the neck, and the GI tract. This history should include information about trouble with swallowing, heartburn, loss of appetite, nausea, vomiting, vomiting of blood, indigestion, unusually frequent bowel movements, changes in bowel habits, rectal bleeding or black and tarry stools, constipation, diarrhea, abdominal pain, food intolerance, excessive belching or passing of flatus, and liver or gallbladder disease. A **physical**

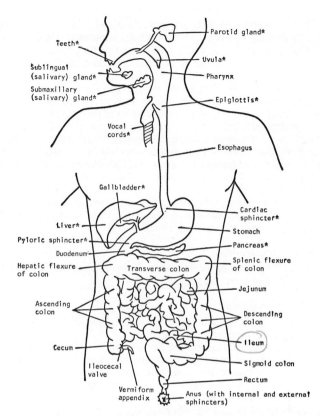

Figure 16-1. Anatomy of the GI tract and associated structures. Asterisks indicate associated structures. *Adapted from* Lewis, C. M. Nutrition: The Basics of Nutrition. Family Nutrition. F. A. Davis Co., Philadelphia. 1977. p. B-75, and Guyton, A. C. Textbook of Medical Physiology. W. B. Saunders Co., Philadelphia. 1981. Sixth edition. p. 784.

examination is also advised, with particular emphasis on inspection, palpation, percussion, and/or auscultation of the areas mentioned above.

Diagnostic tests

The **upper GI series** (UGIS) is an examination of the esophagus, stomach, and beginning of the small intestine using a radiopaque contrast medium (usually barium sulfate in a flavored drink). The purpose of the

UGIS is to detect the presence of ulcers or anatomic defects in the upper GI tract. **IV cholangiography** (IVC), **oral cholecystography** (OCG), and the **gallbladder series** (GBS) are tests for examining the gallbladder and the common bile duct by means of IV or oral administration of a contrast medium that concentrates in the gallbladder. These tests are used to test for gallbladder disease or changes in functioning of the gallbladder. **T-tube cholangiography** is performed during surgical procedures or in the postoperative period to assess for the presence of stones in the gallbladder and common bile duct and to evaluate the patency of the ducts prior to removal of a drainage tube. **Analysis of gastric contents** is accomplished with or without the use of a nasogastric tube (NGT). The NGT is used to withdraw gastric or intestinal contents to (1) observe gastric washings for such acid-fast bacilli as the tuberculosis bacillus, blood, and cancer cells, or (2) to test for pernicious anemia, as evidenced by a lack of hydrochloric acid (HCl) production in response to histamine administration. Tubeless gastric analysis involves the ingestion of blue dye (usually azure A or azuresin [Diagnex Blue]) to test for the presence of HCl.

Common interventions

Rest, changes in diet, medication, and surgical procedures are possible interventions for upper GI problems.

Nursing interventions

Physical 1. Assess comfort, nutrition, and physical signs related to the specific condition.
2. Monitor vital functions, intake and output, and nutritional status.
3. Provide rest, massage, mouth and skin care, and medication.
4. Provide preoperative and postoperative care.
Psychosocial 5. Remove oral and rectal secretions promptly.
6. Control odors with ventilation and/or use of deodorants.
7. Respond to calls for help promptly.
8. Place an emesis basin or bedpan within easy reach.
9. Encourage verbalization of fears and anxieties.
10. Provide attractive meals and small, frequent feedings as indicated.
Educational 11. Assess the patient's and his family's understanding of his condition.
12. Teach the patient and his family about diet, rest, medications, and the changes in life-style needed to prevent recurrence.

Evaluation criteria

Symptoms abate or disappear. Patient is comfortable, rested, and adequately nourished. Vital functions and intake and output are within normal limits. Patient demonstrates knowledge of prevention and treatment appropriate to his condition. Absence of complications. Patient participates in follow-up as needed.

UPPER GI TRACT DEVIATIONS
INGESTION OF POISONS AND FOREIGN BODIES

The development and rupture of esophageal varices (usually subsequent to cirrhosis) and the ingestion of poisons and foreign bodies constitute the bulk of GI emergencies. Ruptured esophageal varices are discussed in Chapter 21. Ingestion of harmful substances or objects is common in children and in adults with decreased levels of awareness and is sometimes seen in persons attempting suicide. Corrosive and noncorrosive poisons include strongly acidic substances, strongly alkaline substances, sleeping pills, ethyl and propyl alcohol, strychnine, insecticides, and poisonous mushrooms. Harmful objects include safety pins and other sharp objects. Psychologic or emotional problems are sometimes etiologically significant.

Symptoms of ingestion of harmful substances or objects include tissue burns (highly acidic or alkaline substances); CNS depression (sleeping pills, ethyl alcohol); selective depression of the nervous system, with decreased cardiorespiratory functioning and increased peristalsis (poison mushrooms); CNS stimulation (strychnine, insecticides); pain; and bleeding. *Complications* include vascular collapse, respiratory obstruction or failure, renal failure, and death. The *diagnosis* is made on the basis of the health history and physical exam.

Common interventions

The focus of treatment is the removal or inactivation of the harmful object or substance and provision of supportive therapy. In addition to the following specific interventions, ventilatory assistance, exchange transfusions, hemodialysis, or peritoneal dialysis may be necessary.

Treatment for ingestion of noncorrosive poisons. Stomach contents are diluted with water or milk. Vomiting is induced with Ipecac syrup. Poisons are adsorbed with medicated charcoal. An NGT is inserted for rapid dilution and removal of substances (gastric lavage).

Treatment for ingestion of corrosive poisons. Vomiting (which causes additional damage to tissues) should be prevented. Oily substances (which may be aspirated, causing lipopneumonia) should not be used.

Treatment for ingestion of foreign bodies. Objects that will not harm the integrity of the tract or cause mechanical obstruction can be allowed to progress through the tract naturally. Foreign bodies can be visualized and removed with a gastroscope or they can be removed surgically.

Nursing interventions

Physical 1. Monitor vital signs, fluid and electrolyte balance (including IV fluids, Foley catheter, and input and output), ABGs, and respiratory status.
2. Help with measures implemented to eliminate the substance.

   3. Provide comfort measures.
   4. Provide preoperative and postoperative care as appropriate.
Psychosocial 5. Be nonjudgmental toward the patient and his family.
   6. Encourage the patient and his family to verbalize their concerns.
   7. Explain procedures and treatment.
   8. Keep the patient and his family informed of any progress.
   9. Refer the patient and his family for counseling as indicated.
Educational 10. Identify the situation leading to ingestion of the harmful substance or object.
   11. Review home safety measures.
   12. Teach the patient and his family about community resources— e.g., the Poison Control Center and counseling facilities.

Evaluation criteria. *See* Overview.

ESOPHAGITIS

Esophagitis is an inflammation of the esophagus. This condition is often associated with a large intake of alcohol, caffeine, or spicy or hot foods and may also be called **heartburn** or **acid eructation**. It is caused by reverse peristalsis, which moves gastric juice to the cardiac end of the stomach, to the esophagus, and possibly to the pharynx, where it may be tasted. The *signs and symptoms* of esophagitis include belching, eructation of acid, and localized discomfort. The *diagnosis* is made on the basis of the health history, physical exam, and esophagoscopy.

Common interventions

The patient should abstain from irritants, use antacids, and eliminate the primary cause.

Nursing interventions

Physical 1. Administer antacids.
   2. Maintain good nutrition with a bland diet.
   3. Provide comfort measures.
   4. Provide preoperative and postoperative care as needed.
Psychosocial 5. Provide emotional support to the patient and his family.
   6. Maintain a restful environment, especially at mealtime.
Educational 7. Instruct the patient to avoid causative or predisposing factors.
   8. Teach the patient about drug and nutritional therapy.

Evaluation criteria. *See* Overview.

ACUTE GASTRITIS

Acute gastritis is an inflammation of the stomach characterized by a sudden onset. This condition is usually related to some dietary indiscretion (rapid eating, overeating, or eating spicy or infected foods), an acute systemic infection, ingestion of alcohol, ingestion of too many salicylates, or uremia. Acute gastritis lasts 2 to 3 days. This condition is *characterized* by a red, swollen mucosa with little acid but much mucus secretion; an uncomfortable feeling in the abdomen; headache; lassitude; nausea and vomiting; hiccuping; a coated tongue; increased saliva production; and possibly colic and diarrhea. The *diagnosis* is made on the basis of the health history, physical exam, gastroscopy, and gastric analysis.

Common interventions

IV administration of glucose and saline solutions may be needed for persistent vomiting. Oral intake should be bland and may be supplemented with antacids. Rest and supportive therapies should be implemented as needed. **Nursing** interventions are the same as for esophagitis (*see above*).

CHRONIC GASTRITIS

Chronic gastritis is a prolonged inflammation of the lining of the stomach. Common causes include chronic uremia, benign and malignant ulcers of the stomach, and cirrhosis of the liver with chronic congestion of the stomach. The early stage of chronic gastritis is *characterized* by thickened and prominantly rugated membranes. Later stages show thinning of the stomach walls and decreased gastric secretions consisting primarily of mucus and water. The *signs and symptoms* of chronic gastritis vary greatly. Included are anorexia or bulimia (binging), heartburn after eating, eructation of gas, a bad taste in the mouth, nausea, and some early morning vomiting. The *diagnosis* is based on the health history, physical exam, gastroscopy, and gastric analysis.

Common interventions

The patient should be provided a diet of easily digested, properly prepared food, which should be well chewed; small, frequent feedings; and specific treatment related to the cause. **Nursing** interventions are the same as for esophagitis (*see above*).

CHOLELITHIASIS AND CHOLEDOCHOLITHIASIS

Cholelithiasis and choledocholithiasis are conditions in which calculi (stones) are present in the gallbladder or the common bile duct (CBD), respectively. These conditions occur most often in overweight, middle-aged, Caucasian women who have had several children (i.e., fair, fat, forty, and fecund). The calculi form from solid constituents of bile—i.e., cholesterol, calcium, bilirubin, and inorganic salts.

These conditions involve an alteration in, or obstruction of, normal bile flow. The *signs and symptoms* include jaundice and various kinds of epigastric distress, such as fullness and belching after meals, heartburn, chronic upper abdominal pain or severe pain in the upper-right abdomen that radiates to the right shoulder, and nausea and vomiting. This distress is more noticeable after a heavy meal including fatty foods. Acute pancreatitis is a possible *complication. Diagnosis* is based on the health history, physical exam, x-rays (OCG and IVC), and laboratory tests. Laboratory tests include a blood test for serum bilirubin, a stool examination for decreased or absent bilirubin and a pale yellow or clay color, and a urine examination for elevated urobilinogen and a dark amber or brown color.

Common interventions

Medical treatment consists of administering liquids initially. Gradually, solid food is introduced and increased as tolerated. The intake of fats should be restricted. The patient should have plenty of rest. Possible **surgical** interventions include cholecystotomy (incision and drainage of the gall-bladder), choledochotomy or choledocholithotomy (making an opening into the CBD and removing stones), and cholecystectomy (removal of the gallbladder) with CBD exploration. Manipulation of the bile duct during exploration necessitates the placement of a T-tube within the CBD to remove the bile (which continues to form in the liver) until swelling in the area subsides and bile flows normally; a T-tube cholangiogram is performed prior to removal of the drainage tube (7 to 10 days postoperatively).

Nursing interventions

Physical 1. Prepare the patient for all diagnostic tests.
2. Implement rest and comfort measures.
3. Administer analgesics as ordered.
4. Monitor fluid and electrolyte status.
5. Observe for signs of infection, inflammation, or perforation if the attack persists.
6. Provide a low-fat diet.
7. Observe and record the color of the stools and the urine.
8. Administer preoperative and postoperative care as needed.
9. Provide appropriate care of the T-tube: maintain gravity drainage, prevent tension on the tubing, observe the skin and dressing for bile drainage, and measure output, noting increases.
Psychosocial 10. Provide emotional support to the patient and his family.
Educational 11. Teach the patient and his family about low-fat diets and the inclusion of essential fats in the diet.
12. Instruct the patient and his family regarding the signs and symptoms of recurrence.

Evaluation criteria.   *See* Overview. Stools and urine are normally colored.

CHOLECYSTITIS

Cholecystitis is an inflammation of the gallbladder. As with cholelithiasis and choledocholithiasis, it occurs most often in overweight, middle-aged, Caucasian women who have had several children. This condition is usually associated with the presence of calculi (stones) in the gallbladder or CBD. *Signs and symptoms* of an acute attack of cholecystitis are severe pain, tenderness and rigidity of the upper-right abdomen, nausea and vomiting, and fever. *Diagnosis* is based on the health history, physical exam, x-rays (OCG and IVC), and laboratory tests.

Common interventions

Surgical treatment consists of cholecystectomy with or without CBD exploration. **Nursing** and **medical** interventions are the same as for cholelithiasis (*see above*).

STOMACH OR GASTRIC CANCER

Stomach or gastric cancer is the seventh leading cause of death in the USA. The ratio of the incidence in males to the incidence in females is 3:2. The average age at which the diagnosis is made is 55 yr. Gastric cancer is related to dietary and social habits; the causes are environmental rather than genetic. Socioeconomic status or ethnicity may be predisposing factors. Persons with blood type A show a greater incidence of this disease. Precancerous states include gastric ulcer, gastric adenoma, chronic gastritis, intestinal metaplasia of the gastric mucosa, and pernicious anemia.

Gastric cancer occurs most often in the antrum and lesser curvature of the stomach. Types of gastric tumors include ulcerative (75% of cases), polypoid (10% of cases), scirrhous (10% of cases), and superficial (5% of cases). Gastric cancer spreads by direct extension, dissemination through the lymph nodes and vascular system, and by peritoneal implantation. *Signs and symptoms* include early vague epigastric discomfort, which may be relieved by belching, use of antacids, and implementation of dietary alterations. The *diagnosis* is made on the basis of the health history, physical exam, x-ray (UGIS), gastroscopy, and biopsy.

Common interventions

Curative interventions include **surgical** resection (which carries a 9.6% 5-yr survival rate) and radiation therapy prior to surgery (radiation therapy makes the tumor more resectable). Palliative interventions include radiation therapy for deep-seated lesions, chemotherapy, and tube feeding (oral or via esophagostomy or gastrostomy). **Nursing** interventions are discussed in Chapter 8.

ESOPHAGEAL STRICTURE

Esophageal stricture is a narrowing of the lumen of the esophagus. It is commonly associated with the ingestion of strongly acidic or alkaline preparations. Children generally swallow such substances accidentally, whereas adults may swallow them intentionally when distraught. Esophageal stricture is caused by inflammation or other changes in the esophageal wall, external pressure, chemical burns, or trauma (e.g., due to swallowing foreign bodies).

Damage to the esophageal wall and tissues forms scars and subsequent narrowing of the lumen. *Signs and symptoms* include severe pain, burns in the esophagus and oral cavity, difficulty in swallowing, and difficult respirations due to edema in the mucosa. *Complications* include possible toxicity and shock and complete closure of the lumen, requiring surgical resection and permanent gastrostomy. *Diagnosis* is based on the health history and physical exam.

Common interventions

Medical interventions include dilution of the harmful chemicals and administration of IV fluids. **Surgical** interventions include removal of any foreign body via esophagoscopy and dilation of the stricture by means of bouginage (pulling increasingly larger dilators or bougies through the affected area).

Nursing interventions

Physical 1. Monitor the patient for shock and pain.
   2. Administer analgesics as ordered.
   3. Monitor respirations and the development of edema.
   4. Assess for signs of toxicity if chemicals are involved.
   5. Keep the pharynx clear of secretions.
   6. Give gastrostomy feedings, if ordered.
   7. Keep the gastrostomy site clean.
Psychosocial 8. Provide emotional support, as children may suffer guilt for exploring or "being naughty" and adults may be emotionally distraught with the same concerns that lead to the suicide attempt.
Educational 9. Teach children and their families how to safely store dangerous substances.
   10. Help adults to verbalize their emotions and tell them where to seek help.
   11. Teach proper preparation and administration of feedings and care of the gastrostomy site to prevent infection.

Evaluation criteria.   *See* Overview. Dangerous substances are safely stored; accidental ingestion is avoided; alternative is found for intentional ingestion of chemicals; and healing and repair are evident.

HIATUS HERNIA

Hiatus hernia is a protrusion of the stomach into the thoracic cavity. This condition may be congenital and may be found incidentally on x-ray examination. The diaphragmatic opening through which the esophagus passes enlarges, allowing the upper part of the stomach to pass into the lower thoracic area.

Symptoms may or may not be present. There is often a feeling of fullness in the lower chest, with a splashing sound audible substernally. Pain and discomfort may be evident in the substernal area due to esophagitis. *Complications* due to the trapped gastric juices in the herniated portion of the stomach include ulceration and hemorrhaging. The *diagnosis* is based on the health history, physical exam, and x-ray of the thoracic area.

Common interventions

Treatment involves surgical replacement of the stomach in the abdominal cavity and suturing of the diaphragmatic opening to prevent recurrence. Either an abdominal or a left-thoracic approach may be used.

Nursing interventions

Physical 1. Provide immediate postoperative care for laparotomy or thoracotomy.
2. Introduce solid foods gradually in small amounts.
3. Minimize the amount of liquids taken with meals.
4. Allow the patient to sit erect for 30 min after eating to promote the passage of food through an edematous site (the edema lasts 2 to 3 days).

Psychosocial 5. Reassure the patient that normal activities and diet can be resumed postoperatively.
6. Provide comfort and supportive measures.

Prevention 7. Prior to surgical repair, reduce the severity of symptoms by introducing the eating techniques described above.

Evaluation criteria.   *See* Overview. Evidence of wound healing.

ANOREXIA NERVOSA

Anorexia nervosa, a syndrome related to aversion to food for other than physical reasons, is usually seen in females 12 to 25 yr of age. Emotional conflict is a predisposing factor. *Signs and symptoms* of anorexia nervosa include hyperactivity, weight loss, and hysteric or obsessive personality. *Complications* include emaciation and nutrition deficiencies. *Diagnosis* is based on the health histry, physical exam, and laboratory studies (electrolyte balance, Hb, and Hct).

Common interventions

Common interventions include administration of nutritional supplements and controlled, supervised provision of nutrients; exploration of contributing emotional and psychosocial factors; and building up the patient's ego and helping her to formulate an adequate support system for the future.

Nursing interventions

Physical 1. Provide a controlled diet and encourage the patient to eat.
2. Monitor dietary intake with a calorie count and dietary recall methods.
3. Provide adequate rest.
4. Minimize physical activities.
Psychosocial 5. Provide diversional activities.
6. Promote interaction with peers.
7. Refer the patient to support groups of people who share this problem.
8. Support verbalization of emotional needs.
Educational 9. Assist the patient in seeking alternative solutions to problems and refer her to other health professionals as needed.
10. Explore new coping mechanisms with the patient.
Prevention 11. Stress a positive self-image.
12. Provide positive feedback for behaviors that demonstrate a good mental health status.

Evaluation criteria.   *See* Overview. Evidence of weight gain; patient has positive self-image.

BULIMIA OR BINGE-PURGE DISEASE

Bulimia is a condition involving overindulgence in food followed by induced vomiting. It is common among young women. As with anorexia nervosa, bulimia may be precipitated by emotional distress. The pathophysiology is the same as that of anorexia nervosa. The *diagnosis* is made on the basis of the health history, physical exam, and laboratory studies (electrolyte balance, Hb, and Hct).

Common interventions

The primary treatment is the provision of psychologic support. In addition, other coping mechanisms for dealing with stress should be taught. Nursing interventions are the same as for anorexia nervosa (*see above*).

OBESITY

Obesity is a state of oversupply of certain nutrients that results in weight gain to a level >20% of that recommended for height, sex, and age. Obesity is prominent in highly industrialized countries, such as the USA, where ~10% of children and adults are considered obese. Factors predisposing to obesity are heredity and emotional factors. Causes include excess intake of food in relation to the energy needs of the body, as evidenced by a weight >20% above the ideal; lack of sufficient exercise in combination with high caloric intake; and metabolic abnormalities.

Symptoms of obesity are overweight and constant eating. *Complications* include metabolic abnormalities, atherosclerosis with associated ischemic heart disease, hypertension, left ventricular hypertrophy, and diabetes mellitus (four times more common in obese than in nonobese individuals). *Diagnosis* is based on the health history and physical exam.

Common interventions

Controlled caloric intake and increased activity are advised for treatment of obesity, along with correction of any contributing physical or psychologic conditions. Gastric stapling may be used to decrease the size of the stomach. Another surgical intervention is intestinal bypass with intraintestinal anastamosis to promote the quick movement of food through the intestine and thereby to prevent absorption of nutrients. Intestinal bypass is a temporary solution that results in great weight loss with chronic diarrhea and carries a potential for regaining the weight if new eating habits are not learned.

Nursing interventions

Physical 1. Provide a controlled-calorie diet.
  2. Provide opportunities for exercise.
  3. Administer supplemental vitamins and minerals as ordered.
  4. Monitor fluid and electrolyte balance.
  5. Monitor vital signs.
  6. Monitor daily weight gain or loss.
  7. Provide preoperative and postoperative care as indicated.
Psychosocial 8. Provide emotional support.
  9. Reinforce positive behaviors.
10. Support the development of an improved self-image.
11. Avoid overreaction to such conditions as anorexia nervosa.
Educational 12. Teach menu planning, using exchange lists.
13. Discuss appropriate cooking methods and mealtime behaviors.
14. Plan follow-up meetings with health personnel.
15. Help the patient set realistic goals, anticipate plateaus, and adapt his or her diet to special occasions or situations.
16. Teach the signs and symptoms of electrolyte imbalance after intestinal bypass.
Prevention 17. Reinforce good eating habits.
18. Stress the importance of regular exercise.
19. Stress the importance of regular evaluation of dietary intake for nutritional adequacy.

Evaluation criteria. *See* Overview. Patient's weight returns to realistic limits and is maintained.

ULCERS

An ulcer is an erosion in the mucosal wall of the stomach, pylorus, or duodenum. Types of ulcers include the following: **Peptic** (an all-inclusive term for erosion of the stomach, the proximal duodenum, or the lower esophagus), **gastric** (erosion of the stomach), **pyloric** (erosion of the pylorus, the opening of the stomach into the small intestine), **duodenal** (erosion of the duodenum), and **stress** (acute gastric erosion resulting from drugs, trauma, or surgery). Ulcers may occur singly or as multiple lesions. They occur most often in the duodenum and less frequently in the stomach, usually near the pylorus. Ulcers occur least often on the pylorus itself.

Predisposing factors include emotional stress and a hurried life-style. Peptic ulcers are caused by psychologic influences (emotional stress and a hurried life-style), especially in young adults or in the early middle years, as stress increases the tone of the vagus nerve, which in turn increases the friability of the gastric mucosa. The cause of gastric ulcers is unknown as yet; possible causes include excess acid secretion in the stomach, with rapid reabsorption and resulting damage to the mucous lining, and destruction of the mucous lining due to reflux of alkaline duodenal contents. Causes of duodenal ulcers include an increased level of acidity of gastric secretions, increased amounts of gastric secretions, and, possibly, vagal involvement. Stress ulcers are caused by severe trauma, serious illness, severe burns (Curling's ulcer), head injuries or intracranial disease (Cushing's ulcer), and ingestion of drugs (salicylates, steroids, or alcohol).

Ulcers entail the loss of the mucosa, submucosa, and muscle layer in areas exposed to acid-pepsin gastric juices. They may be associated with stress, life-style, environmental stress (change of seasons), and use of irritating medications or spicy foods. *Symptoms* include (1) pain that is gnawing or sharp, is localized in the midepigastric area or back, recurs 1 to 3 hr after meals, and is relieved by ingestion of food or alkali; (2) vomiting, with or without nausea, after a bout of pain, which may be related to mechanical obstruction of the pylorus by swelling or scar formation; (3) weight loss; and (4) bleeding. *Complications* include pyloric obstruction, hemorrhaging, and perforation. *Diagnosis* is based on the health history, physical exam, laboratory studies (gastric analysis), x-ray (e.g., UGIS), and gastroscopy.

Common interventions

Medical interventions include control of gastric acidity through the use of sedatives, milk, antacids, and (sometimes) antispasmodics and anticholinergic agents; prevention of complications with bed rest, sedation, and monitoring of vital signs; and provision of psychologic support to alleviate anxiety. **Surgical** intervention is required in 15% of patients to correct complications or to treat intractable pain. Procedures intended to reduce acid production by the stomach include (1) subtotal gastrectomy with gastrojejunostomy — removal of two-thirds to three-quarters of the distal stomach (which has acid-forming cells) as well as the pylorus and the first part of the duodenum, with attachment of the side of the jejunum to the end of the stomach; (2) vagotomy (dividing of the vagus nerve) and removal of the antral part of the stomach, which will reduce acid formation due to vagal and gastrin stimulation; (3) pyloroplasty (division of the pylorus transversely to create a larger opening from the stomach into the duodenum); (4) combined vagotomy and gastrojejunostomy or pyloroplasty, which will reduce acid production and prevent the gastric retention that may follow vagotomy alone; and (5) plication of the stomach (suturing or stapling folds in the mucosa to reduce the surface area in contact with acid and gastrin).

Nursing interventions

Physical 1. Ensure adequate bed rest.
   2. Administer sedatives and sleep medications as ordered.
   3. Provide feedings and medications on time.
   4. Offer frequent, small feedings of bland protein- and fat-containing foods as ordered.
   5. Administer antacids and anticholinergics to relieve discomfort as needed.
   6. Keep the patient hydrated to counter the side effects of anticholinergics.
   7. Monitor vital signs.
   8. Observe the patient for complications (e.g., bleeding, perforation, hematemesis, increased pain, rigid boardlike abdomen, altered vital signs).
   9. Provide preoperative and postoperative care as indicated.
Psychosocial 10. Show interest in the patient.
   11. Reduce anxiety and stress factors.
   12. Help identify causes of tension and frustration.
   13. Suggest psychiatric assistance, if indicated.
Educational 14. Teach the importance of maintaining diet and taking medications as ordered.
   15. Reinforce health teaching and stress the importance of moderate activity, the need for adequate rest, and the dangers of smoking.
   16. Stress the need for alterations in life-style, as indicated.
   17. Stress the need for regular follow-up visits after discharge.

Evaluation criteria. See Overview. Patient reduction in anxiety, altered life-style that promotes healing and lessens stressors, and exploration of options available for dealing with stress.

LOWER GI TRACT OVERVIEW

Anatomy and physiology review

The lower GI tract consists of the area between the ileocecal valve and the rectal area. (*See* Figure 16-1 for a review of anatomic structures, both major and accessory. Chapter 2 contains a review of the physiology of digestion and absorption).

General assessment

The **health history** should have information on the patient's current health status, including a review of nutritional status (changes in eating patterns, weight, and/or food tolerance) and elimination (changes in bowel habits or in the color, odor, or consistency of stools). The past health history includes information on abdominal disorders, surgery, and foreign travel. The review of systems (GI) includes data concerning flatus, nausea and vomiting, and pain. The **physical examination** (abdominal) includes the following: observation for size and shape, a rippling motion on the abdominal surface, guarding, and increased abdominal girth; palpation for masses and rebound tenderness; percussion for resonance; and auscultation for bowel sounds. **Laboratory data** include a CBC and stool examination for occult blood (guaiac test) and ova parasites. A **barium enema** (BE) a may be indicated. This is a study of the lower GI tract, from the ileocecal valve to the rectum, often performed prior to the UGIS and as part of a complete GI work-up. **Enteroscopy** procedures (colonoscopy, sigmoidoscopy, proctoscopy, and anoscopy) are used to visually inspect the rectum and/or colon for bleeding sites, polyps, or anatomic defects (diverticula, strictures, or ulcerations).

Common interventions

Medical interventions include (1) reduction of GI activity through bed rest and either keeping the patient NPO and feeding him intravenously or providing a modified diet (related to the underlying cause), (2) bowel decompression, and (3) medication (antibiotics and steroids). **Surgical** intervention is based on the specific problem and may include ostomy to bypass the obstruction.

Nursing interventions

Physical 1. Maintain nutritional status by providing the diet ordered or monitoring the IV feedings and keeping the patient NPO.
2. Keep drainage tubes patent.
3. Monitor the amount and characteristics of drainage and/or fecal contents.
4. Have a bedpan or bathroom facilities readily available.
5. Provide comfort measures, including elevation of the head of the bed.
6. Monitor vital signs.
7. Assist with preparation for diagnostic procedures.
8. Provide preoperative and postoperative care as needed.
9. Assess for the following complications: changes in the size or shape of the abdomen, the presence of an abdominal mass, pain or guarding, and changes in bowel sounds or resonance.
10. Provide medications as ordered.
Psychosocial 11. Encourage verbalization of feelings and concerns.

12. Keep the patient informed of progress as indicated.
13. Provide ventilation and deodorants as needed.
14. Help the patient and his family to cope with changes in life-style.
Educational 15. Explain tests and treatments.
16. Teach the patient and his family about the appropriate nutritional and drug regimens.

Evaluation criteria

Signs and symptoms subside. Positive nutrition status is maintained or regained. Complications are avoided or rapidly identified and treated. Recurrence is prevented. Patient and family verbalize an understanding of the therapeutic regimen. Patient demonstrates (on follow-up) ability to cope with the necessary alterations in life-style.

LOWER GI TRACT DEVIATIONS

INTESTINAL OBSTRUCTION

An intestinal obstruction is any interruption of the flow of GI tract contents (partial or complete); this is an emergency condition. Predisposing factors include impaired peristalsis, inflammation, and vascular disorders. Causes include mechanical factors (e.g., adhesions, hernia volvulus, intussusception, and tumors), vascular disorders (e.g., mesenteric infarction and abdominal angina), and nervous disorders (e.g., paralytic ileus following bowel surgery).

Symptoms of intestinal obstruction are crampy lower abominal pain, enlargement of the bowel, distension of the abdomen, absence of bowel sounds below the obstruction, early vomiting (in small bowel obstruction), a visible intestinal outline on the abdominal wall, and fecal vomiting (late in the course of the condition). Possible *complications* include perforation of the bowel and fluid and electrolyte imbalance. *Diagnosis* is based on the health history, physical exam, and x-rays.

Common interventions

Medical interventions include monitoring vital signs, recognizing complications, keeping the patient NPO, ensuring adequate hydration (IV administration), and decompressing the intestine with intubation and suction. Tubes that may be used to achieve decompression include the short NGT (Levine); long- and double-lumen tubes, such as the Miller-Abbott tube (10 ft long, with an inflatable balloon); the Dennis or Devine tubes (triple lumen, including suction lumen and air vent); long- and single-lumen tubes, such as the Harris tube (6 ft long, with a metal tip and a mercury-weighted bag to carry the tube into the intestine); and the Cantor tube (10 ft long, with a larger lumen and a mercury-filled bag). **Surgical** treatment is related to the cause (e.g., adhesions, cancer, or a hernia). Surgery may be indicated to relieve the obstruction prior to surgery for removal of the cause.

Surgical procedures include cecostomy (inserting a large tube into the cecum) and colostomy (bringing a loop of colon, with an incision above the obstruction site, up to the skin surface). Types of colostomies include loop, double-barrel, temporary, and permanent, and colostomies may be performed in the ascending, transverse, or descending segments of the colon.

Nursing interventions

Physical 1. Assess the patient for (a) the existence, location, and character of pain; (b) the presence of distension; and (c) the absence of flatus or defecation.
2. Monitor vital signs.
3. Administer IV fluids as ordered.
4. Keep the patient NPO.
5. Monitor fluid intake and output.
6. Examine stools for obvious or occult blood.
7. Monitor laboratory tests (urine, Hb, and CBC) as ordered.
8. Administer analgesics as ordered.
9. Maintain decompression of the intestines.
10. Prepare the patient for surgery as needed.
Psychosocial 11. Reassure the patient regarding the likely outcomes of the procedures.
12. Explain the tests and procedures.
13. Explore fears and anxieties related to the condition and to procedures.
Educational 14. Discuss the purpose of equipment and treatments.
15. Do preoperative and postoperative teaching as needed.
Prevention 16. Monitor signs and symptoms related to causes of intestinal obstruction.

Evaluation criteria. *See* Overview. Flow of intestinal contents is reestablished.

RUPTURED APPENDIX

Ruptured appendix is an emergency condition involving perforation of the appendix, spilling its contents into the peritoneal cavity. This condition occurs when inflammation of the appendix has progressed too far. Incomplete emptying of the veriform appendix results in fecolith (stone) formation and subsequent inflammation. Continued inflammation results in pus formation and eventual rupture. *Symptoms* include low-grade fever, vomiting, loss of appetite, and acute abdominal pain that occurs in waves. In the early stage, this pain may feel like discomfort that could be relieved by having a bowel movement. The pain begins in the upper abdominal area and later localizes in the lower-right quadrant. In the later stage, the pain is more steady, the muscles become rigid, ileus and rebound tenderness are noted, and there is characteristic guarding of the area (the patient lies still and draws his legs up to relieve abdominal tension). *Complictions* of appendicitis include rupture of the appendix and peritonitis. The *diagnosis* is made on the basis of the health history, physical exam, and laboratory studies (an elevated WBC will be noted).

Common interventions

Medical interventions for generalized peritonitis include administration of IV fluids and antibiotics, gastric suctioning, and drainage. **Surgical** interventions include appendectomy prior to rupture and insertion of drainage tubes in the presence of abscess formation or peritonitis.

Nursing interventions

Physical 1. Assess for pending rupture according to the symptoms presented above.
2. Monitor for complications.
3. Provide comfort measures.
4. Keep the patient NPO.
5. Monitor IV therapy.
6. Administer preoperative and postoperative care when indicated (*see* Chapters 9 and 11).

Psychosocial 7. Provide support, reassurance, and information.

Prevention 8. Teach early recognition of the signs and symptoms of acute appendicitis.

Evaluation criteria.   *See* Overview. Absence of pain; wounds heal.

GENERAL AND REGIONAL ENTERITIS

General and regional enteritis (terminal ileitis, granulomatous jejunoileitis, Crohn's disease) involves chronic and relapsing inflammation of a segment of the alimentary tract. It may involve several segments, from the mouth to the anus, and when in the bowel it involves the whole thickness of the bowel wall. The incidence of this disorder appears to be familial and related to ulcerative colitis; it occurs worldwide in people of all ages, but mostly in young adults 20 to 30 yr of age. There is a high incidence among Jews and a low incidence among blacks. The exact cause is unknown; it may be some genetic or hereditary basis or some new environmental factor. There is usually a heavy, edematous, reddish-purple area in the intestine that may have granular spots. *Symptoms* (which result from inflammation, obstruction, and bowel dysfunction) include diarrhea, constipation, abdominal discomfort, cramping, a low-grade fever, and, possibly, retarded growth in children. *Complications* are as follows: a narrowed lumen may cause obstruction, and ulcerations, abscesses, and fistulas may perforate the intestine. *Diagnosis* is based on the health history, a physical exam, BE, and the following laboratory data: decreased Hb or Hct, increased erythrocyte sedimentation rate (ESR), and occult blood in stools.

Common interventions

Medical interventions include alleviation of symptoms, maintenance of good nutrition, administration of antibiotics and antispasmodics, and general supportive therapy. **Surgery** is indicated primarily for complications.

Nursing interventions

Physical 1. Maintain good nutrition.

2. Give antibiotics as ordered to control infection.

3. Give anti-inflammatory drugs as ordered.

4. Prepare the patient for surgery as necessary.

Psychosocial 5. Promote the leading of a productive life.

6. Encourage verbalization of feelings.

7. Explore alternative outlets for feelings.

Educational 8. Teach the patient about the appropriate diet.

9. Teach the patient alternatives for the pursuit of a productive life.

10. Give preoperative instruction, if indicated.

Prevention 11. There are no known preventive measures, but the patient should be prepared for early recognition of symptoms, as this is significant in producing a good outcome.

Evaluation criteria.   *See* Overview. Prompt healing with therapy.

ULCERATIVE COLITIS

Ulcerative colitis is a recurrent inflammatory condition of the colon involving the mucosa and submucosa that is difficult to distinguish from regional enteritis or Crohn's disease of the colon. Factors affecting incidence and etiology are the same as for regional enteritis and Crohn's disease. It is thought that development of ulcerative colitis may be related to bacterial infection, an allergic response, bowel hypersensitivity to trauma or stimuli, and/or emotional instability as characterized by dependence, immaturity, and hypersensitivity to criticism (this factor may cause cholinergic stimulation).

Symptoms include congestion; edema; ulcerations; a slight oozing of blood in the colon that progresses to abscess; frequent passage of stools containing pus, blood, and mucus; possibly liquid feces; weight loss; anorexia; and intermittent mild fever. There are three types of onset. The first is gradual, beginning with crampy pain and passage of scanty and hard stools, blood, pus, and mucus with severe tenesmus (tension and urge to defecate). The second is abrupt, beginning with bloody diarrhea, fever, anorexia, weight loss, liquid or hard stools (depending on the area involved), abdominal tenderness, spasm of the rectum and anus, remissions, and exacerbation. The third is also abrupt, with a rapid and fulminating course that, unless successfully treated, results in death due to toxicity or shock. *Diagnosis* is based on the health history, physical exam, laboratory data (decreased Hb and Hct, increased ESR, and leukocytosis), x-rays (flat plates of the abdomen, BE), sigmoidoscopy, and rectal biopsy.

Common interventions

The patient should be given a high-protein, high-calorie diet to meet normal nutritional needs (the patient may select bland, low-residue foods to control diarrhea). Fluid, electrolyte, and blood should be replaced as needed. Antibiotics should be given for secondary inflammation. Bed rest is advised during exacerbations. Anticholinergics are routinely given to control pain and diarrhea. Supportive measures should be implemented.

Excision of the colon, rectum, and anus with creation of a permanent **ileostomy** may be indicated (the entire procedure may be called an abdominal-perineal resection). This involves opening the ileum onto the abdominal surface and differs from colostomy in that the feces have a more liquid consistency, digestive enzymes are present, and the flow of contents is uncontrolled, so that a collection appliance must be used continuously unless an ileal pouch has been created (this is known as a continent ileostomy, in which there is a reservoir created from the terminal ileum). Colectomy may be indicated for those with long-standing disease because of the high incidence of cancer. This involves removal of a portion or all of the colon and is usually accompanied by a permanent ileostomy.

Nursing interventions

Physical 1. *See* enteritis *above.*
2. For **ileostomy:**
   a. Prevent leakage of fecal contents onto the skin.
   b. Make sure that the appliance fits snugly.
   c. Provide meticulous skin care.
   d. Avoid foods causing gas and odor (e.g., nuts, cauliflower, cabbage, sauerkraut, and broccoli).
   e. Use charcoal, bismuth subgalate, or subcarbonate (given orally or in the appliance) to control odor.
   f. Empty the appliance frequently.
   g. Monitor intake and output and fluid and electrolyte balance.
   h. Administer potassium supplements as indicated.
   i. Assess for signs of shock.
3. For **continent ileostomy,** irrigate the pouch tid or qid; other interventions are the same as for ileostomy, except that no appliance is necessary.
Psychosocial 4. Help the patient adjust to his altered body image and life-style.
5. Assure the patient that usual activities can be resumed.
6. Refer the patient to the Ileostomy Club for peer support and adjustment.

Educational 7. Teach the patient and his family about ileostomy care, avoidance of foods causing gas and odor, the signs and symptoms of fluid and eléctrolyte imbalance, and the need to seek immediate medical attention if diarrhea occurs.

Evaluation criteria.   *See* Overview. Skin is intact, without excoriation; flatus and odor are controlled; patient can care for ileostomy independently; and usual activities are resumed.

DIVERTICULOSIS/DIVERTICULITIS/MECKEL'S DIVERTICULUM

A diverticulum is an outpouching of the bowel mucosa, with or without a muscle tissue covering and mostly in the sigmoid colon. Diverticulosis is a condition in which there is one or more diverticula. Diverticulitis is inflammation of the diverticula. Meckel's diverticulum is a congenital outpouching of the ileum near the cecum, with or without gastric mucosa or pancreatic tissue lining. Diverticula occur anywhere along the GI tract and are acquired. Meckel's diverticulum is developed in embryo; symptoms mimic those of appendicitis.

Predisposing factors are increased pressure in the lumen, ballooning out between muscle fibers where blood vessels pass through the bowel wall, lack of bulk in the diet, and stress. *Signs and symptoms* include bleeding, pain, gas formation with abdominal distension, constipation, and fever (diverticulitis). *Complications* of diverticulosis are perforation, hemorrhage, inflammation (diverticulitis), and abscess formation with fistula to the bladder or other adjacent structures. Complications of Meckel's diverticulum are peptic ulcer with bleeding, perforated ulcer, and possible obstruction by the fibrous connection to the umbilicus. The *diagnosis* is based on the health history, physical exam, and x-rays (a flat plate of the abdomen and a BE, which should be used with caution in acute diverticulitis).

Common interventions

The patient is usually given a high-residue diet, bulk laxatives, antispasmodics, and antibiotics for inflammation. Surgical interventions include excision, bowel resection, and repair of perforations if they do not become walled off by omentum and heal themselves.

Nursing interventions

Physical 1. Provide a high-residue diet.
2. Administer bulk laxatives, antispasmodics, and antibiotics as ordered.
3. Monitor intake and output and vital signs for complications.

4. Provide preoperative and postoperative care as needed.
Psychosocial 5. Identify stressors.
6. Provide reassurance regarding therapeutic outcomes.
Educational 7. Teach the patient about proper diet.
8. Provide instruction in relaxation techniques to reduce stress
9. Provide preoperative and postoperative teaching as needed.

Evaluation criteria. *See* Overview.

APPENDICITIS

Appendicitis is a condition involving inflammation of the vermiform appendix. It is caused by fecolith (stone) or other obstruction of the lumen, by fibrous disease in the bowel wall, or by adhesions. *Signs and symptoms* of appendicitis are acute intermittent abdominal pain that begins in the epigastrum or periumbilic area; spreading of pain to the lower-right quadrant of the abdomen as inflammation spreads to the serosal layers of the bowel close to the peritoneum; guarding of the abdominal muscles, with steady pain; vomiting after the pain starts; anorexia; low-grade fever; a coated tongue and bad breath; and leukocytosis. *Complications* are perforation, abscess formation, and peritonitis. The *diagnosis* is based on the health history, physical exam, and a WBC of 10,000 to 15,000.

Common interventions

Surgical and **nursing** interventions are discussed in the section on ruptured appendix (*see above*). (*See* Chapters 9 and 11 for preoperative and postoperative care.)

PERITONITIS

Peritonitis is an inflammation of the peritoneal lining of the abdominal cavity. This condition may be acute, chronic, primary, or secondary to other conditions. Predisposing factors are inflammations of the GI tract, fallopian tubes, and bloodstream. Peritonitis is caused by toxins entering the cavity from any of a variety of sources and overcoming the peritoneum's ability to localize and combat them. *Signs and symptoms* of peritonitis vary, depending upon the cause. They include localized or generalized pain, rigidity of the abdominal muscles, increased pain with pressure on or movement of the abdomen, nausea and vomiting, low-grade fever, an absence of bowel sounds, and shallow respirations to avoid abdominal movement. *Complications* include circulatory stress due to increased circulating blood volume, increased fluid secretion into the bowel due to fluid retention, air retention related to lack of peristalsis, increased oxygen requirements along with shallow breathing, and eventual fluid and electrolyte imbalance. The *diagnosis* is based on the health history, physical exam, and an elevated WBC.

Common interventions

Medical interventions include IV fluid, protein, and electrolyte replacement; GI decompression; positive-pressure respiratory therapy; administration of antibiotics; and keeping the patient in the semi-Fowler's position or keeping the head of the bed elevated on blocks to pool drainage for localization of the abscess. **Surgical** treatment consists of removal of the cause, when possible, and drainage of the abscess.

Nursing interventions

Physical 1. Assess for the presence of peritonitis on the basis of symptoms presented above, and monitor their status.
2. Provide general comfort measures.
3. Medicate for pain as ordered.
4. Keep the patient NPO and maintain decompression as ordered.
5. Monitor IV therapy and antibiotic administration.
6. Assess the abdomen for rigidity, presence or absence of bowel sounds, and correct placement of the decompression tube.
7. Monitor vital signs, particularly temperature.
8. Monitor fluid intake and output.
Psychosocial 9. Provide support, reassurance, and information as needed.
10. Explain all tests and procedures.
Educational 11. Teach the signs and symptoms of abdominal infection.
12. Teach the patient about diet and relaxation techniques.

Evaluation criteria.   *See* Overview.

RECTAL ABSCESS

A rectal abscess is an accumulation of toxic and purulent materials in an anal crypt, usually following **cryptitis** (accumulation and decay of stool particles trapped in an anal crypt). Predisposing factors are cryptitis, rectal fissure, or rectal fistula; abrasion of local tissues; and entry of virulent organisms through traumatized anal tissue. Cysts form in crypts and extend into the submucosal areas. *Signs and symptoms* of rectal abscess are the presence of a mass in the anal area; localized pain, particularly on evacuation of stools; and, in some cases, purulent drainage. *Complications* include recurrent abscess formation and septicemia. *Diagnosis* is based on the health history and physical exam.

Common interventions

Treatment involves surgical incision and drainage (*see* rectal fistula *below*). **Nursing** care is similar to that for hemorrhoids (*see below*).

PARASITIC INFECTION

Parasitic infection is an infestation of the GI tract with any of the following types of worms: roundworms (*Ascaris*), pinworms (*Enterobius*), *Trichinella spiralis,* and several tapeworm varieties. Incidence is worldwide, including the poorer regions of the USA. *Signs and symptoms* of parasitic infection depend on the type and location of the parasites and may include pain in the abdomen, itching in the anal region, fever, and respiratory symptoms. Serious and even fatal diseases may result if the cause is not eradicated. The *diagnosis* is based on the health history, physical exam, and laboratory evidence of the parasite in stool or other specimens.

Common interventions

Specific medications are given as ordered; thiabendazole is given for trichinosis, and piperazine (Antepar) is given for most other parasitic infections. Supportive measures include provision of proper diet, rest, and hygiene. Antibiotics and analgesics or antispasmodics are given as ordered.

Nursing interventions

Physical 1. Institute those measures presented in the above section.
Psychosocial 2. Implement supportive measures.
Educational 3. Teach the patient about causes and treatments.
Prevention 4. Advise the patient to avoid sources of infestation.

Evaluation criteria. *See* Overview. Eradication of parasite; restoration of well-being.

DYSENTERY

Dysentery is a condition involving intense diarrhea and cramping, primarily of the large bowel. Incidence is worldwide and is especially high in poorer regions that have poorer sanitation and less pure water. Predisposing factors include exposure to infected individuals, crowded and unsanitary conditions, exposure to contaminated food and water, and living in a warm climate (better incubation of causative organisms). Causative organisms include amoebae (*Entamoeba histolytica*) and bacteria (*Shigella*).

Signs and symptoms include intense diarrhea, abdominal cramping, mild to severe fever, and, possibly, blood in the stools. Fluid and electrolyte imbalance may develop, and dysentery can be fatal to the debilitated, the aged, and the very young. The *diagnosis* is based on the health history, physical exam, and laboratory evidence of the causative agent in the stool sample.

Common interventions

Medical interventions include supportive therapy and chemotherapy appropriate to the causative agent.

Nursing interventions

Physical 1. Administer medications as ordered.

2. Provide supportive measures (rest and a nutritious diet).

Psychosocial 3. Reassure the patient regarding therapeutic outcomes.

Educational 4. Teach the patient and his family about the nature of the infection and aspects of therapy.

Evaluation criteria. *See* Overview. Eradication of parasite; restoration of well-being.

PILONIDAL CYST

Pilonidal cysts are hair-containing cysts located at the base of the sacrum. These benign neoplasms are most common in young adult males. Predisposing factors include possible abnormal development in embryo; possible penetration of the skin by hairs, causing formation of sinus tracts; and excessive rubbing from clothing and chairs. An abscess forms as a result of infection of the sinus tracts caused by imbedded hairs.

Signs and symptoms of pilonidal cysts include acute pain, swelling, and discharge. Possible *complications* are recurrence and poor healing. *Diagnosis* is based on the health history and physical exam.

Common interventions

Medical care consists of supportive therapy to completely remove the infection. **Surgical** treatment consists of excision of the abscess.

Nursing interventions

1. Provide supportive measures preoperatively and postoperatively.
2. Provide information about the cause and treatment.
3. Remove hairs in the sacral area to help prevent recurrence.

Evaluation criteria. *See* Overview.

POLYPS

Polyps are benign neoplasms projecting from bowel lumen, either with a stem (pedunculated) or without a stem (sessile). They are the most common tumors of the large bowel. Polyps may be precursors of cancer. *Signs and symptoms* include abdominal discomfort, possible profuse bleeding, and possible intussusception (invagination of one part of the large bowel into another). *Complications* are as follows: polyps may mask a malignant tumor, may serve as a focus for bowel obstruction, and may become malignant. *Diagnosis* is based on the health history, physical exam, and proctoscopy. Treatment consists of **surgical** removal.

Nursing interventions
1. Provide supportive measures for diagnostic, preoperative, and postoperative periods.
2. Encourage routine physical examination, including proctoscopy.

Evaluation criteria. *See* Overview and Chapters 9 and 11.

MALIGNANT NEOPLASMS OF THE COLON

Carcinoma of the large intestine, occurring anywhere from the ileocecal valve to the rectum, is the second most common cause of death in the USA; it is especially common among women. Most cases involve the lower colon. Predisposing factors include a high-fat diet and overnutrition (obesity). A possible correlation exists between low bulk intake and slow transit time (constipation). Metabolic and bacterial end-products may be carcinogenic.

Signs and symptoms vary with location and the type of growth. They include bleeding, change in bowel habits, abdominal pain, weight loss, anorexia, nausea, and vomiting. Possible *complications* are obstruction, metastasis, and death. *Diagnosis* is based on the health history, physical exam, and diagnostic studies, including x-rays of the colon and cytologic studies. About one third of these tumors can be discovered by digital exam.

Common interventions
Medical interventions are the same as those in Chapter 8 for radiation treatment and chemotherapy. **Surgical** treatments for cancer of the colon include resection and colostomy.

Resection involves cutting out the diseased portion of the bowel and anastamosis of the remaining segments. **Colostomy** entails opening some part of the colon onto the abdominal surface to divert feces temporarily or permanently, as with inflammation or obstructive diseases. Single-barreled or end colostomy involves one opening (stoma) on the abdominal surface and is permanent if the portion of the bowel distal to the stoma is removed. Double-barreled or loop colostomy involves two openings on the abdominal surface, the ends of the proximal and distal loops. Loop colostomy may be temporary, with closure at another time; identification of the proximal and distal loops is needed for proper management; and cautery is used to cut into the bowel loop 2 to 3 days after the loop is created.

Nursing interventions
Physical 1. Do not administer laxative and gas-forming foods (roughage, prunes, and fresh fruits).
2. Provide liquids such as tea if diarrhea develops to avoid electrolyte imbalance.

3. Irrigate the colostomy if constipation develops.
4. Control odor by giving charcoal and bismuth subcarbonate orally as ordered and by placing charcoal discs in the collection appliance pouch.
5. Prevent strictures in the stoma through gloved finger dilation prior to irrigations, if ordered.
6. Prevent skin irritation by good hygiene measures and by keeping the skin dry with karaya powder, lightly applied.
7. Empty or change the appliance as needed.

Psychosocial 8. Give support, encouragement, and a realistic appraisal of the situation in the first two stages of adjustment. Adjustment is difficult and depression is common; the phases of adjustment are like those experienced by persons in crisis: shock, defensive retreat, acknowledgement, and adaptation.
9. Encourage interaction with other ostomates, as in an "ostomy club."

Educational 10. Teach self-care techniques at the patient's level of acceptance.
11. Involve the family if this is essential or desired.
12. Tell the patient how to contact an "ostomy club."

Prevention 13. Advise the patient to maintain contact with health care personnel for regular follow-up visits.

Evaluation criteria. *See* Overview. Patient demonstrates independence in self-care activities and adapts to temporary alterations in his situation (such as diarrhea, constipation, or a lack of the proper equipment).

RECTAL/SIGMOID CARCINOMA

Rectal/sigmoid carcinoma is carcinoma of the terminal portion of the large bowel. Mortality from rectal/sigmoid cancer is on the increase. The etiology is the same as for malignant neoplasms of the colon. *Signs and symptoms* include possible changes in bowel habits, bleeding, possible intestinal obstruction, tenesmus, and localized pain. *Complications* and *diagnostic* criteria are the same as for malignant neoplasms of the colon.

Common interventions

Medical treatment is covered in Chapter 8. For cancer of the sigmoid or above, **surgical** treatment is resection with anastomosis of the remaining bowel. For cancer of the anus and terminal rectum, surgical treatment consits of (1) a "pull through" of the bowel through the rectal sphincter as palliative treatment (protosigmoidectomy) and (2) abdominal-peritoneal resection, or anterior-posterior resection, with permanent colostomy.

Nursing interventions

Physical 1. Provide preoperative and postoperative care.
2. Provide colostomy care.

3. Provide cancer treatment (*see* Chapter 8).
4. *See* the nursing interventions for malignant neoplasms of the colon and Chapter 8.

ADHESIONS

Adhesions are fibrous bands of scar tissue that form after abdominal surgery. This abnormal development of massive scar tissue bands occurs in some people but not in others. The reasons are largely unknown, although irritants remaining in the abdomen after surgery are considered causative. *Signs and symptoms* of adhesions are those of obstruction or volvulus (twisting of the bowel around a stationary point). *Complications* include perforation following obstruction or volvulus. The *diagnosis* is based on the health history, physical exam, and x-rays (flat plate of the abdomen).

Common interventions

Treatment is **surgical** removal of the adhesions. **Nursing** interventions are as presented for intestinal obstruction (*see above*).

PARALYTIC ILEUS

Paralytic ileus is a neurogenic or functional obstruction of the bowel that is common after abdominal surgery. Predisposing factors include handling of the bowel during surgery and retroperitoneal surgical procedures. Causes include abdominal and thoracic infections; electrolyte imbalance, especially hypokalemia; and reflex stimulation, inhibiting propulsive activity. *Signs and symptoms* include an absence of bowel sounds, and nausea, vomiting, and absence of flatus postoperatively. *Complications* are the same as for intestinal obstruction. The *diagnosis* is based on the health history, physical exam, and x-rays (flat plate of the abdomen).

Common interventions

Medical intervention consists of decompression with intubation and gastric suction until bowel functioning returns. **Nursing** interventions are the same as for intestinal obstruction (*see above*).

HERNIA

A hernia is a protrusion of an organ through a defect or aperture. There are four main types of hernias: inguinal, femoral, umbilical, and incisional. In **direct inguinal** hernias, the intestine or abdominal contents pass through the abdominal wall in an area of muscular weakness. This is most common in the elderly and is caused by gradually developing weakness in a congenitally deficient area of the wall as a result of intra-abdominal pressure. In **indirect inguinal** hernias, the intestine or abdominal contents pass through the inguinal ring and canal. This is common in male infants and young persons and in men 50 to 60 yr of age. Intra-abdominal pressure may cause the intestines to herniate into the scrotum through the anatomic space available for descent of the testes (from the abdominal cavity after birth). **Femoral** hernias involve a protrusion of abdominal contents through the femoral ring in the groin. This type is most common in females. A femoral hernia begins with a plug of fat forming in the femoral canal; this enlarges to pull the peritoneum into the sac. Femoral hernia carries a high incidence of incarceration. **Umbilical** hernias involve a protrusion of abdominal viscera through the abdominal wall near the umbilicus. Two types of umbilical hernias occur as congenital defects in infants, and a third occurs in obese or multiparous women as a result of a congenital defect. Strangulation and necrosis can result in umbilical hernias occurring at time of birth. **Incisional** hernias involve a protrusion of abdominal contents at the site of previous surgery. The incidence is increasing, probably due to the greater number of surgical procedures being performed. This type of hernia is caused by inadequate healing due to such postoperative problems as inadequate nutrition, extreme distension, and obesity.

Signs and symptoms may include an obvious bulge, localized discomfort, localized swelling, and some degree of intestinal obstruction (e.g., nausea, vomiting, and constipation). *Complications* include incarceration (cannot be replaced in the abdominal cavity), strangulation (blockage of circulation, with resulting necrosis), and complete intestinal obstruction with perforation. *Diagnosis* is based on the health history and physical exam.

Common interventions

Uncomplicated hernias may be reduced with appliances or taping as appropriate for the site and the patient's condition. **Surgical** treatment consists of herniorraphy (repair of the defect), with or without reinforcement of the area with fascia lata or Dacron mesh. **Nursing** interventions are the same as for intestinal obstruction (*see above*).

HEMORRHOIDS (PILES)

Hemorrhoids are dilated veins in the anorectal area internal or external to the hemorrhoidal plexus. They usually occur in adults 20 to 50 yr old. Predisposing factors include the upright posture of humans, with the resulting pressure on the anorectal area; pregnancy; and portal hypertension. Causes of acute enlargement include straining with diarrhea or constipation and venous congestion with CHF or portal hypertension.

Signs and symptoms include an internal or external bulge, severe pain, itching, and bleeding upon evacuation of stools. *Complications* are bleeding, with resulting iron deficiency anemia; strangulation of the vein following prolapse; and thrombosis, with resulting intense pain and edema. *Diagnosis* is based on the health history and physical exam.

Common interventions

Medical interventions include cold-pack applications and elevation of the buttocks to relieve edema, reduction of pressure by treating constipation, relief of pain with application of heat and astringent lotions, and rest in a recumbent position for prolapsed or thrombosed hemorrhoids. The **surgical** treatment is hemorrhoidectomy (excision of varicosed hemorrhoidal veins). Other treatments include rubber band ligation of internal hemorrhoids with a McGivney ligator apparatus and injection of a sclerosing agent at the base of the vein to provide temporary relief by shrinking the contents of the distended vein.

Nursing interventions

Physical 1. Provide a high-bulk diet and sufficient fluid intake to ensure soft, formed stools and to prevent stricture formation.

2. Provide proper hygiene for the operative site.

3. Apply local moist heat to soothe discomfort and promote healing.

4. Provide sitz baths as ordered long enough after surgery to prevent hemorrhage.

5. Monitor vital signs for complications, such as hemorrhage and infection.

6. Monitor urinary output to prevent postoperative retention due to pain in the adjacent area.

7. Administer analgesics as ordered for pain.

Psychosocial 8. Anticipate the sensitivity and embarassment the patient may have because of the location of the condition.

9. Provide matter-of-fact care that is considerate of the patient's need for privacy.

Educational 10. Teach the patient about self-care and proper hygiene, reestablishment of normal bowel habits, and proper diet and fluid intake.

Prevention 11. Prevent constipation and straining at stool.

12. Promote early recognition of the condition and adoption of remedial dietary, activity, and bowel habit modifications.

Evaluation criteria.   *See* Overview. There is prompt healing.

RECTAL FISSURE/RECTAL FISTULA

Rectal fissure (fissure-in-ano) is a longitudinal ulceration on the skin of the anal canal. Rectal fistula (fistula-in-ano) is a sinus tract between the anal canal and the skin outside the anus or from an abscess to the anal canal or perianal area. Rectal fissures result from stretching of tissue and trauma. When chronic, rectal fissure or fistula may be secondary to cryptitis. Formation of an abscess usually precedes fistula formation.

Signs and symptoms of fissures are sharp pain upon defecation and sphincter spasm (in chronic conditions). Fistulas are evidenced by drainage and may heal over and then reopen to drain. Fissures may result in obstipation (no stool passed) due to the desire to avoid the pain of defecation. Fistulas heal slowly, are painful, and may become chronic. *Diagnosis* is based on the health history and physical exam.

Common interventions

Fissures may heal with local dilations, cleansing, and control of constipation. Fistulas may appear to heal without treatment, but they usually close over only temporarily. The fissure tract may be **surgically** excised. The fistula tract is surgically excised and left open to heal by granulation. **Nursing** interventions are the same as for hemorrhoids (*see above*).

CHAPTER 17

ALTERED URINARY FUNCTIONING
Lani Guzman

OVERVIEW

The kidneys and urinary system serve distinct, although related, functions in the body. Kidney functioning is essential for life, a fact that becomes obvious when the multiple functions of the kidneys are considered: regulation of fluid and electrolyte balance, regulation of acid-base balance, excretion of metabolic waste products, regulation of arterial BP, regulation of erythropoiesis, and metabolism of vitamin D. Unfortunately, even the best "artificial kidney" can correct only some of the problems caused by a lack of functioning kidneys; thus, renal failure can be controlled, but not cured. In contrast, the urinary system is much simpler; it serves mainly as a reservoir and conduit for urine from the kidneys to the outside. Although it is less crucial for life, the urinary tract is less well protected from harm and, thus, is commonly affected by a variety of problems.

Essential for life, but dependent on the proper functioning of the rest of the body, the kidneys and urinary system are prone to a variety of intrinsic and extrinsic diseases. Intrinsic diseases and conditions that primarily affect the kidneys and urinary tract include infections, neoplasms, and urolithiasis. Extrinsic diseases and conditions affect the kidneys and urinary tract through their effects on other body systems — for instance, obstruction to urine outflow secondary to enlargement of the prostate, neurogenic bladder, and acute renal failure secondary to hypovolemia. The distinction between intrinsic and extrinsic factors becomes important in designing optimal nursing care for affected patients.

Anatomy and physiology review

Macroscopic anatomy.   The kidneys are bean-shaped organs that sit in the abdomen, outside of the peritoneal cavity, one on either side of the spine. They lie between approximately the 12th thoracic and 3rd lumbar vertebrae, with the left kidney lying slightly lower than the right. The kidneys are protected from physical trauma by their fibrous capsules and by the perinephric fat in which they lie. Each weighs ~150 g.

Blood supply to the kidneys is via the renal arteries, which branch off the aorta and enter the kidneys at the **hilum**, an indentation on the medial border. At rest, the kidneys receive about one fourth of the CO. Renal vein drainage follows the same general pathway to the inferior vena cava. Renal nerves also enter the kidneys at the hilum.

When sliced open from top to bottom, the kidneys reveal two main areas — the outer cortex and the inner medulla. The medulla contains the **renal pyramids**, the apices of which are the **papillae**. The papillae empty into **calyces**, which in turn coalesce to form the **renal pelvis**. The renal pelvis is the beginning of the urinary tract.

Urine formed in the cortex and outer medulla enters the renal pelvis and then the ureter. The ureters serve as the conduits between the kidneys and the bladder. The ureters are narrow, but distensible. Urine flows through the ureters assisted by ureteral peristalsis.

The urinary bladder is essentially a reservoir for urine. It consists mainly of a very flexible muscle, the **detrussor**, which can be passively stretched when distended by urine and which can forcefully contract during micturition. The normal capacity of the bladder is ~400 ml.

The bladder lies between the symphysis pubis and the rectum and seminal vesicles in men and between the vagina and uterus in women. It is supported in place by the levator ani muscle.

Urine enters the bladder from the ureters at the trigone. The ureters enter at an oblique angle, which serves to prevent reflux and thus protect the kidney. Urine leaves the bladder via the urethra — the opening to which also lies in the trigonal area at the base of the bladder. The opening to the urethra is surrounded by muscle fibers forming the internal sphincter. The bladder is largely under parasympathetic nervous system control.

The urethra is the conduit from the bladder to the outside. In females, it is short — ~4 cm (1½ in.) in length — and lies just in front of the vagina. In males, the urethra is longer because it traverses the length of the penis. Immediately below the bladder, it is surrounded by the prostate gland. In males, the urethra serves not only as a conduit for urine but also for seminal fluid.

Microscopic anatomy.   Each kidney is composed of ~1 million functional units called **nephrons**. About 90% of these nephrons lie solely within the renal cortex; the other 10% extend into the renal medulla and are important in the concentration of urine. Each nephron consists of two parts — the **glomerulus**, where the initial filtration of plasma occurs, and the **tubule**, where modification of the filtrate occurs and urine is formed.

The glomerulus consists of a tuft of capillaries surrounded by a hollow capsule known as **Bowman's capsule.** Blood is separated from the capsule by a set of highly permeable membranes that allow filtration of fluid into the capsule. On average ~125 ml of filtrate is formed every minute. In other words, the GFR is normally ~125 ml/min. During the course of the day, ~180 liters of filtrate is formed. Since the average plasma volume is ~3 liters, the entire plasma volume is filtered ~60 times/day.

Exiting Bowman's capsule is the renal tubule. The filtrate flows first through the proximal tubule, then through the loop of Henle, and finally to the collecting ducts. Through a convergent scheme, collecting ducts merge and eventually empty into the renal pelvis.

Blood leaving the glomerular capillaries enters the efferent arterioles and then branches to form the peritubular capillary system. In the juxtamedullary nephrons, the efferent arteriole in which the loops of Henle extend into the medulla, the efferent arteriole also supplies the **vasa recta,** which is a network of thin, hairpin loop capillaries that run parallel to the loops of Henle.

The **macula densa** is that part of the renal tubule between the ascending loop of Henle and the distal tubule that passes between the afferent and efferent arterioles of Bowman's capsule. The area where the macula densa touches the originating glomerulus is known as the juxtaglomerular apparatus. This apparatus is important in the control of renal and systemic arterial BP.

Renal physiology. There are three main processes involved in the formation of urine: filtration, reabsorption, and secretion. By varying these processes, the kidneys are able to regulate urine volume and electrolyte content.

Filtration is the process by which fluid and electrolytes from the plasma enter Bowman's capsule. The membranes separating the two areas are permeable to almost all molecules, except macromolecules such as proteins. In certain diseases, destruction of these barriers may result in large amounts of protein in the filtrate. For the most part, the filtered protein is albumin, because it is a small but concentrated blood protein. Normally, the initial filtrate has the same concentration of electrolytes as plasma.

The GFR is dependent on the balance of forces favoring filtration (capillary hydrostatic pressure) and those opposing it (intracapsular hydrostatic pressure and capillary oncotic pressure). Thus, changes in renal arterial pressure or plasma protein concentration can change the GFR.

Reabsorption is the process by which substances are transported from the renal tubule to the peritubular capillaries. The amount of a substance reabsorbed is specific to that substance. For instance, most metabolic waste products are minimally reabsorbed and, thus, are excreted in the urine. In contrast, metabolically useful substances such as glucose are largely reabsorbed, and their concentration in the final urine is normally zero.

The reabsorption of sodium and water is of extreme importance. Of the 125 ml/min of filtrate formed, 124 ml is reabsorbed under most conditions, leaving 1 ml/min to be excreted as the final urine. If the entire 125 ml/min were excreted, the entire plasma volume would be excreted in ~30 min.

Secretion is, in a sense, the reverse of reabsorption; it is the movement of substances from the plasma to the renal tubule. As with reabsorption, secretion is specific for a given molecular species. In addition, secretion is dependent on the physiologic state of the body. For instance, depending on acid-base balance, hydrogen ions may be secreted. Depending on aldosterone levels, potassium may be secreted. Secretion is also a major route for the excretion of drugs and their metabolites.

General assessment

Health history.   Relevant areas about which information should be obtained in patients with possible diseases of the kidneys or urinary tract are outlined in Table 17-1.

Physical examination.   The kidneys are mainly inspected by palpation. By placing one hand under a supine patient's abdomen and the other hand above, it is possible to palpate the kidneys. Enlargement may indicate hydronephrosis, tumor, or polycystic kidney disease. Tenderness on palpation may indicate acute inflammation. It is important to assess for tenderness at the costovertebral angle by gently striking over the area. Abdominal or renal bruits may be detected by auscultation. These may indicate renal artery stenosis.

There are at least three methods used to assess the amount of urine in the bladder. First, it is sometimes possible to palpate the bladder, particularly if it contains ≥150 ml of urine. However, even a grossly distended bladder may not be palpable if the bladder wall is flaccid. The second method used to assess the amount of urine in the bladder is percussing the bladder's borders. Again, the bladder must contain ≥150 ml of urine to be percussible. Finally, it is possible to estimate the size of the bladder by placing the stethoscope just above the symphysis pubis. A fingernail is then gently drawn across the patient's abdomen, moving from the stethoscope toward the estimated border of the bladder. A loud sound will be heard to the limits of the bladder; beyond the bladder wall, the sound will be much softer.

Digital rectal examination may be indicated in the medical diagnosis of prostatic enlargement.

The external genitalia should be inspected for evidence of inflammation and discharge. If the external urinary meatus is difficult to locate in a female, it can often become more prominent if the patient is asked to cough or bear down.

If the patient requires urinary drainage devices, these should be inspected for evidence of proper functioning. Of particular importance is the condition of the penile skin with the use of condom catheters and the condition of the peristomal skin with urinary diversions.

It is also important to assess other body systems for evidence of abnormalities affecting the renal and urinary tract. Table 17-2 lists some of these important abnormalities and possible interpretations.

Diagnostic tests

Laboratory data. **Urinalysis** is an inexpensive but highly valuable diagnostic test. To be most reliable, a clean, midstream urine specimen should be obtained and examined as soon as possible after collection. Although laboratory analysis may be desired because of its higher degree of quantitative accuracy, rapid qualitative screening may be performed in the clinic or at the bedside by the use of tablets or dipsticks. (Urinalysis findings are presented in Appendix B.)

Bacteriologic studies are important in identifying causes of renal or urinary infection. An optimal specimen for culture and sensitivity is not contaminated by organisms from outside the urinary tract; usable specimens are clean-catch midstream-voided or catheterized specimens. A colony count of >100,000/ml is usually considered to be evidence of significant bacteriuria.

Cytologic studies are best performed on morning urine, collected using a clean-catch technique. These studies are useful in the diagnosis of neoplasms.

Although useful information can be obtained from random single specimens of urine, it is sometimes necessary to obtain a 24-hr collection to quantitate the amount of a given substance excreted or to find an average value when there is significant circadian variation. An optimal collection is free of contamination by toilet paper, feces, or menstrual fluid. During the collection period, urine should be preserved either chemically or by refrigeration, depending on the nature of the test. Important tests carried out on 24-hr urine collections and possible causes of abnormal findings are presented in Appendix B.

Analyses of blood specimens may also help to diagnose renal and urinary disease, since renal failure causes changes throughout the body. Common blood tests used in the diagnosis of renal and urinary disease are presented in Appendix B.

Other. A variety of studies may be carried out to help in the diagnosis of renal or urinary tract disease. The common tests are presented in Table 17-3.

Common interventions

Common interventions for altered urinary functioning encompass medical (drug and diet therapy), surgical, and nursing regimens. General classes of **drugs** used in the management of a variety of renal and urinary tract diseases are presented in Table 17-4. General guidelines for the various related types of therapeutic **diets** are presented in Table 17-5.

TABLE 17-1

Health History

Assessment	Possible abnormalities
Usual pattern of micturition	
Frequency	High residual volume of urine
	Inflammation/infection
	Nervousness
Urgency	Inflammation/infection
Dysuria	Cystitis
	Prostatitis
Nocturia	Primary renal disease
	CHF with edema
	Prostate enlargement
	Drinking fluids late at night
Problems initiating flow, dribbling	Prostate enlargement
Usual urine characteristics	
Color	
Brown, maroon, pink, red	Bleeding due to trauma, neoplasms, transfusion reactions, drugs
Nearly colorless	Large fluid intake
	Interstitial nephritis
	Diuretics
Orange, amber, brown	Concentrated urine secondary to dehydration
	Bile pigments (may indicate hepatic disease)
	Drugs (phenazopyridine)
Odor	Infection
Amount	
Decreased	Dehydraton, renal failure, obstruction
Increased	Overhydration, diuretics
Pain	
Location	Dull ache at costovertebral angle (renal distension, pyelonephritis, ureteral obstruction)
Associated with voiding	Ureteral pain radiating from costovertebral angle to scrotum/vulva (stones, clots)
	Bladder pain
	Constant (urinary retention)
	With voiding (infection)
	Perineal/perirectal pain (prostatitis)
Medications	
Diuretics	For treatment of CHF, hypertension, renal disease
Parasympathomimetics ⎱ Parasympatholytics ⎰	May affect bladder functioning
Antibiotics	For treatment of infections such as streptococci
Nephrotoxins	May damage the kidney

Assessment	Possible abnormalities
Fluid balance	
Weight gain	Fluid retention, renal failure
Weight loss	Diuretics, renal failure
Incontinence	
Frequency	Neurogenic bladder, organic brain syndrome,
Amount	urinary tract infection, prostate enlargement
Related to coughing, sneezing	
Usual diet	
Fluid consumption	High meat intake predisposes to certain types of
Milk, meat consumption	renal stones
History of renal/kidney disease	May predispose to further kidney/renal disease
History of other diseases	Related to development of certain types of renal
Diabetes mellitus	disease
Hypertension	
SLE	
Family history of renal/kidney disease	Polycystic kidney disease

Types of renal and urinary tract **surgery** are outlined in Table 17-6. General **nursing** management of and evaluation criteria for the patient with renal or urinary tract disease are presented in Table 17-7.

DEVIATIONS

A variety of conditions can be life threatening if prompt intervention is not undertaken in patients with impaired renal functioning. However, even with rapid, appropriate therapy, mortality may be high in some conditions since, at best, it is possible to reverse only certain of the problems caused by acute renal disease.

RETENTION

Urinary retention is the abnormal accumulation of urine in the bladder. Because of the variety of problems that can cause acute retention of urine, there is no data on the incidence of retention in the general population. However, the incidence of postoperative urinary retention has been found to be ~13%. The incidence of retention at autopsy, as defined by the presence of hydronephrosis, is between 3 and 4%.

The predisposing factors to urinary retention are advanced age and decreased level of consciousness. Urinary retention may be caused by prostate enlargement, urolithiasis, spinal cord injury, pelvic malignancy, urethral stricture, postoperative conditions, and drugs (e.g., anticholinergics).

TABLE 17-2

Assessment of Other Body Systems

Body system	Abnormalities	Importance
Cardiovascular	Hypertension	May lead to or be caused by renal disease
		Renal artery stenosis
	Hypotension	May lead to acute renal failure
	Elevated pulsus paradoxus, distant heart sounds, elevated jugular venous pressure	Seen in pericarditis, associated with renal failure
Pulmonary	Uremic fetor	Renal failure
	Kussmaul's respiration	Renal failure, diabetes mellitus
	Pleuritic pain, shortness of breath	Renal failure
GI	Anorexia, nausea, vomiting	Renal failure
Skin	Dry, scaly, pallid	Renal failure
	Dry, brittle hair	Renal failure
Musculoskeletal	Weakness, fatigue	Infection
		Renal failure
Neurologic	Decreased level of consciousness, disorientation, altered reflexes	Renal failure
		May lead to neurogenic bladder, incontinence
Immunologic	Elevated temperature	Infection
Fluid balance	Edema, weight gain	Fluid overload, renal failure
	Decreased skin turgor, dry mucous membranes, weight loss, sunken eyeballs	Fluid loss, renal failure

The *signs and symptoms* of urinary retention are absence of voided urine, bladder distension, overflow incontinence, and bladder pain or discomfort. *Complications* include reflux of urine, elevation of intrarenal pressure, hydronephrosis, urinary tract infection, and urolithiasis.

Diagnosis is based on the health history and physical exam. The clinician should determine the underlying cause.

Common interventions

Urinary retention may be treated by urethral catheterization, suprapubic cystostomy, and drug therapy (e.g., cholinergics). **Nursing** interventions are described in Table 17-7.

Evaluation criteria. Patient exhibits adequate urine output, maintains renal functioning, and is free of pain.

ACUTE RENAL FAILURE

Acute renal failure is a rapid decrease in renal functioning, or more specifically in the GFR, which may or may not be accompanied by oliguria or anuria. Since acute renal failure is a syndrome, rather than a disease per se, there are no reliable statistics on its incidence or prevalence within the general population. An estimate of its frequency may be obtained by looking at the frequencies of causes of acute renal failure.

Causes of acute renal failure may be broken down into three general types: prerenal, intrarenal, and postrenal. Specific causes within these categories are presented in Table 17-8.

The *signs and symptoms* of acute renal failure are rising BUN and creatinine levels; altered urinary output with the characteristic urine output during the oliguric phase being <400 ml/day, during the diuretic phase being >400 ml/day, and during the recovery phase returning to normal; fluid retention; weight gain; electrolyte imbalance such as hyperkalemia and hyponatremia; and uremic symptoms including anorexia, nausea, vomiting, asterixis, decreased level of consciousness, convulsions, anemia, acidosis, hypertension, and pruritus. With optimal therapy, 70 to 80% of patients with acute renal failure will survive. However, untreated or inadequately treated acute renal failure can lead to chronic renal failure and cardiovascular *complications* (from fluid overload and hyperkalemia). Of the deaths associated with acute renal failure, 50 to 90% are due to infection. Another possible complication of acute renal failure is drug toxicity, because of a decreased ability to metabolize and/or excrete drugs.

Diagnosis is based on the health history, physical exam, rising BUN and creatinine levels, decreased GFR (usually estimated by creatinine clearance), and urine sodium levels of >20 mEq/liter.

Common interventions

The primary treatment for acute renal failure is dialysis. This is the process of blood purification by diffusion of substances in the blood across a

TABLE 17-3
Diagnostic Studies

Name of test	Procedure	Associated patient care	Possible findings
KUB	Flat plate x-ray of kidneys, ureters, bladder.	No special care required.	Gross malformation of organs. Renal calculi.
IVP	KUB, then injection of radio-opaque dye. Serial x-rays before and after voiding.	Preprocedure Check for iodine sensitivity. NPO or clear liquids for 12 hr before test. Bowel clean-out as ordered. Postprocedure Encourage fluids. Watch for delayed dye reaction.	Altered renal/kidney anatomy. Renal calculi. Postvoiding residual urine.
Retrograde pyelogram	Injection of radiopaque dye into kidneys via cystoscope. Serial x-rays.	Same as for cystoscopy (*see below*). Check for iodine sensitivity.	Confirmation of results of IVP.
Renal angiography	Injection of radiopaque dye into renal vasculature. Vascular access variable; femoral is common.	Preprocedure Same as for IVP. Postprocedure Bed rest for several hr. Observe puncture site for bleeding, check peripheral pulses and vital signs frequently. Watch for delayed dye reaction.	Delineation of renal vasculature; stenosis, trauma, neoplasms.
Renal biopsy	Visualization of kidney by fluoroscopy or ultrasound, then insertion of biopsy needle percutaneously or via open incision.	Preprocedure NPO for 6-8 hr before test. IV line in place. Sedation as ordered. Obtain informed consent. Assess for bleeding disorders, hypertension.	Diagnosis of renal parenchymal disease.

Procedure	Description	Care	Purpose
Renal vein catheterization	Catheterization, usually via femoral vein, under fluoroscopy. Collection of blood specimens.	**Postprocedure** Assess for bleeding (vital signs, pain, hematoma, Hct). Chest x-ray to check for iatrogenic pneumothorax. Bed rest for 24 hr. Encourage fluids. For open biopsy: general postoperative care.	Measurement of renal vein renins.
Voiding cystogram	Bladder catheterization; instillation of radiopaque dye; removal of catheter. X-rays before, during, and after voiding.	Same as for renal angiography. Check for iodine sensitivity.	Ureteral reflux. Ureteral stenosis. Measurement of postvoiding residual urine.
Cystometrogram	Bladder catheterization; instillation of fluid; measurement of intravesicular pressure and correlation with urge to void.	No special care required	Determination of cause of incontinence.
Renal ultrasound	Noninvasive sonography.	No special care required.	Visualization of renal anatomy.
Cystoscopy	Local or general anesthesia. Passage of rigid or flexible cystoscope into bladder via urethra under strict surgical asepsis. May involve ureteral catheterization.	**Preprocedure** NPO. Bowel clean-out as ordered. Sedation as ordered. Antibiotics if at risk of endocarditis. **Postprocedure** Bed rest. General postoperative care. Encourage fluids. Observe for retention, bleeding, infection.	Removal of calculi. Visualization of bladder wall, obtain biopsy specimens.
Renal scan	Injection of radioisotope, usually technetium 99.	No special care required.	Identification of intrarenal masses, renal anatomy.

KUB, kidneys, ureter, bladder; IVP, IV pyelogram.

TABLE 17-4
Medications

Drug type	Indications	Examples	Comments
Diuretics			
Osmotic	Prevent acute renal failure (e.g., following trauma, hemolytic transfusion reaction).	Mannitol	IV only.
Thiazide	Reduce body water (e.g., in edema, hypertension, nephrosis).	Chlorothiazide Hydrochlorothiazide	Monitor CBC, blood chemistries, BUN, creatinine, uric acid, blood sugar. Monitcr fluid balance.
Loop	Same as thiazides.	Furosemide Ethacrynic acid	Potent, rapid-acting. especially when IV. Monitor as for thiazides.
Potassium-sparing	Nephrotic syndrome, edema.	Spironolactone Triamterene	Aldosterone antagonist. Monitor as for thiazides.
Antimicrobials			
Sulfonamides	UTI.	Sulfasoxazole Trimethoprim-sulfamethoxazole	Monitor fluid balance and urinary pH; may precipitate in acid or concentrated urine.
Urinary tract antiseptics	Chronic UTI.	Methenamine mandelate Nalidixic acid Nitrofurantoin	Will not cure acute infections. Often used in people at high risk of recurrent UTI (neurogenic bladder problems, etc.)
		Phenazopyridine	Mild urinary tract anesthetic.
Hypokalemics	Reduce serum potassium (e.g., in renal failure).	Sodium polystyrene sulfonate exchange resin Glucose and insulin	Can be given rectally or orally. Usually mixed with sorbitol. Not immediately effective. Emergency IV therapy in hyperkalemia.
Hyperkalemics	Elevate serum potassium. Adjunctive therapy with loop and thiazide diuretics.	Potassium hydrochloride	Available in a variety of forms, oral and parenteral. Oral forms are irritating to the GI tract and must be diluted. IV forms are very toxic and must be diluted; give no more than 20 mEq/hr,
Cholinergics	Promote bladder emptying in nonobstructive retention, bladder atony.	Bethanechol chloride	Oral or parenteral.

UTI, urinary tract infection.

semipermeable membrane into the dialysis solution. The semipermeable membrane may be synthetic (as in hemodialysis) or biologic (as in peritoneal dialysis). The amount of a given substance that can diffuse across the membrane depends on the concentration of that substance in the dialysate, the concentration in the blood, the time in which the two are in contact, and the permeability of the membrane.

Peritoneal dialysis involves repeated installations and drainages of dialysis fluid into and from the peritoneal cavity. Access to the cavity is via a rigid peritoneal trocar for single-episode dialysis, or via a flexible tube (a Tenckhoff catheter) for repeated dialysis, as in chronic renal failure. Repeated instillation and drainage can be performed manually or with automatic cycling machines. Typically, a peritoneal dialysis treatment in acute renal failure lasts 24 to 48 hr. Continuous ambulatory peritoneal dialysis has been successfully used in patients with chronic renal failure.

Complications of peritoneal dialysis include peritonitis, pain, difficulty draining dialysate, extravasation into other tissues, and atelectasis.

Unlike peritoneal dialysis, **hemodialysis** requires the expertise of a nephrologist and an experienced hemodialysis team. Only rarely will the general medical-surgical nurse be called upon to assist in hemodialysis. This section therefore deals only with the care of the hemodialysis patient at times other than during dialysis.

In hemodialysis, blood is pumped through an external dialysis machine. In patients with acute renal failure requiring hemodialysis, vascular access is usually via large-bore needles placed in an artery and a vein, or two large veins. However, in patients with chronic renal failure who require long-term hemodialysis, it is usually preferable to place either a shunt or a fistula. A shunt is an external Silastic connection between an artery and a vein. During dialysis, the shunt is opened and connected to the dialysis machine. A fistula is an interior arteriovenous anastomosis. During dialysis, large-bore needles are inserted percutaneously into the fistula.

Other treatment modalities in acute renal failure include the use of hypokalemic adjunctive therapy (*see* Table 17-4) and fluid restriction (*see* Table 17-5). During the diuretic phase of acute renal failure, fluid supplementation may be required.

Nursing interventions

Nursing treatment related to the patient with acute renal failure mainly involves the management of the peritoneal and hemodialysis modalities. Nursing management of peritoneal dialysis is described in Table 17-9; hemodialysis in Table 17-10. (*See also* Table 17-7 for general care.)

CYSTITIS

Cystitis is inflammation of the bladder that usually occurs secondary to bacterial infection. Bacteriuria is very common. In adult females, the prevalence rises ~1%/decade; in elderly females, the prevalence is ~10%.

TABLE 17-5

Dietary Modifications for Patients with Renal and Urinary Disorders

Diet modification	Indications	Guidelines	Comments
Low-protein (e.g., 40 g/day)	Renal failure.	Adhere to dietary exchange system to provide required number of grams of protein. Calculate intake of high-protein foods (meats, fish, poultry, dairy products).	Use in renal failure is variable, depending on other therapy (dialysis, etc.). Patient compliance may be a problem, particularly if also on other restrictions.
Sodium-restricted			
Severe (500 mg/day)	Renal failure.	Limit meat, milk. May require distilled water, depending on area. Provide unlimited amounts of fresh, low-sodium fruits and vegetables. Avoid beets, carrots, celery, spinach. Provide low-sodium breads, grains.	Patient compliance may be a problem, particularly if on other restrictions. Degree of restriction depends on disease status and therapy (e.g., dialysis).
Moderate (1,000 mg/day)		May add ¼ tsp salt to day's food or use regular bread; otherwise like severe restriction.	
Mild (3-4 g/day)		Avoid obviously salty foods, salt-processed foods (e.g., canned vegetables).	
Potassium-restricted (e.g., 1.5-3.0 g/day)	Renal failure.	Avoid high-potassium foods (bananas, citrus fruits, potatoes, tomatoes). Limit use of fish, meat, poultry.	Usually prescribed in combination with other restrictions. Patient compliance may be a problem.

Potassium-supplemented	Adjunctive therapy while on potassium-losing diuretics (thiazides, loop diuretics).	Provide opposite of potassium-restricted diet.	Monitor serum potassium.
Fluid-restricted (e.g., 600-800 ml above insensible loss)	Renal failure.	Limit any food that is liquid at body temperature (water, juice, ice cream, soups, etc.)	Degree of restriction depends on other therapy (dialysis).
Fluid-supplemented (e.g., 3,000 ml/day)	Dehydration, renal calculi, following certain diagnostic tests, urinary tract infection.	Increase intake of food that is liquid at body temperature.	Monitor fluid balance.
Low-oxalate	Oxalate urolithiasis.	Avoid high-oxalate foods (tea, cocoa, coffee, cola, beer, beans, spinach).	
Acid-ash	Phosphate- or struvite-containing urolithiasis.	Limit intake of milk products, certain fruits and vegetables; avoid carbonated beverages, chocolate, baking powder/soda. Encourage meats, eggs, most vegetables.	
Alkaline-ash	Uric acid-containing urolithiasis.	Avoid or limit intake of acid-ash foods. Encourage intake of milk, most vegetables, most fruits. Limit meat and protein intake.	Also known as low-purine diet.
Low-calcium (e.g., 400 mg/day)	Calcium-containing urolithiasis.	Avoid milk and dairy products. Limit intake of leafy vegetables and whole grains.	

TABLE 17-6

Renal and Urinary Tract Surgery

General type of surgery	Specific procedure	Definition	Comment
Removal of renal or urinary tract tissue	Nephrectomy	Removal of a kidney,	May be performed to obtain donor kidney; unilaterally for treatment of tumors, injuries, etc.; bilaterally in some cases of renal failure, predialysis, or pretransplant.
	Heminephrectomy	Removal of a portion of the kidney.	
	Nephroureterectomy	Removal of a kidney and associated ureter.	
	Cystectomy	Removal of the bladder,	Used in treatment of bladder neoplasms.
	Prostatectomy	Removal of all or part of the prostate.	Can be performed transurethrally or via open suprapubic or perineal approach.
	Ureterectomy	Removal of one or both ureters.	
Creation of an artificial opening for drainage of urine	Nephrostomy	Opening directly into the kidney.	May be permanent or temporary,
	Ureterostomy	Urinary diversion from ureter to abdominal wall, often via ileal conduit.	Also known as a Bricker procedure.
	Suprapubic cystostomy	Opening above the symphysis pubis into the bladder,	

Creation of access route for dialysis	Shunt formation	Insertion of partially external Silastic arteriovenous shunt.	May be used immediately for hemodialysis.
	Fistula formation	Internal anastomosis of an artery and vein.	Usually allowed to heal for several weeks before it can be used for hemodialysis.
	Tenckhoff catheter placement	Insertion of abdominal catheter for chronic peritoneal dialysis.	
Removal of urolithiasis	Pyelolithotomy	Removal of uroliths from renal pelvis.	Usually can be attempted transurethrally.
	Nephrolithotomy	Removal of uroliths from renal parenchyma.	
	Ureterolithotomy	Removal of uroliths from ureters.	
	Cystolithotomy	Removal of uroliths from bladder.	
Reconstructive procedures	Ureteroplasty	Reconstruction of the ureter.	Performed following trauma; ureteral stents usually placed.
	Ureteroneocystostomy	Resection of the ureter and reimplantation into a new site in the bladder.	Also known as ureterovesicular anastomosis.
	Vesicourethral suspension	Suspension of the bladder neck to the pubis.	Also known as a Marshall-Marchetti procedure. Used in management of stress incontinence in females.
	Colporrhaphy	Repair of the vaginal wall	Used in the treatment of cystocele.
Kidney transplant		Implantation of donor or cadaver kidney.	Donor treated as for nephrectomy. Performed in chronic renal failure as an alternative to dialysis.

TABLE 17-7

*General Nursing Management of the Patient
with Renal or Urinary Tract Diseases*

Patient problem	Nursing measures
Physical needs Alteration in fluid balance	Monitor serum osmolarity, electrolytes, BUN, creatinine, Hct, urine volume, urine sp gr. Monitor body wt, intake and output, vital signs. Physical assessment for signs of dehydration or overhydration.
Altered ability to void	Noninvasive measures (provide privacy for voiding, assist to standing or semierect position if possible, run tap water, pour warm water over the perineum, place patient's hands in water). Use external urinary drainage devices (condom catheter for male patients with incontinence). Change device daily. Observe for signs of skin breakdown. Do not retract the foreskin. Intermittent bladder catheterization as ordered for postoperative urinary retention, certain types of incontinence. In hospital, use sterile technique; at home, may use clean technique. Indwelling bladder catheterization, as ordered. Use smallest possible catheter. Maintain a closed drainage system. Do not clamp catheter for prolonged periods. Ensure free downward urine flow, change the catheter only if contaminated or clogged, avoid contamination of the drainage spout, separate patients with indwelling catheters, clean around urinary meatus at least bid and following bowel movements, using Betadine and soap and water. Maintain ureteral catheterization system as inserted by physician. Manage as for indwelling bladder catheterization. In addition, be extremely careful to prevent dislodging catheter or impeding free downward flow. Maintain suprapubic cystostomy drainage system inserted by physician. Maintain closed drainage system, change dressing daily. Maintain urinary diversion system created by surgeon. Use pouch drainage system, with skin protectants such as karaya as indicated, connect to drainage device at night. Observe for urinary tract infection, peristomal skin irritation, urolithiasis.
Psychosocial needs Anxiety related to disease	Provide sensory level information in preparation for tests, procedures. Allow as much control over situation as possible.

Patient problem	Nursing measures
Change in body image related to disease and/or therapy	Provide emotional support.
Educational needs Lack of understanding About diet	Dietitian consultation. Allow self-choice of meals while in hospital, with supervision. Include family and significant others in teaching about diet.
About medications	Provide written instructions about medications (indications, side effects to watch for, times to take).

Evaluation criteria. Patient is in fluid and electrolyte balance, has adequate urine drainage, is free from infection, and describes self-care in terms of diet, medications, and other therapy.

In males, the prevalence of cystitis is lower because of the longer urethra but rises as men age, with the increased prevalence of prostate-related problems.

The predisposing factors to cystitis include immunoincompetence (advanced age, malnutrition, debilitating disease), diabetes mellitus, prostate enlargement, and pregnancy. Causative factors include fecal contamination of the external urethra, urinary tract instrumentation (including catheterization), and local irritation ("honeymoon cystitis").

The *signs and symptoms* of cystitis include urinary frequency and urgency, burning on urination, cloudy and/or foul-smelling urine, suprapubic pain, positive urine culture, fatigue, and lassitude. Affected patients are usually afebrile and have no increase in WBCs. Cystitis may be *complicated* by spread of infection to the kidneys.

Diagnosis is based on the health history, physical exam, and positive urine cultures.

Common interventions

Treatment consists of antibiotic therapy, depending on culture and sensitivity report, and prophylaxis against recurrence (*see* Table 17-4).

Nursing interventions

Physical 1. Encourage fluids and a high-protein diet.
Psychosocial 2. Provide emotional support.
Educational 3. Teach patients to aid in the prevention of recurrence through such methods as perineal hygiene, voiding after intercourse and frequently during day, and adequate fluid intake.

TABLE 17-8

Causes of Acute Renal Failure

Type	Causative factors	Predisposing factors
Prerenal	Hypovolemia	Increased fluid loss via the skin, GI tract, or kidneys (osmotic diuresis, diabetes insipidus). Decreased fluid intake (NPO, decreased level of consciousness).
	Cardiac failure	Coronary risk factors.
	Shock/trauma	
	Nonselective vasoconstrictor drug therapy (levarterenol, high-dose dopamine, etc.)	
	Cardiac arrest	MI, respiratory arrest.
Intrarenal	Renal vascular obstruction	
	Transfusion reactions	Anemia, surgery.
	Trauma	
	Nephrotoxins (aminoglycosides, heavy metals, organic solvents)	
	Renal parenchymal disease acute tubular necrosis, glomerulonephritis, pyelonephritis)	
Postrenal	Urolithiasis	
	Prostate enlargement	Male, advanced age.
	Tumors	
	Surgical accidents	GU surgery. Poor surgical risk.

Evaluation criteria.   Patient is pain free, has negative urine culture, and states methods to prevent recurrence.

PYELONEPHRITIS

Pyelonephritis is inflammation of the kidneys that usually occurs secondary to bacterial infection. No reliable statistics are available on the incidence/prevalence of pyelonephritis. Pyelonephritis is usually an ascending infection from the bladder; therefore, the predisposing and causative factors are the same as in cystitis (*see above*).

The *signs and symptoms* of pyelonephritis are fever, with shaking chills; pain or tenderness in flank or costovertebral angle; leukocytosis; elevated WBC in the urine; malaise or fatigue; increased frequency or urgency of

TABLE 17-9

*Nursing Management of the Patient Undergoing Peritoneal Dialysis**

Patient problem	Nursing measures
Physical needs Dependence on proper functioning of dialysis catheter	*For rigid trocar:* Ensure that the trocar is securely fastened to the abdomen, allowing little movement. Routine wound care not indicated if duration of dialysis is <48 hr. *For Tenckhoff catheter:* Routine wound care postoperatively. Before each dialysis treatment: clean carefully with Betadine and saline; use strict aseptic technique. If dialysate fails to drain, reposition the patient. Administer heparin in dialysate as ordered to prevent clotting. Monitor catheter insertion site for drainage around catheter, inflammation.
At risk of infection	Strict aseptic technique in handling peritoneal dialysate solution. Check vital signs frequently. Routinely culture dialysate drainage, usually with first exchange and then q 10th exchange during acute dialysis. Observe for signs of peritonitis (fever, elevated WBC, abdominal pain, cloudy dialysis drainage). Observe dialysis fluid for contamination before instillation.
Alteration in fluid and electrolyte balance	Record cumulative intake and output during acute dialysis procedure. By convention, if the patient retains dialysis fluid, positive fluid balance exists; if more fluid drains out, negative fluid balance exists. Administer proper dialysate solution as ordered (1.50 or 4.25% glucose). A higher glucose concentration will cause a greater negative fluid balance. Add potassium to dialysate solution as ordered, depending upon the serum potassium. Weigh patient before each dialysis treatment and then at least q 24 hr, while abdomen is empty of fluid. Monitor serum chemistries, BUN, creatinine, glucose.
Psychosocial needs Maintenance of comfort during procedure	Position in semi-Fowler's position to decrease pressure of dialysate solution on diaphragm. May turn side to side if drainage in inadequate. With continuous ambulatory peritoneal dialysis, little or no activity restriction. Care for back as needed. Administer analgesics as ordered and required.
Anxiety related to dialysis procedure	Explain all procedures, taking into account the patient's physical status. Maintain quiet environment: eliminate extraneous noise, screen unnecessary personnel. Allow uninterrupted rest periods.

**Evaluation criteria.* There is restoration of fluid and electrolyte balance. Patient is free of pain and infection.

urination; burning during urination; and positive urine culture. *Complications* include renal medullary necrosis, chronic pyelonephritis, fulminating sepsis, and death.

Diagnosis is based on the health history, physical exam, WBC, and urine cultures.

TABLE 17-10

Nursing Management of the Patient Undergoing Hemodialysis *

Patient problem	Nursing measures
Physical needs Dependence on proper functioning of vascular access route	Assess for and prevent complications Thrombosis: Check for bruit, thrill. Check for pain. Do not measure BP or draw blood in affected extremity.
	Infection: *AV shunt:* clean with povidone-iodine at insertion site. Apply dry, sterile dressing. Avoid getting site wet.
	AV fistula: immediately postoperatively, apply dry sterile dressing; clean site daily with povidone-iodine. When wound is healed, does not require dressing. Assess for infection or inflammation at venipuncture site.
	Dislodging of AV shunt: Cover with dressing, wrap in gauze. Keep cannula clamps available at all times.
Educational needs Lack of understanding of self-care for vascular access site	Teach patient to avoid carrying heavy items on affected extremity; avoid heat and cold extremes.
	Teach patient how to apply dry dressing and gauze to AV shunt insertion site.
	Teach patient to recognize conditions that require medical consultation (infection, thrombosis, dislodging).

AV, arteriovenous.
*Evaluation criteria.   Vascular access site is functioning properly, and patient describes self-care.

Common interventions

Treatment consists of the administration of antibiotics, including IV systemically active drugs such as the semisynthetic penicillin derivatives.

Nursing interventions

Physical 1. Administer medications as ordered.
2. Provide adequate fluid, as much as 3,000 ml/day.
3. Frequently check vital signs.
4. Institute measures to reduce fever.
Psychosocial 5. Provide emotional support.
Educational 6. Teach patients methods to aid in preventing recurrence, as for cystitis (*see above*).

Evaluation criteria.   Patient is afebrile, free from pain and complications, has negative urine culture, and states methods to prevent recurrence.

GLOMERULONEPHRITIS

Glomerulonephritis is inflammation of the glomeruli. Although the term actually refers to a variety of glomerulopathies, only acute poststreptococcal glomerulonephritis will be dealt with here. The incidence of this disease is correlated with the incidence of streptococcal infections in the population. Males and children are predisposed to glomerulonephritis. The disease is often associated with prior infection with streptococcus (pharyngitis, tonsillitis, etc.).

The *signs and symptoms* of glomerulonephritis include edema, fluid retention (pulmonary edema, ascites, etc.), headache, hypertension, flank pain, weakness, anorexia, nausea, vomiting, and fever with chills. Renal failure may be a *complication.*

Diagnosis is based on the health history and physical exam. Laboratory findings may include hematuria, proteinuria, elevated BUN and creatinine levels, decreased creatinine clearance, elevated C-reactive protein, and elevated antistreptolysin O (ASO) titer.

Common interventions

Glomerulonephritis may be treated with antibiotics (penicillin or related agents) and steroids.

Nursing interventions

Physical 1. Encourage bed rest.
2. Maintain a high-carbohydrate, low-protein, low-sodium diet.
3. Monitor fluid and electrolyte balance.
Psychosocial 4. Provide emotional support.
Educational 5. Teach the patient to avoid infections.
6. Teach the patient to obtain prompt medical attention for possible streptococcal infections.

Evaluation criteria.   Patient is pain free, has negative urine culture, and states methods to prevent recurrence.

BENIGN PROSTATIC HYPERTROPHY

Benign prostatic hypertrophy is noncancerous enlargement of the prostate gland. Prostatic enlargement occurs in almost all men > 50 yr; by age 60, most men have detectable enlargement. However, not all men with detectable enlargement have symptoms. Males are increasingly predisposed to prostatic hypertrophy with advancing age, most likely due to hormonal changes associated with aging.

The signs and symptoms of prostatic enlargement are similar to those seen in urinary retention (*see above*) and include palpable enlargement of the prostate on rectal examination. *Complications* are similar to those seen in urinary retention (*see above*) and also include bladder wall changes (e.g., hypertrophy, diverticuli).

Diagnosis is based on the health history and physical exam (including a rectal examination). Urethral catheterization is useful to check for post-voiding residual. Prostatic cancer should be ruled out.

Common interventions

Medical treatment consists of prostatic massage, treatment of accompanying infection, and catheterization of the urethra in acute retention. **Surgical** treatment includes transurethral resection of the prostate, suprapubic prostatectomy, and retropubic prostatectomy. **Nursing** care of and evaluation criteria for patients undergoing prostatic surgery are described in Table 17-11.

TABLE 17-11

*Nursing Care of Patients Undergoing Prostatic Surgery** *

Period	Type of care	Intervention
Preoperative	Physical	Ensure adequate urine flow. Maintain indwelling catheterization system. Record intake and output. Administer antibiotics as ordered for UTI.
	Psychosocial	Alleviate preoperative anxiety. Provide sensory level information about planned surgery and expected postoperative course.
	Educational	Follow routine preoperative teaching (*see* Chapter 9).
Postoperative	Physical	Observe for possible complications: hemorrhage, UTI, wound infection, inadequate urine flow (displacement of catheters, strictures following catheter removal), urinary incontinence, impotence (rare following transurethral resection).
		Maintain postoperative drainage system. *For continuous bladder irrigation,* use triple-lumen catheter; regulate rate of flow of fluid into the bladder to maintain pink or clear drainage; if drainage is clear, regulate at ~50-100 ml/hr; closely monitor bladder drainage; exercise strict asepsis in changing irrigating solution; otherwise manage as for routine indwelling urinary catheter. *For suprapubic drainage,* maintain dry, sterile dressing over puncture site — change daily; securely tape

Period	Type of care	Intervention
		catheter to abdomen; otherwise manage as for routine indwelling urinary catheter. *Otherwise,* follow routine postoperative care (*see* Chapter 11).
	Psychosocial	Provide emotional support. Alleviate pain and anxiety.
	Education (discharge teaching)	Teach perineal exercises (tense buttock muscles) to help patients control postoperative problems of dribbling, frequency, or burning. Instruct patients to avoid alcohol because it increases burning on urination. For patients requiring long-term suprapubic drainage, teach reasons for drainage, dressing change technique, how to empty/clean drainage bag, signs and management of catheter obstruction, dangers and prevention of UTI, when to seek medical attention (catheter displacement, leakage, obstruction, infection). Advise patients to drink adequate fluids. Inform them that sexual activity may usually be resumed 6-8 wk following surgery.

UTI, urinary tract infection.
Evaluation criteria.   Patient is free of pain, is afebrile, shows adequate urinary output, and describes outpatient self-care.

BLADDER CANCER

Bladder cancer, a malignant tumor of the bladder wall, is the second most common tumor of the GU tract. Males >50 yr of age are particularly predisposed. Prolonged exposure to carcinogens (e.g., industrial aromatic amines, saccharin, and phenacetin) and smoking may be causative factors.

The *signs and symptoms* of bladder cancer may include gross hematuria, which is usually intermittent; infection; obstruction; and indications of metastatic cancer (e.g., weakness or weight loss). *Complications* may include infection, obstruction, hydronephrosis, renal failure, hemorrhage, and metastases.

Diagnosis is based on the health history and physical exam. Laboratory findings are nonspecific. IV pyelogram, cystoscopy with biopsy, urinary cytology, and urinary or plasma carcinoembryonic antigen evaluation may be useful diagnostic tools.

Common interventions

Medical treatment involves radiation therapy and systemic or local chemotherapy (e.g., 5-fluorouracil, methotrexate, doxorubicin, or thiotepa administered systemically or locally). **Surgical** treatment consists of transurethral resection of the bladder or partial or total cystectomy, with urinary diversion (ureterosigmoidostomy or ileal conduit). **Nursing** care of and evaluation criteria for the patient with bladder cancer are described in Table 17-7.

CANCER OF THE PROSTATE

Cancer of the prostate is a malignant tumor of the prostate gland. It is the most common GU tumor in men and is seen in two-thirds of autopsies in men over the age of 80 yr, and in up to 46% of autopsies in younger men. There are ~25,000 new cases/yr. Predisposing factors include advanced age and a positive family history. Causative factors are unknown, but prostate cancer is *not* causally related to benign prostatic hypertrophy.

Affected patients may experience pain and exhibit *signs and symptoms* of urinary obstruction and infection. *Complications* include metastases to bone (pelvis, femur heads, lower spine) and, less commonly, to skin, lungs, and liver. Obstruction, renal failure, and peripheral/dependent edema from pelvic lymph flow obstruction are other complications.

Diagnosis is based on the health history and physical exam, including a rectal examination. Laboratory findings include elevated serum acid phosphatase. Prostate biopsy may be performed transurethrally or via the perineum. Metastatic work-up is also useful.

Common interventions

Curative methods of treatment include radical prostatectomy with lymph node dissection. Palliative measures consist of radiation therapy and hormonal therapy (diethylstilbestrol, surgical orchiectomy, or medical adrenalectomy [corticosteroids]). **Nursing** care of and evaluation criteria for the patient undergoing prostatic surgery are described in Table 17-11.

CHRONIC RENAL FAILURE

Chronic renal failure is a permanent decrease in the GFR to <30 ml/min. There are between 60,000 and 100,000 deaths/yr from chronic renal failure. Predisposing factors consist of advancing age and a positive family history. Causative factors are associated with either **renal disease,** as in acute renal failure, urinary tract infection, cystic kidney disease, renal vascular disease (clots, stenoses), and urinary tract obstruction; **systemic disease,** as in diabetic nephropathy, connective tissue disease (SLE, etc.), hypertensive nephropathy, and dehydration; or **nephrotoxins.**

The *signs and symptoms* of the uremic syndrome include polyuria, oliguria, or anuria; decreased urine sp gr; elevated serum uric acid, urea, triglycerides, glucose; metabolic acidosis; nausea, vomiting, anorexia, GI bleeding, diarrhea, uremic fetor; infertility, decreased libido, impotence, amenorrhea; fatigue, depression, insomnia, peripheral nephropathy; pleuritis, pulmonary edema; osteodystrophy; hypertension, CHF, pericarditis; anemia, bleeding, immunoincompetence; pallor, pruritus, dry skin, decreased perspiration; and retinopathy. *Complications* include hypertension, heart failure, loss of lean body tissue, sodium and fluid retention, coma, and death.

Diagnosis is based on the health history and physical exam. Laboratory findings may consist of elevated serum creatinine and BUN, decreased creatinine clearance, anemia, hyperphosphatemia, hypocalcemia, hypoproteinemia, and metabolic acidosis.

Common interventions

Renal failure may be treated with chronic hemodialysis or peritoneal dialysis or by renal transplantation. The **nursing** care of and evaluation criteria for the patient undergoing peritoneal dialysis, hemodialysis, and renal transplantation are described in Tables 17-9, 17-10, and 17-12, respectively.

POLYCYSTIC KIDNEY

Polycystic kidney is a type of cystic kidney disease in which there is massive kidney enlargement and multiple cyst formation. The estimated incidence is ~1/5,000 population. The disease is transmitted as an autosomal dominant trait, although symptoms may not be manifested until

TABLE 17-12
Nursing Management of the Renal Transplant Patient*

Type of care	Intervention
Physical	Frequently assess fluid and electrolyte balance (intake and output, vital signs, weight, serum electrolytes, osmolarity).
	Carefully monitor urinary drainage system and IV fluid administration.
	Assess for possible rejection (redness, swelling, pain at insertion site; fever; elevated WBC; decreased urine output; weight gain; rising BUN, creatinine levels; edema; elevated BP; anorexia; decreased creatinine clearance; proteinuria).
	Administer medications as ordered (immunosuppressants such as corticosteroids, azothiaprine, cyclophosphamide).
	Observe for infection.
Psychosocial	Assist patient and family/significant others in accepting change in body image, need for long-term medical care.
Educational	Teach patient to recognize signs of rejection, infection, and when to seek medical attention. Teach patient the side effects of medications.

*Evaluation criteria. Patient is free of pain, is afebrile, displays adequate renal functioning (normal BUN, creatinine, creatinine clearance, urine output), and describes self-care.

an advanced age. Males and females are equally affected. The age at which symptoms appear is apparently also genetically determined.

The *signs and symptoms* of polycystic kidney include enlarged kidneys (usually bilaterally), hypertension, uremia, flank pain, hematuria, urinary tract infection, nephrolithiasis, urinary tract obstruction, and nonrenal manifestations (liver cysts, berry aneurysms). *Complications* consist of chronic renal failure and hypertension.

Diagnosis is based on the health history; physical exam; laboratory tests for urinary protein, serum creatinine, and BUN; renal ultrasound; and renal scan.

Nonspecific, symptomatic treatment is usually employed.

Nursing interventions

Physical 1. Administer care for specific manifestations (*see* above sections on chronic renal failure and urinary tract infection).

Psychosocial 2. Provide emotional support during exacerbations.

Educational 3. Provide genetic counseling to patients in childbearing years.

4. Encourage blood relatives of the patient to undergo medical screening for polycystic kidney disease.

Evaluation criteria. Patient is free of preventable complications, demonstrates self-care, and verbalizes the genetic nature of the disease.

NEPHROTIC SYNDROME

Nephrotic syndrome is a clinical syndrome caused by proteinuria and manifested by hypoalbuminemia, edema, and hyperlipidemia. The incidence of nephrotic syndrome in adults is not known with any certainty; the related condition of nephrosis is more common in children. The causative factors include chronic glomerulonephritis, autoimmune disorders, connective tissue diseases (SLE, amyloidosis), systemic diseases (hypertension, diabetes mellitus), toxins, drug hypersensitivity, toxemia of pregnancy, renal transplantation, congenital influences, renal vein thrombosis, and obstruction of the inferior vena cava.

The *signs and symptoms* of the nephrotic syndrome are peripheral edema (usually pitting), hypertension, muscle wasting, hypoalbuminemia, hypovolemia, and hyperlipidemia. *Complications* include chronic renal failure, accelerated atherosclerosis, infection, and protein malnutrition.

Diagnosis is based on the health history, physical exam, renal biopsy, urine protein electrophoresis (to determine type of protein being excreted in urine), and a 24-hr urine specimen (for protein serum electrolytes, protein, triglycerides).

Common interventions

Treatment depends on the underlying cause. Diuretics (thiazides, spironolactone, etc.) and corticosteroids are often used. In emergency situations, it may be necessary to administer IV salt-poor albumin.

Nursing interventions

Physical 1. For patients with edema, encourage bed rest, provide a high-protein diet, apply support stockings or elastic bandages to the extremities, monitor for skin breakdown, measure intake and output of urine, and obtain daily weights.

Psychosocial 2. Provide emotional support.

Educational 3. Teach the patient to avoid infections.

4. Teach self-monitoring of fluid balance and weight.

Evaluation criteria.   Patient is free of complications, has no edema, and describes medications and diet.

UROLITHIASIS

Urolithiasis is the presence of stones or calculi in the urinary tract. This is one of the most common disorders affecting the urinary tract and accounts for ~200,000 hospital admissions/yr. It is more common in men than women and is rare in black individuals. White males with a positive family history are particularly predisposed. Causative factors include a high-calcium diet, immobilization, bone demineralization, hyperparathyroidism, hypervitaminosis D, urinary tract infection (particularly with urease organisms such as *Proteus*), and abnormal urine pH (digestive/absorptive abnormalities, antacid use, acid-base imbalance, and use of carbonic anhydrase inhibitors).

Patients with urolithiasis may be asymptomatic (depending on the size of stones) or may experience pain (ureteral or renal colic) that is usually sharp and may be intermittent. There may be visible stones in the urine, hematuria, frequency of urination, and urinary tract infection. *Complications* may include obstruction or urinary tract infection.

Diagnosis is based on the health history and physical exam. Laboratory tests may include CBC (particularly WBC); urinalysis (particularly for pH, crystals, frank stones); serum chemistry (BUN, creatinine); kidney, ureter, bladder x-ray; IV pyelogram; renal scan; and cystoscopy (may involve ureteral catheterization).

Common interventions

Conservative therapy consists of hydration and treatment of infection. Surgical therapy depends on the location of the stone (ureterolithotomy, pyelolithotomy, cystolithotomy). Mechanical intervention may include cystoscopy with ureteral catheterization, operative nephroscopy, and intrarenal stone manipulation under fluoroscopy. Stone dissolution may be accomplished by irrigation with renacidin or acetyl cysteine.

Nursing interventions

Physical 1. For pain management during the acute stage, administer analgesics as ordered, apply moist heat to flank, and limit activity.

2. During the acute stage, strain urine for stones and encourage fluids.

Psychosocial 3. Provide emotional support.

Educational 4. Teach the patient to prevent stone recurrence by maintaining a high fluid intake, and by restricting his diet according to the type of stone (calcium stone: low-calcium and low vitamin D diet; oxalate stones: low-oxalate diet; uric acid and cysteine stones: alkaline-ash diet).

Evaluation criteria.   Patient is free of pain and states methods to prevent recurrence.

NEUROGENIC BLADDER

Neurogenic bladder is a dysfunction that occurs secondary to altered innervation of the bladder. It may be flaccid or spastic in nature. Causative factors include spinal cord injury, congenital abnormalities (spina bifida), systemic diseases (multiple sclerosis, diabetes mellitus), and tabes dorsalis.

A spastic bladder may be associated with a loss of conscious urge to void, reduced bladder capacity, and frequent incontinence of small amounts. A flaccid bladder may be associated with loss of conscious urge to void, bladder distension, and overflow incontinence. *Complications* may consist of urinary tract infection, urolithiasis, and renal failure.

Diagnosis is based on the health history, physical exam, measurement of postvoiding residual, voiding cystometrogram, cystogram, and cystoscopy.

Common interventions

Treatment may include catheterization (intermittent or continual), cholinergics (bethanechol chloride), or surgery (urinary diversion).

Nursing interventions

Physical 1. Manage the catheterization system according to Table 17-7, which describes altered ability to void.

2. Record intake and output.

3. Encourage mobility to prevent calculi.

4. Encourage oral fluid intake.

5. Institute bladder training. Provide scheduled daytime fluids, no fluids at night. Stimulate voiding at specified time by increasing abdominal pressure, etc. Measure postvoiding residual by percussion, palpation, and/or catheterization. Gradually lengthen times between stimulation for voiding, based on postvoiding residual and frequency of incontinence.

Psychosocial 6. Provide emotional support.

7. Avoid treating the patient like a child (e.g., with diapers).

Educational 8. Teach the patient perineal strengthening exercises (intermittent tensing of buttocks).

9. Teach the patient the importance of fluid intake and mobility.

Evaluation criteria.   Patient is pain free, has negative urine culture, and states methods to prevent recurrence.

URETERAL/URETHRAL STRICTURE

Urethral or ureteral sticture is an abnormal narrowing of the lumen of the urethra or ureters, respectively. The incidence of strictures in the general population is low, but is relatively common following instrumentation or surgery of the urethra or ureters. Factors that predispose to stricture include GU instrumentation, male sex, advanced age, pelvic surgery, and infections (e.g., gonococci). Causes may consist of prostate enlargement, trauma, and tumors.

The *signs and symptoms* of urethral stricture are similar to those of urinary retention and include absence of voided urine, bladder distension, overflow incontinence, and bladder pain or discomfort. Decreased urine output and flank pain in the absence of bladder distension are more symptomatic of ureteral stricture. *Complications* include urinary tract infection and renal failure.

Diagnosis is based on the health history, physical exam, IV pyelogram, retrograde pyelogram, and cystoscopy.

Common interventions

Treatment may consist of catheterization (ureteral or urethral — may require cystoscopy for placement), ureteral dilation, surgery (urethroplasty/ureteroplasty), or urinary diversion. **Nursing** care of and evaluation criteria for patients with altered ability to void are described in Table 17-7.

CHAPTER 18

ALTERED SEXUAL/ REPRODUCTIVE FUNCTIONING

Harriet R. Nussbaum

OVERVIEW

Human sexuality refers to the totality of feelings and behaviors of an individual with regard to gender identity. This complex subject encompasses, but is not limited to, genital responses. The gender/sex roles — female, male, or homosexual — an individual assumes in overt behavior are indicative of one's gender identity. Sexuality is based on the interaction of physiologic, psychologic, cultural, and social forces that shape an individual's self-concept.

In the changing society of western civilization, three basic values associated with the emerging sexual behavior patterns are the **relativistic utilitarian position**, which sanctions a new morality and evaluates sexual actions on the basis of their effects; the **hedonistic position**, which espouses pleasure as the essence of a sexual relationship; and the **absolutistic position**, which postulates reproduction as the primary purpose of sexuality.

Human sexuality encompasses an array of cultural, emotional, and physical components that promote and denote warmth, concern, and a caring relationship. **Reproduction** refers to the time during which physiologic components of the reproductive system are actively capable of producing germ cells, facilitating conception, and supporting fetal development.

Female reproductive capacity commences with menarche at puberty (~ 11 to 12 yr of age) and concludes with menopause (between 40 and 50 yr of age). Male reproductive capacity commences at puberty (~ 13 yr of age) or when ejaculate first contains mature sperm. It may continue into the ninth decade of life, although there is some decrease in sperm production with advancing years.

Female anatomy and physiology review

Anatomic characteristics and functions of the major organs of the female reproductive system are presented in Table 18-1.

Neuroendocrine interactions control the reproductive cycle: the hypothalamus produces releasing and inhibiting factors; the anterior pituitary secretes pituitary gonadotrophins; and endocrine gonads produce gonadal steroids. Hormones may be classified by their cellular action. **Steroids** enter the cell and react with specific proteins. **Peptides** react with cell membrane that has a sensitive receptor site. They need a target cell with the ability to synthesize proteins and change cell membrane permeability. **Follicle-stimulating hormone (FSH)** is a peptide hormone released by the anterior pituitary in response to decreased hormonal messengers from ovaries. It interacts with designated ovarian cells to facilitate specific changes such as secretion of estrogen and maturation of ova (female germ cells). **Estrogen** is a peripheral steroid hormone that causes growth of endometrial cells of the uterus. **Luteinizing hormone (LH)** is a peptide hormone secreted by the anterior pituitary. Its secretion results in ovulation within a few hours. **Progesterone** is a peripheral steroid hormone released by the ovaries while concurrent production of estrogen is maintained. It further stimulates endometrial growth following ovulation. In response to estrogen and progesterone stimulation, the endometrial glands become distorted and enlarged. Ischemia occurs in the absence of fertilization and implantation and results in continual discharge of the endometrial lining (menstruation/menses). **Menstrual and ovarian cycles** are presented in Table 18-2. Fluctuations and changes may result from excessive emotional, physical, or environmental stresses. The number of primary follicles receptive to FSH or LH stimulation decreases after 33 yr of menstrual cycles (usually by 45 yr of age).

Menopause (female climacteric) is the conclusion of the reproductive cycle. It occurs between 40 and 50 yr of age and results from reduction of primary follicles receptive to FSH and LH stimulation. It lasts from several months to several years and may be accompanied by "hot flashes," anxiety, fatigue, dyspnea, and occasional psychotic states, which are sometimes treated with estrogen replacement therapy. Menopause results in atrophy of the female reproductive organs.

Male anatomy and physiology review

Anatomic characteristics and functions of the major organs of the male reproductive system are presented in Table 18-3.

TABLE 18-1
Female Reproductive System

Organ	Anatomic characteristics	Physiologic functions
External genitalia		
Mons pubis/ mons veneris	Located over symphysis pubis; composed of coarse pubic hair, elevated adipose tissue.	Responds to sexual stimulation.
Labia majora	Two bilobate folds of skin, start from mons pubis and extend to perineum; contain sebaceous and sweat glands; outer surface covered with hair after puberty.	Protect labia minora and urinary and vaginal openings.
Labia minora	Two hairless folds of skin situated medially to the labia majora; possess numerous sebaceous glands and sensory receptors.	Protect clitoris and two Bartholin's glands.
Clitoris	Small oval mass of nerve and erectile tissue located below junction of labia minora.	Plays significant role in female sexual excitement.
Vestibule	Boat-shaped region between labia minora containing	
	Urethral orifice	Serves as external opening for excretion of urine.
	Vaginal orifice	Serves as external opening for coitus.
	Hymen	Serves as membranous covering for vaginal opening.
	Skene's glands	Secrete mucus.
	Bartholin's glands	Produce mucoid secretions facilitating lubrication during coitus.
Internal genitalia		
Ovaries/female gonads	Two glands similar in size to two unshelled almonds, found in upper pelvic cavity, bilaterally to uterus.	Produce ova; secrete female sexual hormones.
Fallopian tubes	Two tubes attached to upper portion of uterus; funnel-	Serve as conduits for transporting ova from ovary to

Organ	Anatomic characteristics	Physiologic functions
	shaped opening (infundi-bulum) contains fingerlike projections (fimbriae) that move ova along to uterus after ovulation.	uterus; are sites of fertiliza-tion (upper ⅓ of tube).
Uterus	Inverted pear-shaped organ located in the pelvic cavity between bladder and rectum; composed of **fundus** (dome-shaped upper part), **body** (central part), and **cervix** (lower, narrow part).	Is involved in menstruation, implantation of fertilized ovum, development of fetus (pregnancy), and termina-tion of intrauterine growth (labor).
Vagina	Tubular, muscular organ lined with mucous mem-brane containing glycogen; decomposition of glycogen into organic acids results in acidic environment.	Serves as corridor for menstrual discharge, coital receptacle for penis, and passageway for birth (lower birth canal).

Adapted from Tortora, G. J., R. L. Evans, and N. P. Anagnostakos. Principles of Human Physiology. Harper & Row, Publishers, Inc., New York. 1982. p. 341–350.

Puberty and reproduction are dependent on secretion of **androgens**. Testosterone is the most significant androgenic hormone and serves the following functions: It binds to plasma proteins; converts to dihydrotestos-terone, which activates genetic transcription into new RNA molecule messengers that are then transformed into new cellular enzymes that cause tissue changes; causes differentiation of external genitalia during fetal development; initiates descent of the testes from the pelvic cavity into the scrotum before birth; stimulates development of secondary male character-istics during adolescence (e.g., pubic, facial, chest hair; thyroid cartilage enlargement; increased bone and skeletal growth resulting in the male physique of narrow hips and broad shoulders); stimulates maturation of sperm; and stimulates growth and development of the male sex organs.

Other hormones are also essential in the male reproductive cycle. FSH is secreted by the anterior pituitary and stimulates production and main-tenance of spermatogenesis. **Interstitial cell-stimulating hormone (ICSH)** is secreted by the anterior pituitary. It stimulates production and maintenance of spermatogenesis and activates interstitial cells of Leydig to produce testosterone (negative feedback mechanism). If the testosterone blood level is high, the hypothalamus does not secrete releasing factors necessary for the anterior pituitary to release ICSH and production of testosterone is inhibited. If the testosterone blood level is low, the process is reversed.

TABLE 18-2
Menstrual and Ovarian Cycles

Phase	Time	Physiology of menstrual cycle	Physiology of ovarian cycle
Menstrual	First 1-5 days in a 28-day cycle.	Uterine discharge of 30-70 ml of blood, epithelial cells, tissue fluid, and mucus.	Growth of ovarian follicle into graafian follicle in response to maximal FSH secretion and minimal LH secretion of the anterior pituitary.
Preovulatory	6th-13th day in a 28-day cycle; immediately follows menstruation.	Increase of estrogens; proliferation and repair of endometrium is stimulated.	Maturation of graafian follicle in concert with rising estrogen production, which also provides feedback to anterior pituitary to release abundant amount of LH.
Ovulation	14th day in a 28-day cycle.	Continued growth of endometrium.	Release of ovum by graafian follicle to start journey in fallopian tube; graafian follicle degenerates forming corpus luteum.
Postovulatory	15th-28th day in a 28-day cycle; immediately follows ovulation.	Endometrial preparation awaiting fertilized ovum; drop in estrogen and progesterone levels results in menses.	Increasing amounts of estrogen and progesterone secreted by the corpus luteum stimulate endometrial growth; in absence of fertilization, corpus luteum regresses, decreasing output of estrogen and progesterone.

FSH, follicle-stimulating hormone; LH, luteinizing hormone.
Adapted from Tortora, G. J., R. L. Evans, and N. P. Anagnostakos. Principles of Human Physiology. Harper & Row, Publishers, Inc.,, New York. 1982. p. 351-355.

TABLE 18-3
Male Reproductive System

Organ	Anatomic characteristics	Physiologic functions
External genitalia Scrotum	Superficial fascia and loose skin of abdominal wall that forms a pouch; internally, septum divides scrotum into two sacs, each containing a single testis.	Serves as structural support for testes.
Testes	Paired oval glands, covered by tunica albuginea (white fibrous tissue), which divides each testis into lobules; internal compartments contain several coiled (seminiferous) tubules.	Produce sperm by seminiferous tubules; produce testosterone.
Penis	Composed of **glans** (distal, slightly enlarged region covered by foreskin or prepuce; contains external opening for urethra); and **shaft** (three cylindrical masses of spongelike erectile tissue); **corpora cavernosa** (two lateral masses of tissue with large venous spaces); and **corpus spongiosum** (medially located, contains spongy urethra, and has rich blood and nerve supply).	Serves as organ for excretion of urine; vehicle for introduction of sperm into vagina and genital sexuality; during sexual excitation, penile arterial dilation occurs, with increased blood in venous sinuses resulting in erection; penile arterial constriction results in decreased venous pressure and flaccid penile state.
Epididymis	Highly coiled tube attached to each testis; lies within scrotum.	Serves as sperm maturation and sperm storage site.
Vas deferens	Thicker, less-coiled tail of each epididymis; major portion found in pelvic cavity; enters abdomen through inguinal canal.	Propels sperm toward urethra by peristaltic contractions of muscular layer during ejaculation.

Internal genitalia		
Vas deferens	Lies in pelvic cavity; ascends along posterior margin of testis and encircles top and side of bladder,	As above,
Spermatic cord	Composed of cremaster muscle (band of circular skeletal muscle), autonomic nerves, testicular artery, and veins that drain testes.	Provides structural support of male reproductive system.
Inguinal canal	Small opening in interior abdominal wall.	Provides access to abdominal cavity.
Ejaculatory ducts	~2 cm in length; located posterior to and on each side of the bladder.	Serve as conduits for semen from each vas deferens to prostatic urethra.
Urethra	Tube ~20 cm long that passes through prostate gland and penis.	Serves as passageway for urine, sperm, and liquid portion of semen.
Accessory glands		
Seminal vesicles	Two convoluted pouchlike structures ~5 cm long, located behind bladder,	Secrete alkaline viscous fluid rich in fructose into ejaculatory duct.
Prostate gland	Doughnut-shaped gland about size of chestnut; lies beneath bladder and surrounds upper portion of urethra.	Secretes alkaline fluid into urethra and gives semen milky appearance,
Bulbourethral/Cowper's glands	Situated beneath prostate, on each side of urethra; about the size of a pea.	Secrete mucus for lubrication, giving semen a mucoid consistency.
Semen/seminal fluid	Composed of secretions of seminal vesicles, bulbourethral gland, prostate gland, and sperm.	Contains an average of 50-120 million spermatozoa/ml; if number of spermatozoa is <20 million/ml, male sterility is probable.

Adapted from Tortora, G. J., R. L. Evans, and N. P. Anagnostakos. Principles of Human Physiology. Harper & Row, Publishers, Inc., New York. 1982. p. 339–343.

Fertility declines with age. Spermatogenesis decreases after 50 yr of age and testosterone blood levels decrease after 60 yr of age. Sensual reactions and responses are slower and delayed. Male climacteric is exhibited in a small number of men beyond 60 yr of age. *Symptoms* include weight loss and/or poor appetite; impaired concentration; listlessness, irritability, weakness, and easy fatigability; and decreased libido with loss of potency. *Diagnosis* is based on subnormal blood levels of testosterone (<325 mg/100 ml). Treatment consists of replacement therapy, which causes remission of previous symptoms after 2 mo.

General assessment

Before evaluating a patient's sexual health, nurses must examine their own knowledge, attitudes, values, beliefs, behaviors, and feelings with regard to human sexuality, because these factors influence nursing practice. The health history should emphasize the following components: current health status, including drugs (*see* Table 18-4 for medications that affect sexual ability) and sexuality, e.g., perception of the self as male or female, heterosexual, homosexual, or bisexual; family planning or use of contraceptives (Table 18-5); satisfaction or concerns about current sexual relationships; past health history, especially chronic illnesses (*see* Table 18-6 for conditions that affect sexual function) and obstetric data for females (e.g., the age of onset of menses, educational preparation for puberty, presence or absence of menstrual/gynecologic problems, and history of pregnancies or abortions); relationships within the family and social histories; and review of systems (e.g., GU with gynecologic and mental status). The physical exam should emphasize the GU system and breast and rectal examinations. Diagnostic tests include a Pap smear and serum hormonal levels.

Common interventions

Medical interventions consist of the administration of drugs such as contraceptives. **Surgical** techniques include vasectomy, aspiration/suction, tubal ligation, and abortion.

Nursing interventions

Physical 1. Provide preoperative and postoperative care, as necessary (*see* Chapters 9 and 11).

2. Maintain comfort and privacy.

Psychosocial 3. Encourage the patient to verbalize feelings, attitudes, beliefs, and values related to human sexuality.

4. Explore areas of concern regarding sexual performance, expectations, and functioning.

Educational 5. Increase the patient's knowledge of basic sexual anatomy and physiology.

6. Teach the patient and significant others appropriate contraceptive techniques.

7. Explain (in consultation with a physician) when patients can resume usual routines, including sexual relations, after medical or surgical intervention.
8. Refer patients to appropriate agencies (Planned Parenthood, gay rights organizations, sexual therapist, etc.) as indicated.

Evaluation criteria

Patient and/or family (significant other) demonstrates a greater understanding of human sexuality (e.g., describes personal sexual values, attitudes, and beliefs; describes anatomy and physiology of sexuality and contraception; and states relevant community resources). Patient and/or family demonstrates personal capacity to cope with realities and stresses of sexuality related to physical and psychologic status (e.g., verbalizes anxiety or displays a decrease in previous level of anxiety; discusses personal sexual status with significant others; states options available to meet sexual needs and selects option based on own need; and describes satisfaction with adjusted sexual behavior).

TABLE 18-4
Major Medications Affecting Sexual Ability

Class and use	Effect
Antipsychotics and antidepressants: tranquilizers used in schizophrenia, depression, neurologic problems, enuresis in children.	Changes in libido, altered sexual responsiveness, e.g., inhibition/ depression of ejaculation, amenorrhea, decreased sperm count.
Amphetamines: used for CNS depression, anorexia, narcolepsy, hyperkinetic children.	Impotence, changes in libido — especially decreased in women.
Antispasmodics: used for GI disturbances.	Impotence.
Antiparkinsonians: used for parkinsonism.	Increased sexual feelings and libido.
Cytotoxins: used in cancer and psoriasis.	Sterility, decreased libido and sperm production, impotence, amenorrhea.
Hormonal steroids: used as contraceptives and for deficiency problems.	Decreased libido, depression.

Adapted from Mims, F. H., and M. Swenson. Sexuality: A Nursing Perspective. McGraw-Hill Book Co., New York. 1980. p. 232-233.

TABLE 18-5
Major Contraceptive Measures

Types	Method	Action	Comment
Natural	Coitus interruptus/withdrawal; penis removal prior to ejaculation.	Decreases number of sperm left in vagina.	Popular among adolescents; not considered very effective, as male preejaculate contains sperm; frustrating for both partners.
	Periodic abstinence/rhythm method: capitalizes on regular menstrual cycles and viability of sperm and ova not exceeding 48 hr.	Abstinence from intercourse.	~86% effective; requires abstinence 3 days before and 3 days after ovulation.
Oral	Combination of estrogen and progestogen tablets taken daily for 20-21 days, followed by 7 days without medication.	Suppresses ovulation by altering normal ovarian cycle.	100% effective if taken correctly; variety of side effects contraindicate use in a number of health problems; withdrawal bleeding possible.
	Progestogen.	Produces hostile cervical mucus and endometrium, which inhibit implantation.	97% effective; major discomfort is unpredicted bleeding.
Postcoital	Oral or parenteral administration of high doses of estrogens given within 24 hr after an episode of unprotected intercourse during single menstrual cycle.	Affects implantation process and interferes with transport of ovum.	Most frequently used for rape victims.

	Injection of long-acting progestogen (2-4 times/yr).	Interferes with menstrual cycle; lactation is not suppressed.	Causes amenorrhea; possible delay in fertility after discontinuation; weight increase can result.
Chemical and mechanical barriers	Spermicides: manufactured as jellies, foams, and creams (inserted to cover cervix).	Serve as barrier to sperm penetration; chemical composition decreases sperm viability.	~60-70% effective.
	Condom/sheath/skin prophylactic: placed over penis.	Serves as barrier to sperm by restricting sperm motility into the vagina.	80% effective; provides some prophylaxis against gonorrhea; male responsibility to prevent conception.
	Diaphragm: inserted 2 hr before coitus and maintained in place for a minimum of 6-8 hr (should be used with diaphragmatic contraceptive cream/jelly).	Serves as a barrier to sperm motility and viability.	Requires proper fitting, insertion and removal by woman before and after coitus.
	Intrauterine device (IUD)	Endometrial reaction to foreign body results in hostile environment for sperm implantation.	95-98% effective; should be inserted toward end of normal menses to be certain client is not pregnant; adverse reactions to insertion: syncope/cervical shock in small number of women requires symptomatic treatment and/or immediate removal of IUD.

Types	Method	Action	Comment
Surgical	Vasectomy: permanent severing of vas deferens by surgical intervention.	Permanent barrier to ejaculation of sperm.	100% effective except for first 6 wk after procedure.
	Aspiration/suction: ~ 10-12 days following delay of the expected date of menstruation by any of the following means; endometrial aspiration, menstrual regulation, menstrual extraction, menstrual induction, menstrual planning.	Involves suction or aspiration techniques.	Performed before confirmation of pregnancy; less costly than a therapeutic abortion.
	Tubal ligation: permanent closure of fallopian tubes by surgical intervention.	Permanent barrier to fertilization of sperm in fallopian tubes.	100% effective; will not alter menstrual cycle.
	Abortion: Early first trimester: performed during first 6 wk of gestation; involves cervical dilation followed by trans-cervical aspiration.	Performed under local anesthesia; products of conception are removed by suction.	Documented as safe for termination of early pregnancy.
	Later first trimester: performed during 6th-13th wk of pregnancy; same procedure as early trimester abortion is recommended.	Performed under general anesthesia; includes use of curette for scraping inner uterine walls.	Vital signs monitored for 3 hr after procedure.

		Physically exhausting; requires the following nursing care: check vital signs, measure intake and output, provide for oral and physical hygiene, offer support to patient and family, administer medication as indicated, utilize breathing and relaxation techniques, relate progression of labor.
	Performed under general anesthesia; results in rapid labor and delivery of fetus and placenta within 12 hr.	
Midtrimester: performed after first 22 wk of pregnancy; involves induction of labor by injection of prostaglandin.		

Adapted from Barnard, M. U., B. J. Clancy, and K. E. Krantz. Human Sexuality for Health Professionals. W. B. Saunders Co., Philadelphia. 1978. p. 97–127.

DEVIATIONS

SEXUAL ASSAULT/RAPE

As American society has become more open about human sexuality, attitudes toward sexual assault and rape have changed. Extensive coverage regarding the legal, social, psychologic, and cultural aspects of sexual offenses is given by the press, on television, and in the courts. In the USA, sexual offenses against women are the fastest-growing crimes of violence. In the past, studies were primarily concerned with the victim as "provoker" of the crime, and prevention was suggested by courses in self-defense. Only within the last few years has attention been paid to assisting the victim through this crisis period — especially with her physical, emotional, social, and sexual reactions following the traumatic experience.

According to Woods, **sexual assault** is defined as manual, genital, or oral contact with the genitalia of another person without the consent of that individual. **Rape** is a crime of violence expressed through the sexual act. It is legally defined as "carnal knowledge of a person by force and against that person's will." Even minimal penetration or contact with the labia majora by male genitalia constitutes carnal knowledge. The presence of sperm from an ejaculation or laceration of the hymen is considered to be additional evidence of carnal knowledge. In 1979 the incidence of rape was 34.5/100,000 inhabitants, representing a 12% increase when compared with the rate for 1978, a 31.2% increase when compared with the rate for 1975, and an 84% increase when compared with the rate for 1970. The majority of victims are women between the ages of 15 and 25 yr, although infants and aged persons are also victims. A high percentage of the victims are unmarried and from lower social classes.

Erroneous cultural stereotypes contribute to the picture of the rapist as a virile male who is enticed by a seductive woman and succumbs to sexual frustrations through violent sexual acts. The rapist is seen as a sex fiend with perverted, insatiable desires. Some clinical investigations document rape as an expression of anger and/or power through a sexual act motivated by hostility and control, rather than by passion.

Certain factors within the background of the assailant can contribute to his pathology. He may be a person with psychologic problems — i.e., distrustful and lacking warmth, compassion, empathy, and an intimate, emotionally satisfying relationship with another individual. A small proportion of rapists are psychotic and mentally defective. Cultural misconceptions attribute the availability of pornography, alcohol, and drugs as contributing to the incidence of violent sexual acts.

Rape creates a crisis situation. The biologic and psychologic responses of the rape victim are influenced by demographic factors (e.g., social class, ethnicity, and culture) as well as the personality of the individual and her interpersonal relationships. Table 18-7 summarizes the primary physiologic and psychologic symptomatology of female victims.

Diagnosis is based on the health history, physical exam (noting vaginal penetration or unusual force), and laboratory tests for sperm ejaculate.

Common interventions

Medical treatment consists of the institution of prophylactic antibiotic therapy for VD (penicillin and probenecid). If the victim is allergic to penicillin, spectinomycin can be administered; serial blood tests are required for follow-up, because syphilis is not prevented by this antibiotic. Table 18-5 describes pregnancy prevention. Victims should be referred to a rape crisis center for crisis intervention.

Nursing interventions

Physical 1. Promptly provide the patient with a private and supportive environment.
2. Observe physical appearance, emotional status, mental status.
3. Acquire a nursing history, including circumstances of the offense, description of assailant, details of attack, use of weapons, physical/verbal abuse.
4. Collect objective data, including signs of trauma (emotional, physical, and gynecologic), and specimens of semen, clothing, and pubic hair.
5. Provide comfort measures, including preparation for and support during pelvic examination, water and soap for washing up, mouthwash if desired, juice or other beverage to promote nutrition and relaxation.

Psychosocial 6. Demonstrate empathy for the patient in an extremely traumatic situation.
7. Evaluate situational supports, coping mechanisms, and realistic perception of event.
8. Provide the patient with an opportunity to ventilate her feelings, and prepare for relating the experience to significant others.
9. Offer assistance in decision-making about which significant others to notify and who will notify them.
10. Ensure safe and supportive transportation for the patient to return home.
11. Follow up with a telephone call within 24 to 48 hr and periodically for the first 3 mo to ascertain how the individual is coping and if more intensive counseling is indicated.

Educational 12. Inform the patient of the phases of responses to rape as experienced by other victims (Table 18-8).
13. Refer for follow-up to appropriate community resources – e.g., Community Mental Health Center, Crisis Intervention Center, Rape Crisis Intervention Program, Home Health Agency – for community health nursing visits.
14. Review the physician's instructions regarding medications prescribed; include written instructions to ensure a source of reference for the patient at home.

TABLE 18-6
Chronic Conditions Affecting Sexual Functions

Condition	Sexual effects	Nursing implications
Diabetes mellitus	Male: varying degrees of impotence. Female: dyspareunia, monilial infection, amenorrhea (adolescents).	Attend to sexual needs of patient when planning and working with chronic illness. a. Assess biologic, psychologic, and sociologic influences on sexual functioning. b. Investigate multiple factors that may cause sexual dysfunction; do not assume organicity. Observe for increased incidence of sexual dysfunction with duration of diabetes. a. Uncontrolled male diabetics may experience transient impotence. b. Controlled male diabetics may suffer from permanent impotence. c. Female diabetics may experience decreased vaginal lubrication. d. Fertility disturbances can cause alterations in self-concept (*see* section on fertility). Determine need for genetic counseling regarding disease transmission.
Hypertension	Erectile and ejaculatory problems, libidinal changes.	Advise patient that sexual activity need not be restricted if BP is monitored appropriately; coitus can be resumed following a cerebrovascular accident.

MI	Decreased libido, anxiety, and withdrawal from sexual activity.	Investigate sexually provocative behavior of past MI patient (may be indicative of anxiety about sexuality, resulting in alteration in self-concept) (*see* section on impotence).
		Inform patient that increases in respiratory rate, cardiac rate, and BP are not very different during sexual response cycle than to other forms of exercise.
		Individualize sexual restrictions; gradually resume activity of precoronary state.
		Discuss avoiding overprotective attitude toward sexuality with patient and significant other.
Paraplegia/ quadriplegia	Erectile or ejaculatory problems, altered orgasm, male often infertile, female unaltered fertility.	Stress importance of individualized program to provide optimal sexual gratification.
		Refer for counseling as necessary.
Renal disorders	Impotence, spermatogenic dysfunction, steroidogenic dysfunction.	Be aware that uremia and dialysis therapy may cause feelings of inadequacy and dependency affecting self-concept (*see* section on impotence).
		Renal transplantation may reverse altered sexual functioning.
		Renal failure affects fertility; unusual for male and female patients to achieve conception.

Adapted from Woods, N. F. Human Sexuality in Health and Illness. **C. V. Mosby Co.,** St. Louis, 1979. p. 314-316.

TABLE 18-7
Clinical Manifestations of the Rape Victim

Effect	Description
Physiologic	
Genital injury	Abrasions, lacerations of anal and perineal areas including vagina, cervix, hymen, labia minora and majora; vaginal bleeding; vaginismus and dyspareunia.
Body injury	Trauma, stab wounds, lacerations to face, arms, breasts, other body parts.
Pregnancy	Determine risk factor by assessment of fertility status, e.g., last menstrual period and contraceptive usage.
VD	Evaluate risk factor by collection of laboratory specimens including urethral and cervical smears for gonorrhea and serology for syphilis.
Psychologic	
Initial response	Various degrees of anxiety from moderate to extreme; terror, shock, fear, trembling, anger, crying, exhaustion, and mental fatigue; delays in seeking assistance from police, medical, and psychologic support systems.
Emotional response	Repression of direct anger against rapist by projecting onto medical and police investigations; suppression of anger resulting in self-doubt, guilt, and shame.
Developmental response	Dependent on stage of life cycle and tasks to be achieved, e.g., child and preadolescent especially vulnerable because of undeveloped understanding of sexuality; additional trauma generated by requirement of a pelvic examination; affects future sexual relationships with men.
Sociocultural response	Actively seek support or withdraw from significant others (e.g., parents, husband, close friends, professionals and other social groups). The positive or negative reactions of significant others can markedly influence the victim's adjustment.

Adapted from Hogan, R. Human Sexuality: A Nursing Perspective. Appleton-Century-Crofts, East Norwalk, Conn. 1980. p. 152–160.

Prevention 15. Encourage vigilance at home:
    a. Keep doors locked and curtains on windows.
    b. Vary daily routines.
    c. Leave lights on.
    d. Avoid riding alone in elevators with a stranger.
    e. Develop a trusting relationship with a neighbor.

TABLE 18-8
Phases of Responses to Rape

Phase	Duration	Behavior
I	Several days to several weeks.	Acute distress, shock, disbelief, emotional breakdown, change in normal behavior.
II (outward adjustment)	Several days to weeks after episode.	Return to normal life-style, outwardly composed, "pseudo-adjustment," denial, rationalization, rejection of professional counseling.
III (integration and resolution)	Weeks to months after occurrence.	Consciously seeks to verbalize about experience, resolve her feelings.

Adapted from Woods, N. F. Human Sexuality in Health and Illness. C. V. Mosby Co., St. Louis. 1979. p. 258–259.

16. Encourage the patient to use caution when outdoors:
    a. Plan a route in advance and walk at a steady pace.
    b. Avoid clothing that inhibits movement.
    c. Quickly change direction toward a frequented area if followed.
    d. Scream, if danger is suspected.
    e. Lock car and check back seat before getting into car.
    f. Ride with friends when possible.
    g. Ask taxi driver to wait while entering building.
17. Educate the community — especially high-risk populations — through school, college, and occupational health programs.

Evaluation criteria. See Overview. Untoward effects of crisis have been prevented/minimized. Patient verbalizes phases of rape, procedures and medications prescribed (including side effects, frequency, etc.), and follow-up medical regimen.

GONORRHEA

Gonorrhea ("clap," "drip," "GC") is an acute epithelial infection involving the urethra, cervix, and/or rectum. Other parts of the body may also be involved. It is the most common venereal disease, affecting an estimated 3 million Americans annually, and has its highest incidence among young men (15 to 24 yr of age). Sexually active persons increase their risk of exposure, and males are affected three times as often as females. *Neisseria gonorrhoeae* is the infecting organism and has an incubation period of 2 to 7 days.

Affected males exhibit *symptoms* of urethritis, dysuria, increased frequency of urination, and burning on urination. Females are 40 to 80%

asymptomatic, with the first signs of infection being purulent vaginal discharge, labial tenderness, and low back pain. *Complications* of untreated gonorrhea include fibrosis, causing urethral stricture, and prostatic and epididymis involvement, resulting in sterility from adhesions in males, and cystitis and salpingitis, causing sterility in females.

Diagnosis is based on the health history, physical exam, and positive Gram stain culture for diplococci obtained from the urethra in males and the cervical os in females.

Common Interventions

Medical treatment consists of antibiotic therapy (e.g., procaine penicillin, probenecid, or spectinomycin if the patient is allergic to penicillin. Two cultures should be obtained after treatment is initiated.

Nursing interventions

Physical 1. Offer additional fluids to increase urine output.
   2. Encourage hygienic measures, especially washing hands after urination and defecation.
   3. Relieve discomfort with sitz baths.
   4. Provide pads for excessive drainage (e.g., male, athletic supporter; female, perineal pad).
Psychosocial 5. Provide emotional support and encourage the patient to express his or her feelings.
   6. Maintain a nonjudgmental attitude.
   7. Aid the patient in deciding how to inform his or her partner that the patient has VD (e.g., role playing, writing a note, offering to be available at appropriate time).
Educational 8. Provide the patient with accurate information regarding diagnosis and treatment.
   9. Provide appropriate referrals (e.g., local health department or VD clinic) for follow-up of sexual contacts.
Prevention 10. Educate high-risk populations about gonorrhea, including misconceptions, symptoms, complications, etc.
   11. Stress the importance of regular medical examinations, especially for sexually active individuals.
   12. Emphasize good hygiene – bathing or showering frequently, especially cleaning sex organs before and after coitus.
   13. Stress the importance of early detection and prompt treatment on first sign of symptoms.

Evaluation criteria. *See* Overview. Patient verbalizes symptoms, early diagnosis, and treatment of disease. Plans for follow-up and prevention (including contacts) are implemented.

SYPHILIS

Syphilis ("bad blood," "syph," "lues") is an acute or latent systemic disease resulting from direct contact with infectious lesions. It is the third most common venereal disease and may be congenital or acquired. Sexually active individuals run a high risk of infection. *Treponema pallidum* is the infecting organism.

The primary stage of syphilis is highly contagious and lasts 4 to 12 wk. It is *characterized* by a painless, indurated lesion (chancre) that develops at the site of sexual contact. Healing occurs without generating other symptoms. The secondary stage occurs 1 to 6 mo after exposure, when the spirochetes enter the bloodstream, causing spread of disease in the body. *Symptoms* include solar, palmar, and/or body rash (contagious); loss of hair; sore throat; mucous patches in mouth; weight loss; anorexia; fever; headache; and anemia. The tertiary or latent stage follows 2 to 4 yr of generalized infection with the organism. Progressive system involvement, including the heart and circulatory and nervous systems, ensues.

Diagnosis is based on the health history, physical exam, Venereal Disease Research Laboratory (VDRL) test, *Treponema pallidum* immobilization (TPI) test, and fluorescent treponemal antibody absorption (FTA-ABS) test.

Common interventions

Medical treatment consists of antibiotic therapy, usually with benzyl penicillin in one or more doses as needed. Additional medications may be used, depending on the stage of the disease.

Nursing interventions

1. Refer to gonorrhea (*see above*) for additional interventions.
Physical 2. Isolate the patient for 24 hr after the start of treatment if the patient is in the secondary stage.
Educational 3. Instruct the patient to avoid contact with untreated partners.
4. Administer nontreponemal tests q 3, 6, and 12 mo for patients with primary syphilis.
5. Administer nontreponemal tests q 3, 6, and 12 mo and a serology test annually for patients with secondary stage syphilis.

Evaluation criteria. See Overview. Refer to gonorrhea (*see above*). Isolation is maintained as appropriate.

HERPES GENITALIS

Herpes genitalis is a sexually transmitted disease causing infection of the genital tract. It is the second most common venereal disease, with an estimated 300,000 to 500,000 new cases occurring each year. Between 1960 and 1979 there was a ninefold increase in patient visits to physicians for treatment of genital herpes. Predisposing factors include direct contact with the virus via a break in the skin or mucous membrane (skin-to-skin contact with infected body part). Possible precipitating factors in recurrent disease include local trauma, sunlight, coitus, poor health, and emotional stress. Herpes simplex virus (HSV) type 2 enters the nervous system at the site of infection, usually the sacral or trigeminal ganglia. Classification depends on the stage of the disease. **Primary infection** is described as the first clinical episode, acute phase, absence of antibodies to HSV, most severe outbreak, or lesions that last for 7 to 21 days. **Initial infection** is indicated by the ' presence of HSV antibodies with the appearance of the first clinical symptoms (previous infection was asymptomatic); lesions last for 7 to 21 days. **Recurrent disease** reveals a high antibody titer, at least one previous experience of the disease, decreased frequency and milder symptoms, and lesions lasting for 4 to 10 days.

Symptoms include itching, burning, tingling, and tenderness of the affected area; dysuria; edema; lymphadenopathy; neuralgia; and white, thin discharge. The first eruption consists of a fluid-filled vesicle/papule, which heals spontaneously. The lesion is considered infectious until completely healed. In females the lesions appear on the perineum, vagina, or vulva and may be excruciatingly painful if urine contacts them. In males the lesions appear on the penis, causing urethral discharge, pain, etc. *Complications* include perinatal infections of newborns and a greater risk of developing cervical cancer.

Diagnosis is based on the health history, physical exam, and tissue culture (swabbing infected area and streaking swab on laboratory culture of live tissue cells) that reveals cell destruction, but the virus itself is not seen. A Pap smear (scraping of cells from the infected area and visualizing on a slide) reveals multinucleated giant cells. An antibody titer is used to determine the stage of infection (primary/initial titer is not diagnostic because it reveals past infection).

Common interventions

Medical treatment involves topical use of a newly developed antiviral drug, acyclovir (Zovirax), which decreases symptoms in the initial stage of infection and decreases "viral shedding" in recurrent infection. Sitz baths, warm compresses, and the administration of local anesthetics or analgesics may help to relieve pain.

Nursing interventions

Physical 1. Provide comfort measures, including warm compresses and sitz baths.
2. Administer analgesics as prescribed.

3. Use aseptic techniques and gloves − especially if direct contact is made with oral, genital, or pharyngeal secretions − to prevent herpetic whitlow (HSV infection of fingers).

Psychosocial 4. Encourage the patient and significant others to express fears, anxieties, and concerns about the condition.

5. Provide emotional support to the patient and significant others through an accepting, empathetic relationship.

Educational 6. Instruct the patient and significant others about the disease, epidemiology, pathology, and treatment.

7. Inform the patient about "asymptomatic viral shedding" (absence of clinical symptoms yet capable of transmitting disease), which occurs in < 10% of afflicted individuals and presents serious psychosocial conflicts; e.g., should an afflicted individual kiss or have genital contact with a loved one (child or adult), since disease transmission is possible.

8. Teach the patient about follow-up plans and community resources − e.g., the American Social Health Association has formed an organization called Herpes Resource Center (Box 100, Palo Alto, Calif. 94302), which offers support and information to afflicted individuals.

9. Stress the importance of maintaining a health-promoting life-style, including a well-balanced diet, regular exercise, and periods of relaxation.

Prevention 10. Implement medical asepsis.

11. Provide information to high-risk, sexually active individuals about the course of the disease.

Evaluation criteria. Refer to gonorrhea (*see above*).

PELVIC INFLAMMATORY DISEASE

Pelvic inflammatory disease (PID) is an infection of the pelvic cavity, affecting the fallopian tubes (salpingitis), ovaries (oophoritis), pelvic peritoneum, and pelvic vascular system. It constitutes 15 to 20% of gynecologic admissions in indigent urban areas. Untreated local infections that ascend to the pelvic reproductive organs predispose the patient to the disease. The infecting organisms include *Neisseria gonorrhoeae*, streptococcus, staphylococcus, and tubercle bacilli.

Symptoms include fever, abdominal pain, malaise, vaginal discharge, and leukocytosis. Sterility is a *complication* of an untreated condition.

Diagnosis is based on the health history, physical exam, cervical and urethral smears, hysterosalpingography (tuberculous salpingitis), and laparoscopy that reveals tubal strictures.

Common interventions

Medical treatment of PID depends on the infecting organism, but systemic antibiotics are generally used. Isolation techniques are followed if tuberculous salpingitis is diagnosed.

Nursing interventions

1. Refer to gonorrhea (*see above*) for additional interventions.
Physical 2. Use aseptic technique in providing care.
3. Instruct the patient and other health personnel regarding proper hand-washing, administration of perineal pads, disposal of perineal pads, and proper disinfection (linen, toilet seats, bedpans, eating utensils).
4. Position the patient in semi-Fowler's position to increase drainage.
5. If the patient is febrile, force fluids and administer antipyretic medications as ordered.
Psychosocial 6. Explain the purpose of aseptic techniques to the patient and significant others to alleviate anxiety.

Evaluation criteria. Refer to gonorrhea (*see above*). Aseptic technique is implemented. Drainage within pelvic area is promoted.

VAGINITIS

Vaginitis is an infection of the vaginal canal and is a common occurrence in women; increasing incidence may be stress related. There are three main types of vaginitis: trichomoniasis, moniliasis/candidiasis, and atrophic/senile vaginitis. These three types are discussed below.

Trichomoniasis

Trichomoniasis vaginitis is caused by a change in pH of mucosal secretions, resulting in overgrowth of normal vaginal flora. The causative organism is *Trichomonas vaginalis*, a protozoan. *Symptoms* include vaginal discharge (yellow-brown/yellow-white and malodorous), burning, and itching. *Diagnosis* is based on the health history, physical exam, and bacteriologic examination of a specimen. **Medical** treatment involves the oral administration of metronidazole (Flagyl), but vaginal suppositories of Flagyl are recommended if the infection is chronic. **Nursing** interventions are as follows:

1. Refer to gonorrhea (*see above*) for additional interventions.
Physical 2. Use a vinegar douche followed by medicated suppository, jelly, etc.
3. Provide symptomatic relief (e.g., sitz baths).
4. Emphasize hygienic measures after voiding and defecating.
Educational 5. Educate the patient regarding the diagnosis, treatment, medication, dosage, side effects, etc.
6. Instruct the patient to avoid alcohol during the period of drug administration because, when used concomitantly, Flagyl may cause nausea, vomiting, hot and flushed sensations.
Prevention 7. Instruct the patient to wear cotton underwear and loose-fitting pants to permit natural ventilation.
8. Instruct the patient to wear a loose nightgown/shift without underpants when at home.

9. Encourage relaxation activities for women in highly stressful careers/situations.
10. Instruct the patient about the importance of having his or her sexual partner treated to prevent reinfection.

Evaluation criteria. Refer to gonorrhea *(see above)*. Alcohol is avoided. Proper clothing is worn.

Monilial vaginitis/moniliasis (candidiasis)

Monilial vaginitis is usually associated with poorly controlled diabetes and may follow the use of antibiotics or steroids, which alter the flora of the vaginal tract. *Candida albicans* is the infecting organism. *Symptoms* include itching, reddish irritation because of inflammation of the vaginal epithelium, and discharge of white, cheesy particles. *Diagnosis* is based on the health history, physical exam, and culture of the organism. **Medical** treatment consists of the administration of vaginal nystatin suppositories. If no improvement follows, administration of oral nystatin is recommended. **Nursing** interventions are as follows:

1. Refer to trichomoniasis vaginitis and gonorrhea *(see above)* for additional interventions.
Physical 2. Demonstrate and assist the patient in insertion of the vaginal medication.
Educational 3. Plan for a follow-up culture 4 to 6 wk after completion of the treatment regimen.
4. Instruct the patient to remain recumbent for 30 min after insertion of the medication.
5. Instruct the patient to avoid tampons while taking medication.
6. Advise the use of perineal pads to prevent soiling of clothing.
7. Educate and encourage diabetic patients about controlling disease.
8. Advise abstinence from coitus until infection is controlled to prevent spread and reinfection.
9. Teach the importance of health-promoting activities, including adequate nutrition, fluid intake, and hygienic body care.

Evaluation criteria. Refer to trichomoniasis vaginitis *(see above)*.

Atrophic/senile vaginitis (postmenopausal vaginitis)

Atrophic vaginitis is associated with the absence of estrogen after menopause, which results in atrophy of the mucosa of the vulva and vagina and greater susceptibility to bacterial invasion. *Symptoms* include itching, burning, and vaginal discharge. *Diagnosis* is based on the health history and physical exam. **Medical** treatment consists of topical estrogen therapy and a well-balanced diet high in vitamin C to increase resistance to infection. **Nursing** interventions are as follows:

1. Refer to gonorrhea *(see above)* for additional interventions.
Physical 2. Provide measures to increase comfort (collodial baths, perineal care after urination and defecation).

3. Instruct the patient in the use of medications as prescribed.

Educational 4. Encourage the patient to maintain appropriate nutrition, especially vitamin C intake.

5. Encourage the patient to maintain good hygiene, especially of the perineal area.

Evaluation criteria.   Refer to gonorrhea (*see above*). Well-balanced diet with high vitamin C intake is maintained.

VULVITIS

Vulvitis, an inflammation of the vulva, occurs in conjunction with other systemic or local disorders. Predisposing factors include the presence of VD, dermatologic disorders, poor hygienic practices, diabetes, chronic illness, and advanced age. Vulvovaginitis is related to neurodermatitis, trichomoniasis, moniliasis, idiopathic lichen sclerosis, pediculosis, herpes infections, and pyoderma. Pruritus vulvae of psychosomatic origin may be generated by job or marital problems. *Symptoms* include red, edematous genitalia; vulvar discharge; burning; and pruritus, which increases during urination and defecation. *Diagnosis* is based on the health history, physical exam, vaginal cultures and smears, and blood studies to rule out diabetes.

Common interventions

Medical treatment consists of steroid cream and appropriate medication when the cause is isolated.

Nursing interventions

1. Refer to gonorrhea (*see above*) for additional interventions.

Physical 2. Assess predisposing chemical and physical factors, including perineal soiling, use of contraceptive jellies, perfumes, and antiperspirants.

3. Provide comfort measures.

Psychosocial 4. Assess the patient's mental outlook.

5. Provide supportive care as indicated.

Educational 6. Give instructions regarding proper local hygiene.

7. Advise the patient to avoid excessive washing of the area, use of detergent soaps, and synthetic fibers, which stimulate allergic reactions.

Prevention 8. Advise the patient to keep the area free of irritation by wearing loose clothing; i.e., avoid tight-fitting pants or slacks that restrict natural ventilation.

9. Advise the patient to alternate colloidal baths with warm compresses to stimulate circulation and decrease discomfort.

Evaluation criteria.   Refer to gonorrhea (*see above*). Patient keeps the area clean and dry.

BARTHOLIN'S CYST

A Bartholin's cyst is a dilation of the Bartholin's glands because of an obstruction. It is the most common tumor of the vulvar area and is caused by an infection resulting from *Escherichia coli*, *Staphylococcus aureus*, or *Neisseria gonorrhoeae*. The cyst is often asymptomatic. *Complications* include abscess formation. *Diagnosis* is based on the health history, physical exam, and culture that identifies the infecting organism.

Common interventions

Medical treatment consists of antibiotic therapy. **Surgical** treatment involves incision and drainage.

Nursing interventions

1. Refer to gonorrhea (*see above*) for additional interventions.
Physical 2. Provide symptomatic measures to alleviate discomfort (e.g., compresses and sitz baths).
Educational 3. Teach the patient proper hygiene.

Evaluation criteria. Refer to gonorrhea (*see above*).

PROSTATITIS

Prostatitis is an inflammation of the prostate gland. Chronic nonbacterial prostatitis is more common than bacterial prostatitis. Predisposing factors include urethral stricture and prostatic hyperplasia. Bacteria, viruses, or mycotic organisms carried by the urethra to the prostate are the main causes.

Symptoms include increased frequency of urination, urgency of urination, occasional burning during urination, and perineal discomfort. **Acute bacterial prostatitis** is characterized by the sudden onset of back, rectal, or perineal pain; chills and fever; urinary symptoms as described above; nocturia; and terminal dysuria. Some patients are asymptomatic. Both **chronic bacterial prostatitis** and **nonbacterial prostatitis** may be characterized by any of the above symptoms. *Complications* include septicemia, bacteriemia, pyelonephritis, and epididymitis. Chronic bacterial prostatitis is the primary source of relapsing urinary tract infections.

Diagnosis is based on the health history, physical exam, and culture of the prostatic tissue or fluid.

Common interventions

Medical treatment includes the use of antimicrobial medications for 10 to 14 days, as well as analgesics and bladder sedatives. Tetracycline or trimethoprim and sulfamethoxazole are used for chronic inflammation. Chronic nonbacterial prostatitis is difficult to treat effectively because antimicrobial agents are contraindicated; the use of anticholinergic drugs provides some comfort.

Nursing interventions

Physical 1. Encourage bed rest.
2. Provide comfort measures, including sitz baths, stool softeners, and rectal irrigations with warm saline.
3. Massage the prostate periodically (chronic nonbacterial prostatitis).
Psychosocial 4. Maintain a positive, supportive attitude.
5. Encourage the patient to express his concerns.
6. Aid the patient in discussing his condition with significant others.
Educational 7. Advise the patient to avoid alcohol, coffee, and sexual intercourse during the treatment period.
8. Reassure the patient that his condition is not caused by VD.
Prevention 9. Follow up medically for 6 mo to 1 yr to prevent recurrence.

Evaluation criteria. *See* Overview.

EPIDIDYMITIS

Epididymitis, an infection of the epididymis, may be of hematogenous origin, the result of urinary or prostatic infection that descends to the epididymis, or a complication of gonorrhea. *Symptoms* include soreness along the inguinal canal following the course of the vas deferens, pain in the inguinal and scrotal areas, swelling of the scrotum, pyuria, bacteriuria with chills and fever, and difficulty with walking. *Diagnosis* is based on the health history and physical exam, which reveals an extremely painful and swollen epididymis on palpation.

Common interventions

Medical treatment consists of the administration of antimicrobials, analgesics, and nerve block using local anesthetic infiltration of the spermatic cord during the first 24 hr of onset to relieve pain.

Nursing interventions

Physical 1. Maintain the patient on bed rest.
2. Use scrotal support to increase venous drainage, decrease tension on the spermatic cord, and alleviate pain.
3. During the early stage of infection, apply intermittent cold compresses/ ice packs to the scrotum to relieve pain.
4. During the later stage of infection, apply heat locally or give sitz baths.
5. Monitor pain and use analgesics as necessary.
Psychosocial 6. Refer to prostatitis (*see above*).
7. Refer the patient for follow-up care as necessary.
Educational 8. Avoid sexual activity and lifting until the infection abates (~4 wk)
9. Provide increased fluids to stimulate urinary output.

Evaluation criteria. *See* Overview.

OVARIAN CYST

An ovarian cyst is a benign sac containing semisolid material or fluid, which develops during the ovarian cycle. Cysts may be functional (graafian or lutein cyst), inflammatory, or endometrial. Hormonal activity during the menstrual cycle is a predisposing factor. *Symptoms* vary with the type of cyst. **Graafian cysts** are asymptomatic unless they rupture and hemorrhage. A large number of these cysts cause pelvic pain, uterine bleeding, and dyspareunia. **Lutein cysts** cause local pain and tenderness and amenorrhea. Severe pain may result from ovarian torsion. *Diagnosis* is based on the health history; physical exam, including pelvic exam, which reveals a palpable ovarian cyst; a vaginal smear (high estrogen level and absence of progesterone is indicative of graafian cyst); and laboratory tests, e.g., to evaluate human chorionic gonadotrophin (HCG), which is elevated with lutein cysts.

Common interventions

Medical treatment includes the administration of clomiphene citrate (Clomid) or medroxyprogesterone (Provera), which helps to reestablish the ovarian cycle by stimulating ovulation. **Surgical** removal of the cyst may be necessary to rule out malignancy.

Nursing interventions

Physical 1. Provide comfort measures such as warm douches and pelvic diathermy (heat lamp, warm compresses).
2. Provide pre- and postoperative care if the cyst is removed (*see* Chapters 9 and 11).
3. Inspect vaginal or abdominal dressings for bleeding or foul-smelling discharge.
4. Use an abdominal binder for support (if indicated).
5. Promote vaginal hygiene; note number of perineal pads used; note color, odor, and amount of drainage on pads; and instruct the patient regarding perineal care after voiding and with a change of pads.
6. Provide comfort measures, e.g., back rubs, frequent position changes, rectal tube for flatus.
Psychosocial 7. Encourage verbalization regarding altered self-concept if surgery affects reproductive ability.
8. Provide support to the patient and significant others.
9. Encourage significant others to help the patient work through feelings of loss of femininity.
Educational 10. Instruct the patient about hormonal activity and cystic growth.
11. Inform the patient about self-destruction of graafian and lutein cysts in 2 mo in nonpregnant women.
12 Arrange for a gynecologic evaluation 4 to 6 wk postoperatively.

13. Advise an annual gynecologic examination and close communication with health professionals if irregularities are experienced in menstrual cycle.

Evaluation criteria. See Overview.

POLYPS

Polyps (small, pedunculated growths) are found in both the uterine cavity and cervical canal. These growths are common during the childbearing years. *Symptoms* of uterine polyps include hypermenorrhea, leukorrhea, pelvic pain, intermenstrual bleeding, bleeding without menopause, and a bearing down sensation. Cervical polyps can become infected and may bleed after intercourse. Although polyps themselves are benign, they may undergo malignant changes. *Diagnosis* is based on the health history, physical exam, and visualization by hysterography. A CBC is advisable, especially in the presence of anemia.

Common interventions

Surgical treatment includes polypectomy with microscopic examination to rule out malignancy, electrosurgery, dilation and curettage (D&C), and exploration with the curette for additional polyps or other lesions. **Nursing** interventions are similar to those for patients with ovarian cyst and should be adapted as appropriate.

Evaluation criteria. See Overview.

FIBROIDS

Fibroids (uterine myomas) are common, benign tumors of the uterus and are characterized by connective tissue and unstriated muscle. They most often occur in women >40 yr of age, after menopausal atrophic changes; however, they may occur before the age of 40. Predisposing factors include hereditary influences and stimulation of estrogens. Fibroids occur more frequently in black and nulliparous women. Their cause is unknown. Classification is based on the area of growth in the uterus. The size, location, and structure of the growth influence the *symptoms*, which may include hypermenorrhea, pelvic discomfort, bladder disturbances, and sensations of pressure and bearing down. *Diagnosis* is based on the health history, physical exam, CBC (to detect anemia), vaginal examination under anesthesia with D&C, hysterography, laparoscopy, and hysteroscopy.

Common interventions

No **medical** treatment is required if the patient is asymptomatic. **Surgical** treatment includes a myomectomy (if childbearing capacity can be preserved) or a hysterectomy (if symptoms are severe or multiple tumors are present, especially in middle-aged women).

Nursing interventions

Physical 1. Provide pre- and postoperative care (*see* Chapters 9 and 11).

2. Administer care as for an ovarian cyst (*see above*) and adapt as appropriate.

Psychosocial 3. Encourage verbalization regarding altered self-concept if the uterus is removed.

4. Provide emotional support to the patient and significant others.

5. Encourage the patient to work through feelings of loss of femininity and childbearing potential with support and understanding of significant others.

Educational 6. Stress the importance of health-promoting activities, e.g., adequate nutrition, annual gynecologic examination, etc.

7. Instruct the patient to avoid vaginal entry activities (coitus and douching) for 4 to 6 wk.

8. Advise the patient to avoid heavy lifting, driving a car, and going up and down stairs until the abdominal incision heals.

9. Arrange for assistance with household duties during the postoperative period.

10. Arrange for a postoperative evaluation after 4 to 6 wk.

11. Advise an annual gynecologic examination for high-risk women.

12. Advise all women to report unusual uterine bleeding to a physician or nurse.

Evaluation criteria. See Overview.

CERVICAL CARCINOMA

Cervical carcinoma involves the proliferation of abnormal cells to surrounding tissue. Tables 18-9 and 18-10 describe the classification and

TABLE 18-9
Cervical Intraepithelial Neoplasia Classification System (CIN)

Grade	Diagnosis	Site
I	Mild dysplasia.	Lower third of cervical epithelium.
II	Moderate dysplasia.	Two-thirds of thickness of cervical epithelium.
III	Severe dysplasia.	Undifferentiated, neoplastic cells found near surface.
III	Carcinoma in situ.	Full thickness of epithelium; consists of undifferentiated neoplastic cells.

Adapted from Benson, R. Handbook of Obstetrics & Gynecology. Lange Medical Publications, Los Altos, Calif. 1980. Seventh edition. p. 552–553.

TABLE 18-10
*Summary Classification of Cervical Cancer**

Stage	Description	Five-year survival rate
		%
0	Carcinoma in situ.	95-100
Invasive I	Carcinoma limited to cervix.	84-89
Invasive II	Carcinoma extends beyond cervix (i.e., vagina) but not to pelvic wall.	43-70
Invasive III	Carcinoma found on pelvic wall.	27-43
Invasive IV	Carcinoma involves adjacent organs, i.e., mucosa of bladder/rectum/distant organs.	0-12

*Classification system approved by the International Federation of Gynecology and Obstetrics (FIGO). 1976.
Adapted from Benson, R. Handbook of Obstetrics & Gynecology. Lange Medical Publications, Los Altos, Calif. 1980. Seventh edition. p. 554–566.

staging. This malignancy is most prevalent in women between the ages of 30 and 40 yr. In situ and invasive carcinoma of the cervix are the most common genital tract malignancies in women and the second major site of cancer in women. Predisposing factors include beginning sexual experiences at an early age, early marriage, early childbearing, multiple (especially uncircumcised) sexual partners, multiple pregnancies, low socioeconomic class, and a history of genital herpes. The disease is rare among virgins and Jewish women. The cause is yet unknown. Cell type is usually squamous.

Symptoms depend on the degree of malignancy and may include abnormal vaginal discharge, irregular menstruation, lengthened menstrual cycle, postcoital bleeding, bleeding after douching, leukorrhea, pelvic pain (with pelvic involvement), anemia, anorexia, and weight loss. *Complications* are similar to those of any malignant disease (*see* Chapter 8).

Diagnosis is based on the health history, physical exam, Pap smear (demonstrating abnormal cytology of the cervical epithelium), colposcopy (viewing of cervical lesions by illuminating the area and magnifying the cells 10 to 30 times), Schiller's stain to highlight abnormal epithelium (which rejects iodine stain), and punch biopsy to obtain tissue fragments.

Common interventions

Surgical treatment is based on the extent of the malignancy. Cervical intraepithelial neoplasia (CIN) I and II are monitored by serial cytology q 6 mo or treated by electrocoagulation or cryosurgery (freezing of cervical tissue). For CIN III and carcinoma in situ (CIS) classification, a hysterectomy may be required. Cervical conization may suffice if pregnancy is desired, but the condition must be monitored q 3 mo. A hysterectomy may be necessary at a later date.

Nursing interventions

Physical 1. Administer care as for ovarian cyst (*see above*) and adapt as appropriate.

2. Administer analgesics to relieve pain as indicated.
3. Provide comfort measures, e.g., warm douches.
4. After cryosurgery, note the color, odor, and amount of cervical drainage, and advise the patient to keep a tampon in place for 24 to 48 hr.

Psychosocial 5. Listen to the patient's and partner's concerns.

6. Stress that the disease is treatable.

Educational 7. Advise the patient to report abnormal discharge, irregularities or changes in menstruation, and bleeding after coitus or douching.

8. After cryosurgery, inform the patient that her menstrual period may have a very heavy flow.
9. Advise the patient to abstain from sexual intercourse for 1 to 2 wk after the procedure.

Prevention 10. Advise early detection of high-risk women by means of an annual pelvic examination with Pap smear.

11. Stress the importance of early treatment of vaginitis and cervicitis.
12. Advise male circumcision during infancy.
13. Alert teenagers and young women about the increased risk if coitus begins at an early age or involves numerous sexual partners.
14. Stress the importance of follow-up Pap smear q 6 mo as per physician instructions.
15. Advise the patient to report any drainage to the physician or nurse.
16. Advise males in the use of condoms.
17. Inform the patient of screening programs in the community.
18. Advise prompt treatment of cervical lesions.

Evaluation criteria. *See* Overview.

UTERINE CARCINOMA

Uterine carcinoma is the malignant proliferation of endometrial tissue. Table 18-11 describes the staging and 5-yr survival rate. Postmenopausal women comprise 75% of affected patients. Adenocarcinoma is the most common type of uterine carcinoma, which is the second most common genital malignancy. Predisposing factors include abnormal estrogen balance, obesity, polycystic ovarian disease, hypertension, diabetes mellitus, and prolonged use of exogenous estrogen therapy. *Symptoms* include a previous history of irregular menses, e.g., amenorrhea, hypermenorrhea; postmeno-

TABLE 18-11
Summary Classification of Endometrial Carcinoma*

Stage	Description	Five-year survival rate
		%
0	Carcinoma in situ.	Not available
Invasive I	Carcinoma limited to corpus.	70-75
Invasive II	Carcinoma found beyond corpus, i.e., cervical involvement.	40-50
Invasive III	Carcinoma found outside uterus, not beyond pelvis.	25
Invasive IV	Carcinoma found beyond pelvis, i.e., involvement of other organs, rectum/bladder.	5

*Classification system approved by the International Federation of Gynecology and Obstetrics (FIGO). 1976.
Adapted from Benson, R. Handbook of Obstetrics & Gynecology. Lange Medical Publications, Los Altos, Calif. 1980. Seventh edition. p. 599-604.

pausal vaginal bleeding or spotting; thin, malodorous, yellow/brown discharge; and pain caused by intrauterine infection or uterine enlargement. *Complications* are those of metastatic disease (*see* Chapter 8).

Diagnosis is based on the health history; physical exam (a boggy, enlarged uterus may be palpated in advanced stages), pelvic examination under anesthesia; cytologic examination of uterine, endocervical, and vaginal discharges or aspirations; "jet wash" for endometrial tissue; curettage or endometrial biopsy; hysterosalpingography; and cystoscopy and sigmoidoscopy to rule out spread to other surrounding organs.

Common interventions

Medical treatment is used for patients who are poor surgical risks, or it is used in combination with surgery to arrest foci in the pelvis. Radiation therapies include external irradiation of the primary tumor site and pelvic nodes preoperatively, internal irradiation of the site with radium implants for several days preoperatively, or external pelvic irradiation postoperatively if the patient has advanced disease. **Surgical** treatment may consist of drainage of the infected, distended uterus or hysterectomy (type depends on age, health of the patient, and extent of spread of disease). Abdominal hysterectomy with bilateral salpingo-oophorectomy (removal of uterus, fallopian tubes, and ovaries) or radical hysterectomy with pelvic lymphadenectomy are the options.

Nursing interventions

1. Refer to ovarian cyst (*see above*) for additional interventions.

Physical 2. Institute radiation precautions.

    a. For external radiation treatment, observe skin for redness, desquamation and telangiectasis; do not wash marks from skin; avoid using soap over area (wash only with water); do not use ointments, powders, and lotions; do not apply heat to area either during or after treatment; do not shave area with razor.

    b. For internal radiation treatment, organize nursing activities and frequently rotate nurses to limit the amount of time spent with the patient ($\sim$30 min) and, thus, minimize exposure to radiation; maintain distance from radiation source; give care from head of bed; communicate from door; provide special receptacles for disposal of contaminated linens, dressings, excreta, equipment per individual institutional policy; wear gloves when handling contaminated articles; provide special container for radiation implant if it should become dislodged; use 12-in. forceps to place implant into container.

Psychosocial 3. Provide emotional support; talk frequently from the door to prevent feelings of isolation.

4. Permit visitors for 1 hr/day at 6 ft distance.

Educational 5. Instruct the patient about the use of radiation and skin reactions.

6. Provide and plan for frequent rest periods before and after therapy.

7. Help the patient adjust work/home schedule and obtain assistance.

8. Maintain well-balanced diet; eat small and frequent snacks, drink $\geq$3 liters of liquids/day.

9. Explain the possible occurrence of nausea and vomiting and measures to prevent or treat these symptoms.

10. Instruct the patient to maintain scheduled appointments.

11. Give the telephone number of the nurse/physician to call in an emergency.

Prevention 12. Teach about the need for endometrial biopsy/aspiration before the use of estrogens in postmenopausal women.

13. Obtain periodic vaginal smears.

14. Advise the patient to have a prompt D&C for abnormal menstrual or postmenopausal uterine bleeding.

15. Encourage the patient to have an annual gynecologic examination.

Evaluation criteria. *See* Overview. Radiation precautions are maintained.

OVARIAN CARCINOMA

Ovarian carcinoma is the proliferation of abnormal tissue in the ovary. Table 18-12 describes the staging and 5-yr survival rate. Ovarian carcinoma

TABLE 18-12
Summary Classification of Ovarian Neoplasms*

Stage	Description	Five-year survival rate
I	Carcinoma confined to ovaries.	Surgery alone: 67% Surgery and irradiation: 60% Surgery and chemotherapy: 94%
II	Carcinoma confined to one/both ovaries, with pelvic extension.	Surgery alone: 24% Surgery with irradiation: 60% Surgery with chemotherapy: 75%
III	Carcinoma of one/ both ovaries with metastasis to abdominal organs, e.g., omentum, small intestine.	Surgery alone: 1% Surgery and irradiation: 9% Surgery and chemotherapy: 7%
IV	Carcinoma of one/ both ovaries, with metastasis to other distant sites.	Not available.

*Classification system approved by the International Federation of Gynecology and Obstetrics (FIGO). 1976.
Adapted from Benson, R. Handbook of Obstetrics & Gynecology. Lange Medical Publications, Los Altos, Calif. 1980. Seventh edition. p. 639.

occurs primarily in women between the ages of 40 and 60 yr and is the leading cause of death in women who have genital cancer; 40% of the women with a positive Pap smear are afflicted. Predisposing factors include decreased fertility, delayed childbearing, low parity, and a history of ovarian cysts or endometriosis. *Symptoms* include abdominal distension, urinary frequency, constipation, pain, and hormonal and menstrual irregularities (hypermenorrhea, amenorrhea). However, the disease is often asymptomatic. *Diagnosis* is based on the health history; physical exam that reveals a palpable pelvic mass; x-ray findings of the pelvis, with GI series to rule out colic/gastric metastases; ultrasonography of abdomen and pelvis; laboratory studies, e.g., CBC, urinalysis, electrolytes; cystoscopy; proctoscopy; laparoscopy (inspecting pelvis, lower omentum/diaphragm for metastases); and biopsy of suspect organs.

Common interventions

Medical treatment (used in combination with surgery) consists of chemotherapy and radiation. **Surgical** treatment involves total hysterectomy

and bilateral salpingo-oophorectomy and omentectomy. **Nursing** interventions are similar to those for uterine carcinoma (*see above*).
Evaluation criteria. See Overview.

[Benign prostatic hypertrophy and cancer of the prostate are discussed in Chapter 17.]

TESTICULAR CANCER

Testicular cancer is the abnormal proliferation of testicular tissue. It affects males from 20 to 40 yr of age, with its highest incidence occurring between the ages of 24 and 34. Predisposing factors include undescended testicles, infections, trauma, endocrine disorders, and genetic influences. In its early stage, *symptoms* may include scrotal enlargement, scrotal heaviness, and lower abdominal aching. Symptoms of later stages (metastasis) include lumbar pain, loss of weight, general weakness, gynecomastia, urinary frequency, and dyspnea. *Diagnosis* is based on the health history, physical exam, x-rays of the scrotum and chest to detect masses, IV pyelogram to detect masses, and urine evaluation for gonadotrophins.

Common interventions

Medical treatment consists of radiation of the pelvic area and abdomen (if abdominal involvement is diagnosed) and chemotherapy. **Surgical** treatment includes orchiectomy with nodal dissection.

Nursing interventions

Physical 1. Provide pre- and postoperative care as appropriate (*see* Chapters 9 and 11).
2. Observe the patient for hemorrhage after radical node dissection.
3. Monitor vital signs q 2 to 4 hr, encourage deep-breathing exercises q hr, and turn the patient q hr.
4. Apply elastic bandages to the lower extremities.
5. Use scrotal support and careful positioning to decrease suture tension.
6. Provide for diathermy, e.g., heat lamp.
Psychosocial 7. Encourage verbalization about changes in self-concept, sexuality, and body image.
8. Provide emotional support to the patient and significant others regarding prognosis, self-concept, and treatment.
9. Encourage and facilitate diversional activities.
Educational 10. Teach the patient how to perform a testicular self-examination using the following method: with both hands, examine the testicle between the thumb and first two fingers of the hand for position (lies freely in scrotum), shape (oval), texture (uniform, spongy), size (2 cm thick and 3 cm wide), possible abnormalities (firmness on side and front), and location of epididymis (wirelike structure at back of testis).

11. Stress the importance of performing a monthly testicular self-examination.

Evaluation criteria.   *See* Overview. Patient performs monthly testicular self-examination.

INFERTILITY

Infertility is the lack of pregnancy after 1 yr of normal sexual relations without the use of contraception. Primary infertility precludes a prior history of pregnancy. Secondary infertility follows the achievement of one or more previous pregnancies. Infertility occurs in 10 to 15% of childbearing-age couples. The male partner is infertile in ~40% of childless unions. Certain medications and chronic illnesses can cause infertility (*see* Tables 18-4 and 18-6). In females, contributing factors may be nutritional (hypovitaminosis, decreased protein intake, anemia), endocrine (overactive or underactive pituitary, thyroid, or adrenals), vaginal (infection, congenital anomalies, sperm-inhibiting vaginal fluid), cervical (developmental abnormalities, tumors, cervicitis), uterine (congenital anomalies, tumors, endometrial disorders), tubal (congenital atresia, tubal closure because of infection), ovarian (congenital anomalies, infection, tumors, scarring secondary to endometriosis), psychic (anxiety, severe psychoneurotic conditions such as anorexia nervosa, psychotic conditions such as schizophrenia causing amenorrhea and anovulation), or coital (use of douches, lubricants, or deodorant antiseptics affecting sperm viability). Male infertility may be related to coital factors (incomplete vaginal penetration because of excessive obesity, hypospadias, epispadias, impotence), spermatozoa abnormalities (<30 million active sperm/ml — conception rare; <50 million active sperm/ml — low fertility), testicular deficits (small size, endocrine abnormalities, immunologic difficulties, infection such as mumps, physical and environmental trauma), penile and urethral malformations, prostate and seminal vesicle abnormalities, and epididymis and vas deferens abnormalities. The absence of pregnancy may cause loss of self-esteem manifested by feelings of anger, denial, isolation, guilt, worthlessness, depression, and failure/inadequacy in meeting social/religious/cultural expectations. Women may feel unfeminine; men may feel unmasculine and impotent.

Diagnosis is based on the health history, physical exam, CBC, thyroid function tests, and a urinalysis for 17-ketosteroids. Males may require microscopic evaluation of motility, number, and abnormal formations of sperm, as well as testicular biopsy. Females may require tests for tubal patency, endometrial biopsy, culdoscopy, basal body temperature charts, and postcoital mucus examination.

Common interventions

Medical or **surgical** treatment depends on the cause of infertility. Men may require testosterone or HCG therapy, surgery for congenital anomalies, or ligation of varicoceles. Women may require tubal insufflation or surgical procedures such as myomectomy or plastic repair.

Nursing interventions

Physical 1. Provide comfort measures and pre- and postoperative care (*see* Chapters 9 and 11) as indicated.

Psychosocial 2. Provide emotional support and empathy to the couple regarding this extremely sensitive issue.

3. Assist the couple to verbalize feelings of loss and grief, and support the couple in the resolution of feelings about infertility.

4. Suggest coping strategies for the couple.

  a. Respect wishes of mate regarding returning to pleasurable pattern of sexual relations.

  b. Change usual time, place, and position of intercourse to build new associations and dispel unpleasant memories.

  c. Develop hedonistic philosophy of enjoying sex for its own sake.

  d. Develop close, caring relationship with mate and other significant individuals.

Educational 5. Describe anatomy and physiology of reproductive system, diagnostic tests performed, and treatments prescribed.

6. Serve as a source of information regarding alternatives and community resources, e.g., counseling and national self-help groups (Resolve), adoption, artificial insemination, in vitro fertilization, and surrogate mothering.

Prevention 7. Encourage sexually active populations to seek early medical attention for sexually transmitted diseases.

8. Advise appropriate immunization for mumps, especially for young boys.

Evaluation criteria. See Overview.

ABORTION

Abortion refers to uterine expulsion/removal of a fetus prior to the age of viability. Classifications include **spontaneous abortion** (miscarriage), an involuntary abortion that is threatened, complete, inevitable, or missed, and **induced abortion**, an abortion that is therapeutic/elective and sometimes self-induced. Spontaneous abortions occur most often before menopause and during early adulthood. Therapeutic abortions have increased dramatically since 1973, when the Supreme Court ruled that abortions were legal. The majority of spontaneous abortions result from ovular/fetal abnormalities (60%), e.g., anatomic defects and maternal factors (15%) such as trauma, infections (chronic nephritis, acute infections), poor nutrition, endocrine disorders (hypothyroidism, diabetes mellitus), toxic exposure, uterocervical incompetence or abnormalities, psychologic disorders, and severe emotional shock. Other factors include absence of a chorionic cavity, syphilis, and abnormal placental implantation.

Signs and symptoms vary with the type of abortion. For **threatened**, there is abnormal vaginal bleeding; in **complete** (entire products of conception expelled), a sudden onset of bleeding is followed by pain, which ceases on complete expulsion, while slight spotting continues for several days; in **incomplete** (portions of conception passed) or **inevitable** (impending expulsion of conception), there is continuous bleeding and cramping, moderate cervical effacement, and cervical dilation of >2 cm (rupture of membranes); and in **missed** (pregnancy terminated prior to expulsion of conception for at least a month), the symptoms of pregnancy are no longer visible, there is brownish vaginal discharge, and the uterus becomes smaller. *Complications* include hemorrhage, infection, and infertility.

Diagnosis is based on the health history, physical exam, urine tests that are negative for pregnancy, blood tests that indicate anemia and are negative for HCG, vaginal smears, and ultrasonography.

Common interventions

Medical treatment consists of the maintenance of bed rest until cessation of vaginal bleeding (especially with threatened abortion), and the use of progestogen therapy and sedatives to decrease uterine irritability and bleeding. **Surgical** intervention (D&C) for retained tissue is often necessary.

Nursing interventions

Physical 1. Maintain the patient on bed rest until the bleeding stops (threatened abortion).

2. Instruct the patient to avoid coitus and douches until the bleeding subsides (threatened abortion).

3. Provide prescribed medications.

4. Provide comfort measures, including back rubs and range-of-motion exercises.

5. Provide pre- and postoperative care if D&C is performed (*see* Chapters 9 and 11).

Psychosocial 6. Demonstrate empathy in highly emotional situations, especially if a pregnancy was planned and motherhood/parenthood was eagerly anticipated.

7. Recognize that the patient's feelings of femininity may be related to her childbearing ability. Inability to maintain pregnancy may generate feelings of female reproductive incompetence, resulting in loss of self-esteem and depression.

8. Provide sympathetic support to the patient and significant others through the crisis and grieving period.

Educational 9. Discuss the patient's status, including symptoms, diagnosis, treatment, and prognosis.

10. Discuss the crisis situation and evaluate for coping patterns, situational supports, and realistic perception of the event.
11. Describe alternatives, depending on cause of abortion, e.g., avoiding trauma, adoption, etc.
12. Allow the couple to overcome the mourning period and revitalize former sexual intimacy.
13. Discuss the use of family planning methods for several months, provided there are no anatomic, genetic, or hormonal contraindications to another pregnancy.
14. Provide information about follow-up and community resources.
Prevention 15. Discuss appropriate treatment of maternal disorders before pregnancy.
16. Provide early prenatal care with treatment and supervision of high-risk patients, e.g., diabetic, cardiac, and hypertensive persons.
17. Provide occupational health measures to prevent exposure of child-bearing women to health hazards.
18. Teach communicable disease prevention, especially the avoidance of rubella exposure during the first trimester of pregnancy.
19. Inform the patient about possible surgical intervention to correct incompetent cervix.

Evaluation criteria. *See* Overview.

IMPOTENCE

Impotence is a male's lack of power to achieve or maintain an erection during coitus. Classifications include **primary** (has never achieved erection sufficient for intercourse with partner) and **secondary/situational** (has functioned with erections, then developed difficulties). It is difficult to obtain data regarding impotence, as males do not readily acknowledge the problem. Kinsey reported increasing impotence after the age of 45, and more often after the age of 55. As men enter the seventh decade of life, 27% of white males admit to impotence, 55% at 75 years of age, and 75% at 80 years of age. Causes of primary impotence include inability of the vascular reflex mechanism to provide the cavernous sinuses with a rich blood supply, which causes firmness and hardening; hormonal, endocrine, neurologic, and renal disorders; use of antipsychotic drugs; painful erections; psychologic factors, including societal/familial taboos/restrictions or erections associated with guilt/fear; and early, traumatic sexual encounters. Secondary impotence may result from situational anger, guilt, low self-esteem, or rejection; lack of satisfaction or boredom with partner or work; marital discord; aging; depression; anxiety or physical incapacity after surgery of prostate, colon, or bladder; and hormonal, endocrine, neurologic, renal, and vascular disorders and/or their treatment (*see* Tables 18-4 and 18-6).

Diagnosis is based on the health history, physical exam, and laboratory tests to rule out organic/physiologic disorders. Evaluation of physical ability to achieve erection and interest in sexual intercourse may reveal that there is a complete inability to attain erections and a complete disinterest in coitus; a partial/incomplete erection with minor interest in coitus; a periodic inability to attain erection with minor interest in coitus; erectile ability but absence of sexual gratification from coital ejaculation; or premature ejaculation.

Common interventions

Medical treatment may include psychotherapy to work through psychologic factors; the use of manual stimulation by sexual partner to increase sexual pleasure and penile functioning; or sexual therapy focusing on developing a warm, loving, considerate relationship with open communication (i.e., sharing of concerns and feelings, freedom to discuss pleasurable activities). **Surgical** treatment may involve the insertion of a Small-Carrion device (consists of two sponge-filled silicone rods) in the corpora cavernosa to provide the penis with girth, width, and length simulating an erectile reaction; or the insertion of an inflatable penile prosthesis (consisting of a hollow silicone cylinder) in each corpus cavernosum. A bulb and a reservoir of radiopaque solution are also placed in one scrotal sac. Silicone tubes are connected to all four parts. Squeezing the scrotal bulb causes solution to enter cylinders in each corpus cavernosum and results in an erection. Pressing on a release valve in the bulb causes fluid return to the scrotal reservoir.

Nursing interventions

Physical 1. Provide pre- and postoperative care (*see* Chapters 9 and 11).
    2. Provide comfort measures, including analgesics for pain as ordered.
    3. Provide support for the penis and care in the positioning of a semi-erect penis (if silicone implant is used).
    4. Use aseptic technique to prevent infection.
    5. Observe for urinary retention and reinfection following removal of urethral catheter.
    6. Observe for perineal edema.
    7. Ambulate early (dangle legs on first postoperative evening and walk on first postoperative day).
Psychosocial 8. Provide emotional support to the patient and significant others in this highly sensitive situation.
    9. Encourage the patient and significant others to verbalize their concerns and feelings.
    10. Support continued psychotherapy if feasible.
    11. Arrange a visit with a willing patient who has had similar successful surgery and a positive outlook.
Educational 12. Inform the patient and significant others about the penis remaining in a semierect state following implant with Small-Carrion device.
    13. Encourage the wearing of street clothes and brief-style underwear to

minimize semierect penis by placing the penis in a flat position against the abdomen.

14. Encourage the patient to resume normal life-style, i.e., recreational and occupational activities.
15. Provide the patient with opportunities to assume appropriate self-care activities.
16. Instruct and evaluate the patient's and significant other's ability to manage an inflatable prosthesis.
17. Assist the patient in developing a positive self-concept and attitude toward sexuality.

Evaluation criteria. *See* Overview.

ENDOMETRIOSIS

Endometriosis is the presence of columnar cells of endometrium growing outside the uterus, in the pelvic cavity. It occurs mostly in women between 30 and 40 yr of age and is more common in nulliparous, late-married, and white women. Causes include temporary occlusion of the cervix (causing menstrual flow to pass into the tubes), metaplasia of the peritoneum, and previous surgical intervention (causing uterine trauma). *Symptoms* include dysmenorrhea, pelvic pain (depending on site, e.g., rectal or bladder area), painful defecation (bowel lesions/rectovaginal septum), and hypermenorrhea and shortened menstrual intervals (ovary as site of ectopic endometrium). *Complications* consist of infertility resulting from peritubal and ovarian endometriosis and concealment of bleeding in an ovarian (chocolate) cyst. *Diagnosis* is based on the health history, physical exam, laparoscopy, sigmoidoscopy, and cystoscopy.

Common interventions

Treatment depends on the severity of symptoms, the desire to have children, and the response to previous treatment. **Medical** therapy involves analgesics for pain; endocrine therapy (Danazol or weak androgen) that causes pseudomenopause, but is contraindicated in hirsute women; and irradiation to cause involution of ovarian implants. **Surgical** treatment includes removal of endometrial implants and oophorectomy to stop ovarian functioning and thereby cause involution of endometrial implants.

Nursing interventions

Physical 1. Give general preoperative and postoperative care if surgical intervention is performed (*see* Chapters 9 and 11).
2. Relieve pain with analgesics, comfort measures, and distractors (*see* Chapter 4).
3. Observe for side effects of drugs administered to suppress endometrial implants.

Psychosocial 4. Support the patient and significant others regarding feelings of self-esteem, femininity, body image, and self-concept.

5. Listen to concerns regarding future pregnancies and chronic pain.

Educational 6. Advise the patient to report abnormal bleeding and increased pain.

7. Teach the patient about the administration of medications and their side effects.

8. Stress the importance of an annual pelvic exam during the child-bearing years.

Evaluation criteria. See Overview.

TOXIC SHOCK SYNDROME

Toxic shock syndrome (TSS) is a rare systemic infection that occurs primarily in young women (3/100,000 women) either during or after menstrual periods. The use of tampons — especially those with a mesh, synthetic, sponge-filled bag — seems to predispose individuals to TSS. *Staphylococcus aureus* is the infecting organism. *Symptoms* include a sudden onset of fever, vomiting, diarrhea, a drop in systolic BP (<90 mmHg), and an erythematous macular rash of the palms and soles that desquamates in 7 to 14 days. *Complications* include possible involvement of other body systems, i.e., CNS, cardiopulmonary, GI, and hematologic systems, and kidneys. TSS may occasionally lead to death. *Diagnosis* is based on the health history, physical exam, and laboratory tests that reveal elevated BUN, creatinine phosphokinase (CPK), SGOT, bilirubin, serum creatine, and leukocytosis.

Common interventions

Medical treatment includes fluid and electrolyte replacement, administration of antibiotics, and symptomatic management depending on the body systems involved.

Nursing interventions

Physical 1. Provide comfort measures, e.g., back rubs and range-of-motion exercises.

2. Treat symptomatically, depending on the extent of the system involved, e.g., low-residue diet for hypermotile GI system, etc.

3. Administer antibiotics, noting side effects.

4. Frequently monitor vital signs and fluid status.

Psychosocial 5. Provide emotional support to the patient and significant others.

6. Encourage verbalization of anxieties, feelings, and concerns.

Educational 7. Teach the patient menstrual hygiene, e.g., perineal care, frequent changes of perineal pads.

8. Advise the patient to avoid using tampons for several menstrual cycles.

9. Advise the patient to abstain from the use of synthetic tampons.

Evaluation criteria. *See* Overview. Menstrual hygiene measures are utilized. Tampons are not used for several menstrual cycles.

CHAPTER 19

ALTERED MUSCULOSKELETAL FUNCTIONING

Laurie Verdisco and Sophie Pasternak

OVERVIEW

This chapter focuses on problems concerned primarily with defects of, or trauma to, muscles and bones. The scope is limited to selected problems – those most commonly seen on a general medical-surgical or orthopedic unit. Although patients with musculoskeletal problems require the talents of a multiprofessional team to achieve their optimal level of functioning, this chapter will primarily deal with nursing responsibilities.

Anatomy and physiology review

The **skeletal system**, which consists of 206 bones, provides a supportive structure for the body and is the framework for all body systems. Its components are bones, ligaments, and tendons. The skeletal system provides a surface for the attachment of ligaments and tendons and a storage area for mineral salts. The rib cage provides a bony case for the heart and lungs, and the cranium protects the brain. The skeletal system also maintains a repository for the manufacture of RBCs.

Bone, the hardest tissue in the body, is a living tissue with a need for respiration, assimilation, excretion, reproduction, and response to stimuli. Bone is composed of 30 to 40% collagenous tissue (which provides tensile strength) and 60 to 70% mineral deposits (calcium salts provide compression strength). In addition, an intercellular substance (the matrix) has canals filled with tissue fluids (allowing for transport of oxygen and nutrient material to the bone cells from the blood). The matrix provides for removal of waste products and allows the cells to remain viable in the presence of calcified intercellular material.

Cartilage is fibrous connective tissue composed of chondrocytes and an intercellular substance (matrix). Chondrocytes are arranged singly or in pairs in the lacunae (cavities). Collagenous fibers or elastic fibers may be embedded in the matrix. Cartilage is avascular. Nutrients diffuse through the matrix from blood vessels in the adjacent tissue. Therefore, repair of injured tissue is slow. Perichondrium covers all cartilage except the articular cartilage of synovial joints. Cartilage withstands pressure and pull, allows joints to move with less friction, and absorbs shock to joints during movement. Hyaline cartilage is the most common type of cartilage in the body. It contains collagenous fibers in its matrix, forms the articular surfaces in adult bones, and forms a flexible union of the ribs with the breast bone. Fibrous cartilage is exceedingly tough and contains a heavier bundle of collagenous fibers in its matrix than does hyaline cartilage. It is found in discs that lie between adjacent vertebrae and at the ends of the clavicle, and in areas of insertion of tendons into bone. It reinforces the hyaline cartilage at the knees and hips.

Periosteum is connective tissue that covers bone and extends its fibers into bone. It contains blood vessels, lymphatic vessels, and nerves. The blood vessels enter the bone and become the vessels of the haversian canal.

Compact bone is a hard, dense layer of bony tissue that encases all bone. Compact bone is thickest in the middle of the long bone shaft and gradually becomes thinner as it extends to the articular ends, where it becomes merely a shell. The haversian system allows for the diffusion of fluids and is composed of the lamellae (concentric arrangements of matrix and bone cells); lacunae (small spaces); canaliculi (minute canals that extend from the canal to the lacunae and intercommunicate with each other, penetrating the matrix in all directions); and arteries, veins, lymphatic vessels, and nerves.

Cancellous bone is composed of a meshlike network of spongy bone and contains many more spaces than compact bone. Trabeculae are thin processes of bone between open spaces of cancellous bone that conform to lines of stress, giving bone additional strength. They have intervening spaces filled with red bone marrow, the substance that produces RBCs.

When a fracture occurs, the adjacent soft tissues are also injured. The periosteum is stripped away from the broken ends of bone, and the blood vessel that crosses the fracture site is torn. The **repair process** occurs as follows. First, a hematoma forms in the surrounding tissues and between the broken ends of bone. Then, osteoblasts proliferate at the endosteum and at the stripped edges of the periosteum. A collar of tissue is formed around each bone end. The tissue is differentiated into fibrous connective tissue, fibrocartilage, and hyaline cartilage. Fibrous connective tissue and cartilage form a callus, in which small arteries, capillaries, and veins appear. Bony trabeculae form at the point that has adequate capillary circulation. The collars of bone fragment meet and fuse, and cartilage is replaced by bone.

Bones are classified by shape and structure. Long bones are cylindrically shaped (e.g., humerus), and short bones are cube shaped (e.g., the tarsal bones of the feet). The irregular bones have a variety of shapes (e.g., vertebrae and bones of the skull), and flat bones (e.g., scapula) are flat. The sesamoid bones are nodular and are found in areas where tendon crosses over a bony prominence, causing a friction or rub (e.g., bones of the hands and feet).

Bones have other distinguishing features in addition to their basic structural arrangements. These include elevations or projections that allow for attachments of muscle, articulation of one bone with another, or protection of vital parts. Finally, bone has many depressions, grooves, and openings. Terms used to describe and recognize these features are presented in Table 19-1.

Skeletal ligaments are bands of fibrous tissue that bind together two bones or bony parts. The toughness of the ligament is seen in situations in which a severe, sudden stress results in a fracture of bone rather than in the

TABLE 19-1
Bony Landmarks

Landmark	Example
Projections	
Condyle: a rounded projection on a bone that articulates with another bone.	Femoral condyle.
Crest: a ridge	Upper border of ilium.
Head: an enlarged end of a bone beyond the narrow section called the neck.	Femoral neck.
Process: a distinct prominence of bone.	Olecranon process.
Spine: a marked projection.	Vertebrae.
Trochanter: a very large prominence.	Greater trochanter of femur.
Tubercle: a small, rounded elevation.	Tibial tubercle.
Tuberosity: a large, rounded elevation.	Ischial tuberosity.
Depressions, grooves, openings	
Fossa: a hollow or depressed area in a bone.	Supraspinous fossa of the scapula.
Groove: a shallow, linear depression.	Intertubercular groove on anterior surface of humerus.
Foramen: a natural opening or passage in a bone.	Foramen magnum.

tearing of the ligament. Ligaments are composed of closely packed, collagenous, elastic fibers that are either white or yellow, usually run in the same direction, and occasionally fuse with the fibrous wall of a joint. Ligaments serve to hold articular joints together during motion, permit desired motion of a joint and limit motion in another direction, and constrain bones that must remain together to function. Types of ligaments, their specific characteristics and functions, and examples of each, are listed in Table 19-2.

Tendons are composed of very dense collagenous tissues that extend directly from muscle and are usually attached to bone. They possess great tensile strength and provide a connection through which the pull of muscle can pass without being diminished. In tendons, fiber bundles are aligned in a close, compact, and parallel arrangement. Certain tendons are surrounded by a tendon sheath, which is lined with a synovial membrane. These sheaths are found in the flexor tendons of the hands and feet and provide a moist, smooth surface through which the tendon may move easily. Tendons differ considerably in appearance according to the muscle to which they are joined. They may be broad and flat (when part of a broad, flat muscle) or cylindrical cords (when part of a long, slender muscle). A broad, flat, tendinous sheet that is arranged in the form of a ribbonlike expansion is called an aponeurosis.

Skeletal muscles are described as "striated" because of their appearance under the microscope, and as "voluntary" because of their response to volitional control. The body, or belly, of the muscle lies between the points of origin and insertion. Origin is the fixed end or attachment of the muscle; insertion is the place of attachment of the muscle to the bone that it moves. Some of the descriptive features used to characterize muscles are included in Table 19-3. Posture is maintained through partial contraction of many muscles; movements of parts of the body or the whole body are facilitated by contraction of muscles. **Muscle fibers** vary in length and thickness and are grouped into parallel bundles called fasciculi, which seldom extend continuously from one end of the muscle to the other. These fibers are multinucleated, each containing a large number of myofibrils embedded in a semifluid matrix called sarcoplasm. Myofibrils exhibit cross-striation, or alternating light and dark bands in muscle tissue. Actin is a protein that acts with myosin particles and is responsible for contraction and relaxation of muscles. **Sarcolemma**, a plasma membrane that invests every striated muscle fiber, functions as a semipermeable membrane between the potassium-rich interior of the fiber and the sodium- and chloride-rich exterior. It transmits stimuli so that the entire fiber contracts as a unit and contributes tension to the muscle. **Endomysium** is a delicate network of fibrous tissue that surrounds each muscle fiber. It attaches muscles to adjacent fibers holding capillary and nerve fibers in relation to it. **Perimysium** is a slightly denser connective tissue that covers muscle fibers that are bundled together into a large unit called muscle fasciculi. It provides a pathway for nerve fibers and blood vessels. **Epimysium** is the outermost connective tissue, which encases the entire muscle and gives each muscle its

TABLE 19-2
Specific Ligaments: Functions and Characteristics

Types	Characteristics	Function	Example
Capsular (most common)	Surround the articulating ends of bones that form the joint. Fuse with the fibrous covering of bone.	Permit motion in certain directions.	Hips, knees.
Accessory Extrinsic	Extend from one bone to another. Bind bones together. Are located outside the joint capsule.	Provide more stability to the joint.	Collateral ligaments of knees.
Intrinsic	Cross the joint cavity within capsule. Are composed of short bands.	Provide stability to the joint.	Ligamentum teres of hip.

TABLE 19-3
Descriptive Features of Muscles

Muscle type	Function or description
Abductor	Draws away from median plane.
Adductor	Draws toward median plane.
Biceps	Has two heads.
Brevis	Is short.
Deltoid	Is triangular in outline.
Extensor	Extends a joint.
Flexor	Flexes a joint.
Interosseous	Is between bones.
Levator	Elevates the structure into which it is inserted.
Latissimus	Is a broad structure.
Longus	Is a long structure.
Magnum	Is great.
Pronator	Serves to pronate.
Quadriceps	Is four headed.

own characteristic shape and form. Muscles are highly vascular, each type having its own pattern of distribution of blood vessels. One set of blood vessels or a series of blood vessels enters at different locations into the muscle. Arteries are carried from the epimysium to the substance of the muscle by the perimysium. They are subdivided so that capillaries are carried to each muscle fiber by the endomysium. Capillaries are designed to provide each fiber close contact with one or more capillaries. Shortening and/or the development of tension in muscle tissue is referred to as **contraction**. Tonus is a slight, continuous contraction of muscle, which aids in maintaining posture. Isotonic contractions shorten the muscle without an appreciable change in the force of the contraction. Isometric contractions do not result in an appreciable change in distance between the muscle's origin and insertion. A twitch is a brief contraction in response to a single stimulus. A sustained contraction without an interval of relaxation is referred to as tetanic. Treppe is a gradual increase in the extent of contraction following repeated stimulations.

A **joint** is defined as an articulation (or as the place of union or junction) between two or more bones of the skeleton. The joints of the skeletal system may be classified as fibrous, cartilaginous, or synovial. Examples, description, and movements of each type of joint are presented in Table 19-4.

General Assessment

Below are only a few examples of why a complete **health history** should be obtained and how components of the health history are directed specifically to musculoskeletal complaints.

The most frequent complaint (**reason for contact**) associated with musculoskeletal problems is pain. The specifics of the pain should be explored with the patient and recorded in the **current health status**. The location and the pattern of the pain is of particular importance. The pain may be localized or may radiate to other areas (which could be a significant clue in identifying the problem). For example, the patient may state the pain is in the buttock and radiates down the leg, which may indicate the problem is in the low back. The onset of the pain is significant. Was it sudden pain or pain caused by trauma? Acute joint pain rarely begins at rest; if it does, a systemic problem may be suspected. Attention should also be given to the pain and its progress. Is it a long-standing, chronic type pain that had an insidious onset (started with an ache and progressed over time to severe discomfort or even to an acute state)? Did the pain start in one joint, clear up, and then appear in another joint (migratory pain)? The quality of the pain gives an important clue as to origin: vascular, neurologic, musculoskeletal. A "pins and needle," burning, or numb feeling may be neurologic, whereas a sharp, deep-throbbing, aching type of pain (depending on location) is usually associated with a serious bone or joint disease. What aggravates the pain, and what makes it better? Does rest make it subside? Does it only hurt when the patient climbs stairs or is in motion? Microtrauma to muscles often begins when the patient is at rest; muscle pain caused by cold begins at rest and goes away with warmth. "Night pain" is significant: it can be a manifestation of a bone tumor, a beginning sign of ankylosing spondylitis or a spinal cord tumor, or a factor in diagnosing carpal tunnel syndrome, which becomes worse at night.

Other common complaints associated with musculoskeletal problems include stiffness, weakness, swelling, warmth, and redness. For each complaint, data related to location, mode of onset, duration, quality, aggravation, and relieving circumstances would be asked.

Focusing on the patient's exercise habits (**current health status**) can provide specific data related to musculoskeletal injuries. For example, a patient who is a jogger may complain of pain in the knee or ankle joint or in the lower part of the leg. There may be no gross deformities, swelling, or warmth. There may be point tenderness, and on x-ray, one might discover a shin split or hairline fracture of the ankle. Also, specific exercises or participation in sports may be helpful in identifying the mechanics of injury, and better enable one to make a more accurate diagnosis.

The **past health history** will provide specific data related to birth defects or skeletal deformities; developmental problems, such as difficulties in motor coordination or gait; joint problems involving pain, limitation, or arthritis; problems with motor weakness, cramping, spasm, or muscle atrophy; infections; spinal problems; or neurologic involvement. Any of the above could relate to the problem the patient is currently experiencing.

There are several musculoskeletal diseases that have a genetic relationship (e.g., club foot and scoliosis). Therefore, in the **family history**, it is important to ask questions related to specific diseases. Information concern-

TABLE 19-4
Types of Joints

Joints	Location or example	Description	Movement
Fibrous			
Syndesmosis	Distal tibiofibular junction.	The intervening fibrous tissue forms an interrous membrane or ligament.	None.
Cartilaginous			
Synchonrosis	Developing bones.	The epiphysis and the diaphysis are united by hyaline cartilage.	None.
Symphysis	Symphysis pubis; bones of the vertebral column.	Fibrous cartilage binds the two bones together.	Slight.
Synovial			
Plane	Bones of wrist and articular process of adjacent vertebrae.	Articulating surfaces are almost flat.	Limited amount of sliding.
Trachoid (pivot)	Radius and ulna.	Pivotlike process of one joint serves as a pin while other bone and its ligaments form a circle enclosing the pin.	Rotation.
Hinge	Knee, elbow, ankle.	Convex surface articulates with concave surface.	Flexion and extension.

Spheroid (ball and socket)	Hip and shoulder.	Rounded head fits into a deep socket.	Free movement in all directions.
Condylar	Between carpals and radius.	A rounded projection accommodated by an ellipsoid socket.	Movement along two axes.
Sellar (saddle)	Between carpal bone and first metacarpal of the thumb.	Concave-convex surface of one bone fits into convex-concave surface of second bone.	Some free movements; limited rotation.

ing family relationships is equally important because, frequently, patients with musculoskeletal problems must be dependent on others for assistance and support. An assessment of the situation may indicate that the family is unwilling or unable to cope with the needs of the patient. The treatment plan may have to be altered or other means established for the patient's rehabilitation.

The **social history** is very important. For example, patients experiencing musculoskeletal problems are frequently under treatment for a long period of time. Consequently, there may be concerns related to employment and finances. Also, the outcome of the disease or trauma may leave the patient with a deformity or limitation of motion that would require a change in occupation or a return to the same occupation with adjustments made.

In doing the **review of systems**, the nurse should remember that musculoskeletal complaints may relate to other systems. For example, a complaint of joint pain could be a mechanical problem, a bursitis, a neurologic problem, vascular insufficiency, or an early sign of multiple myeloma. Complaints of malaise and fever (**general health status**) with joint pain could relate to the joint, but could also indicate a systemic disease. Many medications used to treat joint problems cause GI distress. Patients with a history of peptic ulcer or dyspepsia may not be able to tolerate a number of the anti-inflammatory drugs.

During the patient assessment, the **physical examination** skills used are primarily inspection and palpation. The equipment needed includes a tape measure, goniometer, and reflex hammer. The environment should be well lighted and ventilated. If the room is exceptionally cold, the patient may not be relaxed, and tests of joint or muscle activity may produce inaccurate results. The physical exam begins at the first meeting with the patient. Observations should be directed to how the patient walks (posture, gait — size of steps, arm swing, balance, start and stop, heel strike), stands (on one leg or two, one shoulder higher than the other), sits (straight, on one buttock, stooped forward, changing positions frequently), grasps examiner's hand (firmly, limply, with discomfort), moves about the room (with ease or discomfort), climbs on and off the examining table (independently, requires assistance, favors a body part, difficulty with specific movements), and wears out shoes (lateral or medial aspect of sole, heels, scuffed toes). The examiner should always compare one side of the patient's body with the other. Each body area should be inspected and palpated for deformity (shortening, angulation, rotation, etc.), symmetry, abnormal movements (tremors, fasciculations, instability, etc.), swelling or masses (fluid, inflammation, blood, tumors), skin (color, temperature, ecchymoses, abrasions, blebs, scars, etc.), edema, varicosities, and tenderness. Bones and joints are examined specifically for active and passive range of motion (ROM), crepitus, and tenderness. Muscles are examined by (1) observing for size, symmetry, atrophy, hypertrophy, spasm, and contractions; (2) palpating for masses, tone, strength, tenderness, consistency, and ruptures; and (3) testing muscles in pairs, positioning limbs symmetrically, inspecting contours at rest and in contraction, relaxing limbs and passively moving them through ROM (slight muscular resistance can be felt), testing strength with and without gravity and resistance (movement should be smooth and steady), and measuring and comparing both limbs for circumference and strength. Specifics of inspection, palpation, and ROM that should be considered for each joint are listed in Table 19-5. For an accurate examination, the patient should be undressed.

The more common **laboratory tests** are listed below. Specific implications of findings are described in Appendix B. Hematology tests include RBC, Hb, Hct, WBC, differential WBC, platelets, and erythrocyte sedimentation rate (ESR). Blood chemistry analysis includes calcium, alkaline phosphatase, phosphorus, acid phosphatase, potassium, creatinine, protein electrophoresis, SGOT, uric acid, and creatine phosphokinase (CPK). Urinalysis includes microscopic examination and evaluation of creatine, calcium, and Bence Jones protein. Synovial fluid is examined for its appearance, WBC, percentage of neutrophils, possible mucin clots, bacteria, and crystals. **X-rays** are some of the most important diagnostic tools in determining musculoskeletal alterations. Regardless of the problem, three basic views are obtained — anteroposterior (AP), lateral, and oblique. In addition, special views or x-ray procedures may be needed to make a more accurate diagnosis. Table 19-6 lists special x-ray procedures, their indications, and nursing interventions after the procedure. The principal nursing responsibility is patient education before the procedure. **Special diagnostic tests** other than those listed in Table 19-7 will be presented in the sections where they specifically apply. Once again, the major nursing responsibility is the education of the patient for the procedure.

Common nursing interventions (general)

Physical needs include prevention of complications; prevention of pressure areas, in particular those caused by the equipment used; observations relative to neurologic, sensory, motor, and vascular impairment of extremities; and positioning, alignment, and ambulation. Because physical needs are related to the pathophysiology, body part involved, and the treatment, the nursing interventions are included with specific treatments and/or problems.

The nature of musculoskeletal problems elicits multiple **psychosocial** responses from patients, many of which relate to patients' past experiences and ability to cope. **Body-image interventions** are based on the fact that patients may fear or be threatened by loss of a body part, function, sexuality, deformity, independence, role in family, job, etc. This fear may be sustained or distorted by equipment being used, inability to maintain or carry out personal hygiene, pain, family interactions, etc.

1. Provide an opportunity for the patient to verbalize his fears.
2. Reinforce strengths.
3. Keep the patient informed of progress.
4. Explain equipment.

TABLE 19-5
Joint Assessment

Joint	Inspection	Palpation	ROM/muscle strength
Temporomandibular (patient sitting)	Symmetry, swelling, deformity, abnormal movements, skin.	Just in front of the tragus of each ear; with fingers on joint, ask patient to open and close jaw, and check for crepitus, tenderness, abnormal movement.	Open and close mouth, side to side movement, clench jaw and try to open.
Neck (patient sitting)	Symmetry, swelling, deformity, abnormal movements, skin.	Trapezius and paravertebral muscles for tenderness, joint for crepitus and abnormal movements.	Flexion: touch chin to each shoulder and chest, touch ear to shoulder. Extension: touch head to back. Repeat against resistance.
Hands (patient sitting) Fingers	Dorsal and palmar surfaces. Skin, fingernails, symmetry, atrophy (particularly thenar eminence), swelling (loss of normal skin folds over joints is subtle evidence of swelling of the interphalangeal joints; absence of grooves between the joints when making a fist indicates swelling of the metacarpal phalangeal joints).	Each joint for pain, tenderness, irregularities, swelling or spongy feeling, abnormal movements.	Extend all fingers, flex all fingers, abduct and adduct the fingers, oppose each finger with the thumb, grasp and squeeze two of the examiner's fingers, make circle with thumb and index finger (examiner tries to pull apart) to test thenar muscle.

Wrist	Dorsal and volar surfaces; skin, asymmetry, atrophy, swelling, deformity.	Ulnar and radial styloids.	Extension: have patient place hands in "prayer position," then lift up elbows. Asymmetry noted by difference in height of elbows or the angle between extensor surface of forearm and dorsum of hand. Flexion: bend wrist down, repeat against resistance, compare extremities.
Elbow (patient sitting)	Skin, symmetry, swelling, deformity, atrophy.	Medial and lateral epicondyles for tenderness or crepitus; olecranon process, olecranon bursa, epicondylar lymph nodes.	Flexion and extension of elbow: observe carrying angle with arm extended for symmetry, pronation and supination of forearm. Repeat against resistance.
Shoulder (patient sitting)	Skin, symmetry, swelling, deformity, atrophy.	All four joints (sternoclavicular, acromioclavicular, glenohumeral, scapulothoracic).	Active: flexion and extension, abduction and adduction, internal rotation and external rotation, circumduction. Passive: passive ROM (abduction, internal and external rotation) is tested by having the patient place hands behind neck with elbows pointing out (external rotation and abduction), and clasp hands behind back and move them up in

Joint	Inspection	Palpation	ROM/muscle strength
			between shoulder blades (internal rotation and abduction). Smooth, rhythmic movements should be observed, and asymmetry should be easily detected. Repeat against resistance.
Hip (patient standing)	All aspects listed in general rules in Overview and look for leg shortening by placing index finger on lateral aspect of iliac crest (level of fingers should be even).		
(patient standing)	Posture; gait: painful (antalgic), gluteus medius limp (muscles contracting on the same side as weight bearing to keep the pelvis from tilting to the opposite side), Trendelenburg's gait (a prominent sag on the side of the weakened muscles or nerve as patient takes a step).		
(patient supine)	Position of hip with patient flat. (With swelling or irritation of the joint there will probably be 30–45° of	Femoral head, superficial trochanteric bursa (posterior lateral surface of greater trochanter).	Flexion and extension, abduction and adduction (stabilize the pelvis to assure true hip motion vs. motion

	flexion, external rotation, and abduction. This is the position that provides for maximum room within the joint capsule.)		from other joints), internal and external rotation. Repeat all the above against resistance. (Note: All ROMs tested with the hip in both 90° flexion and full extension.)
Knee (patient sitting)	Skin, symmetry, atrophy, swelling, deformity.	Place hand over patella, flex and extend knee, and feel patella slipping into patello-femoral groove or crepitus. Extend and feel along inferior patella line at joint space for subluxation of patella. If subluxation is present, the patient will not allow the test to be performed (positive apprehension test). Flex to 30° and apply pressure between patella and femur (tenderness). Flex and feel along joint line for irregularities. Then rotate tibia and extend knee to test for lateral meniscus lesion. Place hand with thumb behind knee. Control distal tibia with other hand and force extremity into valgus. Feel abnormal movement at joint line (medial	Flexion and extension, varus and valgus. Repeat against resistance. Specifically test anterior and posterior cruciates, medial and lateral collateral ligaments.

Joint	Inspection	Palpation	ROM/muscle strength
		and/or lateral instability). Flex to 90°, fix foot, apply a push-pull movement to knee (anterior and posterior stability). Rotatory instability also can be tested using this position. Feel behind knee for a popliteal or Baker's cyst.	
(patient supine)	Flexion contracture: have patient flex knee and pull firmly to chest. Note degree of flexion and position of the other extremity.	Flex knee, place thumb and index finger on either side of joint space. Hold heel (other hand), rotate lower leg and foot laterally; then extend knee. A click will be heard if a torn meniscus is present (McMurray's sign). Flex knee. Milk medial aspect of knee using an upward movement. Tap lateral aspect of knee. A bulge will appear in the hollow medial to the patella if small amount of fluid is present (bulge test). Extend leg, press firmly on thigh and briskly tap patella. Click is heard if fluid is present (ballottement test).	Flexion and extension, internal and external rotation, sliding of femur on tibia. Repeat against resistance.

Feet and ankles (patient sitting)	Skin, symmetry, atrophy, swelling, deformity.	Extend knee and compress suprapatella pouch with one hand and feel each side of patella over the area of the tibiofemoral joint space. Feel suprapatella pouch on each side of quadriceps for bogginess, thickening, fluid, tenderness. Feel Achilles tendon for nodules, tenderness; anterior talofibular, fibulocalcaneal, tibiofibular, medial deltoid, and ligaments for tenderness. Stress joint in varus and valgus positions for integrity of lateral and medial ligaments. Place foot in plantar flexion and try to pull forward (anterior stability). Feel ball of foot, including metatarsals and metatarsophalangeal joint.	Plantar flexion (ankle), dorsiflexion (ankle); inversion and eversion (forefoot); flexion and extension (metatarsophalangeal and interphalangeal joints).
Back (patient standing)	All areas previously mentioned under general rules in the Overview. Curvatures	Feel spinous processes (tenderness, motion). Place two fingers on two spinous	Performed with the pelvis stabilized. Bend to side (lateral bend), bend back

Joint	Inspection	Palpation	ROM/muscle strength
	of cervical, thoracic, and lumbar regions; level of shoulders and iliac crest,	processes and have patient bend forward. Fingers should move apart (indicates joint movement). Observe paravertebral muscle spasm.	(extension), bend forward (flexion), twist to one side and then the other (rotation). Repeat against resistance.
(patient supine)		Flex one knee and hold to abdomen, lower opposite leg on table. Pain indicates sacroiliac involvement. Straight leg raise until discomfort; dorsiflex foot. Discomfort intensifies if the sciatic nerve is involved.	

ROM, range of motion.

TABLE 19-6
Special X-Ray Procedures

X-ray procedure	Indication	Nursing interventions postprocedure
Arteriography	Posttraumatic injuries, bone tumors, soft tissue masses.	Maintain bed rest until next day. Monitor BP, arterial pulses of involved extremity, the presence or absence of numbness or tingling of extremity, movement of extremity, signs of bleeding or the presence of hematoma (groin, axilla), temperature. Limit exercise activity for ~4 hr.
Arthrography	Injury to shoulder, hip, knee, soft tissue.	Monitor as above.
Bone scan	Early detection of tumors, infection, ischemia.	None.
Myelogram	Herniated nucleus pulposus, pressure on nerve root or spinal cord.	Maintain bed rest as per physician's orders (12–24 hr). Position patient in bed according to contrast media used. Monitor BP, pulses, temperature, movement of extremities, muscle strength.
Scanogram	Leg length discrepancy.	None.
Tomograms	Joint abnormalities, lesions in medullary canal or cortices, nonunions, foreign bodies.	None.

5. Attend to the patient's personal hygiene, identifying those aspects important the individual, e.g., hair, makeup, etc. Allow the patient to participate in self-care regardless of the time required.
6. Involve the patient in activities that afford a sense of accomplishment and support self-image.
7. Encourage verbalization of concerns with family, employer, etc.

TABLE 19-7
Special Diagnostic Tests

Test	Description/definition and indication	Nursing observation after procedure
Bone marrow aspiration	Microscopic evaluation of bone marrow for multiple myeloma, tumor, infection.	Bleeding at aspiration site. Pressure dressing over aspiration site.
Electromyography	Electrical potential of each muscle. Detection of muscle denervation; level and site of nerve injury; dystrophies, myopathies.	Bleeding or hematoma at needle site.
Joint aspiration	Microscopic evaluation of joint fluid. Decrease pressure in joint capsule to relieve pain.	Infection. Bleeding at aspiration site. Pressure dressing over aspiration site.

Patients frequently experience **separation**. Because treatment may extend for a significant period of time, the patient may experience fear of rejection; isolation; loss of position in family, work group, school, etc.; and isolation from personal objects of importance.

1. Encourage social and work contacts, use of phone, writing letters, etc.
2. Plan the day so that school or office work can be accomplished. Encourage participation.
3. Adjust visiting hours if needed.
4. Encourage socialization with other patients.
5. Incorporate personal objects into the patient's environment.

Factors contributing to **regression/depression** include seeing oneself as worthless, helpless, nonproductive; fear of dependency, physical limitation, loss of control of environment, becoming a burden; concerns about losing family, housing, job; and financial concerns.

1. Help patients enhance their sense of dignity and self-respect.
2. Recognize physical changes due to age and/or the condition, and provide activities that the patient can participate in with a sense of accomplishment.
3. Allow the patient to make decisions; provide choices.
4. Help patients recognize preferences and maintain a sense of control.
5. Encourage patients to verbalize fears.
6. Explain what can be expected from the treatment and environment.
7. Provide an opportunity for the patient to participate in self-care.

8. Discuss involvement with social service regarding housing and financial concerns.
9. Encourage the patient to maintain contact with family and friends.

Evaluation criteria. Complications of immobilization are prevented. Skin is free of pressure areas caused by equipment. Neurosensory, motor, and vascular functioning are intact. Extremities are free from swelling. Proper position is maintained during the healing process. Equipment is functioning properly. Patient is pain free and comfortable. Patient and family verbalize an understanding of the disease, drugs and their side effects, and the long-range program. Patient verbalizes good self-image. Patient is productive and verbalizes a sense of accomplishment. Social and work ties are maintained. Therapeutic regimen is implemented effectively. Independence is achieved. Proper ambulation techniques are demonstrated. Medications are taken as prescribed. Family is involved in care. Patient returns for follow-up care and evaluation.

Common nursing interventions (nutrition)

Most patients admitted for major elective orthopedic surgery are sufficiently nourished to sustain a week of decreased nutritional intake postoperatively. However, severely debilitated and malnourished patients need carefully planned nutritional therapy preoperatively to decrease the risks of surgery. Patients who have sustained severe multiple injuries may have been healthy and well nourished before their accident. However, the major catabolic response to trauma places a great demand on their available fat and protein reserves, which become exhausted or depleted within 2 to 5 wk. Their body reserves of protein and fat are usually sufficient to carry them for a week or more without any serious consequence.

Obesity, the result of an imbalanced diet, affects the musculoskeletal system by aggravating osteoarthritis, which often affects the weight-bearing joints; placing a strain on the arches of the feet, causing flat feet; increasing the tendency to produce calluses, corns, and bunions; and causing increased joint pain and deformity for patients with bowlegs (genu varum) and knock-knees (genu valgum).

Increases in all essential nutrients are needed for wound healing in the postoperative patient. A diet high in protein, vitamins, iron, and calcium is essential for healing fractures. (Refer to Chapters 2, 11, and 12 for further details on nutrition and wound healing.)

Common nursing interventions (drugs)

For some patients, especially the elderly, having even very simple or therapeutic procedures may require a variety of medications because of multisystem medical diseases. The nurse must be knowledgeable about all the medication administered. The most commonly used **analgesics** (listed in order of their frequency of use and in reverse order related to the severity of pain) are aspirin, acetaminophen (Tylenol), propoxyphene (Darvon), and narcotics. (Additional data about analgesics may be found in Chapter 4.) A variety of **antibiotics** may be used for their bacteriostatic and/or bactericidal effects and their spectrum of action (broad or narrow). These anti-infective agents are used prophylactically for patients who are considered poor risks for major surgery, have a history of infections, undergo extensive major surgery, or have contaminated wounds due to trauma. These agents are used therapeutically for patients who develop infections in any part of their bodies.

A complication of immobility is the formation of a blood clot within the deep veins. **Anticoagulants** are used to prevent the extension of a blood clot and the formation of other emboli and thrombi. **Anti-inflammatory drugs** are basically used for inflammation of joints. Some of the medications used for specific symptoms of disease include aspirin, sodium salicylate, phenylbutazone, indomethacin, and corticosteroids for rheumatoid arthritis; aspirin, sodium salicylate, acetaminophen, and propoxyphene for osteoarthritis; and allopurinol, colchicine, and phenylbutazone for gout. Because anti-inflammatory medications are generally given for a prolonged time, the nurse must be alert for many types of side effects. General side effects may range from nausea and vomiting to abdominal pain, and from GI distress to internal bleeding. Skin rash and dizziness may also occur. Specific reactions to allopurinol may include some of the above side effects, as well as chills, fever, and blood dyscrasias. Colchicine may cause nausea, vomiting, and diarrhea. Corticosteroids can produce a variety of side effects. Those of most concern for the patient with an orthopedic problem include decreased resistance to infection, delayed wound healing, and osteoporosis. **Muscle relaxants** are administered to reduce tension, fears, and anxieties; relieve acute muscle spasm caused by sprains and traumatic injuries; and treat inflammatory conditions of the skeletal muscles. Some of the muscle relaxants currently used are diazepam (Valium), carisoprodol (Soma), and methocarbamol (Robaxin). Some of the side effects of these drugs include drowsiness, skin rash, light-headedness, mental confusion, dizziness, fatigue, and ataxia.

Nursing interventions and observations involved with medication administration should be accurately documented in the patient's chart and reported to the physician.

1. Note the progression of symptoms following the administration of a specific drug.
2. Observe the patient for side effects before continuing to administer the drug.
3. Know medications that patients are receiving and food they are eating, because certain drugs are incompatible with other drugs and foods (e.g., antacids decrease the amount of absorption of antibiotics; aspirin and anticoagulants can have a cumulative effect in prolonging blood clotting and therefore should not be used together; and milk and dairy products interfere with the absorption of tetracycline).

Evaluation criteria.   Medication is received on time as prescribed by the physician. Appropriate food is given with specific medications. Medications are compatible. No side effects or adverse reactions are experienced. Patient's symptoms have subsided and/or disappeared with medical therapy. Medications are consistent/compatible with the laboratory data received.

Common nursing interventions (plaster casts)

Plaster of paris is dehydrated gypsum. When reconstituted with water, plaster recrystallizes into solid gypsum. Plaster receives its strength from the long, thin, interlocking crystals that form as the plaster dries. The heat felt by patients during the application of plaster is created by the chemical reaction in reconstitution. Plaster casts are used to immobilize a part of the body after reduction of a fractured bone and/or dislocated joint until the damaged tissue has healed, to support and protect an injured part of the body during the healing process, and to support and rest part of the body after an operation until healing occurs. Casts are also used to provide rest and prevent movement of joints (as in tenosynovitis), to correct deformities (e.g., contracture of joints), and to provide a traction force such as in the treatment of fracture of the humerus with a hanging arm cast. Before a cast is applied, the health team should explain why the cast is being applied, and what occurs during the application of the cast. The patient's cooperation is particularly essential because it is necessary to maintain a specific position to allow for the proper maintenance of alignment of a part during the application of the cast. The patient should understand how the cast will appear when it is finished and how to cope with limitations. The patient's skin should be examined for redness, acne, abrasions, and pressure areas. It can be helpful to introduce the patient to someone who has a similar cast. While the cast is drying, certain precautions should be observed.

1. Keep the cast uncovered and all surfaces exposed. Before the cast obtains its maximum strength, the excess water must disappear by evaporation from the surface of the cast. The rate of evaporation depends on the humidity present, the temperature, and the circulation of air around the cast.
2. Turn the patient with a body jacket regularly q 1 to 2 hr until the cast is dry.
3. Handle the cast with the palms of the hands and not the fingers. The fingers may cause an indentation that can lead to a pressure area.
4. Support the extremity on pillows to avoid stress on joints (e.g., hips and knees).
5. Support an affected lower extremity on a pillow so that the heel is free from pressure.

Several principles are related to the proper fitting of a cast. A cast should fit properly — smoothly and snugly, without ridges and pressure. A loose cast is ineffective and may cause irritation in areas where the edge of the cast rubs against the skin. A tight cast will cause constriction (*see below:* compartmental syndrome). A cast with ridges will cause a friction point. A cast should be only as thick or heavy as is essential for it to be effective; a thin cast may be adequate. A thick cast gives additional strength, but a heavy, thick cast is very tiring for patients to wear and carry. The amount of padding under a cast is related to the need. A thin layer of sheet wadding over the stockinette may be adequate. Extra padding permits expansion to occur without constriction of the extremity within the cast, if swelling is anticipated. Padding over bony prominences is essential to prevent decubiti. The patient should be discharged with a cast that has a smooth, polished surface, because casts are worn for many weeks. The cast is trimmed and the edges are covered by fastening the stockinette neatly with plaster. The edges of the cast should be covered with moleskin if a stockinette is not used. The edges of the cast are bound in order to prevent crumbs of plaster from falling inside the cast. Basic types of plaster casts and a guide to their positioning and rationale are presented in Table 19-8. Although a plaster cast does serve an important function, unfortunately it can be responsible for the development of serious complications in a relatively short period of time. A summary of these complications and their causes is listed in Table 19-9.

1. Establish base-line data so that evaluation is meaningful.
2. Check circulation and compare the affected and unaffected extremities carefully and frequently.
3. Report untoward signs to the physician immediately. (Table 19-10 discusses circulatory assessment, signs to report, and possible causes.)
4. Investigate complaints of pain. Localized pain or a burning sensation may indicate a pressure sore. Pressure sores over bony prominences are difficult to heal because of poor blood supply to the area. Once a full-thickness ulceration develops, the pain and burning sensation will no longer exist because the nerve ending will have become deadened.
5. Advise the physician if pressure areas are suspected.
6. Examine the skin underlying the cast edges.
7. For patients in body jackets, observe for cast syndrome. (Symptoms are similar to those of paralytic ileus. The condition occurs because of pressure on the mesentery, or it may be psychologic in nature.)
8. Give the following written and verbal discharge instructions to any patient in a cast and also to the caregiver at home:
   a. Inspect the skin under the cast edges for irritation.
   b. Maintain the skin in good condition.
   c. Keep the plaster dry at all times.
   d. Observe toes and fingers for swelling and circulation.
   e. Elevate the extremity if swelling of toes or fingers occurs.

f. Call the physician or return to the clinic for persistent swelling of toes or fingers despite elevation of extremity; numbness or loss of feeling; inability to move toes or fingers; blueness of toes or fingers; severe pain; a break in the cast or softness of the cast; drainage on the cast and/or offensive odor; or a foreign object in the cast.

Evaluation criteria. Casted area is free of pressure, cast lacks indentations or ridges, is neatly trimmed at its edges, fits snugly, and has a smooth, polished surface. Skin along the cast edges is free from pressure. Patient is able to cope with his limitations, verbalizes an understanding of the purpose for the cast, performs those self-care activities that can be managed alone, and anticipates those needs that cannot be managed alone (e.g., the patient with an upper extremity cast needs assistance with cutting meat, etc., and the patient in a body cast needs assistance in bathing lower extremities).

Common nursing interventions (traction)

Traction can be defined as pulling on a body part or extremity while the body acts as a countertraction, pulling in the opposite direction. Traction is used as part of the preoperative or postoperative treatment plan or as a specific method of treatment. The general purposes of traction are to attain and maintain a reduction of a fracture or, in some instances, a dislocation; to correct a deformity or prevent or reduce contractures of joint muscles or pressure on joint surfaces; to decrease or overcome muscle spasm; and to immobilize the body or body part. Important data for each patient in traction are the reason for the type of traction, specific alignment of traction equipment and/or body part, possibility of removing traction and need for interim manual traction, whether or not the patient is allowed to move or turn and to what extent, and specific functioning of the traction (which frequently is modified or adapted to the individual patient's problem).

Adherence to specific guidelines will maximize the benefits of traction: Traction is **continuous** unless otherwise indicated. Ropes are in grooves of pulleys; rope ends are taped back on the rope to safeguard against the knots' slipping. Weights hang free. Patients are instructed not to tamper with or release the traction. Traction is carefully observed during each shift. Traction must have **countertraction**. Traction of the lower extremity requires elevation of the foot of the bed, with the head of the bed flat or minimally elevated. Cervical traction requires elevation of the head of the bed; the body's sliding down provides countertraction. Traction follows an **established line of pull**, which directly relates to the position and alignment of the body part involved. Line of pull is set by the apparatus attached to the patient and the placement of the first pulley. It is determined by the physician and is maintained by the nurse throughout daily care. Traction is **free from friction**. Friction is eliminated when all ropes are on the pulleys and all weights are hanging free, the hook holding the weight bag is not

TABLE 19-8

Plaster Casts: Basic Types, Positioning, and Rationale

Type	Positioning	Rationale
Short arm cast (extends from hand or fingers to elbow)	Elevate in sling so that forearm is upright. Secure sling to Balkan frame or IV pole. Support arm in sling when ambulating.	Assist venous return by gravity.
Long arm cast (extends from hand or wrist to axilla)	Elevate arm on one or two pillows. Place pillow so that hand is also supported if not incorporated in plaster.	Assist venous return. Prevent wrist drop.
Long arm hanging cast (extends from midportion of upper extremity to wrist, with elbow in 90° flexion)	Keep head of bed elevated at all times for a constant pulling force. Do not support the cast itself with pillows.	Provide traction on distal fragment. Assist venous return.
	Support wrist portion of cast with a collar-cuff sling. Pad neck with felt or foam rubber.	Support wrist and provide traction. Prevent pressure on neck.
Shoulder spica (incorporates the trunk, shoulder, and upper extremity)	Position on unaffected side. Support back by placing pillows along entire length of cast.	Promote comfort.
Body jacket (extends from shoulder to iliac crest) or Minerva jacket (a body jacket with a headpiece)	Position on either side. Support back by placing pillows along entire length of cast. Prone if permitted. Turn with arm extended down along the body or fully extended up over the head. Place pillow under abdomen.	Promote comfort. Prevent injury to the extremity. Promote comfort.
Hip spica (incorporates trunk or part of trunk and lower extremities)	Supine: Place pillows under legs encased in plaster to support contours of cast.	Prevent stress at the joints.

	Intervention	Rationale
Single spica (includes trunk and one extremity)	Place small pillow or pad under lumbar region.	Prevent anterior portion of cast from pressing on abdomen or chest.
Double spica (includes trunk and both extremities)	Support uncasted extremity with pillow.	Prevent pressure on heels.
One and a half spica (includes trunk and one leg entirely and extends to knee on other leg)	**Prone:** Turn patient as a unit toward unaffected side.	Avoid twisting patient in cast.
Mini-spica (includes lower part of trunk and one leg to the knee)	Keep patient's arm down along side of body or extended up over his head during turning.	Prevent injury to arm.
	Place pillows in position for chest and abdomen.	Provide comfort.
	Keep toes of foot encased in plaster from touching the mattress by extending plaster on foot 1½" to 2" beyond toes, positioning patient so that foot hangs over edge of mattress, or placing a pillow or sandbag under leg to elevate foot.	Prevent pressure on toes from weight of cast.
	Support unaffected extremity with pillow.	Clear toes of mattress.
	Side: Position on unaffected side. Suspend casted extremity with a muslin sling attached to Balkan frame.	Provide comfort and prevent pressure on affected extremity. Ensure safe position.
	Support entire back with pillows.	Provide comfort. Maintain alignment.

TABLE 19-9

Plaster Casts: Complications and Their Causes

Complication	Cause
Pressure under cast	Application of cast over acned skin, abrasions, or reddened areas. Irregularities under cast because of loose or wrinkled stockinette, uneven padding, overlapping felt, or uneven inner surface of cast. Insufficient padding of bony prominences. Indentations resulting from handling damp cast with fingers rather than palm of hand. Flattened heel caused by damp cast resting on hard surface. Foreign objects falling into cast and becoming embedded in skin.
Pressure along edges of cast	Rough edges irritating underlying skin. Cast edges not beveled, creating pressure ridges on underlying skin. Improper positioning or support of cast resulting in cast edges at opposite end of cast digging into patient's skin. Inadequate padding along edges of cast, e.g., on Achilles tendon.

caught on the bed frame or on the bed gatch, snap hooks are not resting on the bed frame, knots in the rope are not caught in the pulleys, and linen is not resting on the ropes.

There are three main types of traction: manual, skin, and skeletal. In **manual** traction, force is applied to the body part by the hands pulling to extend or realign a limb. It is a temporary measure usually used to reduce a fracture and maintain alignment until a cast or other traction can be applied. In **skin** traction, force is applied by directly pulling on the skin and soft tissue. Buck's extension is one type of skin traction that is also a part of Russell traction. An adhesive material such as moleskin or a treaded foam rubber appliance is held in place on the extremity with an elastic bandage. A foam rubber boot may also be used. A traction cord is attached to the spreader of the apparatus at one end and a weight at the other, which puts tension on the tissues. The traction force is applied over a large area of skin (for example, the entire lower leg) so that it spreads the load and is more efficient and comfortable. More than 2 to 3 kg (5 to 7 lb) of pull on the skin or a tight elastic bandage or boot strap can occlude small blood vessels and cause skin necrosis. Details of Russell traction will appear under the section on treatment of fractured hips. Fitted appliances such as a head halter and pelvic belt traction are other types of skin traction. The appliance should fit snugly, distributing the pressure evenly over the largest possible skin

TABLE 19-10

Circulatory Assessment and Untoward Findings for Patients in Plaster Casts

Assessment	Untoward effect	Possible cause
Toes and fingers	Swelling	Dependency of extremity, venous obstruction, lack of exercise.
Nail beds	Blue, white, cold	Venous or arterial obstruction.
Movement of toes and fingers	Pain on passive movement	Ischemia of flexor muscles.

surface, and be applied symmetrically to avoid rotation. In **skeletal** traction, force is applied directly to the skeleton. This is usually accomplished by inserting a Kirschner wire or Steinmann pin directly through the bone, or Crutchfield or Vinke tongs or a halo apparatus into the bone. A traction cord is applied to a spreader at one end and weight on the other end, thus exerting pull on the bone.

The major **nursing** objectives for any patient in traction, regardless of type, are to keep the patient comfortable and free from complications, and at the same time maintain the traction in proper functioning order so that maximum benefits may be obtained. In order to achieve this, the nurse must understand the purposes and the principles of traction (*see above*). In addition the nurse must establish and record base-line data for evaluation of the following parameters:

1. Skin: Inspect for open or bruised area, dermatitis, circulatory problems, drainage, unusual color, and size of the involved area. Discuss observations with the physician. Skin problems can contraindicate the use of skin traction.
2. Neurovascular status: Check and record, comparing limbs for temperature, color, capillary perfusion of nail beds, movement and sensation of extremities, and presence or absence of pulses.
3. Pain: Note location, quality, quantity, and alleviating or aggravating manifestations. Discuss with the physician any pain that is out of proportion to the problem.
4. Position of extremity in traction: Observe and record the alignment of the extremity. Maintain the extremity in the position of its original placement.

Finally, the complications of immobility and equipment failure should be prevented. The three main complications of traction are immobility (*see* Chapter 7), pressure, and problems at the pin site. **Pressure** is the major complication caused by traction equipment.

1. Heel: For patients in Buck's extension or Russell traction, place the leg on a pillow with the heel free. Make certain that the pillow does not bunch up under the knee and cause pressure in the popliteal space.
2. Malleoli: Have the spreader for skin traction wide enough for straps to clear the malleoli. Do not place the elastic bandage holding the traction straps over the malleoli.
3. Achilles tendon: Check skin traction frequently for slippage and bunching in the area of the Achilles tendon. Rewrap when necessary.
4. Shaft of tibia: With skeletal traction, prevent pressure caused by the yoke resting on the tibia by checking to see that the bar holding the traction has not slipped. Consult with the physician before adjusting the traction bar. (The line of pull may have to be reestablished to take the pressure off the shaft of the tibia). Maintain the same degree of gatch and/or elevation of the foot of the bed as was set up initially.
5. Peroneal nerve: Prevent foot drop. Check that the elastic bandage holding skin traction on the leg is not too tight. Check that the extremity in skin traction is not externally rotated, causing pressure on the peroneal nerve. Observe for complaints of pain, tingling on the dorsum of foot and anterior surface of the leg, difficulty in pulling up the great toe, and inversion of the forefoot. If symptoms are detected, release the elastic bandage from the area over the fibula head and notify the physician.
6. Sacrum: In skeletal traction, pull on the lower extremity causes friction on the sacrum and lower back area. Minimize this by checking the area frequently and providing good skin care.
7. Scapula: Reduce pressure on the scapula when skeletal traction to the upper extremity pulls the arm off the bed. Press down on the mattress and massage the scapula.
8. Occipital region: Reduce pressure/friction from the halo traction. Massage occiput (have the patient turn 45 degrees if possible; otherwise, push down on the mattress and reach under the area).
9. Chin: Reduce friction from the head halter's rubbing against the skin. Pad the entire halter with a small piece of silk to prevent friction. Maintain symmetric pull and prevent rotation of the apparatus.

The major complications at the **pin sites** are infection and thrombosis.

1. Check daily for signs of infection, which may result from slippage of an area of nonsterile pin into the bone and may be indicated by the presence of excessive drainage (in particular, pus), pain, redness, and swelling. Some serous drainage is common because of irritation from the pin.
2. Check for venous thrombosis in a lower extremity (e.g., pain, swelling, and edema with discoloration below the pin site).
3. Notify the physician if any of the above occur.
4. Protect the entrance and exit sites of pins (considered surgical wounds) in the following manner:

a. Cleanse entrance and exit sites daily with hydrogen peroxide to remove accumulated drainage, which could clog the pin sites and create a medium for bacteria, and expose pin sites to air, *or*
b. Cleanse the pin sites as above with hydrogen peroxide or Betadine and then cover with a Betadine dressing, *or*
c. Cover the pin sites with a sterile dressing at the time of insertion and leave alone, unless there is evidence of infection.

Common nursing interventions (balanced suspension)

Balanced suspension is frequently used in combination with traction of a lower extremity. This device, consisting of a Thomas splint and Pearson attachment, supports a body part and overcomes the force of gravity. A variation of a Thomas splint can be used to attain the same results. Balanced suspension serves several functions. It helps to maintain an elevation that can be higher and more dependable than that provided by a pillow, thus enhancing the return of venous and lymphatic flow with gravity assistance. It provides support for an extremity and helps maintain correct alignment. It permits greater mobility of the patient while maintaining alignment of the involved extremity. It provides a means of exercise for the involved extremity by mobilizing the Pearson attachment, and it facilitates nursing care because the patient is more mobile.

The major **nursing** objectives are the same as for any patient in traction. Unfortunately, the equipment easily becomes nonfunctional and requires frequent checking by the nurse.

1. Maintain proper balance of the apparatus at all times. The apparatus should rise when the patient lifts up in bed. Suspension that falls to the bed is not balanced.
2. Observe the groin and thigh for pressure. Pressure in the groin can be alleviated by increasing the weight on the rope holding the ring portion of the Thomas splint. Pressure on the thigh or groin can be alleviated by shifting the overhead pulley slightly in the opposite direction from the pressure.
3. Keep the apparatus entirely free from the bed except for the ring portion of the Thomas splint which should rest lightly on the bed.
4. See that the supporting swaths provide even tension and support and are wrinkle free to prevent skin breakdown.
5. Place the Pearson attachment at the knee to provide for knee flexion, which controls rotation and prevents stretching of the cruciate ligaments and posterior capsule. Pressure in the region of the fibula head because of external rotation or bunching of the splint mattress in the popliteal region could damage the peroneal nerve.
6. Check for the proper alignment of the extremity so that the patella is perpendicular to the ceiling. There may be a slight degree of external rotation; however, marked external rotation can be controlled by placing a small towel roll along the lateral aspect of the lower leg.

7. Place a foot support so that the foot is kept in dorsiflexion. Inspect the sole of the foot for pressure areas.
8. Observe for pressure on the heel or in the region of the Achilles tendon.

Frequently, patients in traction/balanced suspension have sustained a severe traumatic injury and experience pain, particularly pain on motion. They are apprehensive and often confused. At the time they are placed in traction/balanced suspension, patients may not be fully conscious of what is happening to them. The equipment used is frightening not only to patients but to family members and other visitors. Family members are frequently reluctant to touch or even go near the patient for fear of causing further distress. Patients also are reluctant to move any part of their body or have anyone come near their bed. Often, the patient and family demonstrate their **anxiety** by frequently requesting help from the nursing staff. The following suggestions can help patients and their families to cope with the fears and anxieties of traction/balanced suspension.

1. Explain the purpose of the traction, the alignment that is desired, how to move and the importance of movement, what to expect in terms of pain or areas of potential pressure or discomfort, the need for medication, and how care will be approached (bathing, eating, toileting, etc.) Discuss traction/balanced suspension before its application whenever possible.
2. Determine if the patient's complaints are physiologically based or stem from anxiety. Frequently, patient complaints are manifestations of apprehension and can be alleviated by explanations of what is happening and why. Use knowledge of developmental stages in planning interventions. (For example, young adults may be experiencing fears of distortion of body image or an inability to function in a sexual capacity or to provide in the future for the needs of a family. Elderly patients may be experiencing feelings of becoming a burden to others or of loss of independence.)
3. Convey a willingness to listen and acceptance of the individual. The physical care of patients in traction/balanced suspension is often complex because such patients do have difficulty moving and may require the assistance of more than one person. Attempt to maintain eye contact. Patients in cervical traction or head halters cannot make eye contact with a person who is not positioned properly. Check to see that patients have call bells within reach and let them know that their call will be answered.
4. Handle the equipment carefully. Appear knowledgeable and competent. Seek information about the equipment before approaching the patient. Handle the equipment and the involved extremity carefully. Bumping or abruptly moving the bed or the equipment, especially if the patient has a fresh fracture, can cause pain.

5. Provide appropriate activities to alleviate boredom and keep the patient motivated. (For example, a young, athletic individual may be very restless and need activities. If the problem involves a lower extremity, set up a series of physical activities that can be performed with the upper extremities. Incorporate the patient's usual activities into the hospital regimen to alleviate boredom.)

6. Promote sleep. Discuss the patient's usual sleeping positions and the restrictions of the traction/balanced suspension. Try to find a position that is comfortable, then medicate for sleep as needed.

Evaluation criteria. Patient is comfortable and relaxed in the equipment, is pain free, describes the purpose of the equipment, participates in self-care, and verbalizes anxieties. Patient sleeps through the night, communicates needs, and has minimal signs of boredom. Complications are minimized. Proper alignment of the extremity is maintained, and the neurovascular supply is adequate. Skin is free of pressure areas. Patient complaints are evaluated and resolved. Pin sites are free of infection. Immobilization is not impeding patient's progress. ROM to all unaffected extremities is maintained. Nutrition is adequate, and base-line data are established, recorded, and continuously evaluated. Equipment is maintained in proper functioning order. Traction is continuous; countertraction is maintained; equipment is free from friction; and suspension is balanced.

DEVIATIONS

COMPARTMENTAL SYNDROME

Compartmental syndrome, a condition in which increased pressure compromises the circulation and functioning of tissues within a closed space, occurs relatively infrequently, but can be devastating to the patient. It affects the hands, the feet, the buttocks, and, more often, the forearms and legs. Compartmental syndromes can occur wherever tissue is surrounded by a limited envelope. The basic problem is too large a volume in too small a space. Decreased compartmental volume may result from closure of fascial defects and traction. Increased compartmental volume may result from bleeding, fluid loss from capillaries, infiltrated IV fluid, fractures, muscle exertion, surgical revascularization, burns, snake bites, and orthopedic surgical techniques such as tibial osteotomies and Hauser procedures. Externally applied pressures such as air splints, compression dressings, casts, Bryant's traction, arterial tourniquets, and lying on a limb may also cause compartmental syndrome.

There are four limiting envelopes that may surround a compartment: the epimysium (the sheath of connective tissue that surrounds a muscle), the fascia (the fibrous tissue between the muscles, forming the muscle sheath), the skin, and casts or dressings. Compartmental syndrome begins when capillary perfusion ceases. Increased compartmental content or decreased compartmental size causes edema, which leads to tissue pressure. The increased tissue pressure causes more edema and a resultant ischemia. The end result is progressive death of muscles and nerves.

Pain is the earliest *symptom* and appears to be out of proportion to the patient's problem. It is a vital clue to the onset of locally insufficient blood flow. Pain on passive stretch of intracompartmental muscles is an indication of inadequate blood flow, as is tenderness of the compartment on palpation. Pallor may be symptomatic, depending on the degree of circulatory compromise. Absence of a pulse may not be a valid sign; frequently the pulse is present. Neuromuscular sensory loss is specific to the involved area. If the compartmental syndrome is not detected and treated early, the following *complications* can occur: persistent hypesthesia and dysesthesia, persistent motor weakness, infection, myoglobinuric renal failure, contractures, amputation, and death.

Diagnosis is based on the health history, positive clinical findings, and elevated tissue pressure.

Common interventions

The goal of treatment is to minimize neurologic deficit by promptly lowering the tissue pressure to a normal level so that blood flow will be restored. Methods of treatment include removal of externally applied pressure (i.e., casts, dressings, air splints) and surgical decompression.

Nursing interventions

Physical 1. For all patients at risk for compartmental syndrome, careful observation, establishment of base-line data, and continuous assessment are of utmost importance. Time is an important factor, because early recognition of the problem can prevent a devastating outcome for the patient.

2. Be alert for constant piercing pain that appears to be out of proportion to the problem, frequent requests for pain medication without relief, and pain that increases on passive stretch of the involved extremity.

3. Check for an extremity that appears pale. Monitor the pulse. (The pulse may be present or absent. If the underlying problem is a vascular injury, there will be no pulse.) Check for capillary perfusion.

4. Palpate the involved compartment for tenderness.

5. Ask the patient to extend his toes to test for motor function of the lower extremity. (A patient can wiggle his toes without anterior compartment function by using his flexor and then allowing his toes to spring back.)

6. Demonstrate what is to be done to make it easier for the patient to follow, when testing motor function of an upper extremity.

7. Use light touch or two-point discrimination, which are better quali-

fiers than pinprick, when testing sensation. (Methods of testing specific nerves are listed in Table 19-11.)

8. Institute the following measures if a patient is at risk:
    a. Assign the same nurse to make frequent observations and record findings on a flow sheet.
    b. Evaluate findings at the end of each shift. The nurse who has been caring for the patient should make rounds with the nurse coming on duty. They should perform the tests together and validate each other's findings to ensure greater continuity.
    c. Elevate the extremity. Elevation may prevent the beginning of a compartmental syndrome; however, once the syndrome has started, elevation above the level of the heart should be avoided to maintain local arterial pressure.
    d. Evaluate symptoms or changes in symptoms and report them immediately. Time is critical: A few hours can make a big difference in the outcome.

Psychosocial. 9. Attempt to become acquainted with the patient and build his trust and confidence. Patients experiencing symptoms of a

TABLE 19-11

Methods of Testing Specific Nerves for Compartmental Syndrome

Nerve	Sensory*	Motor
Radial	Test web space between thumb and first finger.	Ask the patient to touch each finger to his thumb.
Median	Test distal surface of index finger.	Ask the patient to touch his fourth finger to his thumb, making a circle, or to make a "scratching" motion with his index finger.
Ulnar	Test distal end of little finger.	Ask the patient to abduct his fingers or produce a "key pinch" motion.
Peroneal	Test web space between first and second toes.	Ask the patient to dorsi-flex his ankle and extend his toes.
Tibial	Test medial and lateral surfaces of sole of foot.	Ask the patient to plantar flex his ankle and flex his toes.

*Use light touch or two-point discrimination.

compartmental syndrome are often frightened as they, too, recognize that their pain is out of proportion to the problem.

10. Take the time to assess each patient accurately. When being tested for motor and sensory function, the patient is in pain and may be fearful of moving the extremity or may not be able to discriminate between touch and pain.

11. Explain all procedures and why they are essential, because frequently checking the extremity may alarm the patient.

Evaluation criteria. *See* Overview. Symptoms or changes in symptoms reported immediately. Extremity assessed every shift.

FAT EMBOLISM

Fat embolism is a syndrome characterized by "self-limited" pulmonary disease that usually occurs ≤3 days after a fracture. It results from skeletal trauma and is seen most frequently in patients with fractures of bones that contain marrow fat, such as the long bones of the extremities, the pelvis, the ribs, and the sternum.

Two theories exist regarding the pathophysiology of fat emboli. The mechanical theory hypothesizes that minute fat globules are released from the marrow of the fractured bone and enter the circulation through the venous system and migrate to the lungs. The metabolic theory holds that minute fat globules combine with platelets and other blood products to form an embolus, which travels through the blood system to the lungs.

Insidious *symptoms* that occur within the first 24 hr include signs of confusion, restlessness, and irritability; elevated temperature and pulse; and headache. In addition to the above symptoms, tachypnea, dyspnea, and petechial rash on the chest, shoulders, and in the conjunctiva are more suggestive of fat embolus.

Diagnosis is based on the health history, physical exam, ECG changes, chest x-ray, and laboratory findings of a PO_2 <60 mmHg, elevated serum lipase, platelet count <150,000/mm^3, and the presence of fat in the urine.

Common interventions

The patient should be treated for shock by the maintenance of an adequate airway, the use of oxygen for respiratory distress, and replacement of blood and fluids. Oxygen is used to maintain adequate PO_2 levels. Drug therapy may include corticosteroids or IV alcohol, dextran, or heparin.

Nursing interventions

Physical 1. Monitor vital signs and temperature closely.

2. Observe for changes in the patient's behavior.

3. Be alert to the insidious signs of fat embolus; observe for petechial rash.

4. Report observations promptly to the physician and record observations accurately in the nursing notes.

Psychosocial 5. Be aware that trauma patients have many fears and anxieties because of the sudden, severe stress situation that they are experiencing; acute pain associated with their trauma; multiple procedures and treatments they are encountering that they cannot fully comprehend in spite of explanations given to them; and nebulous physical changes.

Evaluation criteria. *See* Overview. Symptoms of fat emboli recognized early. Changes in patient's behavior recognized early and reported to physician.

CONTUSION

A contusion is a bruise or injury to a body part without a break in the skin, causing soft tissue hemorrhage into the adjacent tissues. Contusions may result from trauma (a blunt force or blow) and may develop anywhere in the body, in persons of all age groups.

Symptoms include pain, swelling, and tenderness over the site, and discoloration of skin in the area (local hemorrhage). *Complications* include abscess formation and infection.

Diagnosis is based on the health history and physical exam. Treatment consists of the application of cold, wet compresses or ice to the involved part; immobilization of the injured part; application of heat after 24 hr; and the administration of antibiotics in some instances. Surgery is contraindicated because problems usually resolve spontaneously. Healing time depends on the individual.

Evaluation criteria. *See* Overview.

STRAIN

A strain is defined as excessive stretching, overuse, or misuse of a muscle or group of muscles, resulting in a tear of the muscle fibers or involvement of the tendon. Strains can be classified as acute or chronic and may affect any muscle in all age groups of individuals. Acute strains may result from sudden trauma. Repeated use of a muscle beyond normal capacity may cause chronic strains. Overexertion or overstretching of part of a muscle may contribute to a strain.

Symptoms of acute strain include pain, limitation of motion, tenderness over the site, swelling, and ecchymoses. Symptoms of chronic strain include pain, limitation of motion, and tenderness over the site. Chronic strain can result in weakness of the involved area.

Diagnosis is based on the health history and physical exam. Common interventions include immobilization, cold compresses or ice, analgesics, and heat after the first 24 to 28 hr.

Evaluation criteria. *See* Overview.

SPRAIN

A sprain is an injury to the joint capsule or ligaments surrounding the joint, causing overstretching or tearing of the tissues. Persons of all ages may be affected. Sprains may occur in any joint, but the most common sites are the ankles, knees, cervical region (whiplash injury), and lower back region. Trauma and a sudden, twisting injury are the usual causes.

Symptoms include pain, swelling, limitation of motion, tenderness, and ecchymosis over the area. *Diagnosis* is based on the health history, physical exam, and x-ray. Common interventions include immobilization, elevation, wet compresses or ice, compression dressing using an elastic bandage, and analgesics.

Evaluation criteria. See Overview.

DISLOCATIONS

A dislocation is an injury resulting in complete disruption of a joint so that the articulating surfaces no longer have contact. Persons of all age groups may be affected. Dislocation may occur in any joint, but most commonly occurs in the jaw, shoulders, elbows, wrists, fingers, hip, knees, ankles, and toes. Trauma or excessive stress (usually a twisting force) to the bones near the joint may result in dislocation. *Symptoms* include pain, swelling, deformity, loss of motion, and neurovascular impairment. *Complications* include nerve injuries. *Diagnosis* is based on the health history, physical exam, and x-ray (two planes). Common interventions consist of either manual or surgical (open or closed) reduction; elevation; wet compresses or ice; immobilization with splints, casts, or traction; analgesics; and an exercise program once healing has occurred.

Evaluation criteria. See Overview.

SUBLUXATION

Subluxation is an injury resulting in a partial dislocation. The characteristics and treatment of subluxations are similar to those of dislocations, but usually require less time to heal (*see above*).

FRACTURE

A fracture is a break in the continuity of bone causing damage to the soft tissue and adjacent structures. Classification is according to **anatomic location** (proximal, middle, distal third of the shaft; supracondylar; subtrochanteric); **direction of the fracture line** (transverse, spiral, oblique); **type** (displaced or undisplaced, complete or incomplete, comminuted — many splinters or fragments, butterfly — shape of fragment, segmental — sections, impacted — one piece forced into contact with another, compression — caused by pressure, pathologic — caused by disease); and whether it is **closed** or **open** (skin intact or broken).

Fractures may occur in any bone, in persons of all age groups. Fractures may be caused by (1) trauma from a direct blow to the body, rotation or torsion movement, or prolonged or excessive stress or strain, or (2) pathologic causes such as bone tumor and decalcified bone or faulty metabolism.

Symptoms include pain, swelling, deformity, movement at the site, muscle spasm, tenderness, loss of function, an area that is warm to the touch, neurovascular impairment, and a bruise. *Complications* include neurovascular impairment, limitation or loss of functional ability, malunion, nonunion, and infection.

Diagnosis is based on the health history, physical exam, and x-rays that may include more than one plane and views of joints above and below the injured part.

Common interventions

Medical treatment consists of manipulation, closed reduction, immobilization (plaster casts, traction), and analgesics. **Surgical** treatment may include open reduction and internal fixation with use of a nail and plate, rod, wire, screw, or intramedullary rod. A replacement prosthesis or compression device may also be used.

Nursing interventions

Nursing assessment and interventions are related to circulation, neuromuscular/sensory systems, position, etc. For details, refer to plaster, traction, compartmental syndrome, fat emboli, preoperative care (*see* Chapter 9), and postoperative care (*see* Chapter 11).

FRACTURED HIPS

Intracapsular fractures of the head and neck of the femur are contained within the joint capsule. They are classified by anatomic location (subcapital, transcervical, basilar neck) and type (impacted, stable, unstable). **Extracapsular fractures** occur outside the joint capsule, most commonly between the greater and lesser trochanter. They are classified by anatomic location (base of neck, intertrochanteric, subtrochanteric) and type (nondisplaced, stable, unstable).

Fractured hips are rare in young people (except from severe force). Women are affected more often than men. Persons between 60 and 90 yr of age are most vulnerable. Both intracapsular and extracapsular fractures occur as a result of trauma. Intracapsular fractures can be the result of a minor injury, e.g., a twisting force, missing a step on uneven ground, or stepping off a curb. They can also be due to a blow to the shaft of the femur. Extracapsular fractures usually occur after a fall, either because of a direct blow to the femur or trochanter or indirectly by a forcible pull on the muscles that insert on the trochanter.

Symptoms include external rotation, shortening, swelling, ecchymosis, and pain on motion. These symptoms are more pronounced in extracapsular fractures and may not be apparent in impacted fractures. The patient may be walking despite a fractured hip. *Complications* of intracapsular fractures include nonunion, aseptic necrosis, infection, and loss of the previous level of ambulation because of the fracture, the patient's age, and/or systemic disease. Complications of extracapsular fractures include loss of the previous level of ambulation related to the fracture, the patient's age, and/or systemic disease; infection; shortening of the extremity; fat emboli (subtrochanteric); thromboembolic disease; and death. *Diagnosis* is based on the health history, physical exam, and AP and lateral x-rays.

Common interventions

The optimum treatment would be to take the patient to the OR and immediately reduce the fracture. This is not always possible as elderly patients frequently have multiple medical problems that must be evaluated before surgery can be performed. Intracapsular fractures are treated with closed reduction with internal fixation, open reduction with internal fixation, a replacement prosthesis, and/or traction. Extracapsular fractures are treated with open reduction with internal fixation and/or traction, which could be followed by a plaster cast.

Nursing interventions for persons with hip fractures are discussed in Table 19-12.

RHEUMATOID ARTHRITIS

Rheumatoid arthritis is a chronic systemic inflammatory disease involving the body's connective tissue. The inflammatory process occurring in the synovium includes edema, vascular congestion, and vascular infiltration, which result in thickened synovium. Rheumatoid arthritis occurs more frequently in females than males and can occur at any age; however, it usually begins between the age of 20 and 50 yr and is seen most frequently during middle age and later life. Although the cause is unknown, several theories suggest that it is an autoimmune disease, genetic, or caused by a virus. The disease usually takes the following course: Inflammation of the synovium occurs. Granulation tissue proliferates and spreads over the articular cartilage to form a pannus. Swelling of synovium distends the joint and stretches the capsule and collateral ligaments. The results of this process interfere with normal joint motion, and continuation of this process erodes the subchondral bone. The proliferation and destruction of the synovial membrane are followed by joint destruction and deformity. Remissions and exacerbations are *characteristic*.

The clinical picture of rheumatoid arthritis may be extremely variable. Onset is usually insidious but may be abrupt. Constitutional *symptoms* include fatigue, weakness, fever, and weight loss. Joint symptoms include stiffness on arising in the morning or after prolonged inactivity; swelling due to soft tissue thickening, fluid, or bony overgrowth; joint swelling (usually symmetric); and swelling of another joint. Joints commonly involved include the proximal interphalangeal joints of fingers, metacarpophalangeal joints, metatarsophalangeal joints, and those of the wrists, knees, elbows, ankles, shoulders, and spine. Pain on motion, tenderness, subcutaneous rheumatic nodules, cold and clammy hands, and smooth and shiny skin in the extremities are other symptoms. *Complications* include flexion contracture, unstable or dislocated joints, ankylosis, atrophy of muscle, deformities, and disabilities.

Diagnosis is based on the health history, physical exam, and laboratory tests that reveal elevated ESR, positive rheumatoid factor, and poor mucin precipitation in the synovial fluid. X-rays show narrowing of the joint space, damaged articular cartilage, and bony erosion.

Common interventions

The treatments for rheumatoid arthritis are diverse and numerous. The evaluation of treatment may be difficult because of spontaneous remissions and exacerbations. The primary goals are to reduce inflammation and pain, preserve joint function, and prevent deformity. A basic program of **medical** treatment includes several measures. The duration of **rest** depends on the severity of the disease or the occurrence of remission. (Patients with systemic and articular involvement may require complete bed rest, whereas other patients with milder involvement may only need 2 to 4 hr/day of rest). **Immobilization** of involved joints provides rest for inflamed joints, relieves spasm and pain, and prevents deformity. **Exercise** is recommended to preserve joint motion and maintain muscle strength and endurance. An exercise program should be part of the patient's daily activities and be performed within the limits of pain. The use of heat or analgesics before exercising may help to alleviate some discomfort and relax muscles, thus allowing the patient to carry out the prescribed exercises. The exercise program may need to be altered if pain persists for 1 to 2 hr after the exercises. **Drug therapy** may include the following: salicylates, which are used for their analgesic and anti-inflammatory effects and are prescribed in large dosages depending on the patient's tolerance and need; indomethacin (Indocin) and phenylbutazine (Butazolidin), anti-inflammatory agents; gold salts; corticosteroids; and chloroquine.

Surgical intervention may be necessary to correct deformities, improve function, or alleviate pain. Various operative procedures are available, including osteotomies (to correct deformities); arthrodesis (to stabilize a joint); arthroplasties of the hips, knees, elbows, and shoulders (to improve motion); and synovectomy (to relieve pain).

Nursing interventions

Understanding the patient's personality and reaction to the disease is an important component of the assessment. The effects of arthritis may be more devastating emotionally than physically. Anxiety and emotional stress may be due to fears of crippling, loss of mobility, confinement to a wheelchair existence, burden to the family, and loss of employment. The patient's

TABLE 19-12
Nursing Management of Patients with Hip Fractures

Assessment/intervention	Rationale
Preoperative Establish base-line data regarding the following: History of medical problems (cardiac, respiratory, renal)	Aids in further evaluation of progression of symptoms. The patient's age coupled with trauma and immobility could cause major problems (pneumonia, bladder infections, labile BP).
Vital signs	Bleeding from fracture can cause shock. Patients who have major fluctuations in BP may develop a stroke.
Pain	Failure to immobilize the hip properly will cause pain and muscle spasm, which prevent rest and will easily fatigue the elderly patient.
Swelling of the thigh	This may not be an early sign. If care is not taken in transferring a patient from stretcher to bed, a non-displaced fracture can become displaced. An intertrochanteric fracture can bleed up to 2 liters of blood into the soft tissue before it is detected.
State of orientation	Confusion and disorientation are frequently precipitated by trauma. However, the patient could also have sustained a head injury at the time of the trauma.
Condition of the skin	A decubitus ulcer may have formed because, when patients fall at home and are afraid to move, several days can elapse before they are found.
Intake and output	Dehydration may be a major problem for the above patient. An IV may have been started in the ER at a slow rate to prevent the patient from going into CHF. The rate of flow may change during the transfer to the unit and must be checked. Bladder distension and overflow incontinence are common problems following a fractured hip.
Prepare unit for traction (bed board, hard mattress, Balkan frame, and trapeze)	Provide for easier mobility of the patient.

Assessment/intervention	Rationale
Maintain Russell traction	
Elevate extremity on two pillows	Maintain proper flexion at the hip and knee.
	Decreases edema.
Hold knee sling wide apart by a spreader over the patella	Decreases pressure in the popliteal region and over the peroneal nerve.
Check that elastic bandage holding Buck's extension in place is not constricting	Prevents occlusion of the small blood vessels and skin necrosis.
Prevent slipping of the elastic bandage. It may need to be reapplied frequently and the skin inspected	Will bunch around the Achilles tendon and dorsum of foot causing pressure and skin breakdown. Achilles tendon has a poor blood supply, which makes healing difficult.
Place no more than 2–3 kg (5–7 lb) of weight on the skin	Prevents occlusion of the small blood vessels and skin necrosis.
Maintain neutral alignment or minimal external rotation of the extremity	External rotation is more apt to occur with the extremity in extension. Flexion provided by the Russell traction may not be enough to keep the leg in position. May need a towel roll along the lateral aspect of the leg. Peroneal nerve curves about the neck of the fibula and runs superficially over the fibular head. Pressure in this area because of external rotation can cause a foot drop. This will occur more rapidly in an extremity that is very thin and has little muscle padding.
Prevent complications of immobilization	If complications occur, they could impede surgery or affect the patient's ability to ambulate later.

Postoperative

Continue observations as stated preoperatively	Aids in accurate assessment of patient's progress.
Positioning	
For replacement prosthesis with a posterior or lateral posterior approach, prevent flexion, adduction, and internal rotation of the extremity	Prevents dislocation. These are the positions used to dislocate the hip at the time of surgery. Extremes of these positions can cause the prosthesis to dislocate.
For replacement prosthesis with an anterior approach, prevent external rotation of the extremity.	This approach is used for patients with Parkinson's disease.

Assessment/intervention	Rationale
With internal fixation, maintain internal or external rotation of the leg (depends on the type of fracture), extension, and abduction.	Maintain hip in the position of the reduction. Forcing the extremity into other positions will cause pain and stress on the fracture site.
Before turning patient, place pillow between his legs, then turn patient onto the nonoperative side, supporting the hip and knee in neutral alignment.	Prevents dislocation or stress at the fracture site.
Put all unaffected extremities through ROM exercises.	Maintains muscle tone and prepares patient for ambulation.
Begin patient ambulation (weight-bearing, nonweight-bearing, or partial weight-bearing gait).	Gait used will depend on the fracture and the patient's ability to use an ambulatory aid and the physician's recommendation.
Decrease fear/anxiety	
Provide opportunity for patients to verbalize.	Encourages independence vs. dependence.
Encourage family to bring familiar objects from home; environment is unfamiliar and often a source of fear.	Promotes orientation. Elderly patients are often confused or disoriented.
Provide detailed and consistent instructions.	Prevents confusion when things are done differently each day — especially for elderly patients.
Encourage participation in self-care.	Prevents regression.
Provide experiences that give patient a feeling of success and accomplishment; it is most important that the initial transfer from bed to chair go smoothly.	Decreases anxiety. Increases self-confidence and feeling of accomplishment.

knowledge of the course of the disease and the results of the prescribed medical treatment are essential in the management. Denial or acceptance of the disease may not only affect motivation to follow the recommended course of treatment, but also may affect the patient's life-style.

Physical 1. Encourage bed rest or planned rest periods.
2. Maintain proper body alignment to include use of splints or braces to immobilize the extremity, and prevention of flexion and rotation of the extremity.
3. Administer medication as prescribed.

4. Observe for side effects of the medication.
5. Supervise and/or assist the patient with a planned exercise program.
6. Observe the effects of the exercise program on the patient's tolerance and pain.
7. Encourage the patient to be as independent as possible with activities of daily living.
8. Handle involved limbs gently, avoiding jerky movements.
9. Provide good skin care.
10. Maintain an adequate diet and fluid intake.
11. Provide assistive devices for activities of daily living, e.g., long-handled shoehorn, pick-up scissors, modified eating utensils, long-handled brushes, etc.
12. Provide appropriate preoperative care (see Chapter 9).
13. Provide postoperative care, including general care (see Chapter 11), maintenance of appropriate position of the extremities, and maintenance of the prescribed exercise program.

Psychosocial 14. Repeat information about the disease several times over the long course of treatment to dispel anxieties related to crippling and disabilities.
15. Approach the patient with a positive attitude, sensitivity, and understanding of the problems.
16. Provide continual emotional support and reassurance.

Educational 17. Instruct the patient to observe the following directions:
    a. Maintain proper body alignment.
    b. Prevent deformities by using splints and braces, following the prescribed exercise program, and using a firm, flat mattress.
    c. Maintain drug therapy.
    d. Observe for side effects of medications.
    e. Avoid fatigue by taking planned rest periods.
    f. Control pain by taking salicylates, applying moist heat, using a heating pad, and wearing warm clothing.
    g. Maintain normal body weight.
    h. Maintain good posture.
    i. Continue full ROM of all joints.

Evaluation criteria. See Overview.

OSTEOARTHRITIS

Osteoarthritis is a slowly progressing noninflammatory joint disease that is characterized by the degeneration of articular cartilage and bony overgrowth at the margin of the joints. This condition is also referred to as degenerative arthritis, hypertrophic arthritis, and degenerative joint disease. It most commonly affects middle-aged and older populations and is more frequent in women than men. Weight-bearing joints, particularly the hips and the knees, are most frequently involved. However, the cervical, thoracic, and lumbar spine may also be involved. Predisposing factors include advanced age, female sex, obesity, heredity, joint injury, joint infection, and congenital deformities.

The earliest osteoarthritic changes occur in the articular cartilage with erosion of the chondrocytes, which may be a result of mechanical stress. The degeneration and disappearance of the articular cartilage causes joint space narrowing. Formations of rough, thick, irregular bone occur as the disease progresses. Osteophytes form at the joint margins. Movement of these rough, irregular joint surfaces causes pain and stiffness. (Heberden's nodes, which occur in the interphalangeal joints of the fingers, are also a form of osteoarthritis.)

Symptoms vary according to the progression of the disease process and the extent of movement of the involved joints. Tenderness is noted on palpation of the joint area. Pain, the primary complaint, may begin as a vague ache and increase as the disease progresses. It increases with excessive movement and damp, cold weather, and it may occur during rest in later stages of the disease. Stiffness may be gradual and vague at the onset, but it increases as the disease progresses and may cause marked limitation of movement. It occurs after periods of rest but is relieved with a moderate amount of movement of the joint. Stiffness may be a result of protective splinting against pain and may be manifested by limited rotation of the joint. Swelling is minimal at the onset, but may cause malalignment of the extremity in later stages. The patient may feel crepitus during motion in the later stages. Fatigue also occurs in later stages of the illness. *Complications* include contractures and deformities. Varus and valgus deformities in the lower extremity can result in marked instability of the knee joints.

Diagnosis is based on the health history and physical exam that detects the limited rotation of the joint, crepitus on motion, and tenderness on palpation of the joint area. X-rays may disclose narrowing of the joint spaces, malalignment of the joints, or spur formation on the marginal surface of the joint.

Common interventions

Conservative **medical** therapy may include any of the following: Drug therapy (analgesics, anti-inflammatory drugs, muscle relaxants); moist heat for relief of pain; mild exercise to maintain muscle tone, decrease muscle spasm, and prevent muscle atrophy; immobilization of the joint during the acute phase by use of splints and braces for joints, a cervical collar, and corsets for the spine; the use of assistive devices in walking (such as canes, crutches, or walker) to decrease weight bearing on the involved joint; a low-calorie diet for weight reduction of the obese patient; or planned rest periods to alleviate overuse of involved joints.

Indications for **surgery** include failure of conservative therapy to relieve pain adequately, incapacitation and/or curtailment of activities of daily living, and inability of a wage earner to work. Reconstructive measures (arthrodesis, arthroplasty, osteotomy, or partial or total replacement of a joint) may improve joint motion, relieve pain, and correct deformity.

Nursing care is similar to that for patients with rheumatoid arthritis (*see above*).

GOUT

Gout is a metabolic disease manifested by an excess of uric acid in the blood (hyperuricemia). The highest incidence (90 to 95%) occurs in males in the fifth decade of life; another 5 to 10% of the afflicted are postmenopausal women. The great toe is the most common site; other sites are the ankles, wrists, knees, fingers, and any other toes. Primary gout is the result of an inborn error in metabolism. Secondary gout is an acquired disease associated with an illness that leads to excessive formation of uric acid, such as leukemia, polycythemia vera, or multiple myeloma. It may also result from decreased renal excretion of uric acid because of chronic renal insufficiency. Predisposing factors of acute gouty arthritis include local or general trauma to the body, surgery, strenuous exercise, excessive use of alcohol, a diet high in purines, a starvation diet, and the use of certain drugs causing elevated levels of serum uric acids (e.g., thiazide diuretics, low doses of salicylates, and some hypertensive medications).

Persons suffering from gout have limited solubility of uric acid and its salts; an excessive quantity of urates in the circulating blood and body fluids; and urate deposit in the tendons, bursae, cartilage, joints, epiphyseal bone, and the kidneys. Acute attacks are the result of an inflammatory reaction because of a sudden precipitation of urate crystals in the joint cavity.

Symptoms of acute gout include a sudden attack without warning, accompanied by swollen, red, indurated joints; tense skin that is hot, shiny, and dusky; and severe joint pain that progressively worsens. Chronic gout is characterized by the presence of tophi (deposits of urates) in tissue and around joints and tendons. *Complications* include local tissue necrosis and proliferation of fibrous tissue from tophi, resulting in joint damage and chronic disability, renal dysfunction, and hypertension and cardiovascular accidents.

Diagnosis is based on the health history, physical exam, elevated serum uric acid, urate crystals in synovial fluid, and the presence of tophi on x-ray.

Common interventions

1. Encourage bed rest with immobilization of the involved area in an acute attack.
2. Apply local heat or cold.
3. Maintain a low-purine diet.
4. Encourage high fluid intake to prevent precipitation of urate crystals.
5. Administer drug therapy in acute attacks.
   a. Give narcotics for pain relief.
   b. Give colchicine q 1 to 2 hr until pain subsides. Give no more than 8 to 10 doses within 24 hr and stop medication if the patient develops diarrhea, nausea, or vomiting. Give colchicine IV prn.
   c. Administer corticosteroids.

Nursing interventions

Physical 1. Observe the condition of the skin — particularly the joints — for redness, induration, swelling, and dusky color.
2. Document and report to the physician any untoward signs.
3. Maintain the patient on a low-purine diet. A low-calorie diet should also be provided if the patient is overweight.
4. Monitor the fluid intake and output to ensure a high fluid intake.
5. Administer medications on time.
6. Observe for toxic effects of medications and report these to the physician immediately so that the medication can be changed.
Psychosocial 7. Provide opportunities for the patient to verbalize fears and concerns that may evolve from suddenness of attack without warning, severity of pain, anticipation of future attacks, or possible disabilities that may require alterations in life-style and work.
8. Teach patients about the disease and long-term plan of treatment that will help to prevent exacerbations and disabilities.
Educational 9. Advise patients to avoid strenuous exercises.
10. Advise patients to avoid excessive use of alcohol.
11. Advise patients to avoid fasting.
12. Instruct patients to return to the clinic or physician's office for follow-up care.

Evaluation criteria. *See* Overview. Patient is maintained on low-purine, low-calorie diet and has ≥ 2 liters of fluid daily.

OSTEOCLASTOMA

Osteoclastoma is a very aggressive giant cell tumor arising from osseous tissue. Although considered a benign tumor, osteoclastoma has a tendency to become malignant. It occurs after the epiphyseal plate closes, and is seen mostly in young adults, rarely after the age of 35 yr. The common sites are the distal radius, distal femur, and proximal tibia. The etiology is unknown. *Symptoms* include pain that is worse at night and increases with activity, swelling over the site, moderate tenderness at the site, and limited movement if the tumor extends into a joint. *Complications* include pathologic fractures. *Diagnosis* is based on the health history, physical exam, x-ray, and Craig needle biopsy (tumor cells contain acid phosphatase). Treatment consists of curettage and bone graft, and amputation if malignant cells are found. **Nursing** care is described in the Overview and Chapters 8, 9, and 11.

OSTEOID OSTEOMA

Osteoid osteoma is a benign tumor arising from osseous tissue. It occurs most often in the 20- to 30-yr age group and is more common in males than females. Common sites include the long bones (tibia and femur) and the small bones of the hands and feet. The etiology is unknown. *Symptoms* include pain that is mild at first, becomes very severe, is worse at night, and is relieved by aspirin; swelling at the site; and pronounced tenderness on palpation. *Diagnosis* is based on the health history, physical exam, and x-ray that reveals nidus surrounded by an area of sclerosis. Surgical excision is the usual treatment. **Nursing** care is described in the Overview and Chapters 9 and 11.

CHONDROMA

Chondroma is a benign tumor arising from cartilaginous tissue and is found in the metaphyseal region. It may occur in persons from childhood to the age of 50 yr. It may have its onset during the growth period but may not become apparent for years. Common sites are the fingers and toes; the long bones and innominate bone are less common sites. The etiology is unknown. *Symptoms* include the presence of a slowly progressing mass and deformity. *Complications* include pathologic fractures and malignant changes (can develop into a chondrosarcoma). *Diagnosis* is based on the health history, physical exam, and x-ray that discloses an oval, well-circumscribed lesion with calcific stippling. Biopsy is contraindicated because the cells spread easily. Treatment consists of excision and curettage of the tumor, bone grafting, and radical resection for lesions of the long bones and pelvis. **Nursing** care is described in the Overview and Chapters 9 and 11.

ANEURYSMAL BONE CYST

An aneurysmal bone cyst is a type of benign superperiosteal giant cell tumor arising from vascular tissue or bone. It most often occurs between the ages of 10 and 50 yr. It may affect any bone but occurs most commonly in the metaphysis of the long bones or the arches of the vertebrae. The etiology is unknown. *Symptoms* include pain, a palpable mass, limitation of motion, and spinal cord or nerve root involvement (when the vertebrae are involved). *Complications* include pathologic fractures. *Diagnosis* is based on the health history, physical exam, and x-rays. Treatment consists of curettage and filling the area with bone graft, radiation therapy, or a combination of the above techniques. **Nursing** care is described in the Overview and Chapters 8, 9, and 11.

OSTEOGENIC SARCOMA

Osteogenic sarcoma is a type of malignant tumor arising from osseous tissue. It is the most frequently seen bone tumor and is usually fatal. It usually affects people between 15 and 30 yr of age, and men are affected more often than women. Common sites are the area near epiphyseal plate, the lower femur, and the upper tibia. Predisposing factors include Paget's disease, irradiation of bone, and osteochondroma. *Symptoms* include pain and swelling; nonmobile, soft parts over the tumor; and thin and glossy skin over the area. *Complications* include pathologic fractures and death.

Diagnosis is based on the health history, physical exam, x-ray, and Craig needle biopsy. Medical treatment consists of cytotoxic drugs and radiation, which may help local symptoms. The tumor sometimes is radiosensitive. Surgical treatment requires amputation or disarticulation, depending on the location of the lesion. **Nursing** care is described in the Overview and Chapters 8, 9, and 11.

CHONDROSARCOMA

Chondrosarcoma is a primary or secondary malignant tumor arising from cartilage. Affected patients are usually under the age of 30 yr with primary disease and above 30 yr with secondary disease. Men are affected more often than women. Common sites of primary chondrosarcoma are the knees, hips, shoulders, pelvis, and trunk. Secondary disease affects the upper end of the humerus, the ribs, and the innominate bone. The etiology is unknown. Pain is usually worse at night. If the tumor develops in the knees, flexion contracture and swelling near the joint may occur. The disease may be fatal. *Diagnosis* is based on the health history, physical exam, x-ray, and Craig needle biopsy. Amputation or disarticulation and wide resection are the usual methods of treatment. **Nursing** care is described in the Overview and Chapters 9 and 11.

FIBROSARCOMA

Fibrosarcoma is a type of malignant tumor arising from connective tissue. It occurs most often in middle age and affects the long bones, ribs, skull, vertebrae, and mandible. The etiology is unknown. *Symptoms* include pain that is worse at night and swelling. Metastasis to the lungs may ensue. *Diagnosis* is based on the health history, physical exam, x-ray, and biopsy. Treatment consists of amputation and/or cytotoxic drugs. **Nursing** care is described in the Overview and Chapters 8, 9, and 11.

MULTIPLE MYELOMA

Multiple myeloma is a malignant tumor that arises from bone marrow and invades cancellous bone. It is most common in men between the ages of 40 and 60 yr. The etiology is unknown. *Symptoms* include pain, nerve root involvement with lesions in the vertebral area, tenderness on palpation of the involved site, and secondary anemia. *Complications* include pathologic fractures, spinal cord or nerve root compression, leukopenia (late stage), and death. *Diagnosis* is based on the health history, physical exam, x-rays, and laboratory studies for Bence Jones protein in the urine (positive), serum globulin (increased), albumin (globulin ratio reversed), and CBC (anemia, leukopenia [late stage], and immature myocytes). Methods of treatment include chemotherapy, irradiation, and surgery for pathologic fractures. **Nursing** care is described in the Overview and Chapter 8.

EWING'S SARCOMA

Ewing's sarcoma is a highly malignant tumor arising from bone marrow. It usually affects persons under 30 yr of age and may occur in any bone, in the diaphyseal region. The etiology is unknown. *Symptoms* include pain that is worse at night, tenderness on palpation, skin that is red and edematous and contains dilated veins, elevated temperature, elevated WBC, and anemia. *Complications* include pathologic fractures and metastasis through the lymphatics and bloodstream to other bones (skull, vertebrae, ribs) and the lungs (late sign). Death may result. *Diagnosis* is based on the health history, physical exam, x-rays, and CBC (decreased RBCs and increased WBCs). Methods of treatment consist of irradiation and/or cytotoxic drugs. **Nursing care** is described in the Overview and Chapter 8.

OSTEOPOROSIS

Osteoporosis is a common metabolic disorder that involves both mineral and protein matrix components and results in diffuse reduction of bone density. It is most common in postmenopausal women, men over the age of 50 yr, and Caucasians. The specific cause of generalized osteoporosis is unknown. However, contributing factors include estrogen deficit, lack of androgenic steroids in males, catabolic hormone excess (as in Cushing's disease), prolonged use of corticosteroids, liver disease, immobilization, inadequate diet, and chronic diseases such as malignant tumors and collagen disease.

Various pathophysiologic changes are associated with osteoporosis. Disturbance of normal osteoblastic and osteoclastic balance occurs, and mineral and protein matrix components are diminished. Trabeculae are decreased in numbers and width, marrow spaces are widened, and bone mass is decreased. *Symptoms* of osteoporosis include pain, localized tenderness when a fracture occurs, and decreased body height when multiple vertebral fractures occur. *Complications* include kyphosis, fractures after minor trauma, compression fractures of the vertebrae, and renal calcification in immobilized patients. *Diagnosis* is based on the health history (including diet and activities) and physical exam. Laboratory tests of serum phosphorus may disclose slightly increased levels in postmenopausal women and low levels in patients with Cushing's disease. Urine calcium may be increased. X-rays may reveal concavity of both upper and lower portions of the vertebrae and compression fracture of the vertebrae with anterior wedging.

Common interventions

1. Administer analgesics to relieve pain.
2. Use a supportive device (corset or brace) for vertebral fractures.
3. Encourage a proper diet with moderate to high protein content.
4. Supplement intake of calcium and vitamin D.

5. Encourage weight reduction in obese patients.
6. Administer gonadal hormones.
7. Initiate an exercise program to strengthen muscles as well as to improve posture.

Nursing interventions

Physical 1. Handle extremities carefully when changing the patient's position.
2. Exercise noninvolved extremities if the patient is on best rest.
3. Maintain an adequate diet with high protein content and increased calcium intake.
4. Monitor fluid intake and output.
5. Maintain immobilization of the spine with a corset or brace for patients with fractured vertebrae.
6. Administer medications on time.
7. Provide an assistive walking device to prevent injury.
Psychosocial 8. Allow the patient to verbalize concerns regarding pain, changes in body image, and fear of fractures.
9. Teach the patient about the disease process, prescribed treatment, and measures taken to minimize or prevent fractures.
10. Advise the patient to avoid any weight gain (if obese).
Educational 11. Warn the patient about hazards that can contribute to falls (wet or waxed floors, scatter rugs).
12. Apply the brace or corset properly.

Evaluation criteria. *See* Overview. Patient maintains high-protein diet, increased calcium intake, and adequate fluid intake.

PAGET'S DISEASE

Paget's disease is a slowly progressive, chronic disease of the skeleton that results in thickened, enlarged bone, causing abnormal structure and skeletal deformities. It affects more men than women and usually appears after the age of 40 yr. Its etiology is unknown but there may be a familial tendency.

The disease is initially *characterized* by decalcification and softening of the bone. Deposition of calcium follows. New bone formation and erosion increase, causing abnormal regeneration of osseous tissue. Abnormal skeletal structural changes occur, resulting in thickened, enlarged, and deformed bones. The skull becomes enlarged in the advanced stages. *Symptoms* consist of dull, aching, bone pain often associated with weight bearing; bowing of the tibia anteriorly and bowing of femur laterally; and enlarged temporal arteries. The patient stands with the head held forward. *Complications* include microfractures; pathologic fractures; kyphosis; neurologic deficits secondary to vertebral compression; osteogenic sarcoma; headaches, dizziness, and impaired hearing related to temporal bone involvement; and visual disturbance.

Diagnosis is based on the health history and physical exam (including enlarged temporal arteries). Laboratory tests reveal elevated alkaline phosphatase and hypercalcemia if the fracture occurs and the patient is on bed rest. The disease may be first discovered on routine x-ray examination, which may reveal coarse, bony trabeculae; mottled increase of bone density; thickened and enlarged cortex of the long bones; minifractures; and transverse pathologic fractures.

Common interventions

No specific treatment for Paget's disease is known. Treatment is supportive and symptomatic. Drugs are used to reduce pain by producing anti-inflammatory and analgesic effects (e.g., acetylsalicylic acid and indomethacin). The pathologic process of the disease may be affected by lowering the serum calcium level with drugs such as mithramycin and calcitonin. Fluid intake should be increased and a low-calcium diet provided. Physical activity should be maintained.

Nursing interventions

Physical 1. Provide a diet low in calcium.
2. Encourage adequate fluid intake.
3. Administer medications as ordered.
4. Observe patients for side effects of medications.
5. Control pain with analgesics and other pain-relieving measures (*see* Chapter 4).
6. Handle the extremities gently.
7. Encourage the patient to be active if no fracture is involved.
Psychosocial 8. Assist the patient and family to deal with changes in body structure.
9. Approach patients with support and assurance to help reduce their anxieties.
Educational 10. Instruct patients to return to the clinic or physician's office for follow-up care.

Evaluation criteria. *See* Overview. Patient maintains low-calcium diet.

HAMMER TOE

Hammer toe is a flexion deformity involving the proximal interphalangeal joint. The metatarsophalangeal joint may be subluxed. This condition can occur in adolescence and early adulthood and is more common in women than men. It may occur with rheumatoid arthritis and clawfoot. It may be congenital/hereditary or acquired from wearing shoes that fit incorrectly and cause undue pressure over joints. Hammer toe involves a flexion contracture of the proximal interphalangeal joint with extension or slight hyperextension of the distal interphalangeal joint. A painful callus forms over the dorsal surface of the involved joint. *Diagnosis* is based on the health history (family history is significant), physical exam, and x-rays of the foot.

Common interventions

Conservative **medical** treatment for mild symptoms may include passive stretching exercises, removal of the callus, use of a pad to protect the joint from shoe pressure, and changing to properly fitted shoes. **Surgical** intervention for severe symptoms may include arthrodesis of the interphalangeal joint in a straight position or resection of the proximal phalanx if a metatarsophalangeal dislocation exists.

Nursing interventions

Assessment of patients undergoing a surgical procedure for a foot problem requires base-line data so that ongoing evaluation will be significant. However, neurovascular assessment of the toes may be complicated by the presence of a wire inserted in the toes, a bulky dressing or plaster boot allowing only the tips of the toes to be exposed, or discoloration of the toes as a result of the solution used in preoperation preparation.

Physical 1. Observe the toes for color, temperature, sensation, movements, and swelling.
2. Observe the dressing or cast for excessive drainage.
3. Provide routine postoperative care (*see* Chapter 11).
4. Maintain elevation of the foot with pillows, and elevate the foot of the bed so that the foot is higher than the knee.
5. Keep bed clothes off the toes with the use of a foot cradle. For patients who have pins inserted in the toes, cover the pins with tape.
6. Apply ice packs to the foot as prescribed (first 24 to 48 hr).
7. Administer pain medication as ordered.
8. Instruct patients to use walker, crutches, or cane.
9. Instruct patients operated on for hallux valgus or hammer toes to walk on the heels.
10. Report to the physician any untoward changes in the toes, significant swelling, or extensive drainage.
Educational 11. Advise the patient to wear properly fitted shoes. (Patients with a wire inserted into their toes may need to cut an old pair of shoes to accommodate the pins and swelling.)
12. Provide cast care when indicated (*see* section on plaster casts).

Evaluation criteria. *See* Overview. Patient ambulates well with crutches, cane, or walkerette; guards against bumping toe with inserted pins; and wears properly fitting shoes.

HALLUX VALGUS

Hallux valgus is a deformity of the great toe characterized by an acute angulation of the metatarsophalangeal joint. The great toe deviates laterally and may lie over or under the adjacent toe. This condition is most common in young women and may occur in patients with rheumatoid arthritis. Predisposing factors include short, narrow, pointed shoes; tight stockings or shoes; and high-heeled shoes. Hallux valgus is *characterized* by a bony enlargement that appears on the medial side of the metatarsal head. Bursae (bunions) develop over the bony enlargement. These bursae sometimes become inflamed. *Symptoms* include deformity of the great toe, tenderness over the metatarsophalangeal joint, and a painful great toe. *Complications* include degenerative arthritic changes. *Diagnosis* is based on the health history (including the type of footwear used), physical exam, and x-rays.

Common interventions

Conservative **medical** therapy consists of a properly fitting shoe with a wide forefoot. The medial border of the shoe near the metatarsal head may need to be slit if the bursa is inflamed. A bunion pad may be useful to relieve shoe pressure. Several **surgical** procedures are available to remove the exostosis, realign the great toe by removal of bone, transfer tendons, or osteotomize the first metatarsal shaft. The most common surgical procedures currently used are the Keller procedure, bunionectomy, the Silver procedure, and the McBride procedure. **Nursing** care is similar to that for hammer toes (*see above*).

PES PLANUS

Pes planus (flatfoot) is a deformity of the foot characterized by the flattening of the longitudinal arch on weight bearing, outward rotation of the heel, and lateral deviation of the forefoot. It is common in children but is also seen in adults. Predisposing factors include familial tendencies, relaxed muscles and ligaments, faulty posture, obesity (may lead to overstretching of muscles and ligaments), trauma, standing or walking on hard surfaces for prolonged periods of time (e.g., policeman, mailman), improper shoes, rheumatoid arthritis, and abnormal development of tarsal and metatarsal bones.

Pes planus develops when muscular fatigue and weakness place a strain on the ligaments. Strained ligaments and the weakened muscles cannot prevent the arches from flattening and contribute to flatfeet. Body weight is displaced medially, causing excessive strain on the feet during weight bearing. *Symptoms* may include pain in the longitudinal arch, pain in the forefoot from wearing improper shoes, fatigue associated with weight bearing, tenderness or callus formation under the first metatarsophalangeal joint, awkward gait, and marked wear of the soles of the shoes on the medial sides. *Complications* include knock-knees. *Diagnosis* is based on the health history (family history is significant), physical exam, and x-rays of the feet.

Common interventions

Conservative **medical** treatment may include an exercise program to strengthen the muscles of the legs and feet, longitudinal arch supports, properly fitting shoes, weight reduction if a problem of obesity exists, correct posture in standing and walking, and rest periods if pain and tenderness exist. **Surgical** intervention is recommended if conservative measures have not alleviated the symptoms. Procedures include triple arthrodesis. **Nursing** care is similar to that for hammer toes (*see above*).

CARPAL TUNNEL SYNDROME

Carpal tunnel syndrome occurs when the median nerve is compressed within the carpal tunnel, causing a progressive deformity of the hand and wrist. It is more common in women 40 to 50 yr of age, and in a dominant extremity. Etiologic factors include trauma, inflammation, osteoarthritis, bony deformity, hypertrophy of the volar ligaments, a soft tissue mass, and thickening of the flexor tendon sheaths. *Symptoms* include a history of pain, numbness, tingling, and paresthesias occurring at night or after manual activities such as writing. Motor and sensory loss along the distribution of the median nerve is also common. Symptoms can be reproduced by holding the wrist in flexion. Motor and sensory impairment is a *complication*. *Diagnosis* is based on the health history, physical exam, and electromyographic studies. Medical treatment consists of placing a splint on the wrist in neutral alignment during the day and night if possible. Antiinflammatory drugs are also used. Surgical decompression is another means of treatment. Refer to trigger finger (*see below*) for **nursing** care.

DUPUYTREN'S CONTRACTURE

Dupuytren's contracture is a fibrous contracture of the palmar surface causing a flexion contracture at the metacarpophalangeal joint and sometimes the proximal interphalangeal joints. It is more common in adult males, persons between the ages of 50 and 70 yr, and Caucasians. The most common sites are the ring finger and little finger. Although the exact cause is unknown, there appears to be a familial tendency. The condition is aggravated by trauma. *Symptoms* include functional disability (limited extension of the fingers) and deformities such as thickening (formation of a fibrous band) of the palmar skin and underlying fascia, small nodules near the distal palmar crease, and severe flexion contracture, which is often bilateral and symmetric. The flexed fingers may interfere with the ability to perform activities. Thickening of the fascia occludes circulation, causing skin atrophy and poor healing postoperatively. *Diagnosis* is based on the health history and physical exam. Surgical resection of the involved palmar fascia is the usual treatment. Refer to trigger finger (*see below*) for **nursing** care.

GANGLION

A ganglion is a cystic lesion that is most commonly found in or about a tendon sheath or joint capsule, but can be found anywhere in the hand. Females are more susceptible than males. The condition affects persons from adolescence to 50 yr of age and frequently occurs following trauma. It is caused by protrusion of synovial tissue into the tendon sheath or joint capsule. *Symptoms* include pain or discomfort in the region of the tendon or joint, weakness of the fingers or wrist, swelling, and increased pain on motion. Associated *complications* include temporary functional impairment. Recurrence is common. *Diagnosis* is based on the health history and physical exam. Treatment consists of aspiration of fluid and injection of hydrocortisone or surgical excision and immobilization. Refer to trigger finger (*see below*) for **nursing** care.

TRIGGER FINGER

In a trigger finger, during flexion and reextension, there is a sudden snapping sensation of the finger. The finger becomes locked in flexion and is unable to be actively reextended. It is most common in the ring or middle finger. Familial tendency appears to be a predisposing factor. It may be congenital, since it is found in infants. Acute, severe, or repetitive trauma may lead to trigger finger. *Symptoms* include a thickened ligamentous sheath, swelling and the formation of nodules on the sheath, a snapping sensation on movement, the finger and thumb lock in flexion and cannot actively release, and an aching type of pain. The condition may interfere with daily activities. *Diagnosis* is based on the health history and physical exam.

Common interventions

Medical treatment consists of anti-inflammatory drugs, cortisone injections into the sheath, and immobilization. **Surgical** excision is indicated when medical therapy fails.

Nursing interventions

1. Preoperative care consists of the following:
    a. Assess pain and the sensory and motor components of ulnar, median, and radial nerves (*see* compartmental syndrome).
    b. Assist the patient with activities of daily living.
    c. Provide an opportunity for the patient to express fears or anxieties.
    d. Teach the patient the preoperative and postoperative routines.
2. Postoperative care consists of the following:
    a. Assess the color, movement, sensation, and temperature of each finger.
    b. Elevate the extremity, placing the hand higher than the elbow.
    c. Apply ice as directed (usually in the first 24 to 48 hr).
    d. Check the dressing for drainage, and the splint (if applied) for proper positioning.
    e. Evaluate pain and medicate as needed.
    f. Encourage movement of all fingers when possible.
    g. Ambulate with the extremity elevated.
    h. Assess general postoperative parameters and report unusual findings.

3. Educational and discharge planning and follow-up consist of the following:
   a. Evaluate the patient's ability to perform activities of daily living and assist the patient in adapting to changes.
   b. Provide an exercise program to strengthen muscles.
   c. Instruct the patient in the use and care of the splint, if required after discharge.
   d. Discuss important observations — e.g., swelling, discoloration, pain, numbness, tingling, decreased motor ability, etc. — and report to the physician.
   e. Caution the patient to avoid lifting heavy objects for at least 2 to 3 mo.
   f. Assist patients in making follow-up visits to a clinic or physician's office.

Evaluation criteria. See Overview. Postoperatively, ulnar, median, and radial nerves are intact; circulation to extremity is good; fingers are not swollen; and splint is in proper position.

LOW BACK PROBLEMS

Congenital anomalies and herniated discs are common problems that lead to low back pain. **Lumbosacral transitional vertebrae** (also referred to as **sacralization**) are a result of an overdeveloped transverse process, which forms a joint or a complete bony union with the sacrum. **Spondylolysis** is a defect in the pars interarticularis. **Spondylolisthesis** is a defect in the pars interarticularis causing the slipping forward of one vertebral body on the other. **Herniated nucleus pulposus** (HNP) results from a defect in the annulus fibrosus; the soft, jellylike center (nucleus pulposus) protrudes into the neural canal and causes pressure on the nerve root. Spondylolisthesis is frequently seen in adolescents. Herniated discs are usually seen in persons between 30 and 50 yr of age, but can occur in younger age groups. Predisposing factors include congenital anomalies and degenerative changes. Any of the following factors can contribute to low back problems: repeated stress to the area, trauma, congenital anomalies, tumors, metabolic diseases, infections, degenerative disease, inflammatory processes, and vascular problems.

Symptoms of lumbosacral transitional vertebrae are severe pain and changes in mobility. Spondylolysis and spondylolisthesis are characterized by occasional back pain. However, when slippage becomes severe enough to cause pressure on nerve roots, symptoms similar to a herniated disc present. The symptoms of HNP are many and varied and may include tilting gait, sciatic pain (first in buttock then radiating down the leg, intensified by bending forward, sneezing, coughing, straining), muscle spasm, tenderness over the intervertebral space, flattening of the lumbar area, and muscle weakness (sensory deficit and atrophy may be present). L3,4 disc herniation causes weakness and atrophy of quadriceps, diminished knee jerk, and numbness along the anteromedial thigh and knee. Herniation of the L4,5 disc results in weakness on dorsiflexion of the foot and great toe and difficulty in walking on the heels. Usually there is no atrophy or reflex changes. Numbness along the lateral aspect of the leg and web space of the great toe may occur. Pain in the sacroiliac joint, hip, lateral leg, and thigh is common. L5, S1 disc herniation causes weakness on plantar flexion of the foot and great toe. Patients may experience difficulty in walking on the toes. There may be atrophy of the gastrocnemius and soleus muscles. The ankle jerk is diminished or absent. Numbness may occur along the back of the calf, lateral heel, foot, and toe. Pain over the sacroiliac joint, hip, posterolateral thigh, leg, and heel is also symptomatic. *Complications* include paresthesia, drop foot, and bowel and bladder dysfunction.

Diagnosis is based on the health history, physical exam, and electromyelography. Laboratory tests include CBC, ESR, serum calcium and phosphorus, alkaline phosphatase, and urinalysis. X-ray studies may include AP, lateral, and oblique views of the lumbar and thoracic spine; myelogram; discogram; and CAT scan.

Common interventions

Medical treatment may include any of the following: bed rest, traction, lumbosacral corset, exercise, a firm mattress or bed board, heat, or muscle relaxants. **Surgical** therapy may include laminectomy, disc removal and spinal fusion, or chemonucleolysis (injection of an enzyme into the disc). Table 19-13 (*see* p. 606-610) describes the **nursing** care of patients with low back problems.

Evaluation criteria. *See* Overview. Postoperatively, bowel and bladder functioning is intact, and patient can apply brace correctly and ambulate without difficulty.

TABLE 19-13

Nursing Interventions for Patients with Low Back Problems

Nursing intervention	Rationale
On admission establish baseline data	For ongoing evaluation.
Assess the following factors	
Mobility	
Tilting gait (tilts away from disc).	Pressure on nerve root may affect gait.
Drop-foot gait.	Pressure from the disc can cause pressure on the sciatic nerve, which may cause either a decrease in or absence of function of the anterior tibial or peroneal muscles.
Ability to move from stretcher to bed, etc.	Splinting muscles and guarding to immobilize the lower back area and decrease pain may be evident.
Pain	
Location, extent, radiation, duration, number of episodes, causes, and effective measures in alleviating.	Pressure on the sciatic nerve will cause pain in lower back region radiating down leg to foot and ankle.
Functional abilities	
Test lower extremities for dorsiflexion of ankle, pulling up of great toes, and paresthesia.	Pressure on nerve roots can affect motor ability.
Changes in bowel and bladder habits.	Pressure on nerve roots can affect the sympathetic and parasympathetic nervous systems. Sudden loss of function can be considered an emergency. If not corrected, permanent damage can result.
Patient's understanding of	
1. Body mechanics (ask the patient to describe how he picks up, reaches for, and lifts heavy objects).	Improper body mechanics are a major cause of lower back pain.
2. Previous treatment (bed rest, medication, corset, heat, and exercise).	Conservative treatment frequently is not effective because the patient does not understand what is supposed to be done (e.g., the patient assumes that bed rest means

Nursing intervention	Rationale
	short periods of rest in between caring for children and household chores).
3. Current treatment/hospitalization (conservative treatment, myelogram, surgery.)	The patient's expectation may be different from the physician's treatment plan.
4. Pelvic traction: fit snugly around the waist and hips; place straps along lateral aspects of the legs and attach to a spreader; attach 6.8–9.0 kg (15–20 lbs) of weight; check skin for areas of breakdown.	Immobilization decreases muscle spasm. If improperly applied, areas of friction can occur.

Position
    On back (jackknife or beach chair). On side (pillow between legs; hips and knees flexed).

These positions decrease pressure on the sciatic nerve. When the patient is lying flat with lower extremities extended, the sciatic nerve is taut.

Fear and anxiety
    Determine the level of anxiety. Provide opportunity for the patient to talk.

A patient who has been coping with pain for long periods of time can be frustrated or fearful of becoming permanently disabled and may exhibit demanding or irritating behavior.

Preoperative care*

Explain that back pain will not disappear immediately following surgery.

Inflammation and edema must subside first. Muscle spasm can also cause pain.

Explain that pain will be present at the bone graft site (iliac crest).

Inflammation and edema at the bone graft site must subside first. (In most instances, this takes longer).

Administer pain medication promptly to be effective.

Ineffectiveness or delay will predispose to muscle spasm, exhaustion, and lack of participation in self-care.

Evaluate effectiveness of pain medication.

See above.

Nursing intervention	Rationale
Position and turn the patient to provide the opportunity to practice proper techniques for	
1. Lying on back. (Buttocks directly under shoulders, pillow under knees, foot of the bed elevated 30–45°.)	Pressure is taken off sciatic nerve. Hyperextension of the spine is prevented.
2. Log-rolling. (Place a pillow between his knees; place arm on side to which the patient is turned, over the head, or straight down along the side; ask the patient to extend his leg on the side to which he is turning and flex his hip and knee of the other leg. Guide the hips and shoulders as the patient pushes down on his heel and reaches for the side rail to help pull onto side.)	Shoulders and hips move in the same plane to avoid twisting the spine.
3. Getting on and off bedpan. (Log-roll onto the side, place fracture bedpan against the patient's buttocks, ask the patient to roll onto the bedpan, and place small pillow or folded/rolled towel in lower back region.)	Provides comfort.
Teach the patient the proper technique to get in and out of bed. (Roll onto his side and push up with his hands until he reaches a sitting position. At the same time swing his legs down.)	Prevents stress on the low back area.

Postoperative care‡
Observe the following
    Pain and positioning (*see* preoperative care above.)

Drainage (Position the patient on his back immediately after	The body acts as a pressure dressing. Both soft tissues and bone in

Nursing intervention	Rationale
surgery. Note drainage on dressing.)	the lumbosacral area are very vascular, and there is significant blood loss during surgery.
Check wound suction apparatus to be sure that it is functioning properly and that the patient is not lying on the tube and obstructing flow.	A suction catheter is inserted into the wound to prevent formation of a hematoma.
Vital signs (Check and record q 30 min until stable, then qid.)	Complication of surgery is hypovolemic shock. The aorta or vena cava can be nicked accidentally. Vascular injuries may not be apparent for several days.
Circulation (Check nail beds for color and perfusion, note rate of capillary return, evaluate dorsal pedis pulse and note changes.)	Vascular problems can result from surgery.
Monitor Hb and Hct.	Extensive blood loss can occur. Low levels can affect ability to ambulate.
Movement and sensation (Ask the patient to dorsiflex his ankle and pull up great toe.)	Hematoma can form in the disc space and cause symptoms.
Use light touch to determine areas of decreased sensation of lower extremities.	Paresthesias along the lateral aspect of thigh (lateral femoral cutaneous nerve) immediately after surgery may result from position on operating table and disappear quickly.
Abdominal distension Bowel (Auscultate for bowel sounds, palpate abdomen.)	Retroperitoneal bleeding at the time of surgery may lead to paralytic ileus.
Bladder (Observe for distension, palpate bladder.)	Overdistended bladder may cause a temporary loss of muscle tone.
Closed-space infection (Evaluate unusual complaints of persistent back pain, sometimes leading to abdominal or groin pain. Muscle spasm increases with the slightest movement.)	Infection may occur in the area where the disc was removed.

Nursing intervention	Rationale
Teach the patient the following	
Apply brace when in supine position. While lying on side, place steel stays on either side of spine, then roll the patient onto brace. Fasten in front.	When supine, all organs in abdominal cavity are in proper alignment and brace will offer greater support.
Use walker with wheels initially.	Walker provides greater feeling of security and helps maintain balance.
Educational	
Instruct and/or review with the patient the prescribed ambulation techniques, range-of-motion exercises, and medications.	An informed patient will make an easier transition from hospital to home and will be motivated toward greater independence.
Prevention of injuries	
Caution the patient against wearing long robes and slip-on type shoes.	Certain types of clothing can be hazardous and can impede ambulation.
Alert the patient to safety hazards in the home and environment.	Icy or wet surfaces, uneven surfaces, scatter rugs, and electric cords should be avoided. Stairs and curbs should be approached with caution.
Instruct the patient to use the proper size chair and to sit down the easiest and safest way.	The height of the seat should allow the patient to sit with his ankles, knees, and hips at a 90° angle. Feeling the seat of the chair against the back of the legs before sitting aids positioning in the chair.

*See Chapter 9 for general preoperative nursing care.
‡See Chapter 11 for general postoperative nursing care.

Evaluation criteria. Patient ambulates with proper gait, has good range of motion in all unaffected extremities, discusses safety hazards, has minimal anxiety, verbalizes fears, and shows no evidence of complication of immobilization.

CHAPTER 20

ALTERED NEUROLOGIC FUNCTIONING

Aurora Villafuerte

OVERVIEW

This chapter will present concepts related to the acute and ongoing care of the patient with altered neurologic functioning. Increasingly, these patients are found in general hospitals rather than specialized neurologic units. In addition, with the aging population, the nurse is very likely to encounter patients in the ongoing phase of these conditions in the home and the community.

Anatomy and physiology review

Nerve cells. The nervous system, together with the endocrine system, functions in controlling all body activities including transmitting, processing, and storing information.

Nerve cells are composed of neurons and neuroglia. **Neurons** are highly specialized cells that function primarily as impulse transmitters. They have three major components: cell body (main part); dendrites, which transmit impulses to the cell body; and axons, which transmit impulses away from the cell body. Neurons can also be classified according to functions: sensory (afferent) neurons transmit impulses to the spinal cord and brain, and motor (efferent) neurons transmit impulses away from the spinal cord to muscles and glands. The **neuroglia** (glial cells), which are composed of connective tissue cells, primarily support and connect nerve cells to blood vessels and serve as a defense or protective mechanism.

Impulse transmission occurs at a synapse, which is the point of contact between neurons, or between a neuron and muscle or glandular cells. An impulse is conducted when action potential in a presynaptic neuron travels distally down the axon and releases a neurotransmitter from vesicles at the presynaptic terminal. The neurotransmitter diffuses to the postsynaptic membrane and causes an excitatory or inhibitory reaction.

The nervous system has three major components: the central (brain and spinal cord), peripheral (cranial and spinal nerves), and autonomic (sympathetic and parasympathetic) nervous systems.

Central nervous system. The CNS consists of the brain and spinal cord. Their coverings consist of the cranial bones (brain), vertebrae (spinal cord), and the meninges (brain and spinal cord). The meninges are made up of three layers of membrane: dura mater, arachnoid, and pia mater. The dura mater is a tough, semitranslucent, inelastic membrane composed of the outer (periosteum of the skull bone) and inner dura. The arachnoid is a delicate cobwebby membrane that lies between the dura and the innermost layer of the meninges (pia). The pia mater is a transparent layer that adheres to the outer surface of the brain and spinal cord and contains blood vessels that nourish neural tissue.

The divisions, structures, and functions of the brain are described in Table 20-1. The reticular activating system begins in the lower brainstem, extends upward through the mesencephalon and thalamus to be distributed throughout the cerebral cortex. The reticular activating system controls the overall degree of CNS activity, wakefulness, sleep, and the ability to direct attention to specific areas of consciousness. **Blood** is supplied to the brain via the vertebral and internal carotid arteries. The vertebral arteries supply the posterior portion of the cranial cavity: brainstem, caudal part of diencephalon, cerebellum, occipital lobes, and parts of the temporal lobes. The vertebral arteries unite to form the basilar artery, which bifurcates into two posterior cerebral arteries. The internal carotid is the major source of blood supply to the eye and cerebral hemisphere (including most of the diencephalon). Each internal carotid artery gives off an ophthalmic artery and posterior communicating artery and then divides into the middle and anterior cerebral arteries. The vertebral and internal carotid arteries are joined by communicating arteries at the base of the brain to form the circle of Willis. Venous blood empties into the sinuses of the dura mater, which are drained by the internal jugular veins, which return venous blood to the heart. The **ventricles** consist of a series of four cavities within the brain. There are two lateral ventricles (one in each hemisphere), which communicate with the third ventricle by means of the interventricular foramen (foramen of Monro). The third and fourth ventricles are united by a narrow channel (aqueduct of Sylvius). The fourth ventricle opens into the subarachnoid space and is continuous with the narrow central canal of the medulla and spinal cord. The CSF formed at the choroid plexus of each ventricle flows through the communicating channels into the subarachnoid space (between the arachnoid and pia mater) to surround the brain and spinal cord. It is eventually absorbed into the venous circulation. The CSF protects the brain and spinal cord by acting as a shock absorber. The **spinal cord**, which originates at the foramen magnum, extends down the vertebral canal to approximately the second lumbar vertebrae. The spinal cord consists of 31 segments, each of which gives rise to a pair of spinal nerves. There are 8 pairs of cervical, 12 thoracic, 5 lumbar, 5 sacral, and 1 coccygeal spinal nerves. The spinal cord provides conduction pathways to and from the brain and functions as a center for reflex actions.

Peripheral nervous system.   The peripheral nervous system consists of nerves and ganglia. The nerves are divided into two main groups: cranial nerves and spinal nerves. **Cranial nerves** consist of 12 pairs of nerves that emerge from under the surface of the brain. They are numbered according to the order in which they arise (from front to back) and named according to function and distribution (Table 20-2). The cranial nerves conduct impulses between the brain and various structures in the head, neck, thoracic, and abdominal cavities. These impulses may be motor (efferent fibers), sensory (afferent fibers), or mixed (motor and sensory). Thirty-one pairs of **spinal nerves** originate in the spinal cord and are numbered according to the spinal column at which they emerge from the spinal cavity. Each spinal nerve consists of a dorsal (sensory) root and a ventral (motor) root. The dorsal root consists of the sensory or afferent fibers whose cell bodies are located in the spinal ganglion within the intervertebral foramen. The sensory fibers transmit impulses from sensory receptors in the body to the spinal cord. The ventral root consists of motor or efferent fibers whose cell bodies are located in the gray matter of the spinal cord. The motor fibers transmit impulses from the spinal cord to the muscles and glands of the body. The spinal nerves are composed of a sensory dendrite (which comes from a cell body located in the ganglion on the posterior root in the spinal cord) and a motor axon (which originates from a cell body located in the anterior gray column of the cord). The spinal nerves, which serve as two-way conduction paths between the periphery and the spinal cord, perform the general functions of making possible both sensations and movements.

Autonomic nervous system.   The ANS is primarily concerned with involuntary or autonomic function. Its motor neurons convey impulses to the visceral effectors such as the smooth muscle, cardiac muscle, and glandular epithelium. Its center is located in the hypothalamus, brainstem, and spinal cord. The ANS is divided into the sympathetic and parasympathetic nervous systems. The locations, origins, and functions of these systems are discussed in Table 20-3.

General assessment

A complete neurologic examination is not always possible in emergency situations. The patient's immediate needs are met first. Base-line data are

TABLE 20-1
Structures and Functions of the Brain

Divisions	Structure	Function
Cerebrum	Two hemispheres are divided by a deep groove (the longitudinal fissure), are not completely separated from each other, but are joined in the inferior surface by a structure composed of white matter (the corpus callosum). The cerebral cortex or gray matter on the surface of the cerebrum is marked by sulci (convolutions). The raised ridges are called gyri (convolutions). Each cerebral hemisphere is divided into four lobes.	Consciousness, mental processes, sensations, emotions, and voluntary movements. All mental functions and essential motor, sensory, and visceral functions are also included.
	Frontal lobe	Primarily concerned with personality and the expression of emotion, performance of higher intellectual function, motor aspects of vocalization, and voluntary motor control.
	Parietal lobe	Receptive area for fine sensory stimuli; integration and correlation of sensory information.
	Temporal lobe	Primary auditory receptive area. Involved in hearing, memory, and recognition of written and spoken word.
	Occipital lobe	Primary receptive area for vision.
Cerebellum	The second largest part of the brain. Lies under the occipital lobe of the cerebrum. Consists of an outer layer of gray matter and an interior layer of almost white matter. Separated from the cerebral hemisphere by the tentorium (a tough, tent-shaped sheet of meninges).	Controls balance and coordination.

Diencephalon	
Right thalamus	Consists of a rounded mass of gray matter located deep inside the right half of the cerebrum.	Serves as a relay station for sensory impulses to the cerebral cortex.
Left thalamus	A similar mass inside the left half of the cerebrum.	Serves as a relay station for sensory impulses to the cerebral cortex.
Hypo-thalamus	Located under each thalamus and above the midbrain. It forms the floor and part of the walls of the 3rd ventricle. It includes the optic chiasm and the stalk of the pituitary, linking the nervous system to the endocrine system.	Acts as the major center for controlling the ANS and, therefore, most internal organs (control of heart rate, constriction and dilation of blood vessels, etc.). It is also involved in the regulation of body temperature, control of appetite, maintenance of water balance and wakefulness, and transmission of impulses to lower autonomic centers.
Brainstem	
Midbrain	Short segment located between the pons and diencephalon. Composed of a number of ascending and descending pathways.	A reflex center for pupillary reflexes and eye movements, mediated by the 3rd and 4th cranial nerves, respectively.
Pons	Located between the midbrain and medulla. Consists almost entirely of tracts linking the various parts of the brain and includes the nuclei of the 5th–8th cranial nerves.	Serves as a conductive pathway. Contains a portion of the respiratory control mechanism.
Medulla	Lies below the pons. Connects with the spinal cord at the foramen of magnum. Contains a number of reflex centers. Contains nuclei for the 9th–12th cranial nerves.	Vital reflex centers (cardiac, vasomotor, and respiratory). Nonvital reflexes (vomiting, coughing, sneezing, and swallowing).

TABLE 20-2
Cranial Nerves and Their Functions

Number/name		Function
1st	Olfactory	Smell
2nd	Optic	Vision
3rd	Oculomotor	Eye movements, pupillary constriction and accommodation
4th	Trochlear	Eye movements
5th	Trigeminal	Mastication, sensations of the face, oral and nasal mucosa, and the cornea of the eye
6th	Abducens	Eye movements
7th	Facial	Taste, facial expression, lacrimation, salivation
8th	Acoustic	Hearing, balance
9th	Glossopharyngeal	Taste, salivation, swallowing, control of BP and heart rate
10th	Vagus	Swallowing; movements of soft palate, pharynx, and larynx; sensory to pharynx and larynx; parasympathetic to thoracic and abdominal viscera
11th	Spinal accessory	Shoulder movement, turning of head
12th	Hypoglossal	Tongue movement

then obtained for future comparisons of any changes that may occur. Baseline information is also important in detecting the presence or absence of residual deficits after neurosurgery and in determining the patient's ability to perform self-care activities.

Health history. Four components of the health history are especially important. The **current health status** is used to determine the specific complaint (onset, symptoms, duration, etc.), the patient's elimination status (especially incontinence), and any medications the patient is taking. The **past health history** reviews any injuries (especially head trauma), surgery, and previous medications (unless listed above), e.g., anticoagulants, diuretics, tranquilizers, and oral contraceptives. The **family history** is concerned with any familial illnesses, especially epilepsy and migraine. The **review of systems** should include the following: head (injury, headache), eyes (vision changes), ears (bleeding, vertigo, hearing changes), nose (bleeding), mouth (bleeding, voice changes), musculoskeletal (ambulation, range of motion), and neurologic (unconsciousness, seizures, etc.).

Physical examination. A physical exam should be performed on all body systems, especially cardiovascular, respiratory, and GU, which could

TABLE 20-3

Divisions of the Autonomic Nervous System: Locations, Origins, and Functions

Division	Location/origin	Function
Sympathetic nervous system	Preganglionic fibers emerge from thoracolumbar segment of spinal cord. Postganglionic fibers are distributed to heart, smooth muscles, and glands.	Increase cardiovascular response (tachycardia, BP, cardiac contractility), dilate pupils, decrease peristalsis, regulate temperature, raise blood sugar, increase secretion of sweat glands, and stimulate thick salivary secretions. Epinephrine released from the adrenal medulla increases the above responses.
Parasympathetic nervous system	3rd, 7th, 9th, and 10th cranial nerves. Sacral area of spinal cord.	Constrict pupils, slow heart rate, stimulate watery salivary secretions, and relax bladder and rectal spincters.

complicate the neurologic condition. A neurologic exam assesses cerebral functioning, cranial nerves, cerebellar functioning, motor system, sensory system, and reflex status. The **equipment** for a neurologic exam are discussed in Table 20-4. Examination of **cerebral functioning** focuses on the patient's mental status and level of consciousness (LOC). The purpose of determining mental status is to evaluate the presence of organic brain disease. Relevant deviations include changes in intellectual performance, emotional behavior, and communication. Observations include physical appearance (body build, size of head, grooming, facial expression), motor activity and coordination, and attitude. The adequacy of the patient's LOC is evaluated, and changes or elicited responses are described accurately. The patient should be assessed in terms of orientation to time (day, month, year), place, and person. (Disorientation with cerebral deterioration occurs in the

TABLE 20-4
Purposes and Use of Equipment for Neurologic Exam

Equipment	Purpose (test for)	Nerve/system tested
1. Vial or test tube containing coffee, peppermint, cloves or tobacco	Olfaction	Olfactory
2. Snellen chart; newsprint	Visual acuity	Optic
3. Ophthalmoscope	Papilledema	Optic
4. Penlight or flashlight	Pupillary response	Oculomotor
5. Wisp of cotton; safety pin	Sensation of touch	Trigeminal/sensory system
6. Test tube with hot and cold H_2O	Temperature sense	Trigeminal/sensory system
7. Vial or test tube containing sugar, salt, vinegar, lemon, or quinine	Various senses of taste	Facial
8. Watch and tuning fork	Hearing and vibration	Acoustic/sensory system
9. Tongue blade	Strength of tongue	Hypoglossal
10. Tape measure	Muscle size	Motor
11. Reflex hammer	Reflexes	Sensory

order listed.) The various states of consciousness are discussed in Table 20-5. The tests and abnormal findings related to **cranial nerves** are listed in Table 20-6, **cerebellar functioning** in Table 20-7, and **motor system** in Table 20-8. Preparation for evaluating the patient's **sensory system,** involves determination of his LOC (patient cooperation is necessary for accurate results) and explaining the necessity of the patient closing his eyes during all components of the exam. All tests are performed bilaterally in the upper and lower extremities. It is important to assess whether sensory changes are dimensional in distribution, involve only one side of the body, or are confined to the peripheral nerves. Primary and cortical and discriminatory sensation are tested (Table 20-9). Deep, superficial, and abnormal **reflexes** also are evaluated. Deep reflexes are tested by tapping a tendon or bony prominence briskly with a reflex hammer. A sudden stretching and contraction of the muscles will be evoked (Table 20-10). Superficial reflexes are tested by stroking the skin with an object that is moderately sharp (*see* Table 20-10). Tests for abnormal reflexes are listed in Table 20-11.

Diagnostic tests. A variety of invasive and noninvasive procedures are performed to confirm data obtained in the health history and physical exam. Important nursing responsibilities are explanation of the procedures to the patient and/or significant others and posttest monitoring for altered neurologic functioning. The most common tests, their purposes, nursing care, and complications are outlined in Table 20-12. Other tests include brain scan (used to detect brain tumors), ultrasound (used to detect displacement of central structures of the brain by a mass lesion), and electromyography (used

TABLE 20-5

States of Altered Consciousness

State	Description
Alert	Is aware of self and environment. Responds appropriately to stimuli. Is awake.
Lethargy	Exhibits minimal disorientation to time and sometimes to place and person. Is slightly disoriented to time and person.
Obtundation	Exhibits mild to moderate reduction in alertness, lessened interest in environment. Has slower response to stimulation.
Stupor	Is a condition of deep sleep. Is arousable only by vigorous and repeated stimuli.
Coma	Has no response to external stimuli. Has no verbal response. May exhibit decorticate or decerebrate posturing. Reflexes absent.

TABLE 20-6
Cranial Nerve Assessment

Cranial	Test/purpose	Method	Abnormal finding
1st	Sense of smell	Test each side separately. Have patient close eyes. Ask patient to identify familiar odors such as tobacco, coffee, or cloves.	Loss of smell.
2nd	Visual acuity	Have patient read from newspaper or Snellen chart.	Decreased acuity.
	Visual fields	Have patient cover eye not tested and focus on object. Move finger or cotton applicator into patient's field of vision. (90 degrees would indicate over and side of head; 0 degrees, point straight ahead.) Have patient say "now" when finger or cotton is seen. Test each eye separately.	Absence of blink reflex; decreased field of vision.
	Ophthalmoscopic	Look at blood vessels, optic disc, and periphery of retina.	Nicked or distorted vessels; choking or atrophy of disc.
3rd, 4th, and 6th	Eye movement test	Ask patient to follow examiner's finger as it is moved in all directions of gaze.	3rd: Ptosis and dilation of pupils. 4th: Inability to look up, down, and medially with affected eye. 6th: Inability to look laterally with affected eye.
	Size, shape, and equality of pupils		Unequal in size. Irregular shape.
	Pupillary accommodation reflex	Check constriction of pupils as patient changes focus from a distant or close object.	Delayed or absent constriction.
	Pupillary light reflex	Check both direct and consensual response to light.	Absence of direct pupil reflex in affected eye and of consensual pupil reflex in unaffected eye.

5th	Sensory		
	Light touch, blink response/corneal reflex	Have patient close eyes. Touch forehead, cheek, and jaw with a wisp of cotton. Touch cornea lightly with wisp of cotton.	Increased or decreased sensation; absent blinking.
	Pain	Apply pinpricks to above areas, first with dull, then sharp, end.	Increased or decreased pain.
	Temperature	Apply hot and cold water to above areas.	Increased or decreased sensation.
	Motor		
	Masseter and temporal muscles	Palpate muscles with jaws tightly clamped. Note strength of muscle contraction.	Weak or absent contraction.
	Maxillary reflex	Tap middle of chin with reflex hammer while mouth is slightly opened.	Unable to close mouth.
7th	Sensory	Have patient protrude tongue. Place sugar then salt on anterior part of tongue. Have patient identify taste.	Impaired taste.
	Motor		
	Strength of eyelid muscles	Check for symmetry of face. Have patient attempt to open eyes (against pressure on eyelids). Note patient's ability to wrinkle forehead, smile, frown, and raise eyebrows.	Asymmetry. Paralysis of facial muscles.
8th	Cochlear-hearing	Ask patient to identify whispered voice or ticking watch from a distance.	Inability to hear sound.
	Weber test (lateralization)	Place tuning fork on patient's forehead or top of skull. Ask to describe if sounds equal.	Louder sound in one ear (conductive loss).
	Rinne test		
	Bone conduction	Place activated tuning fork over mastoid process until sound no longer heard.	Sound heard longer by bone than air conduction.
	Air conduction	Place activated tuning fork ~1 in. from ear.	

Cranial	Test/purpose	Method	Abnormal finding
9th and 10th	Glossopharyngeal Motor-pharyngeal gag reflex	Touch each side of pharynx with tongue depressor or applicator stick.	Absence of gag reflex.
	Sensory-taste (posterior third of tongue)		Loss of taste.
	Vagus Motor	Test soft palate for symmetry when patient says "ah." Stroke each side of uvula.	Deviation from midline.
11th	Trapezius muscle Sternocleido-mastoid muscle	Palpate shoulders while shrugged against resistance. Palpate muscle for strength.	Failure of muscles to contract.
12th	Tongue Atrophy or tremor	Have patient protrude tongue.	Deviation of tongue toward involved side.
	Strength	Have patient move tongue from side to side against a tongue depressor.	Diminished or absent movement on affected side.

TABLE 20-7
Test for Cerebellar Functioning

Evaluate balance and coordination.

Tests:

1. Touch finger to nose (alternate hands) first with eyes open, then with eyes closed.
2. Touch finger to nose and to examiner's finger with eyes open.
3. Touch finger to thumb rapidly.
4. Pat knees rapidly with palm and back of hands.
5. Run heel down shin.
6. Stand erect with feet together (eyes open, then closed).

Note:

Presence or absence of ataxia, posture, ability to gauge distances, and swing of arms.

to record the electrical activity of muscles in order to detect abnormalities, such as neuromuscular disorders and peripheral nerve damage). Relevant **laboratory tests** include serum electrolytes (to determine the presence of metabolic problems), glucose, circulating blood cells, and CSF.

Common interventions

General treatment consists of measures to prevent irreversible brain damage.

1. Establish an adequate airway via intubation (cuffed endotracheal tube), suction, tracheostomy, and/or ventilatory support.
2. Support circulation.
   a. Provide IV infusion of 50 ml of 50% glucose.
   b. Take blood specimens to determine the cause: blood gases, CBC and electrolytes, BUN, liver function, and toxicology tests (to determine levels of barbiturates, narcotics, alcohol, and other pharmacologic agents).
   c. Aspirate gastric content (to rule out drug ingestion).
   d. Observe cardiac rhythm.
   e. Observe for any evidence of bleeding.
3. Begin a more detailed neurologic examination.
4. Maintain adequate nutrition.
   a. Keep the patient NPO, if comatose.
   b. Administer IV fluids to provide calories (e.g., dextrose in water).
   c. Restrict fluids to prevent cerebral edema.
   d. Provide tube feedings (nasogastric, gastrostomy) as ordered.
   e. Advance diet as tolerated (pureed, soft, to regular).

TABLE 20-8
Tests for Motor System*

Test	Procedures
Muscle size	Measure upper arms, thighs, calves. Inspect and palpate for size and atrophy. Compare muscles of hands, and observe for wasting, fasciculation, and fine tremors. *Note*: Fasciculations (present in lesions of lower motor origin).
Muscle tone	Test resistance to passive movement. Observe for spasticity, rigidity, or flaccidity.
Involuntary movement	Observe presence of irregular twitchings and choreiform movement.
Muscle strength	Test for flexion, extension, and other movement, without resistance and then with resistance. Indicate diminished strength or weakness.

*All major joints are tested for flexion and extension first without resistance and then with resistance. The examiner should observe for equality.

Medications used for patients with altered neurologic functioning range from over-the-counter drugs to highly sophisticated experimental drugs. The brain is highly sensitive to drugs. Therefore, extreme caution must be taken in evaluating the effects of these drugs, particularly in the elderly. More commonly used drugs and their desired effects are listed in Table 20-13.

Brain surgery may be required to remove brain tumor or scar tissue, evacuate hematomas, aspirate fluids from cysts, drain an abscess, obtain a specimen of brain tissue for biopsy, relieve intracranial pressure, treat vascular malformation (such as repair of an aneurysm), or remove foreign bodies such as bone fragments. Craniotomy is an opening or operation on the cranium or skull. The approach depends on the location of the lesion (i.e., left temporal, left frontal, or suboccipital craniotomy). Preoperative preparation (*see* Chapter 9) includes obtaining base-line data for assessment, continuing the patient on anticonvulsants and steroids as ordered, questioning the use of narcotics (which mask clinical signs and depress the respiratory system), and shaving the patient's head (in OR). Immediately after surgery, the patient may be brought to the ICU. Postoperative care (*see* Chapter 11) should focus on neurologic and musculoskeletal status, safety precautions, and potential complications. Neurologic data include establishing a base line and assessing LOC, pupillary reaction to light, motor strength, sensory status, deficits of cranial nerves (especially 2nd, 7th, 9th,

TABLE 20-9
Tests for Sensory System

Test	Procedure
Tests for primary forms of sensation	
Superficial tactile sensations	With a wisp of cotton, touch hands, forearms, upper arms, trunk, thighs, lower legs, and feet. Compare sensitivity to cotton on one side with opposite side. Check also sensitivity of proximal to distal.
Superficial pain	With a sharp object (safety pin) do the same procedure as above.
Temperature	Use test tubes with hot and cold H_2O, and touch various parts of the body.
Sensitivity to vibration	Test ability to feel vibration of tuning fork held over the bony prominences, such as wrist, elbow, shoulder, hip, knee, shin, and ankle.
Deep pressure pain	Apply pressure to Achilles tendon, calf, and forearm muscles, and note sensitivity.
Motion and position	Grasp toes, thumbs, and finger between index finger and thumb. Ask patient to indicate direction of movement and final position of the digit.
Tests for cortical and discriminatory sensation	
Two point discrimination	Use two safety pins to touch various parts of the body simultaneously. Ask patient if he is being touched by one or two points. (The distance by which the patient can differentiate one from two point varies for different areas of the body.)
Point localization	Ask patient to locate spot where he was touched with his eyes closed.
Stereognostic function	Place in patient's hands, familiar objects (such as a coin and keys) and ask him to identify objects.
Extinction phenomenon	Touch two points simultaneously using identical areas on opposite side of body. With eyes closed, patient should be able to identify which side was touched.

TABLE 20-10
Tests for Deep and Superficial Reflex Status

Reflex	Site of stimulus	Normal response	CNS segment
Deep reflexes			
Biceps	Biceps tendon	Contraction of biceps	C5-6
Brachioradials	Styloid process of radius	Flexion of elbow and pronation of forearm	C5-6
Triceps	Triceps tendon above the olecranon	Extension of elbow	C6-8
Patellar	Patellar tendon	Extension of leg and knee	L2-4
Achilles	Achilles tendon	Plantar flexion of foot	S1-2
Superficial reflexes			
Upper abdominal	Above umbilicus	Umbilicus moves up and toward area being stroked	T7-9
Lower abdominal	Below umbilicus	Umbilicus moves down	T11-12
Cremasteric	Inner aspect of thigh	Testicles elevate	T12, L1
Plantar	Lateral aspect of foot	Flexion of toes	S1-2

C, cervical; L, lumbar; S, sacral; T, thoracic.
Adapted from Erickson, R. Essentials of Neurological Examination. SmithKline Corp., Philadelphia. 1974. p. 39-45.

TABLE 20-11
Tests for Abnormal Reflex Status

Reflex	How elicited	Response
Babinski	Stroke lateral aspect of sole of foot.	Extension or dorsiflexion of big toe in addition to fanning of all toes.
Chaddock	Stroke lateral aspect of dorsum of foot.	Dorsiflexion of great toe and fanning of other toes.
Gordon	Squeeze calf muscles.	Same response.
Oppenheim	Stroke anteromedial tibial surface.	Abnormal extension of great toe.

Adapted from Erickson, R. Essentials of Neurological Examination. SmithKline Corp., Philadelphia. 1974. p. 46.

10th, 12th), signs of increasing intracranial pressure, seizure activity (administration of drugs as ordered), and CSF leaks. The patient's head should be elevated 30 degrees to promote venous drainage. The musculoskeletal status should be monitored for motor changes, and range-of-motion exercises should be provided. Pull sheets should be used to move patients with suboccipital craniotomies; patients should *not* be pulled by their arms. Safety precautions are very important, especially if seizures occur. Potential *complications* include pulmonary embolism, seizures, infection, increased intracranial pressure, and cerebral edema.

Nursing interventions

Specific nursing interventions for cranial nerve deficits are discussed in Table 20-14. General nursing interventions for the unconscious patient are as follows:

Physical 1. During the acute phase, assess rate, depth, type, and rhythm of respirations.
2. Assess abnormal breathing patterns (Cheyne-Stokes respiration, central neurogenic hyperventilation, apneustic breathing, ataxic breathing, cluster and posthyperventilation apnea, and Kussmaul's respiration).
3. Assess breath sounds to detect rales and rhonchi and quantity and quality of secretions.
4. Assess the odor of the patient's breath: acetone in diabetic coma and prolonged starvation; bitter almond in cyanide poisoning; and musty smell in hepatic coma.
5. Assess the color of nail beds and mucous membranes.
6. Obtain and assess arterial blood gases.

TABLE 20-12
Common Diagnostic Tests

Test	Purpose	Nursing care	Complications
Lumbar puncture (insertion of needle into subarachnoid space in 4th lumbar vertebral space)	Obtain CSF for examination, e.g., bacterial studies (VD) and chemical tests (glucose, protein, cells). Measure pressure of CSF. Administer anesthetics. Inject air or contrast media (after removal of CSF), e.g., pneumoencephalography or myelography.	Maintain aseptic technique. Maintain bed rest for ≥24 hr. Obtain permit.	Tentorial herniation, especially in increased ICP. Infection and headache.
Angiography (injection of radiopaque contrast media into carotid or femoral artery)	Visualize arch of aorta, origins of carotid and vertebral systems into the cranial cavity. Diagnose conditions such as aneurysms, vascular malformations, occluded arteries and veins, abscesses, and tumors.	**Preangiography** Obtain permit. Premedicate as ordered. Keep NPO, except for medications such as steroids. Assess neurologic status (pupillary reaction, motor strength, LOC). Monitor vital signs. **Postangiography** Assess vital signs and neurologic status (LOC, pupillary reaction, motor strength). Assess for bleeding. Apply pressure dressings over puncture site, and notify physician immediately, if bleeding occurs. Apply ice bags to carotid artery. Check pedal pulses and report any changes.	Vascular spasms from too high concentration of contrast media. Occlusions. Embolization of clots on catheter tips. Neurologic deficits (worsening of the condition). Bleeding from the puncture site (especially if anticoagulation therapy is in use). Hypotension. Allergic reaction (skin rash, nausea, and vomiting). Compression of airway from hematoma in carotid angiography.

Procedure	Purpose	Nursing considerations	Complications
Pneumoencephalogram (injection of air or O$_2$ into lumbar subarachnoid space)	Visualize ventricular and cisternal systems. Detect conditions such as brain lesions, cerebral atrophy, and hydrocephalus.	Keep on bed rest for 24 hr as ordered. Withhold PO feedings if patient is nauseated, vomiting, or lethargic. Keep siderails up to protect patient from injury. Monitor closely for development of complications. Monitor vital signs and LOC. (See angiography.)	Severe headache, nausea, and vomiting. (See angiography.)
Myelogram (injection of air or contrast media into spinal subarachnoid space, followed by x-rays)	Visualize abnormalities of spinal cord (e.g., tumor, herniated disc, other lesions). Detect specific level of lesion.	See angiography.	See angiography.
EEG (recording of electrical activity of brain)	Diagnose types of seizure activity, brain tumors, abscesses, other lesions, coma, and state of impaired consciousness. Establish criteria for brain death.	Withhold anticonvulsants (tend to diminish EEG abnormalities) and sedatives (may alter brain wave patterns). Reassure that procedure is painless and will not receive electric shock. Remove paste after procedure.	None.
CAT scan (noninvasive radiologic technique that obtains cross-sectional view of body)	Calculate differential absorption of x-ray by tissues in continuous slices. Diagnose malignant and benign lesions, abscesses, cysts, and vascular problems (MI, subdural hematoma, arteriovenous malformation, and aneurysms).	No special preparation.	None.

TABLE 20-13
Commonly Used Drugs

Classification	Desired effects
Anticonvulsants	Control seizure activity.
Barbiturates	Sedate the patient; prophylactically control seizures (usually with an anticonvulsant).
Psychotropic agents	Potentiate CNS depressants; utilize tranquilizer or antidepressant properties.
Narcotics	Relieve pain without loss of consciousness and reflex activity.
Nonnarcotics	Relieve pain; reduce fever.
Antimicrobials	Treat and prevent infections.
Anticoagulants	Prevent thrombosis.
Steroids	Maintain normal plasma glucose concentration; reduce or prevent cerebral edema; provide anti-inflammatory effect.
Antihypertensives	Reduce the risk of severe hypertension and the incidence of stroke.
Cathartics	Induce defecation; prevent constipation.
Vitamins	Provide adequate nutritional needs. (Also, vitamin B complex is indicated in the presence of polyneuritis.)
Antianemics or hematopoietics	Eliminate the cause of, or provide symptomatic relief for, anemia.

7. Prevent aspiration of secretions and vomitus. Position the patient in a lateral or semiprone position if there is no cervical injury. Avoid Trendelenburg's position.
8. Insert an airway if there is evidence of airway obstruction.
9. Continue to observe and report any significant respiratory changes: hyperventilation may result in respiratory alkalosis, and hypoventilation may result in respiratory acidosis.
10. Avoid narcotics (e.g., morphine sulfate may depress the respiratory center).
11. Apply principles of respiratory care (*see* Chapter 14).
12. Assess vital signs serially (if known hypertension, should be considered in evaluating BP). Changes may indicate increasing intracranial pressure (ICP) (rise in BP, slowing pulse, slowing respiration); intracranial hemorrhage and hypertensive encephalopathy (increased

BP); internal bleeding (decreased BP); or hypoglycemia and/or hypertension (full, bounding pulse).

13. Maintain adequate circulation.

14. Replace blood loss if the patient is in shock (whole blood, albumin, or other colloids).

15. Administer mannitol (hyperosmotic agent) IV as ordered if ICP is evident.

16. Record fluid intake accurately. Fluids are usually restricted to 1,500 ml for first 24 hr to prevent cerebral edema.

17. Elevate the head of the bed 30 degrees to promote venous drainage.

18. Apply antiembolic stockings to prevent thrombophlebitis.

19. Assess LOC; pupil shape, size, equality, and reaction to light; seizures; elevated temperature (measured rectally); and CSF leak.

20. Protect the patient from injury. Side rails must be up at all times; padded if seizure is apparent.

21. Administer other therapeutic measures to prevent complications.
    a. Administer antipyretics (if temperature is elevated), anticonvulsants, and steroid therapy as ordered.
    b. Use a hypothermia blanket as ordered.

22. Maintain adequate nutrition status with a high-protein and high-calorie diet.

23. Assess gag and swallowing reflexes, vomiting, and bowel sounds.

24. Administer feedings via a nasogastric (NG) tube.

25. Record fluid intake accurately (especially if the patient is on tube feedings and IV fluids at the same time).

26. Assess for the presence of lacerations, contusions, swelling, and deformity (in traumatic injury).

27. Assess motor functioning: presence or absence of voluntary or spontaneous movement, unusual movements (hiccuping, sucking, or yawning), posturing of limbs (decorticate or decerebrate), and Babinski's sign (positive response may indicate malfunction of pyramidal tract).

28. Maintain correct body alignment: position the patient laterally; turn the patient q 2 hr (hemiplegic patients should not be turned on the affected side for more than 20 min at a time); use pillows, trochanter rolls, and footboard to prevent deformities; and use turning sheets to position the patient properly.

29. Perform passive range-of-motion exercises (if not contraindicated, they should be initiated early to prevent joint deformities).

30. Assess for disturbances of bladder functioning (such as incontinence or urinary retention).

31. Assess the color and sp gr of the urine.

32. Insert a Foley catheter or perform intermittent catheterization as ordered. (Tape Foley catheter to lower abdomen, in male patients, to prevent the development of a fistula at the penoscrotal juncture.

TABLE 20-14

Cranial Nerve Deficit and Implications for Nursing Care

Cranial nerve	Deficit	Nursing care implications
1st (olfactory)	Anosmia	Teach patient about loss of defensive mechanism. Check food intake.
2nd (optic)	Decreased visual acuity	Remind patient to use his glasses. Use appropriate lighting. Orient to environment.
	Limited field of vision (homonymous hemianopsia)	Teach patient to scan, turn head, and place object on unaffected side.
3rd, 4th, and 6th (oculomotor, trochlear,	Limited motion of eye, dyplopia, pupil abnormalities	Teach patient to move head. Tape eyes shut. Investigate possibility of head trauma or drug abuse.
5th (trigeminal)	Cornea will dry and ulcerate (sensory)	Provide eye care. Tape eyes shut. Make sure eye is closed before applying patch. Apply tear drops as ordered.
7th (facial)	Paralysis of facial nerves	Observe for delayed forms of paralysis. Check for food intake.
8th (acoustic)	Decreased or loss of hearing (cochlear)	Assist patient in activities of daily living.
	Balance problems (vestibular)	Protect patient from injury if patient has problem with ambulation.
9th (glossopharyngeal) and 10th (vagus)	Absent or diminished gag reflex, difficulty swallowing	Position patient to prevent aspiration. Suction to maintain patent airway.
11th (spinal accessory)	Decreased or absent contraction of trapezius and/or sternocleido-mastoid muscles	Assess ability to shrug shoulder (important to use of assistive devices in quadriplegia).
12th (hypoglossal)	Atrophy of tongue	Check for food intake.

Change Foley catheter at weekly intervals or according to the protocols of the institution.)

33. Monitor for urinary tract infection.
34. Provide thorough perineal care.
35. Assess normal elimination pattern, incontinence of stool (loss of sphincter control), and fecal impaction.
36. Check stools for occult blood.
37. Administer stool softeners or suppositories as ordered.
38. Record all bowel movements.
39. Assess skin breakdown (especially on bony prominences), presence of rash, and color (reddish hue or cyanosis).
40. Prevent skin breakdown (*see* Chapter 12).
41. Provide oral hygiene at least q 4 hr to prevent parotitis, sordes, and aspiration of crusts. Change airway daily if the patient has an endotracheal tube.
42. Administer mouth care with the patient's head elevated and turned to the unaffected side, so that the affected side is uppermost.
43. Instill water or a solution of half-strength hydrogen peroxide and water with a catheter tip syringe (glass syringe should not be used).
44. Use a padded tongue blade to keep the mouth open.
45. Suction immediately after instilling the solution to prevent aspiration.
46. Apply cold cream around the patient's lips to prevent drying of skin around the mouth.
47. Have at least two people perform mouth care.
48. Provide a bite block to protect the patient's teeth and tongue (in cases where comatose patients grind their teeth).
49. Administer eye care to prevent complications such as corneal ulceration, which may eventually lead to blindness if corneal reflex is absent.
50. Cover the eye with an eye shield and instill methyl cellulose (0.5 to 1.0%) to the affected eye as ordered.
51. Remove contact lenses (ideally these should be removed in the ER).
52. Give appropriate care if the patient has an artificial eye.
53. During the long-term phase, when the patient regains consciousness, consult a physiatrist to evaluate motor disabilities, institute appropriate measures (such as use of assistive devices and daily exercises in physical therapy department), refer the patient to occupational therapy, and continue to assess progress and institute measures to prevent complications.
54. Institute a bladder training program for patients with neurogenic bladder. Cystometrogram is used to determine if the bladder is spastic (upper motor neuron bladder) or flaccid (lower motor neuron bladder). For upper motor neuron bladder, use "trigger areas" to initiate voiding (e.g., stroking the inner thigh, stimulating the rectum digitally, and pulling pubic hair), or encourage straining or Credé's

maneuver, if the patient has not voided in 2 hr. For lower motor neuron bladder, use the Credé's maneuver. Teach the patient self-catheterization if intermittent catheterization is indicated for long-term care.

55. If the patient remains in a coma, continue assessment of all body systems (especially neurologic and respiratory), and institute measures based on changes in the patient's status. Emphasis should be placed on respiratory care, including chest physiotherapy, to prevent respiratory complications (which usually cause death) and on physical therapy (to prevent contractures and other deformities).

Psychosocial 56. Maintain the dignity and worth of the patient by explaining all procedures, providing privacy, and avoiding all unnecessary conversations. (It is assumed that sense of hearing is the last of the senses to go and the first to return when the patient regains consciousness.)

57. Provide tactile stimulation (especially if sensory deficit is evident) by touching the patient or holding his hand.

58. Provide support and understanding to the family (inability to communicate with the patient may produce anxiety among family members).

59. Respect the family's wishes with regard to religious beliefs or practices and, in the event of impending death, make spiritual help available on the request of the family.

60. During the ongoing phase, help the patient adjust to his disability by considering the following factors: loss of body image, loss of a body part, and stages of grief and grieving.

61. Encourage the patient and family to verbalize fears and concerns.

62. Help the patient establish realistic goals. Emphasis should be placed on the patient's strengths, rather than on limitations.

63. Assist the family and significant others to adapt to the patient's disability.

64. Use a team approach to meet psychosocial needs of the patient; regaining normal functioning is a long and tedious process.

Educational 65. Discuss the patient's condition, especially if remissions are anticipated.

66. Review complications.

67. Consider safety factors (e.g., crossing the street for patients with hemianopsia).

68. Provide information about diet, medications (dosage, drug interactions), treatments, and exercises.

69. Make the patient and family aware of resources, such as the Myasthenia Gravis Foundation, Parkinson's Foundation, or stroke club.

70. Instruct the patient and family to report any unusual signs and symptoms.

71. Emphasize the importance of keeping appointments with the physician to evaluate the condition.
72. Refer the patient to a visiting nurse service before discharge.

Evaluation criteria

Respiratory status: no respiratory distress, cyanosis, or complications; blood gases within normal limits; and chest x-ray normal. *Neurologic status*: alert and oriented to time, place, and person; pupils equal, round, and reactive to light and accommodation; no evidence of other cranial nerve deficits; no seizures; temperature within normal limits; no CNS leak from nose or ears; and no toxic effects of drugs. *Cardiovascular status*: vital signs within normal limits, no signs of fluid and electrolyte imbalance, and no thrombophlebitis. *Nutrition status*: intake adequate; no difficulty swallowing, choking, or aspiration; appropriate diet provided; proper positioning maintained during meals; no hypoproteinemia or vitamin deficiency; and no excessive weight loss or weight gain. *Musculoskeletal status*: no motor deficits or contractures, muscle tone normal (no flaccidity or spasticity), self-care activities demonstrated, standing and wheelchair transfers demonstrated, and no injuries sustained during ambulation. *Elimination status*: no urinary incontinence, retention, or infection; output adequate; self-catheterization demonstrated; normal pattern of elimination; no fecal impaction or incontinence; and foods high in roughage included in diet. *Integumentary status*: skin integrity maintained; no complications related to inadequate oral, eye, or perineal care; no injuries sustained related to sensory loss; and skin warm to touch. *Psychosocial status*: dignity maintained in all aspects of care (even in unconscious state), support and understanding communicated to the family, realistic goals stated by both the patient and family, verbalization of the nature of the disease, verbalization of concerns about any changes in life-style related to permanent disability, verbalization by the patient and family about the significance of taking medications as prescribed, verbalization and demonstration by the patient and family regarding exercises prescribed by the physical therapist and the use of assistive devices, verbalization by the patient and family about measures to prevent complications, and verbalization by the patient and family about the importance of keeping up all future appointments with a private physician or outpatient clinic.

DEVIATIONS

INCREASED INTRACRANIAL PRESSURE

Increased ICP is a result of acute changes in dynamic forces affecting the intracranial contents. It is caused by cerebral edema, increased volume of CSF, hydrocephalus, intracerebral mass lesions (abscess, tumors), blood clots, and blockage of venous outflow. Precipitating factors include changes in intrathoracic pressure (tracheal suctioning producing bronchospasm and coughing), postural changes, hypoxia, and the Valsalva maneuver. Other suggested factors include isometric muscular contractions, emotional upset, body position, and turning in bed.

According to the Monro-Kellie hypothesis, the cranial cavity, a rigid container, has restricted volume. Any increase in the volume of one of the intracranial contents (CSF, blood, brain tissue) must be at the expense of one or both of the others. A diminished volume of one is met with a compensatory increase in the others. ICP rises when the capacity of the compensatory mechanisms is exceeded.

An increase in ICP in the normal brain is asymptomatic because autoregulation of cerebral blood vessels maintains a relatively normal blood flow. Lesser changes in ICP in a damaged brain may cause cerebral ischemia because of impaired autoregulation. Larger pressure changes produce symptoms related to compartmental herniation — mass lesions or brain hernias obstruct tentorial incisura or foramen magnum. Early *signs and symptoms* include headache, nausea and vomiting, lethargy, diplopia, and papilledema. As ICP continues to rise, there is increased BP, bradycardia, pupillary changes (unilateral pupil dilation), deepening coma, and the following changes in motor response: ipsilateral hemiplegia, decorticate or decerebrate posturing, and Babinski's sign. *Diagnosis* is based on the health history, physical exam, blood studies (blood gases, glucose levels), and CAT scan.

Common interventions

Medical treatment consists of hyperventilation (to decrease CO_2 levels), drug therapy (steroids or mannitol), and ventricular puncture. **Surgical** treatment involves the removal of the mass or hematoma.

Nursing interventions

1. *See* Overview.
Physical 2. Maintain a patent airway and provide for adequate oxygenation (*see* Chapter 14).
3. Assess the patient's neurologic status, particularly for the presence of 3rd cranial nerve palsy.
4. Assess the patient's cardiovascular status for increasing systolic pressure, widening pulse pressure, and decreasing pulse rate.
5. Prevent flexion of the neck and isometric muscular contraction.
6. Advise the patient to avoid the Valsalva maneuver when defecating.

Evaluation criteria. See Overview. No ipsilateral hemiplegia, decorticate or decerebrate posturing, or Babinski's sign. Valsalva maneuver avoided.

HEAD INJURY

Head injury (craniocerebral trauma) is damage to the brain as a result of traumatic injury. There are two classifications: closed (blunt head injuries) and open. **Closed head injuries** are *characterized* by no injury to the skull, or only a linear fracture. They may result from sudden acceleration or deceleration of the head. Temporary loss of consciousness and gross brain damage may result, depending on the severity of cerebral tissue damage. In the case of a concussion, there is no significant degree of damage to the brain, but it may result in transient functional impairment. A contusion (bruising of brain tissue) results in destruction of brain tissue and may be accompanied by laceration, swelling, hemorrhage, and herniation. Common sites for contusions are the frontal and temporal lobes. **Open head injuries** involve exposure of brain tissue or meninges. The dura mater, leptomeninges, and brain tissue may be injured by a sharp instrument or projectile that penetrates the skull. Open head injuries can be classified as skull fractures (simple and compound) and penetrating injuries. A simple depressed skull fracture means that the cranium is intact and a fragment of fractured bone is depressed inward to compress or injure the underlying brain substance. A compound fracture means that the pericranial tissues are torn and there is direct communication between the lacerated scalp and the cerebral substance through the depressed or comminuted fragments of bone and lacerated dura. A penetrating injury occurs when the cerebral tissue is injured by a bullet or fragments, causing necrosis and hemorrhage.

There are ~3 million head injuries each year, resulting in 30,000 deaths. These injuries occur at any age, adult men are most frequently affected, and their incidence is high in the military. Head injuries are often caused by automobile and motorcycle accidents (most common cause of head injury), falling objects, gunshot wounds, and sharp instruments or projectiles. Precipitating factors include driving under the influence of alcohol, participation in contact sports, anticoagulants, and altered LOC, often related to drugs prescribed for medical conditions (e.g., diazepam, phenytoin, phenobarbital).

In a head injury, the cerebral substance is contused or lacerated. Hemorrhage (meningeal or intracerebral) may occur in conjunction with localized swelling of cerebral tissues. Certain biochemical changes accompany head injury: acetylcholine and lactate are elevated in the CSF during the first days, sodium is retained, and sodium and nitrogen are lost. Most of the symptoms of severe head injury, both general or focal, depend on highly reversible changes in the brain and may be multiple or varied. Generalized *symptoms* include altered LOC (drowsiness, confusion, and coma [duration depends on site and severity of injury]). A coma of short duration indicates a concussion. Prolonged coma (which may last for hours or days) indicates edema, hemorrhage, contusion, or laceration of the brain. If a coma is prolonged over several days or weeks, it is reflective of the fact that the brain or brainstem is severely contused. Generalized symptoms also include altered vital signs (indicative of increased ICP), which may include a decreasing pulse rate, rising BP, and slow and deep respirations; elevated temperature; pupillary changes; papilledema; seizures; headache; and dizziness. Focal neurologic signs include hemiplegia, cranial nerve palsies, and aphasia. Other symptoms include CSF leak from the nose (rhinorrhea) or ears (otorrhea); bleeding from the scalp, nose, or mouth; and hemothorax, broken rib, or fractured femur (from other injuries).

Infectious *complications* of head injuries include meningitis and brain abscess. Vascular complications include intracerebral hemorrhage and extracerebral (intracranial) hemorrhage, which may be epidural or subdural. In the epidural form (temporal or parietal region), which occurs within minutes or hours, there is rupture of the middle meningeal artery, temporary loss of consciousness followed by a lucid interval, and temporal lobe herniation. The subdural form, which occurs within days or weeks, is venous in origin and maybe acute or chronic. Acute subdural (extracerebral) hemorrhage may cause herniation. The sequelae of head injuries may include posttraumatic seizures, postconcussion syndrome, psychoses and mental disturbances, and hydrocephalus.

Diagnosis is based on the health history, physical exam, blood studies (blood gases, electrolytes, glucose, CBC), lateral cervical spine x-ray, chest x-ray (to determine pneumo- or hemothorax), skull x-ray (to define fractures), CAT scan, cerebral angiography, lumbar puncture (contraindicated in ICP), and EEG.

Common interventions

Medical treatment involves the maintenance of adequate cerebral perfusion via intubation (endotracheal tube), tracheostomy, and ventilatory assistance; control of hemorrhage via pressure or elevation (from scalp or elsewhere) and nasal packs (nose and mouth); maintenance of fluid balance via blood and IV fluids based on patient's needs; and drug therapy using steroids, antibiotics (open, contaminated wounds), tetanus toxoid (open head injuries), and anticonvulsants. **Surgical** treatment consists of surgical exploration (burr holes) and evacuation of hematoma.

Nursing interventions

Physical priorities in the acute phase are the respiratory, cardiovascular, and neurologic status. (*See* Overview.)

Physical 1. Suction the patient via the oral route (nasal suctioning may be contraindicated if a skull fracture is evident).
2. Apply principles of care if the patient is on ventilatory assistance and tracheostomy care (*see* Chapter 14).
3. Assess the head wound for further bleeding.

4. Identify any developing trend of neurologic status (if deterioration is evident, notify the physician immediately).
5. Test drainage from nose and ear for glucose (positive results indicate CSF).
6. Elevate the patient's head 30 degrees.
7. Obtain the patient's temperature rectally and control hyperthermia as appropriate.
8. Assist the patient with activities of daily living if hemiplegia is present.
9. Maintain orders for bed rest, especially if the patient is on close observation. Explain carefully to the patient the significance of bed rest.
10. Avoid restraints if the patient becomes restless. Keep side rails up at all times. Apply appropriate restraints if the patient is extremely agitated.
11. Report large amounts of urinary output (posttraumatic diabetes insipidus may occur with contusion of the hypothalamic area).
12. Assess bowel sounds. (Immediately after injury, the patient may have an NG tube attached to suction for abdominal distension.)
13. Maintain strict aseptic technique when handling any type of wound to prevent infection.
14. Apply a cold compress if periorbital edema is present.
15. In the long-term phase, direct care toward meeting physical and psychologic needs of patients with neurologic sequelae.
Psychosocial 16. Have the physician explain the possibility of neurologic deficits.
Educational 17. Refer the patient to a physical therapist for assistive devices if indicated.
18. Discuss with the family any alternative means of communication if the patient is aphasic.
19. Educate the public about alcohol abuse.
20. Educate the public about the importance of safe driving.

Evaluation criteria. *See* Overview. Lungs clear and free of secretions. Fluid restriction maintained. No evidence of wound infection or periorbital edema.

SPINAL CORD INJURY

Spinal cord injury/trauma (SCI) is injury to the nerve roots or substances of the spinal cord resulting from severe trauma to the spine. Approximately 200,000 Americans have SCI, and ~ 10,000 new cases occur each year. The majority of patients are men, ≤30 yr old. The mortality rate is ~20% for patients with quadriplegia in their first year of care.

SCI is caused by trauma resulting from falls, diving accidents, automobile accidents, gunshot or stab wounds (direct injury to the cord), industrial accidents, and athletic activities. A major precipitating factor is alcohol intoxication.

During SCI, shearing or squeezing of the spinal cord results in destruction of the gray and white matter with a varying degree of hemorrhage, mainly in the vascular area. Edema occurs, causing swelling and compression of the nerve tracts, followed by necrosis. These changes occur at the level of injury and one or two segments above and below the injury. The result may be a complete or incomplete transection of the cord. *Symptoms* are related to the level of lesion. In a complete transection of the cord, there is loss of all voluntary movements below the lesion (paralysis), loss of sensation below the lesion (anesthesia), and loss of reflex functioning of all spinal segments below the lesion (spinal shock or areflexia). (All skeletal muscles are affected: bowel, bladder, autonomic control, and sexual functioning.) Incomplete transection of the cord involves a variable degree of motor and sensory loss below the level of lesion. Functional impairments (arising from lesions at various levels) are as follows: cervical 1-7, quadriplegia (respiratory functioning is compromised, especially at C1-C4 level); thoracic 1-12, paraplegia; lumbar L1-L2, paraplegia; cauda equina (below L2-S5), cauda equina syndrome (flaccid paralysis and sensory loss of the lower extremities, loss of sensation, paralysis of bladder and rectum). Immediately after the injury there is respiratory distress, neck pain, and signs of spinal shock (hypotension, bradycardia, loss of temperature control, flaccid paralysis, bowel distension and paralytic ileus, and absence of perspiration below the level of injury). After initial flaccidity, heightened reflex activity (hyperreflexia) occurs over a period of 1 to 6 wk in most cases, although varying degrees may last for years. This hyperreflexia is characterized by spastic paralysis, flexor spasms, automatic bladder (neurogenic bladder), reflex defecation, profuse sweating, piloerection, and paresthesias (burning, stabbing pain in lower back, abdomen, and buttocks). *Complications* include respiratory failure, pneumonia, atelectasis, orthostatic hypotension, thrombophlebitis, urinary tract infection, pyelonephritis, renal failure, renal and bladder stones, autonomic hyperreflexia, pressure ulcers, osteoporosis, fecal impaction, and infected sores.

Diagnosis is based on the health history, physical exam, chest x-ray, lateral spine x-ray, and myelogram.

Common interventions

Medical treatment consists of respiratory assistance and immobilization of the injured spine via cervical stabilization traction board or improvised board with sandbags, etc., to stabilize the neck (site of accident) or via skull traction with Gardner-Wells tongs, Crutchfield tongs, or halo traction brace. Other medical treatments include drug therapy (corticosteroids), physiotherapy (muscle reeducation and use of braces and other assistive devices), and occupational therapy. **Surgical** treatment consists of decompressive laminectomy and fusion.

Nursing interventions

Physical priorities in the acute phase are the respiratory, cardiovascular, and neurologic status. (*See* Overview and Chapters 14 and 15.)

Physical 1. Apply principles of respiratory care for patients with a tracheostomy or assisted ventilation. (Usually indicated for patients with high cervical injury.)

2. Assess for hypotension or bradycardia and report findings.

3. Assess sensory status and deep tendon and superficial reflexes.

4. Administer steroids as ordered to reduce swelling of spinal cord tissue.

5. Assess for bowel sounds. (Initially, an NG tube is inserted and attached to suction to prevent abdominal distension.)

6. Assist the patient during mealtime and feed him slowly to prevent choking and aspiration related to enforced immobilization.

7. Maintain orders for immobilization while providing nursing measures. Position the patient's limbs in proper alignment. Keep hands and wrists in a functional position for patients with quadriplegia because correct positioning during the early stages of injury will determine the ultimate posture. Keep the patient's head and spine in alignment during turning.

8. Prevent or control GU problems. (SCI patients are particularly susceptible to GU complications.) Implement measures presented in the Overview. Maintain acidity of the urine (test pH and provide cranberry juice, vitamin C, and urinary antiseptics as ordered).

9. Maintain precautions to prevent injury to the skin because of sensory loss. (Monitor the patient carefully for burns if using a heat lamp for a pressure ulcer.)

10. Administer injectable medications above the level of injury to ensure adequate absorption (oral route is preferable).

11. Inspect tong sites for evidence of bleeding or infection and provide care as ordered.

12. During the long-term phase, continue with active physical rehabilitation (reconditioning and progressive resistance exercises, use of braces and other assistive devices for ambulation, and mastery of activities of daily living).

13. Implement measures to prevent further complications as follows:
    a. For autonomic hyperreflexia, monitor for and report immediately elevated BP, bradycardia, severe throbbing headache, and profuse diaphoresis above injury level; obtain orders for ganglionic blocking agents to relieve symptoms; and identify trigger mechanisms (e.g., distended bladder and bowel, fecal impaction, and decubitus ulcer) and carry out appropriate measures to remove these stimuli.
    b. For spasticity, assess for spastic contractions (e.g., adduction or hip flexion), and protect the patient from injury when severe

spasms occur; administer muscle relaxants as ordered and monitor for side effects; and provide other measures to relieve spasms, such as physical and hydrotherapy. (Rhizotomy had also been done to relieve spasms. Spasms aggravate other complications and may promote deformities of the hips, knees, and ankles.)

   c. For pain, refer the patient to the physician if pain persists so that appropriate measures can be implemented, such as nerve block or chordotomy (*see* Chapter 4).

   d. For neurogenic bladder, reinforce the patient's understanding with regard to long-term management of the GU tract. (*See* Overview regarding a bladder retraining program.)

Psychosocial 14. Reassure the patient that a productive life is possible.

15. Encourage the patient to participate in his care after the acute phase.

16. Keep the patient occupied to prevent boredom during the long period of rehabilitation. (Make available radio, television, and suitable reading material. Provide prism glasses during the period of enforced immobilization. Encourage friends and relatives to visit, and guide their approach to further facilitate adjustment.)

17. Explore feelings related to sexuality. (Explain the limitations of sexual function and available alternatives.)

18. Encourage the patient to join a local or national organization for SCI patients.

Educational 19. Before discharge, teach the patient catheterization, bladder and bowel training, and measures to prevent complications, especially bladder problems and pressure ulcers, and to report them immediately.

20. Reinforce the physical therapist's teachings with regard to exercises and the use of assistive devices.

21. Refer the patient to a visiting nurse service to evaluate his home so that it can be adapted to a wheelchair occupant.

22. Refer to social service to secure special devices for patients with quadriplegia.

23. Make sure that a lightweight collapsible wheelchair is ready before discharge.

24. Discuss the possibility of driving an automobile fitted with a hand control to provide mobility (especially if the patient plans to return to work).

25. Refer the patient to a vocational counselor if appropriate.

Prevention 26. Teach the public, firefighters, and paramedics how to recognize obvious signs of injury to the spinal cord and how to provide preventive and supportive treatment at the accident.

27. Educate the public about the causes of SCI.

Evaluation criteria. *See* Overview. No associated head injuries, sensory function regained, no hyperreflexia or paresthesias. No evidence of autonomic hyperreflexia. No paralytic ileus. Ambulation with braces and/or crutches for patients with paraplegia, wheelchair locomotion for patients with quadriplegia, no permanent deformities in paralyzed limbs, and no flexor spasms. No infection or bleeding on tong sites. Adaptation to present life-style evident, and verbalization of feelings of sexuality and ways of coping.

MENINGITIS

Meningitis (leptomeningitis) is an infection of the pia mater and arach-noid, including the subarachnoid space and the CSF. The three most common types of bacterial meningitis are meningococcal meningitis, pneumococcal meningitis, and *Haemophilus influenzae* meningitis. Menin-gitis, which is prevalent worldwide, occurs mostly in the autumn, winter, and spring. It is slightly more predominant in males than in females. *H. influenzae* meningitis usually affects children. Meningococcal meningitis affects children, adolescents, and adults. Pneumococcal meningitis is more predominant in the very young and in adults >40 yr of age.

Almost any of the pathogenic bacteria can cause meningitis. The most common are *Neisseria meningitidis* (meningococcal), *Diplococcus pneumoniae* (pneumococcal), and *H. influenzae*. Less frequent causative bacteria are *Staphylococcus aureus*, *Streptococcus*, and *Enterobacteriaceae* such as *Escherichia coli* (neonates), *Pseudomonas*, *Klebsiella*, and *Proteus mirabilis*. Predisposing factors include upper respiratory tract infection; infections in the lungs, middle ear, mastoid or paranasal sinuses; trauma (penetrating head injuries, skull fractures); brain abscess; lumbar puncture; neurosurgical procedures (ventriculoperitoneal shunts); and therapy with immunosuppressive agents.

Bacteria gain access to the meninges via the bloodstream or other avenues, causing an inflammatory reaction of the pia, arachnoid, ventricles, and adjacent structures. Vascular congestion of the meningeal vessels follows. Purulent exudate then forms in the subarachnoid space and increases rapidly over the base of the brain, cranial and spinal nerve sheaths, and the perivascular spaces of the cortex. As the infection progresses, the pia and arachnoid become thickened and adhesions may form, causing hydrocephalus, cranial nerve palsies, and damage to the auditory nerve. If infection is controlled at an early stage, no residual change may occur in the arachnoid. In fulminating cases, vasomotor collapse associated with adreno-cortical necrosis (Waterhouse-Friderichsen syndrome) may occur. Death results from the effects of overwhelming infection (bacteremia), brain swell-ing, and cerebellar herniation. *Symptoms* of meningitis include high fever, severe headache, nausea and vomiting, seizures, altered LOC (lethargy, stupor, coma), photophobia, petechial or purpuric rash (meningococcus), and signs of meningeal irritation, including nuchal rigidity (resistance to passive flexion of neck), Kernig's sign (resistance to attempts to fully extend the leg when the hip is flexed), and Brudzinski's sign (flexion of the knee and hip when the neck is flexed). The most common *complications*, which are due to injury of the nervous system, include convulsions, hydrocephalus, personality changes, ocular palsies, deafness, and flaccid paralysis. There may also be respiratory complications, bacteremia, and cerebral edema.

Diagnosis is based on the health history; physical exam; cultures of CSF (cloudy, purulent, elevated WBC), blood, nasopharyngeal secretions, and wounds; BUN and serum electrolytes (to determine hyponatremia); skull and chest x-rays; and CAT scan (if brain abscess is suspected).

Common interventions

Medical treatment consists of drug therapy with antibiotics, steroids (recommended for overwhelming meningococcal sepsis), anticonvulsants (to control seizures), and osmotic diuretics (for cerebral edema). Supportive medical treatment consists of airway maintenance, parenteral administration of fluids, and strict isolation (depends on the microorganism).

Nursing interventions

Physical priorities in the acute stage are the respiratory, cardiovascular, and neurologic status. (*See* Overview.)

Physical 1. Provide appropriate care if the patient is on assisted ventilation (*see* Chapter 14).
  2. Observe for signs of ICP and meningeal irritation.
  3. Maintain seizure precautions.
  4. Monitor central venous pressure if indicated.
  5. Monitor IV therapy (for fluid replacement and for antibiotics).
  6. Maintain fluid balance because dehydration and hyponatremia may occur.
  7. Monitor output accurately (especially if the patient is receiving an aminoglycoside antibiotic).
  8. Assess for petechial hemorrhages.
Psychosocial 9. Explain all care to the patient and family, especially if on isolation.
Educational 10. Instruct the patient to seek consultation if evidence of residual disability is present.
  11. Teach the patient ways to increase his resistance to infection.
Prevention 12. Apply strict aseptic technique for patients undergoing invasive procedures.
  13. Institute proper therapy for patients with acute and chronic infection (e.g., of the sinus).
  14. Avoid situations where there is overcrowding.
  15. Build up resistance to infection (e.g., nutrition, rest).

Evaluation criteria. See Overview. Patient able to breathe independently, without respiratory aids. No signs of meningeal irritation, seizures, headache, or injury. No evidence of flaccid paralysis. Patient and family verbalize nature of disease and reason for isolation, and participate in diversional activities.

ENCEPHALITIS

Encephalitis is an inflammation of the brain substance. Viral forms of encephalitis include epidemic encephalitis (von Economo's encephalitis, encephalitis lethargica), herpes simplex encephalitis, and arbovirus (*ar*thropod-*bo*rne) encephalitis (includes equine encephalitis). Encephalitis occurs in all parts of the world. It may occur at any age, but is most common in childhood, adolescence, and early adult life. It is also characterized by geographic and seasonal incidence. Encephalitis is caused by microorganisms (viruses, bacteria, fungi, and parasites). Viruses gain entrance to the body via the following routes: transmitted to humans by mosquito bite or tick (arbovirus), and person to person (droplet infection). Precipitating factors include infectious diseases (mumps, measles, chickenpox) (postinfectious encephalitis follows these infectious diseases), and vaccination against smallpox, rabies, and pertussis (postvaccinal encephalitis).

Encephalitis involves widespread degenerative changes of nerve cells accompanied by cellular infiltration in both the gray and white matter, meninges, and perivascular spaces of the brain. The lesions may affect massive areas of the cerebral hemispheres, as is often seen in equine encephalitis. The cerebellum and spinal cord may also be involved.

Symptoms of encephalitis include fever, headache, nausea and vomiting, seizures, confusion, drowsiness, stupor, coma, signs of meningeal irritation, photophobia, hemiparesis, aphasia or mutism, and cranial nerve palsies. Death or residual deficits occur in two-thirds of patients infected with Eastern equine encephalitis. Residual deficits include memory impairment, personality changes, hemiplegia, recurrent seizures, deafness, and speech disorders.

Diagnosis is based on the health history, physical exam, viral studies of CSF, blood culture, EEG, CAT scan, and brain biopsy (to confirm diagnosis).

Common interventions

Medical treatment is symptomatic, and may involve physiotherapy and drug therapy: adenine arabinoside (Ara-A) is the recommended treatment for herpes simplex encephalitis.

Nursing interventions

Physical priorities of care are the respiratory, neurologic, and cardiovascular status. (*See* Overview.)

Physical 1. Assess for signs of increasing ICP.
2. Assess for signs of meningeal irritation.
3. Maintain seizure precautions to prevent injury (e.g., provide a quiet environment).

4. Apply restraints as appropriate if the patient becomes hostile and aggressive.

Psychosocial 5. Provide the family with information regarding the progress of the disease, especially if the patient has neurologic sequelae such as motor disabilities, aphasia, and personality changes.

6. Approach calmly if the patient becomes hostile.

7. Provide the patient with diversional activities during the day (in rehabilitation phase) as patients have alterations of sleep pattern.

Prevention 8. Prevent arbovirus-type encephalitis by eradicating breeding places of mosquito.

Evaluation criteria. See Overview. No signs of meningeal irritation, seizures, aphasia, or cranial nerve palsies. No injury sustained if hostile or aggressive. Sleep pattern back to normal.

BRAIN ABSCESS

A brain abscess is a collection of pus in the substance of the brain tissue secondary to an acute purulent infection. It is relatively rare and constitutes <2% of patients referred for intracranial surgery. A brain abscess may occur at any age, although it is more common in the first to the third decades of life (due to high incidence of mastoid and nasal sinus disease at this period). It affects males slightly more than females.

The most common microorganisms involved in the development of a brain abscess (vary with the site of the abscess) are *Streptococcus* (spread from lung), *Staphylococcus* (consequence of penetrating head trauma or of bacteremia), *Enterobacteriaceae* (*E. coli* and *Proteus*), and *Bacteroides*. Primary sources of infection occur as direct extension of infections of the paranasal sinuses (especially frontal and sphenoidal), middle ear, or mastoid. Infections may also occur secondary to compound skull fractures, intracranial surgery, or the suppurative processes in the lungs (lung abscess or bronchiectasis) or heart (acute bacterial endocarditis). Other sources of infection include upper respiratory tract infection, tonsils, abscessed teeth, osteomyelitis, and infected pelvic organs. Congenital heart disease (tetralogy of Fallot) is a precipitating factor.

An early reaction to bacterial invasion of the brain results in suppurative encephalitis. At this stage, pus formation is not visible. Within a few days, pus appears in the center of the abscess. Macroglia and fibroblasts then proliferate to form a wall of granulation tissue. Because the wall is not of uniform thickness (thinner on its deeper parts), brain abscesses tend to spread deeply into the white matter, produce a chain of abscesses, and, in some cases, rupture in the ventricles. This inflammatory process is usually accompanied by edema of the cerebrum.

Early *symptoms* (which may improve with antimicrobial therapy) include headache, chills and fever (in some cases), nausea and vomiting, drowsiness and confusion, focal or generalized seizures, and speech disorders. Late symptoms include recurrent headache, focal or generalized seizures, altered LOC (drowsiness, stupor, and coma), signs of increased ICP, and focal neurologic signs (depending on the location of the abscess): frontal lobe (headache, impairments of mental functioning, hemiparesis), temporal lobe or parietooccipital lobes (aphasic disturbances, especially anomia, and homonymous hemianopsia), cerebellar (headache in postauricular region, nystagmus, intention tremor, ataxia). *Complications* include recurrence of abscess, focal epilepsy, and residual neurologic deficits.

Diagnosis is based on the health history, physical exam, studies of CSF (lumbar puncture may be dangerous if there is evidence of increased ICP), blood cultures, CAT scan, EEG, and skull and chest x-rays.

Common interventions

Medical treatment for the patient with a brain abscess includes drug therapy with antibiotics (penicillin and chloramphenicol given pre- and postoperatively), mannitol (IV) followed by dexamethasone (for ICP), and anticonvulsants. **Surgery** is delayed until the abscess is firmly encapsulated (as confirmed by CAT scan). Progression of ICP, however, may necessitate surgical intervention regardless of stage of abscess. Methods of treating an abscess include aspiration of abscess and drainage, complete removal (if superficial and encapsulated), and aspiration and injection of antibiotics into the abscess (if deep).

Nursing interventions

Physical priorities of care are the respiratory, neurologic, and nutrition status. (*See* Overview.)

Physical 1. Monitor the patient for side effects of steroid and antibiotic therapy.
2. Monitor and record output accurately, especially if the patient is on mannitol.
Educational 3. Instruct the patient with regard to the side effects of antibiotic therapy, especially if continued for several weeks.
4. Instruct the patient with regard to prescribed anticonvulsant medications.
5. Encourage the patient to consult the physician if signs of recurrent abscess occur.
Prevention 6. Eliminate foci of infection.
7. Advise correction of cardiac deformity following successful treatment of a cerebral abscess in a patient with a congenital heart disease.

Evaluation criteria. See Overview. Verbalization of the importance of preventing any kind of infection that may contribute to recurrence of brain abscess.

GUILLAIN-BARRÉ SYNDROME

Guillain-Barré syndrome is an inflammatory disease of unknown cause involving primarily the peripheral and cranial nerves. It affects children and adults of all ages, is slightly more common in the third and fourth decades of life, and affects males and females equally. It occurs in all parts of the world and in all seasons.

The cause of Guillain-Barré syndrome is unknown; however, current theories suggest an antoimmune reaction or a viral etiology. Precipitating factors include vaccination (swine influenza, antirabies), surgical procedures, Hodgkin's disease, and viral infection: upper respiratory tract and GI infection (usually precedes the onset of symptoms by 1 to 3 wk).

Guillain-Barré syndrome involves infiltration of perivascular lymphocytes in the spinal and cranial nerves, causing inflammation and edema along with demyelination and degeneration. Nerve conduction is then interrupted, producing paralysis.

Clinical *characteristics* may vary. In mild forms, for example, weakness is confined to the legs, with the arms only slightly affected. The rate of recovery also varies, often within a few weeks or months. In a majority of cases, normal functioning is restored. In some patients there may be residual motor deficits. The onset of *symptoms* usually develops after the respiratory and GI infection have subsided. Initially, muscle weakness develops symmetrically over a period of several hours to several days. Muscle weakness ascends rapidly to the trunk, upper extremities, and muscles innervated by cranial nerves, producing total paralysis. Respiratory failure may occur if the respiratory muscles are severely affected. Paralysis is usually flaccid. The following cranial nerves may be involved: 7th (facial) (the most commonly affected, resulting in facial paralysis), 9th (glossopharyngeal), 10th (vagus), and 12th (hypoglossal). Involvement may result in difficulty in swallowing, masticating, and talking. Sensory changes may also occur, including paresthesias (pain is rare), muscle tenderness to moderate or deep pressure, loss of position and vibration sense, and diminishèd or absent deep tendon reflexes. Autonomic disturbances include fluctuations in BP and the development of sinus tachycardia. Urinary retention may also occur. *Complications* include respiratory failure, complications related to immobility, cardiac abnormalities (due to autonomic dysfunction), and hyponatremia (rare).

Diagnosis is based on the health history, physical exam, and diagnostic studies of the CSF. CSF examination shows albuminocytologic dissociation (increase in protein content without an increase in cell count).

Common interventions

Methods of treatment are generally supportive with respiratory assistance (ventilator, tracheostomy); drug therapy with steroids (therapeutic usefulness is controversial, some physicians advocate use) and antibiotics (respiratory complications); and physiotherapy. Plasmapheresis has been used experimentally with reports of dramatic improvements.

Nursing interventions

Physical priorities of care in the acute phase are the respiratory, neurologic, and cardiovascular status. (*See* Overview.)

Physical 1. Monitor signs of impending respiratory failure.
2. Measure vital capacity.
3. Monitor blood gases.
4. Monitor BP and report any fluctuations.
5. Monitor for tachycardia.
6. Evaluate the patient's muscle strength and tone.
7. Institute measures to prevent deformities (*see* Chapter 7).
8. Consult occupational and physical therapists as appropriate.
9. Assess for urinary retention.
10. Continue rehabilitative measures during the long-term phase. (When rehabilitation centers are available, patients may be transferred to the rehabilitation unit for extensive therapy.)
Psychosocial 11. Devise alternative means of communication during the acute phase when the patient is unable to communicate.
12. Reassure the patient and family that chances of recovery are excellent.
13. Encourage verbalization of feelings of anger and frustration.
Educational 14. Instruct the patient to report any abnormal changes (*see* symptoms *above*) because of the potential for a relapse.
Prevention 15. Build up resistance to infection since Guillain-Barré has been closely associated with disease of viral origin.

Evaluation criteria. *See* Overview. No evidence of cranial nerve deficits or sensory changes. No tachycardia, BP within normal limits. No evidence of muscle weakness. Verbalization of ways of dealing with anger and frustration, use of alternative means of communication during acute phase, and gradual participation in performing activities of daily living as condition permits.

BRAIN TUMORS

Brain tumors (intracranial tumors, intracranial neoplasms) are abnormal growths that occupy space within the cranial cavity. There are two classifications of brain tumors. **Primary** brain tumors arise from cells of the CNS, and may be benign or malignant. Metastasis to other parts of the body is rare. The characteristics of the different types of primary tumors are listed in Table 20-15. **Secondary** brain tumors arise from metastatic lesions from the lungs, breast, skin (melanoma), GI tract, kidney, liver, thyroid, uterus,

TABLE 20-15

Type, Origin, Sites, and Clinical Characteristics of Primary Tumors

Type	Origin	Sites	Characteristics
Gliomas	Glial cells	Cerebral hemispheres (adults), cerebellum (children).	Most common form of intracranial tumor. Infiltrates the brain tissue.
Glioblastoma multiforme	Undifferentiated cells,	Cerebral hemispheres (frontal lobes).	Highly malignant, rapidly growing. Presence of hemorrhage. More common in males.
Astrocytoma	Astrocytes.	Cerebrum, cerebellum (children and young adults), optic nerve and chiasm, and brainstem (pons and hypothalamus).	Slow-growing tumor. Undergoes cystic formation.
Oligodendroglioma	Oligodendrocytes.	Cerebral hemispheres (frontal lobes).	Rare. Grows slowly. Tendency to calcium formation.
Ependymoma	Ependymal cells lining the ventricles.	Ventricles (4th [most common site], 3rd, and lateral), and spinal cord (caudal part).	Slow growing. May obstruct CSF flow.
Medulloblastoma	Round undifferentiated cells.	Cerebellum, roof of 4th ventricle.	Common in children. Rapidly growing. Highly malignant,
Meningiomas	Arachnoidal cells (arachnoidal villi).	Predilection for sites near the venous sinuses. Most common sites are convexity of cerebral hemispheres, parasagittal region, sphenoidal ridge, anterior fossa (olfactory groove or sella turcica), posterior fossa (rare).	Extracerebral. Benign (not invasive into brain parenchyma). Slow growing. Often invade cranial bones.

Acoustic neuroma (schwannoma, neurofibroma)	Sheath of 8th nerve (Schwann's cells).	Vestibular division of 8th cranial nerve. Smaller tumors are located within auditory canal. Larger tumors may extend to posterior fossa and lie in angle between cerebellum and pons (cerebellopontine angle).	Grows slowly. Compresses 5th (trigiminal) and 7th (facial) nerves, as well as cerebellum and brainstem. Obstructs CSF flow.
Pituitary adenoma	Arise from cells of anterior pituitary. Three types of cells (see below).	Anterior lobe of pituitary (adenohypophysis).	Benign. Rare in childhood and adolescence. Each type of adenoma produces endocrine dysfunction or visual problems.
Chromophobic adenoma	Chromophobe cells.		Most common type of pituitary adenoma. Compresses pituitary (hypoituitarism), optic chiasm (bitemporal hemianopsia), and hypothalamus (diabetes insipidus).
Eosinophilic adenoma	Eosinophil cells.		Causes hyperpituitarism (giantism or acromegaly). Compresses optic chiasm, causing bitemporal hemianopsia.
Basophilic adenoma	Basophil cells.		Small tumor. One of the causes of Cushing's syndrome. Confined to sella turcica.

ovary, pancreas, prostate, etc. Metastases are multiple. Secondary brain tumors are most common in the cerebral hemispheres and cerebellum. They may invade the skull. The onset of neurologic deficits is rapid. It is estimated that 11,000 people die from primary tumors each year; 22% from intracranial metastasis. Although these tumors affect all age groups, the majority occur in adult life, most often in the fifth decade. In childhood, the peak age is between 5 and 10 yr. Both sexes are equally affected, but there is a sex preference in some types (glioblastoma is common in men; meningioma and acoustic neuroma, in women). There is no known cause of brain tumors, but they may be congenital or hereditary (rare). Other theories suggest trauma (head injuries), infection, metabolic diseases, carcinogens, and exposure to radiation as the causative agents.

Progressive enlargement of the neoplasm causes elevated ICP, swelling of tissue (vasogenic edema), and displacement of brain tissue, leading to uncal herniation. Infiltration or destruction of neurologic structures occurs.

Symptoms are variable, depending on the nature, size, and location of the lesion. Generalized symptoms are related to the effects of increased ICP and focal signs to localized destruction or compression of brain tissue. Generalized symptoms include headache, vomiting, papilledema, seizures, alterations in vital signs, and altered cerebral functioning (lethargy, confusion, and personality changes). Focal or localizing signs include hemiparesis or hemiplegia, visual field defects, aphasia, ataxia, hearing loss, and seizures (Jacksonian). Respiratory *complications* include respiratory failure and respiratory infection. Postoperative complications may involve shock, increased ICP, cerebral edema, neurologic deficits (speech disturbances, motor deficits, sensory deficits, visual disturbances, personality changes), seizures, hyperthermia, wound infection, periocular edema, thrombophlebitis, diabetes insipidus, and urinary disturbances (incontinence, retention). In addition, there may be complications related to radiation therapy (cerebral herniation with the first dose of radiation, nausea, vomiting, alopecia) and/or bone marrow suppression (related to chemotherapy).

Diagnosis is based on the health history, physical exam, CAT scan, skull x-rays, lumbar puncture (contraindicated in marked ICP), EEG, and cerebral angiography.

Common interventions

Medical treatment consists of radiation therapy and drug therapy with steroids, osmotic agents (acute treatment of uncal herniation), anticonvulsants, analgesics, and chemotherapy (for metastatic brain tumor) with nitrosoureas (carmustine [BCNU], lomustine [CCNU], semustine [Methyl-CCNU]), vincristine sulfate (Oncovin), methotrexate (Amethopterin), and procarbazine (Benzamide). **Surgical** treatment may involve complete or partial removal of the tumor or biopsy. For malignant tumors, surgery, radiation, and chemotherapy may be used in combination or separately.

Nursing interventions

General physical priorities are the neurologic, respiratory, and cardiovascular status. (*See* Overview and Chapter 8.)

Physical 1. Establish base-line data.
2. Assess and report signs of increased ICP and localizing signs.
3. Administer medications as ordered and observe for side effects (especially tapering doses of steroids).
4. Elevate the patient's head 30 degrees to promote venous drainage.
5. Monitor the blood count if the patient is on chemotherapy and radiation therapy.
6. Assess for nausea and vomiting. Administer antiemetic medications as ordered.
7. Monitor IV fluids closely if the patient is on fluid restriction.
8. Provide range-of-motion exercises if the patient has hemiplegia.
9. Assist with ambulation if the patient has problems with balance and coordination as well as visual disturbances.
10. Plan rest periods if the patient is experiencing extreme fatigue.
11. Encourage the patient to participate in activities of daily living.
12. Monitor urine output closely if the patient is on osmotic agents.
13 Advise the patient not to strain when defecating to prevent increased ICP.
14. Position the patient as ordered postoperatively to prevent pressure on the operative site.
Psychosocial 15. Provide an alternative means of communication if the patient is aphasic.
16. Reassure patients undergoing radiation therapy that loss of hair is temporary. Provide a wig, if they so desire, to maintain their body image.
17. Provide emotional support to the family if the disease is terminal.
Prevention 18. For prevention and early detection, report symptoms early so that diagnostic tests can be done and treatment initiated immediately, and avoid exposure to radiation.

Evaluation criteria. See Overview. No headaches or other signs of increased ICP. Blood count normal, no seizures. No nausea or vomiting. Alternative means of communication provided (if aphasic).

TRANSIENT ISCHEMIC ATTACKS

Transient ischemic attacks (TIAs ["little strokes"]) are temporary episodes of focal neurologic dysfunction due to cerebral ischemia. The risk of TIAs is higher in the older age group, with men affected twice as often as women. Prevalence is high in people with hypertension, diabetes, and cardiovascular diseases. It is estimated that 35 to 60% of patients with a TIA will have a completed stroke within a 5-yr period.

It is suggested that impairment of arterial supply to a specific area of the brain is caused by microembolism from an ulcerated plaque (carotid bifurcation or vertebral basilar arteries), emboli from the heart (e.g., patients with prosthetic heart valves, bacterial endocarditis), stenosis of extracranial or intracranial arteries, transient systemic hypotension, which may compromise intracranial circulation (e.g., acute MI, blood loss, use of certain medications), and cerebral vasospasm (result of hypertension and acute migraine attacks). Precipitating factors include diseases that increase blood viscosity (polycythemia, thrombocytopenia), cardiac arrhythmias, hypoglycemia, and anemia.

The process of a TIA involves ulceration of an atheroma, aggregation of platelets, formation of a thrombus, subsequent occlusion of an artery, or embolization of fibrin platelets. Characteristic *symptoms* include focal dysfunction, which may last a few seconds to minutes and occasionally as long as 24 hr. There is an absence of neurologic deficits after episodes. The most common sites of stenosis and occlusion are the origin of the internal carotid artery, common carotid artery, and basilar vertebral arteries. Symptoms that are focal rather than generalized vary depending on the major arteries involved. Symptoms of internal carotid artery involvement include transient blindness or blurring of vision, contralateral weakness or numbness, headache (supraorbital or temporal), confusion, and aphasia. Symptoms of vertebral basilar artery involvement include vertigo (may be related to changes in head and neck positions), unilateral or bilateral numbness or weakness, diplopia, homonymous hemianopsia, dysarthria, dysphagia, occipital headache, nausea and vomiting, and transient alteration of consciousness (rare). Other symptoms may include bruits (carotid bifurcation), diminished or absent arterial pulsations, unequal BP between the two arms, and emboli of fibrin platelets or cholesterol in the retinal artery (fundoscopic examination). *Complications* include completed stroke, intracranial hemorrhage (related to anticoagulation therapy), and neurologic deficits (related to angiography).

Diagnosis is based on the health history, physical exam, blood studies (blood sugar, cholesterol, lipid profile, prothrombin time, activated partial thromboplastin time), angiography, ECG, Holter monitoring, CAT scan, lumbar puncture, and (in special cases) ophthalmodynamometry (measurement of retinal artery pressure) and Doppler ultrasonography (measurement of blood flow in the supraorbital region).

Common interventions

Medical treatment consists of drug therapy with anticoagulants (heparin, warfarin sodium [Coumadin]) and antiplatelet drugs (aspirin, dipyrimadole [Persantine]). **Surgical** treatment may involve an endarterectomy (recommended for patients with extracranial stenosis and ulcerated plaques in carotid artery), which is the excision of atheromatous plaque in the innermost lining of an artery. A bypass operation (anastomosis of the external carotid with branches of the middle cerebral artery) may also be performed.

Nursing interventions

Physical priorities are the neurologic, cardiovascular, and musculoskeletal status. (*See* Overview).

Physical 1. Assess the cranial nerves: 3rd (oculomotor), 4th (trochlear), 6th (abducens), 7th (facial), 9th (glossopharyngeal), 10th (vagus), and 12th (hypoglossal).

2. Assess for bruits.

3. Check BP in both arms.

4. Assess for any signs of bleeding in stool, urine, skin, and mucous membrane.

5. Encourage bed rest during the first few days of the attacks.

Psychosocial 6. Explain to the patient and family the nature of the attacks.

Educational 7. Instruct the patient to consult the physician if symptoms last >24 hr.

Prevention 8. Teach the importance of early recognition and treatment of TIA.

9. Teach ways of preventing atherosclerotic disease and injury when such attacks occur.

Evaluation criteria. See Overview. Absence of focal signs. Arterial BP maintained at a normotensive level in both arms; no signs of bleeding in skin, stool, urine, or mucous membrane; absence of bruits. Absence of hemiparesis, no injuries sustained as a consequence of the attacks.

CEREBROVASCULAR ACCIDENT

Cerebrovascular accident (CVA [stroke, apoplexy]) is a sudden onset of neurologic deficits resulting from insufficient blood flow to an area of the brain. There are three major types of CVA. **Thrombotic** CVA is occlusion of a cerebral artery by a clot or thrombus that forms inside an artery, usually secondary to atherosclerosis. **Embolic** CVA is occlusion of a cerebral artery by a fragment of clotted blood, air, fat, or tumor, originating elsewhere in the body (often the heart). **Hemorrhagic** CVA is rupture of an artery as a result of weakness of the wall of the artery, causing bleeding into the brain tissue or surrounding spaces.

Stroke is the third leading cause of death in the USA, with 400,000 people stricken every year. Two-thirds of those who survive have some kind of disability. Acute strokes occur 44% more frequently in males than in females. Strokes are caused by vascular occlusion (thrombosis, embolism) and cerebral hemorrhage. Precipitating factors (risk factors) include prior stroke, hypertension, heart disease (coronary artery disease, MI, arrhythmias, CHF, prosthetic heart valves, bacterial endocarditis), and diabetes mellitus (accelerates progression of arteriosclerosis). Other risk factors are smoking, age, obesity, family history of stroke, oral contraceptive agents, high-cholesterol diet, and stress.

During **cerebral ischemia**, blood supply to the brain is interrupted, tissue hypoxia develops and brain metabolism is altered, infarction or necrosis occurs if tissue hypoxia is prolonged, and widespread destruction of nerve cells and fibers (in a large area of infarction) occurs. Edema follows as a result of changes in vascular and membrane permeability, and may cause increased ICP. During **cerebral hemorrhage** blood leaks directly into the brain tissue, ventricles, or subarachnoid space. Clotted blood displaces a part of the brain tissue or may compress surrounding tissue. If massive hemorrhage occurs, midline structures are displaced, leading to herniation, coma, and death. Later, the clot is absorbed slowly over a period of weeks or months, and replaced by a scar or a cavity filled with yellow serous fluid.

The neurologic deficits depend on the location and the site of the infarct or hemorrhage. In thrombotic strokes, TIAs (warning signs) may precede the onset of severe paralysis by a few hours or days, occurring during sleep or on arising in the morning. In embolic strokes, the onset is sudden (usually no warning signs) and not related to activity. In hemorrhagic strokes, the onset is sudden, occurs during waking hours, is associated with activity or exertion, and the patient may have severe headaches and nausea and vomiting. Other premonitory symptoms include dizziness, drowsiness, and confusion. *Symptoms* may be characterized as generalized or focal. Generalized symptoms (more common in cerebral hemorrhage) include headache, vomiting, seizures, loss of consciousness, nuchal rigidity, fever, increased BP, alterations in respiratory pattern, bradycardia, and urinary and fecal incontinence. Focal neurologic deficits (related to the area of infarct or hemorrhage) include motor deficits (hemiparesis or hemiplegia), sensory deficits, visual disturbances (homonymous hemianopsia, diplopia), and disorders of higher cortical function: language impairment (aphasia), visual-spatial perception and constructional abilities, attention and consciousness, intelligence, memory, emotional behavior, and personality. *Complications* may include atelectasis, aspiration pneumonia, risk of a second stroke (with thrombotic stroke), and intellectual deterioration. Secondary complications related to motor deficits are contractures, shoulder subluxation, and decubitus ulcers.

Diagnosis is based on the health history, physical exam, cerebral angiography, CAT scan, ECG, lumbar puncture, and blood tests for fasting blood sugar, cholesterol, triglyceride profile, and coagulation profile.

Common interventions

Medical treatment consists of drug therapy with anticoagulants for non-hemorrhagic strokes in acute phase (low-dose heparin therapy, warfarin), antiplatelet aggregation drugs (aspirin, dipyrimadole), antiedema drugs (steroids, dehydrating agents), vasodilators (controversial), and antihypertensive medications (indicated for hemorrhagic stroke). An extensive rehabilitation program of physiotherapy and speech and occupational therapy may also be instituted. **Surgical** treatment consists of evacuation of a hematoma or the procedures used for TIA (*see above*).

Nursing interventions

Physical priorities in the acute phase include the respiratory, neurologic, and cardiovascular status. (*See* Overview and Chapters 14 and 15.)

Physical 1. Suction the patient as necessary.
  2. Monitor and record BP and pulse rate. Obtain BP on the unaffected side, if the patient has hemiplegia.
  3. Monitor for signs of cardiac complications, such as arrhythmias.
  4. Administer anticoagulants as ordered and observe for side effects. (Be aware that drug interactions can occur with anticoagulation therapy. Monitor activated partial thromboplastin time and prothrombin time.)
  5. Monitor fluid intake, especially if the patient is receiving a high-protein feeding.
  6. Teach the patient to place food on the unaffected side if facial paralysis is present.
  7. Encourage the patient to feed himself, but supervise closely to prevent choking.
  8. Weigh the patient weekly or as appropriate.
  9. Turn the patient q 2 hr to his unaffected side.
  10. Provide passive range-of-joint motion to all extremities. (Educate the patient or family members to perform some of the exercises.)
  11. Prevent shoulder subluxation by using a sling when the patient is walking or transferring only (should not be used all day since elbow and shoulder contractures may develop), and by supporting the patient's arms on pillows when he is sitting in a chair.
  12. Prevent hip contracture by supporting the patient's hips with a trochanter roll from his iliac crest to midthigh, and by aligning his legs with his body and in full extension.
  13. Prevent wrist contractures by using a rolled cloth alternately with a splint to maintain the patient's hand in a functional position, and by extending his wrist and positioning his fingers flat.
  14. Prevent leg contracture by supporting the patient's leg with a trochanter roll or pillow to prevent outward rotation.
  15. Prevent foot drop and heel pressure by using supportive devices such as a footboard, cradle, and pillow.
  16. Prevent injury if there is impaired sensation.
  17. During the long-term phase, correct deformities that have occurred and retrain the patient to achieve maximum independence. (Rehabili-

tation after a stroke requires a multidisciplinary approach. Specific needs in the long-term phase relate to perceptual disorders, language impairment, potential emotional problems, and impairment of mental functioning.)

18. Refer the patient to a speech therapist for any language problems.

Psychosocial 19. Explain to the patient and family about the stroke syndrome.

20. Explain to the family the anticipated changes in the patient's behavior and emotions.

21. Allay the patient's anxiety if he is unable to communicate by using other means of communication.

22. Encourage independence and allow the patient to take on responsibilities for self-care activities.

23. Encourage the patient to join a stroke club in the community.

Educational 24. Teach the family how to provide appropriate nursing care to prevent the complications of immobility.

25. Teach the family how to provide range-of-motion exercises and how to use any necessary assistive devices.

Prevention 26. Take appropriate measures to reduce factors that contribute to the risk (*see above*).

Evaluation criteria. *See* Overview. No evidence of bleeding related to anticoagulation therapy; verbalization of side effects of antihypertensive medications. Balance regained, demonstration of standing and transferring techniques, demonstration of active exercises. No marked weight loss.

SUBARACHNOID HEMORRHAGE

A subarachnoid hemorrhage (SAH) is a clinical syndrome that occurs as a result of blood leaking into the subarachnoid space, primarily from a ruptured aneurysm, and is characterized by acute onset of neurologic deficit. Approximately 26,000 persons suffer an SAH annually in the USA and Canada. SAH (from ruptured aneurysms) occurs mostly in previously healthy, young, and middle-aged adults. It is rare in childhood. Approximately 50% of all fatal CVAs in patients <45 yr are caused by ruptured aneurysms. The majority (~60%) of those affected are women.

SAH may be caused by rupture of an intracranial aneurysm (most common cause), intracerebral hemorrhage, intracranial trauma, arteriovenous malformation, primary (glioblastoma) and metastatic tumors of the brain (metastatic cancer from lung and breast), blood dyscrasias and bleeding disorders (sickle cell anemia, leukemias, hemophilia, and iatrogenic anticoagulation with warfarin compounds), and septic emboli (mycotic aneurysm). Precipitating factors include hypertension, polycystic kidney disease, coarctation of the aorta, vigorous exercise (although SAH can occur at rest or when a person is involved in light activity), and emotional stress.

The mechanism of SAH involves dilation of an artery (aneurysm) resulting from a congenital defect in the internal elastic lamina of the vessel wall and degenerative changes of the vessel wall. These congenital (berry or saccular) aneurysms are located at the bifurcations of cerebral arteries. Approximately 85% arise from the anterior portion of the circle of Willis. The most common sites are the junction of the anterior communicating artery and the anterior cerebral artery, the junction of the internal carotid artery and the posterior communicating artery, and the middle cerebral artery. Enlargement may occur gradually over a period of time (believed to be precipitated by hypertension and other hemodynamic forces), and may cause symptoms by compressing cerebral tissue and cranial nerves, or by rupturing and bleeding into the subarachnoid space, resulting in sudden onset of neurologic deficits.

Prior to rupture, most patients are asymptomatic. Some patients, however, may experience prodromal *symptoms* such as pain above the eye and a generalized, mild headache as a result of a small leak from the aneurysm. After rupture occurs, the onset of symptoms is rapid. There is sudden onset of severe headache and alteration in LOC (from mild confusion, disorientation, and drowsiness, to coma). Signs of meningeal irritation include nuchal rigidity, Kernig's sign (resistance to attempts to fully extend the leg when the hip is flexed), Brudzinski's sign (flexion of the knee and hip when the neck is flexed), and photophobia. Other symptoms include generalized seizures, autonomic disturbances (fever, nausea and vomiting, chills, tachycardia), retinal changes (subhyaloid retinal hemorrhages, papilledema), and focal neurologic signs (depend on the site of lesion), including hemiparesis, aphasia, and the following visual disturbances: 3rd (oculomotor) nerve palsy (ptosis, diplopia, dilation of pupil), homonymous hemianopsia (compression of optic nerve), and 6th (abducens) nerve palsy (affected eye turns medially). The patients are usually graded according to the severity of symptoms, with lower grades indicating a more favorable outcome (Table 20-16). *Complications* include recurrent bleeding (common between the 7th and 10th day after initial bleeding); vasospasm (narrowing of an artery), possibly resulting in cerebral ischemia; hydrocephalus (ventricular dilation due to blockage of CSF pathways by blood); subdural hematoma; and cerebral edema. Other complications include respiratory distress, pneumonia, atelectasis, thrombophlebitis, GI bleeding, and neurologic deficits (motor, speech, or visual disturbances).

Diagnosis is based on the health history, physical exam, lumbar puncture (CSF is grossly bloody and xanthochromic, elevated pressure and protein content), cerebral angiography, EEG (diffusely abnormal after rupture), CAT scan, and skull x-rays (evidence of pineal shift as a result of hematoma).

Common interventions

Medical treatment consists of respiratory support to prevent hypoxic cerebral damage, complete or strict bed rest (4 to 6 wk if surgery is not indicated), and "aneurysm precautions" (to reduce unnecessary stimuli to a minimum). For aneurysm precautions, the patient is placed in a single room, darkened, without telephone, radio, or television; there is strict limitation of

TABLE 20-16
Description of Clinical States Used to Grade Patients with Subarachnoid Hemorrhage

Grade I	Grade II	Grade III	Grade IV	Grade V
Alert	Alert	Drowsiness or confusion	Stupor	Deep coma
Minimal headache	Mild to severe headache	Nuchal rigidity	Nuchal rigidity	Decerebrate rigidity
Slight nuchal rigidity	Nuchal rigidity	Mild focal deficit	Mild to severe hemiparesis	
No neurologic deficit	Minimal neurologic deficit (third nerve palsy)		Possible decerebrate rigidity	

visitors and restriction of all mild stimulants (including coffee, tea, and tobacco); and a stool softener is used to prevent straining during a bowel movement (which may cause increased ICP). A sign should be placed on the patient's door to alert personnel that aneurysm precautions are in effect and to prevent unnecessary entry. Medical treatment may also involve fluid restriction and drug therapy with sedatives (to sedate lightly, lower BP, and control seizures), anticonvulsants, corticosteroids, antihypertensive agents, antifibrinolytic agents, and antipyretics. **Surgical** treatment may involve a craniotomy and clipping of an aneurysm (7 to 14 days after the initial bleeding); wrapping of an aneurysmal sac in a fine-mesh gauze, muscle, fascia, or plastic coating; ligation of the carotid artery; or surgical evacuation of the hematoma.

Nursing interventions

Physical priorities are the respiratory, neurologic, and cardiovascular status. (*See* Overview and Chapters 9, 11, and 14.)

Physical 1. Institute aneurysm precautions.
2. Elevate the head of the bed 30 degrees to promote venous drainage.
3. Administer sedatives as ordered to keep the patient quiet.
4. Monitor the patient's temperature. (Obtain axillary temperature.)
5. Observe the patient frequently for the development of new headaches or neurologic deficits in order to detect rebleeding or other complications.
6. Administer antihypertensive medications and antifibrinolytic agents as ordererd. (Observe for side effects.)
7. Restrict fluid intake as ordered (usually 1,500 to 1,800 ml).
8. Keep a strict recording of patient intake. (Overhydration can raise ICP.)
9. Ensure complete bed rest (may be modified depending on the patient's condition).
10. Anticipate the patient's needs and assist him with activities of daily living. (The patient may have impaired communication.)
11. Remind the patient to avoid excessive physical strain.
12. Offer the patient a bedpan or urinal. If the patient is extremely agitated, consult the physician regarding the use of a bedside commode. (Caution the patient to avoid straining while defecating.)
Psychosocial 13. Allay the patient's anxiety by explaining the importance of aneurysm precautions.
14. Enlist the family's cooperation in maintaining a quiet environment.
15. Minimize situations that may precipitate emotional stress.
Educational 16. Instruct the patient regarding the need to continue physical therapy if neurologic deficits are evident.
17. Teach the patient ways to avoid sneezing and coughing.
Prevention 18. Promote early recognition and treatment.

19. Identify patients with unruptured aneurysms.
20. Advise the patient to avoid strenuous physical activity and emotional stress.

Evaluation criteria. *See* Overview. Absence of headache, aneurysm precautions maintained, absence of restlessness or agitation. No evidence of rebleeding. Bed rest maintained, patient quiet and resting comfortably, no coughing or sneezing. Bedpan, urinal, commode used as directed; no straining. Verbalization of importance of minimizing unnecessary stimuli, family visiting one at a time, verbalization of the importance of avoiding strenuous activity once discharged.

CONVULSIVE DISORDERS

Convulsive disorders (epilepsy, seizure disorders) are paroxysmal disorders of the nervous system possibly due to excessive and abnormal discharge of cerebral neurons, which produce a sudden disturbance of brain functioning such as alterations in consciousness, motor, sensory, and autonomic functioning, as well as in behavior. The term **epilepsy** implies chronicity and recurrence of seizures; it is a symptom of brain dysfunction. Seizures are classified as generalized or partial. **Generalized seizures,** which arise from deep midline structures in the brainstem or the thalamus, include tonic-clonic seizures (grand mal), absence seizures (petit mal), myoclonic seizures, and akinetic seizures. **Partial (focal) seizures,** which arise from a specific cerebral area, include simple seizures (motor symptoms [Jacksonian] and sensory symptoms [somatic sensory]) and complex seizures (complex partial seizures [psychomotor or temporal lobe seizures]). In the USA, the prevalence rate is 2% of the population. Seizure disorders occur at any age, with the highest incidence occurring in the age group <5 yr (usually associated with acute febrile illness). Approximately 90% of all epileptic patients experience their initial seizure before the age of 20 yr.

Idiopathic (primary) epilepsy has no known cause. Symptomatic (secondary) epilepsy may be caused by structural (e.g., brain tumor, abscess, infarct, posttraumatic scars) or biochemical (e.g., electrolyte imbalance, drug overdose) problems. There is a genetic predisposition to epilepsy. Precipitating factors include alcohol, loss of sleep, flickering light, physical and emotional stress, electric shock, excessive fatigue, menstruation, excessive hydration, abrupt withdrawal of anticonvulsant medications, and hyperventilation.

The exact cellular mechanism that initiates epilepsy is not known. Small groups of injured, hyperexcitable neurons arising in any part of the cerebrum or cortical, subcortical, and brainstem centers (epileptogenic focus) initiate the seizure activity. It is postulated that local biochemical changes or abnormal synaptic input causes high-frequency discharges. The resulting discharge spreads itself to normal neurons in adjacent areas of the brain via neural pathways. If the epileptic focus is deep within the reticular activating system, the ensuing extensive discharge will spread within the subcortical structures and be transmitted symmetrically to the cerebral hemispheres. A generalized centrencephalic seizure results, characterized by a sudden loss of consciousness, tonic-clonic convulsion, signs of ANS hyperactivity (tachycardia, increased BP, salivation, pupillary dilation, etc.), temporary cessation of vital functions, or death due to respiratory arrest, cardiac abnormalities, or some unknown cause (rare instances). Focal seizures spread transcortically or via subcortical pathways (limbic system).

There is a discontinuity of *symptoms* in epilepsy, with varying intervals between attacks (minutes, hours, days, months, or years). The wide variety of clinical presentations, duration, and symptoms are presented in Table 20-17. *Complications* of convulsive disorders include status epilepticus (generalized seizures occur without recovery between attacks; a medical emergency caused frequently by abrupt withdrawal of anticonvulsant drugs), and brain damage (related to hypoxia or repeated falls). Other complications include severe craniofacial injury (related to akinetic seizures), compression or fracture of the spine (related to violent muscular movement), fractures of the skull or limbs, burns, airway obstruction, and aspiration.

The health history plays an important function in the *diagnosis* of epilepsy. The patient should be asked about precipitating factors, aura, ictal and postictal experiences, and frequency. The observer should check for aura, pattern, duration, and postictal experience. The diagnosis is further facilitated by the physical exam, urinalysis, EEG, CAT scan, skull x-rays, lumbar puncture, cerebral angiography, and blood studies of the patient's CBC, fasting blood sugar, electrolytes, BUN, and serum drug levels.

Common interventions

Medical management of status epilepticus involves establishing an adequate airway (oral airway, endotracheal intubation, O_2 therapy, assisted ventilation); providing appropriate therapy for the metabolic cause (e.g., glucose for hypoglycemia, calcium for hypocalcemia); and administering IV diazepam (Valium) (drug of choice if no specific cause), anticonvulsants (maintenance dose), and/or general anesthesia if necessary. Anticonvulsant drug therapy includes phenobarbital (Luminal), phenytoin (Dilantin), primidone (Mysoline), and carbamazepine (Tegrotol) for focal and grand mal seizures; ethosuximide (Zarontin), trimethadione (Tridione), and valproic acid (Depakene) for absence (petit mal) seizures; and diazepam (Valium) and clonazepam (Clonopin) for myoclonic seizures. **Surgical** treatment may involve removal of structural epileptogenic lesions (neoplasms, brain abscess, cortical scars, arteriovenous malformation, the anterior portion of the temporal lobe [temporal lobe epilepsy], or damaged cerebral hemispheres [hemispherectomy] for intractable seizures). Other surgical procedures (still experimental) include callosal commisurotomy, stereotactic ablation of selected diencephalic areas, and cerebellar stimulation.

TABLE 20-17

Types of Seizures: Onset, Duration, and Characteristics of Ictal and Postictal Phases

Type	Age of onset	Duration	Ictal phase	Postictal phase
Generalized Tonic-clonic seizures (grand mal)	Childhood and adult life.	2-5 min.	May or may not be preceded by an aura. Sudden loss of consciousness.	Unconsciousness for a variable period of time. Confusion and disorientation on awakening. Headache. Stiffness and soreness. No recollection of attack.
		Tonic phase; 10-15 sec.	Tonic contraction of muscles: moan or cry (spasm of vocal cord), apnea, cyanosis, tongue biting, pupils dilated, incontinence.	
		Clonic phase; 1-2 min.	Gradual transition phase: mild generalized trembling, rhythmic violent muscular contraction, eyes roll, excessive salivation with bloody froth in mouth, rapid pulse and profuse sweating, deep inspiration (end of clonic phase). Terminal phase: All muscles are relaxed. Breathing quiet. Pupils react to light.	

Absence seizures (petit mal)	Between 4-12 yr.	5-20 sec.	Sudden onset; no aura. Interruption of ongoing activities. Lapse of consciousness ("absences"). Blank stare accompanied by blinking of eyelids. Ends rapidly with resumption of normal activity. Hyperventilation may precipitate attack. ≥50 episodes/day.	None.
Myoclonic seizures	Childhood, middle and late adult years.	Intermittently every few sec.	Sudden, brief muscular contraction that may be generalized or confined to face or trunk, one or more extremities, individual or groups of muscles. Repetitive or single; around the hours of sleep or on awakening.	None.
Akinetic seizures	Between 2-5 yr.	Sec.	Brief loss of postural muscle tone ("drop attacks"). Patient falls to the floor. Occur many times a day.	None.

Type	Age of onset	Duration	Ictal phase	Postictal phase
Partial (focal) seizures				
Simple: motor	Any age.	Sec to min.	Occur without loss of consciousness. Originate in motor cortex. Begin with a tonic contraction of contralateral thumb and then spread to the hand, arm, face, and foot (Jacksonian march). Electrical discharges may spread to deep structures, resulting in loss of consciousness and generalized convulsive movement. Head and eyes may turn to side opposite irritative focus (adversive seizure).	Paralysis of an extremity (Todd's paralysis). May last from min to hr. Aphasia (transitory).
Simple: sensory	Any age.	Sec to min.	Originate from foci in the post central gyrus. Described as "pins and needles," numbness, or burning sensation. In most cases, the onset is in the lip, fingers, and toes. May also spread (like motor seizures) to become generalized tonic-clonic seizures. Special sensory symptoms include visual, auditory, olfactory, gustatory, and vertiginous sensations.	None.

| Complex partial seizures (psycho-motor or temporal lobe) | Children or adults, | 1-2 min. | Aura (alterations in psychic functions). Hallucinations (visual, auditory, olfactory, and gustatory). Perceptual illusions. Cognitive disturbances (feeling of increased familiarity with environment: déjà vu phenomenon). Visceral sensations. Affective symptoms (fear and anxiety). Behavioral automatisms include lip smacking, chewing, swallowing, inappropriate acts, habitual acts (driving a car, etc.), and violence and aggression. | Confusion and amnesia. |

Nursing interventions

Physical priorities include the respiratory, neurologic, and cardio-vascular status. (*See* Overview and Chapter 14.)

Physical 1. For status epilepticus, establish a patent airway and adequate oxygenation (suction as necessary, oral airway, endotracheal intubation, O_2 as ordered, or assisted ventilation).

   2. Observe and record seizure activity.

   3. Protect the patient from injury by maintaining seizure precautions.

   4. Assist with the administration of drugs to maintain a seizure-free status.

   5. Have all anticonvulsants available and ready for use.

   6. Monitor the effects of anticonvulsant therapy once treatment begins.

   7. Monitor for signs of cardiovascular collapse (especially during IV administration of anticonvulsant medications).

   8. Observe and regulate the IV flow rate of prescribed medications.

   9. Prepare equipment to give cardiorespiratory assistance if necessary.

   10. For general care, maintain a patent airway and adequate oxygenation by loosening all the patient's tight clothing, turning him to his side, and suctioning him to prevent aspiration.

   11. Observe the patient during the ictal phase. Note and record aura or warning sign, LOC, motor activity (parts of the body involved, type of movement, progression from one part of the body to other parts), incontinence of urine and feces, and duration.

   12. Observe the patient during the postictal phase. Note and record behavioral changes (confusion, disorientation, amnesia), weakness or paralysis of an extremity, speech (garbled speech or transient aphasia), injury, and vital signs (avoid taking temperature orally).

   13. Protect the patient from injury during the seizure by remaining with him, providing for privacy, protecting his head if he is not in bed, avoiding the use of restraints, not inserting a padded tongue blade between his teeth if they are tightly clenched, and using padded siderails.

   14. Administer anticonvulsant drugs as ordered and monitor serum anticonvulsant drug levels; signs of acute drug toxicity (CNS toxicity, GI disturbances, and allergic manifestations); signs of chronic drug toxicity (CNS toxicity, allergic manifestations, gingival hyperplasia, endocrine disturbances, hematologic and immunologic effects, renal toxicity, and hepatic dysfunction); and adverse drug reactions, which may occur when two or more anticonvulsants are administered concurrently or between anticonvulsants and drugs administered for other conditions.

   15. Administer phenytoin (Dilantin) with meals to prevent gastric distress.

   16. Caution the patient about alcohol consumption.

17. Provide good oral hygiene and teach the patient to massage his gums daily to minimize gingival hyperplasia.
18. Assess for constipation (common problem).
Psychosocial 19. Encourage the patient to seek psychotherapy to help overcome feelings of inferiority complex and self-consciousness.
20. Advise the family members not to be over solicitous and over-protective.
21. Provide support by encouraging the patient to participate in recreational activities as well as contact sports (if not contraindicated).
22. Encourage parents to keep children in school as long as the seizure is well controlled.
23. Encourage the patient to seek the services of the Epilepsy Foundation or other special agencies in the community.
Educational 24. Teach the patient about compliance with the prescribed drug regimen and the complications that may occur with noncompliance, the importance of frequent measurements of serum drug levels and other blood studies, reporting toxic effects of anticonvulsant drugs, possible drug interactions, and maintaining a regular activity of sleep and recreation.
25. Teach the patient and family what to do if a seizure occurs.
26. Remind the patient to keep all scheduled appointments with the physician or seizure clinic during drug adjustments.
27. Advise the patient with regard to long-term follow-up care for repeat EEG and neurologic examination.
28. Educate members of the family as well as the public about their attitude toward the patient with epilepsy.
Prevention 29. Ensure that the proper diagnosis is made through screening programs and that the appropriate intervention is taken.
30. Eliminate any aggravating or precipitating factors.
31. Educate the public with regard to preventing causative factors such as lead poisoning, infections, and head injuries.
32. Advise the patient to avoid activities such as high climbing, horseback riding, diving, and swimming without supervision.
33. Prevent seizures by use of anticonvulsants.
34. Advise the patient to wear a medical alert bracelet.
35. Advise the patient to wear a helmet to prevent injury from repeated falls.

Evaluation criteria. *See* Overview. Plasma concentration of anticonvulsant drugs within therapeutic range, no injuries sustained during seizures. No cardiac abnormalities related to drug therapy. No gastric distress related to drug therapy, no excessive consumption of alcohol. Absence of rash, gingival hyperplasia prevented or minimized, no bruises. No constipation. Normal life maintained (e.g., working, sports, etc.) demonstration of coping mechanisms.

MULTIPLE SCLEROSIS

Multiple sclerosis (MS [disseminated sclerosis]) is a chronic degenerative disease characterized by demyelination of multifocal areas of the CNS. The usual onset is between 20 and 40 yr of age (late 50s and 60s in some people). More women are affected than men. MS is more prevalent in temperate climates, particularly in the northern latitudes (northern Europe, Canada, and northern USA), and rare in the tropics. There is a familial tendency (may be related to exposure to a common environmental agent), and the average duration is >25 yr.

The exact cause of MS is not known. The two major theories that are being pursued suggest viral infections and alterations in the immune system as causative factors. Predisposing factors include trauma, pregnancy, infection, and emotional stress.

Initially, inflammation and destruction of myelin sheaths (demyelination) occur during MS. These areas of demyelination are scattered irregularly in white matter of the brain and spinal cord (especially the brainstem, cerebrum, cerebellum, optic nerves, and chiasm). Peripheral nerves are not affected. Later, proliferation of microglial cells leads to the formation of sclerotic plaque or scar to replace damaged myelin. Transmission of nerve impulses is then blocked or reduced.

Signs and symptoms vary, depending on the area involved. They may be transient, and they tend toward remissions and exacerbations. During the early stage, symptoms include weakness in one or more extremity, paresthesias (numbness and tingling sensations), visual disturbances (nystagmus, diplopia, partial or total loss of vision in one eye [optic neuritis], blurred vision), bladder dysfunction (frequency and urgency), vertigo, vomiting, facial paralysis (with brainstem involvement), ataxic gait, intention tremor of the arms and legs, and emotional lability: euphoria (probably due to frontal lobe lesions) or depression and irritability (response to the disabling features of MS). During the advanced stage, symptoms include dysarthria (scanning speech), spasticity and hyperreflexia, paraplegia, dysphagia, and bladder incontinence and retention. Other symptoms include seizures, muscle spasms, low back pain, and burning sensation in lower extremities. *Complications* include aspiration pneumonia, urinary tract infection, and constipation.

Diagnosis is based on the health history, physical exam, CSF exam (gamma globulin [increased], mild pleocytosis [increased lymphocytes]), evoked visual response, CAT scan, and myelography.

Common interventions

There is no specific treatment for MS but intervention generally consists of supportive measures via physical therapy, psychotherapy, and respiratory support (during periods of exacerbation). Drug therapy may consist of the administration of ACTH or steroids (to inhibit inflammatory response), muscle relaxants (to relieve flexor spasms), anticholinergics (to reduce urinary frequency and urgency), urinary tract antiseptics and antibiotics (for urinary tract infection), and anticonvulsants.

Nursing interventions

Physical priorities include the neurologic, respiratory, and musculo-skeletal status. (*See* Overview.)

Physical 1. Assess visual acuity, diplopia, and sensory loss.
    2. Instruct the patient to wear an eye patch if diplopia is present.
    3. Protect the patient from injury if a seizure occurs.
    4. Administer steroids and anticonvulsants as ordered and monitor for side effects.
    5. Protect the patient from exposure to respiratory tract infection.
    6. Provide respiratory support during the late stage of the disease.
    7. Assess changes of motor status.
    8. Refer the patient to a physiatrist or physical therapist for appropriate rehabilitative measures as the disease progresses (e.g., transfer techniques and assistive devices).
    9. Administer muscle relaxants as ordered.
    10. Encourage fluid intake of ~2,000 ml unless contraindicated.
    11. Provide a soft or pureed diet if swallowing becomes difficult.
Psychosocial 12. Help the family to understand the changes in the patient's personality and to provide the patient with the necessary support.
    13. Help the patient to understand that living with MS requires significant changes in life-style and that goals should be realistic.
    14. Encourage the patient to live and work to capacity despite limitations.
    15. Encourage the patient to participate in hobbies and interests but to avoid fatigue.
    16. Encourage the patient to seek support from the National Multiple Sclerosis Association.
Educational 17. Teach the patient about measures to prevent complications, drug therapy, safety measures to prevent injury, and avoiding extremes of hot and cold.

Evaluation criteria. See Overview. Neurologic changes observed and reported, verbalization of measures to prevent injury, absence of injury. Independent breathing without respiratory support. Family verbalizes changes in patient's personality and changes in life-style.

PARKINSON'S DISEASE

Parkinson's disease (shaking palsy, paralysis agitans) is a progressive disorder of the CNS characterized by muscular rigidity, tremors, and slowness of movements. The most frequent onset is between the ages of 50 and 65 yr. It is a fairly common neurologic disorder among older age groups, and it is rarely encountered in the juvenile. Parkinson's disease is slightly more common in men than in women, and a familial tendency is claimed by some authorities. An estimated 500,000 people are affected with Parkinson's disease.

In most cases, the cause of Parkinson's disease is unknown. Other causes relate to a variety of diseases and conditions of the nervous system, such as encephalitis, arteriosclerosis, carbon monoxide and manganese poisoning, cerebral trauma, brain tumor, and high doses of drugs such as phenothiazine derivatives and reserpine. Biochemical studies suggest that there is an imbalance of the dopaminergic and cholinergic neurochemical systems by underactivity or overactivity of one or the other. Precipitating factors are suggested to be trauma, exposure to cold and emotional stress, and overwork. However, there is no convincing evidence to support this.

In Parkinson's disease, selective depletion of dopamine, a neurotransmitter substance, occurs in the corpus striatum (caudate nucleus, putamen, and pallidum). This striatal dopamine depletion correlates with the degree of loss of pigmented cells in the substantia nigra. The greater the cell loss in the substantia nigra, the lower the concentration of dopamine in the striatum and the more severe the degree of Parkinsonism.

The classic triad of Parkinsonian *symptoms* is tremors, rigidity, and akinesia. Other symptoms include masklike expression, stooped posture, festinating gait, and disturbances of the ANS (salivary drooling, seborrhea, thermal paresthesias, orthostatic hypotension, urinary bladder dysfunction, and constipation). *Complications* include aspiration pneumonia, weight loss, dehydration, decubitus ulcer, and accidental fractures. *Diagnosis* is based on the health history and physical exam.

Common interventions

Although there is no known treatment, **medical** interventions are symptomatic and may include physical and drug therapy with levodopa; levodopa and carbidopa combination (Sinemet); anticholinergic agents (trihexyphenydyl [Artane], cycrimine [Pagitane], procyclidine [Kemadrin], biperiden [Akineton], benztropine [Cogentin]); antihistamines (used as adjuncts to the more potent drugs for anticholinergic and sedative effects), including diphenhydramine (Benadryl), orphenadrine (Disipal), and chlorphenoxamine (Phenoxene); and antiviral agents, e.g., amantadine (Symmetrel). **Surgical** treatment may involve stereotactic surgery: placement of a lesion in either the ventrolateral nucleus of the thalamus (to reduce tremor) or the globus pallidus (to reduce rigidity).

Nursing interventions

Physical priorities include the nutrition, cardiovascular, and musculoskeletal status. (*See* Overview.)

Physical 1. Assess dietary habits to determine the need for supplemental high-calorie foods.

2. Provide measures to prevent choking and aspiration: supervise closely during meals but encourage self-feeding, and suggest pureed or NG feedings if the patient has difficulty swallowing.
3. Prevent dehydration by monitoring intake accurately.
4. Weigh the patient at least once a week to monitor weight loss or gain.
5. Monitor for cardiac irregularities (e.g., tachycardia or palpitations).
6. Monitor for orthostatic hypotension (change position slowly when getting the patient out of bed).
7. Assess motor status (tremors, rigidity, etc.) and contractures.
8. Provide passive range-of-motion exercises.
9. Encourage the patient to practice speech exercises.
10. Assist the patient in ambulation.
11. Incorporate safety factors in all activities to prevent fractures.
12. Assess the patient's mental status and report any significant changes.
Psychosocial 13. Make family members aware that patient withdrawal and depression may be due to the limitations of the disease.
14. Encourage socialization with others and participation in activities outside the home. (While in the hospital, the patient should be encouraged to participate in group exercises with other patients with Parkinson's disease.)
Educational 15. Teach the patient and family about compliance and significance of drugs as prescribed, adverse reactions of drug therapy, drug interactions with levodopa therapy, prevention of complications (e.g., respiratory, fractures), maintaining the desired weight, and the importance of follow-up care either in the outpatient clinic or in a physician's office.
16. Instruct the patient to contact the American Parkinson Disease Association for educational materials (home exercises, aids, and other equipment).
Prevention 17. Teach the patient to avoid trauma, stress, fatigue, cold, etc.

Evaluation criteria. *See* Overview. Absence of respiratory complications resulting from aspiration, absence of dehydration, adequate intake, weight within normal limits. Absence of tachycardia, palpitations, and orthostatic hypotension. Absence of tremors, rigidity, etc.; speech clear, loud, and resonant; gait more normal. Absence of hallucinations. Absence of dryness of mouth. Active participation in group exercises, more active socialization with others.

MYASTHENIA GRAVIS

Myasthenia gravis (MG) is a chronic neuromuscular disease character-ized by weakness of voluntary (skeletal) muscles, particularly those innervated by the cranial nerves. The prevalence of MG is estimated to be from 1 in 10,000 to 1 in 50,000 of the population. MG is generally not hereditary, and it affects all races and both sexes. The onset is rare during the first decade and after 70 yr of age. The peak of onset is between 20 and 30 yr. Under the age of 40, MG is two or three times more common in women than men. Both sexes are equally affected in later life. Transient MG may occur in infants born to myasthenic mothers. For patients with thymomas, MG is more common in men and older people (50 to 60 yr of age).

The etiology of MG is unknown. One theory suggests that an autoimmune mechanism at the neuromuscular junction is responsible for the functional disorder of the muscles. The following factors support this theory: (1) The thymus, a common site of MG, is involved with the development of cell-mediated immunity, and thymic cells with acetylcholine nicotine receptors may be injured by a virus causing antibody formation. (2) MG is closely associated with other autoimmune diseases: SLE, rheumatoid arthritis, polymyositis, and thyroid dysfunction. (3) There is an occurrence of transient MG in infants born to myasthenic mothers, which strongly indicates the presence of circulating antibodies. Predisposing factors include hormonal changes (menstruation, pregnancy, disturbance in thyroid functioning), emotional stress, excessive physical activity, infection (respiratory), diarrhea, and fever.

MG is a defect in neuromuscular transmission. Transmission of nerve impulses at the neuromuscular junction is believed to be impeded by a decrease in the number of acetylcholine receptor sites on the postsynaptic part of the neuromuscular junction and by circulating antibodies that block acetylcholine receptors.

Characteristic *symptoms* of MG include excessive fatigue accompanied by weakness of involved muscles (improves with rest), weakness (which varies, depending on the muscles involved, and which is usually more pronounced at the end of the day), normal sensory status and tendon reflexes, slight muscular atrophy, and a tendency toward remission and exacerbations. Early stage symptoms include ptosis (often the first symptom), ocular palsy, diplopia, limitation of facial movement giving rise to a snarled appearance on smiling, a hanging jaw (because of weakness), difficulty in chewing, difficulty in swallowing (dysphagia), nasal speech, and difficulty in raising the arms above the head. In the advanced stage, all muscles are involved, including the bowel and bladder sphincters, but especially the intercostal, diaphragm, and abdominal muscles (causing respiratory difficulty). *Complications* include aspiration pneumonia, upper respiratory tract infection, and myasthenic crisis, which is a sudden increase of muscular weakness accompanied by acute respiratory distress. Precipitating factors to myasthenic crisis include emotional stress, infection, and inadequate doses of anticholinesterase. Another complication of MG is cholinergic crisis, which is an increased myasthenic weakness accompanied by acute respiratory difficulty that is caused by an overdose of anticholinesterase. Symptoms of cholinergic crisis include nausea, vomiting, pallor, sweating, salivation, diarrhea, miosis, and bradycardia.

Diagnosis is based on the health history; physical exam; laboratory studies of CSF, urine, and blood, measurement of receptor antibodies, and electromyography (shows a decrease of muscle response after repetitive nerve stimulation); chest x-ray (to detect enlargement of the thymus); and pharmacologic tests (anticholinesterase) with edrophonium (Tensilon) (IV), neostigmine (Prostigmin) (IM), or curare (rarely used).

Common interventions

Medical treatment consists of drug therapy with anticholinesterase drugs, such as neostigmine (Prostigmin) (high doses may produce cholinergic crisis) and pyridostigmine (Mestinon); and with corticosteroids (e.g., prednisone) simultaneously administered with anticholinesterase and administered with potassium supplement and antacids. Medical treatment may also include plasmapheresis (plasma exchange). Pheresis is the separation of blood into its individual components for the removal of selected components. **Surgical** treatment involves thymectomy (removal of the thymus).

Nursing interventions

Physical priorities of care include the respiratory, neurologic, and musculoskeletal status. (*See* Overview and Chapters 7 and 14.)

Acute phase (cholinergic or myasthenic crisis)
Physical 1. Establish a base line and continue to assess changes in respiratory status to detect impending crisis.
  2. Have ventilatory aids ready at the bedside.
  3. Maintain a patent airway (endotracheal intubation or tracheostomy may be indicated).
  4. Make arrangements for possible transfer to the ICU.
  5. Follow instructions carefully with regard to the administration of anticholinesterase drugs. (Usually withheld while the patient is on ventilator.)
  6. Observe and record accurately the patient's response to drug therapy.
  7. Assess pupil size (miosis is a sign of cholinergic crisis).
  8. Observe and report side effects of steroid therapy.
  9. Cover the patient's eye with an eye patch if diplopia is present.
 10. Assess muscle strength.
 11. Provide adequate rest.
Long-term phase
Physical 1. Avoid exposure to persons with an upper respiratory tract infection.
  2. Build up the patient's general resistance.
  3. Continue to provide periods of rest.
  4. Adjust the diet to the patient's needs: food should be soft or semisolid.

5. Assess for side effects of drugs.

Psychosocial 6. Establish an alternative means to communicate, especially if the patient has a tracheostomy.

7. Foster independence when the patient regains muscle strength.

Educational 8. Teach the patient and significant others regarding the disease (course, including remissions, exacerbations, and complications) and drugs that may interfere with neuromuscular transmission.

9. Teach the patient about the importance of avoiding factors that may precipitate a crisis, recognizing signs and symptoms of crisis, and wearing an identification bracelet.

10. Teach the patient how to use portable suction.

11. Inform the patient about community resources, such as the Myasthenia Gravis Foundation.

Prevention 12. Instruct the patient to avoid activities that may increase fatigue and to avoid exposure to persons with upper respiratory tract infections.

Evaluation criteria. *See* Overview. During the **acute phase** the following factors are important. Patient able to breathe independently without respiratory aids; response to drug therapy observed and recorded. Side effects of steroid therapy observed and recorded; no evidence of diplopia. Strength returned to normal or almost normal in involved muscle; no evidence of fatigue. During the **long-term phase**, the following factors are important. No evidence of upper respiratory tract infection. Patient less dependent on others; alternative means of communication established; signs and symptoms of cholinergic crises verbalized.

MUSCULAR DYSTROPHY

Muscular dystrophy refers to a group of progressive degenerative diseases of the skeletal or voluntary muscles characterized by symmetrical weakness and atrophy. There are three major types (mixed and rare types also occur): Duchenne's or pseudohypertrophic, facioscapulohumeral (Landouzy-Déjèrine), and limb-girdle. Muscular dystrophy is a genetically transmitted disease. Although the cause of progressive degeneration of muscle fibers is unknown, biochemical studies suggest abnormality of muscle surface membrane. (How a membrane defect leads to the development of muscle degeneration is not known.)

Muscular dystrophy is primarily a muscle disease; the spinal neurons and their axons in the roots and the peripheral nerves are normal. The loss of muscle fibers is thought to result from recurrent segmental necrosis with phagocytosis or from progressive atrophy. There is regeneration of residual fibers after necrosis. Small fiber regeneration may be due to gradual failure of the metabolism. Large fiber regeneration contributes to muscle hypertrophy (pseudohypertrophy) in the early stages. There is replacement of muscle fibers by fat cells and connective tissue in the late stages of the dystrophic process.

General *characteristics* of muscular dystrophy are symmetrical muscular weakness and atrophy, with the limb-girdle muscles (shoulder and pelvic) more severely affected, and the muscles of the hands often the last to be affected. Progression is more rapid if clinical signs appear earlier. Pseudo-hypertrophy may or may not accompany the disease, and sensation remains intact. *Complications* include pneumonia, contractures, scoliosis, fractures, cardiac failure, and obesity.

Diagnosis is based on the health history, physical exam, electromyography, muscle biopsy, ECG (arrythmias), and chest x-ray (cardiomegaly). Serum enzyme determination is especially useful as a diagnostic tool in the early stages of the disease process. An elevated creatine phosphokinase level is clinically significant in confirming the Duchenne's type of dystrophy and in detecting its female carriers. Other diagnostically significant findings are increased serum levels of aldolase, lactic dehydrogenase, SGOT, and several other enzymes. Muscle metabolism is indicated by high and low urinary outputs of creatine and creatinine, respectively. Because high levels of creatine and low levels of creatinine are found in many neuromuscular diseases, they confirm muscle wasting but do not indicate a particular disorder.

Common interventions

There is no known specific treatment for muscular dystrophy; however, medical treatment tends to be symptomatic (bracing and tendon-lengthening procedures) and supportive (physical, occupational, and respiratory therapy).

Nursing interventions

Physical priorities of care include the respiratory, musculoskeletal, and cardiovascular status. (*See* Overview and Chapter 14.)

Physical 1. Assess for signs and symptoms of respiratory insufficiency and infection.
2. Administer antibiotics as ordered.
3. Provide aggressive chest physiotherapy.
4. Advise the patient to avoid prolonged bed rest.
5. Refer the patient to a chest physiotherapist to provide instruction regarding diaphragmatic breathing exercises, the use of any prescribed respiratory equipment, and postural drainage techniques.
6. Assess muscle strength to detect changes and initiate appropriate intervention.
7. Prevent injuries (fractures and sprains) by providing safety measures.
8. Prevent contractures by having the patient ambulate as much as possible, providing range-of-joint-motion exercises, and applying night splints as prescribed.
9. Collaborate with the physical therapist with regard to the prescribed exercise program, including stretching exercises, ambulation, and transfer techniques.

10. Consult an occupational therapist to assess the patient's functional abilities and to assist the patient with activities of daily living, recreation, and vocational training.
11. Provide adequate support for the patient's spine and pelvis, such as prescribed braces or a corset, when the patient becomes wheelchair-bound.
12. Assess for signs and symptoms of cardiac failure (late stage), thrombophlebitis, and edema.
13. Consult a dietitian with regard to caloric intake and a well-balanced diet to prevent obesity.
14. Encourage frequent change of position to prevent urinary stasis.

Psychosocial 15. Assist the patient and family to avoid overprotection.
16. Assist the patient and family to cope with physical and emotional problems imposed by the disease.

Educational 17. Provide instruction to the patient and family regarding respiratory care (especially proper humidification and prompt treatment of minor respiratory tract infections) and physical therapy.
18. Communicate changes in the patient's therapeutic regimen to other patient care providers (physicians, public health and school nurses, and therapists).
19. Advise the patient to return to the local Muscular Dystrophy Association clinic for periodic reevaluation.

Prevention 20. Advise the family to seek genetic counseling regarding detection of carriers (creatine phosphokinase determination) and amniocentesis during pregnancy to determine the sex of the fetus.
21. Advise the patient and family about self-help devices for home care, such as grab bars, raised chairs, toilet seats, mechanical lifts, etc.

Evaluation criteria. *See* Overview. Proper technique demonstrated for diaphragmatic breathing and postural drainage. Independent walking with braces, adequate support for spine and pelvis provided. Pulse rate within normal limits, no evidence of cardiac failure. Active participation in school and recreational activities, genetic counseling sought, services sought from Muscular Dystrophy Association and other community agencies.

AMYOTROPHIC LATERAL SCLEROSIS

Amyotrophic lateral sclerosis (ALS) is a progressive degenerative disease that affects the motor neurons of the brain and spinal cord. ALS is also known as motor neuron disease and Lou Gehrig disease. There are three forms, based on the initial site involved: (1) Progressive bulbar palsy (motor cells of the medulla oblongata) affects the muscles of face, jaw, tongue, pharynx, and larynx. (2) Progressive muscular atrophy (degeneration of motor neurons in the spinal cord) affects muscles of the trunk and extremities. (3) ALS (corticospinal involvement) usually accompanies atrophy of the bulbar and trunk muscles. ALS is relatively common, occurring in 1.4 per 100,000 persons. It affects all races (high incidence in Guam), and it affects males twice as often as females. It occurs between 50 and 70 yr of age, with a 3- to 5-yr life expectancy after onset (some 10 to 20 yr, but rare). The cause of ALS is unknown. Current theories suggest that ALS is related to a slow viral infection, an autoimmune disorder, or a genetic predisposition. Other suspected agents include trauma, electric shock, spinal anesthesia, and a trace metal imbalance.

The pathophysiologic basis of ALS includes loss of nerve cells (anterior horn cells of the spinal cord and motor nuclei of the lower brainstem), which results in secondary atrophy of muscles. Degeneration of the corticospinal tract also occurs, resulting in loss of myelin, but this is thought to be secondary to the neuronal and axonal loss.

During the early stages of ALS, weakness is asymmetrical. *Symptoms* include difficulty with fine finger movements, slight atrophy or weakness of the muscles of the hands, thick and monotonous speech, atrophy of the tongue, and muscle cramping and twitching. As the disease progresses, weakness becomes symmetrical, with weakness and atrophy of the hands and forearms, slight spasticity of legs, hyperreflexia, muscular fasciculations, and weakness and atrophy of other muscles: upper arm and shoulder girdle, those innervated by brainstem (pharyngeal, laryngeal, tongue, and neck), and, eventually, the trunk and lower extremities. During the advanced (terminal) stage, there is generalized weakness and atrophy, with complete aphagia, bulbar palsy, and quadriplegia. *Complications* include aspiration pneumonia, paralysis of accessory muscles of respiration, and complications resulting from immobility.

Diagnosis is based on the health history, physical exam, and neurologic exam, which should show intact mental status, sensory status, and extra-ocular muscles. Electromyography shows fibrillations and fasciculations. There will be a slight increase (between 45 and 95 mg/100 ml) in protein in the CSF, a decreased output of creatinine, and a slightly increased output of creatine. A spinal x-ray and myelography should be performed to rule out other diseases. There is no specific treatment. **Medical** interventions are supportive and symptomatic.

Nursing interventions

Physical priorities of care include the neurologic, respiratory, and nutrition status. (*See* Overview and Chapters 2 and 14.)

Physical 1. Assess cerebral functioning, cranial nerves (especially 7th, 10th, 11th, and 12th), motor status (muscle size, tone, strength, and involuntary movement), sensory status, and reflexes.

2. Maintain a patent airway. (Suction the patient prn and use aseptic techniques. Turn the patient q 2 hr. Administer O_2 as ordered. Provide mechanical ventilatory support, if indicated [for respiratory failure]. Monitor blood gases.)

3. Assess swallowing ability and provide a diet as tolerated (soft or pureed foods as the disease progresses).

4. Assess motor status.
5. Provide range-of-motion exercises to all limbs.
6. Refer the patient to a physical therapist for assistive devices, such as a wheelchair or walker, when ambulation becomes difficult.
7. Assist the patient with activities of daily living.

Psychosocial 8. Observe for depression and emotional lability (which are expected behaviors).

9. Establish an alternative means of communication when speech becomes impaired. (Instruct the patient to use extraocular muscles as a code to communicate: "Blink twice if answer is no; once if answer is yes.")

Educational 10. Teach the family members or significant others the skills needed for home care.

11. Emphasize continuity of care from the hospital to home.
12. Familiarize the patient and significant others with community services like Home Health Service.

Evaluation criteria. *See* Overview. Changes in neurologic status documented and reported. Airway patent, blood gases within normal limits, chest x-ray clear. Patient using alternative means of communication.

HUNTINGTON'S CHOREA

Huntington's chorea (Huntington's disease [HD]) is a progressive hereditary disorder of the CNS characterized by choreathetosis and mental deterioration. HD affects all races, with the prevalence rate estimated at 10/100,000. It is more common in males than in females. The onset occurs in the 4th and 5th decades, some before the 20th year, and some in childhood. The disease progresses slowly over a 10- to 20-yr period. HD is caused by an autosomal dominant genetic defect. Each child (male or female) has a 50% chance of inheriting the disease from either parent with the HD gene. A precipitating factor is levodopa, which should not be administered to patients at risk of developing the disease.

HD involves atrophy in the caudate nucleus and putamen of basal ganglia and in the gyri of the frontal and temporal lobes of the cerebral cortex. Recent studies of neurochemical changes suggest a deficiency of the neurotransmitters gamma aminobutyric acid (GABA) and acetylcholine (ACh). The normal balance between GABA, ACh, and dopamine is disrupted, resulting in excess dopamine. It is postulated that choreiform movement in HD may be due to increased sensitivity of striatal receptors to excess dopamine.

Early (insidious) *symptoms* of HD include emotional disturbances exhibited by apathy, indifference, listlessness, fits of anger, irritability, memory loss, poor judgment, neglect of personal hygiene and other responsibilities, severe depression, and hallucinations. As the disease progresses, physical symptoms (which in some instances, may precede emotional disturbances) involve involuntary movements such as tics, jerks, and spasms in the muscles of the face, tongue, neck, and arms. Movements gradually become exaggerated, with all parts of the body (especially the trunk, arms, and legs) in constant, uncontrollable motion. During sleep, movements may diminish or cease. Other symptoms include slurred speech, difficulty with swallowing, unsteady gait, and loss of bladder and bowel functioning. There are no periods of remission. The major *complication* is death, which may result from respiratory complications (pneumonia), dysphagia, heart failure, or suicide.

Diagnosis is based on the health history, physical exam, and CAT scan (in advanced cases), which shows atrophy of the caudate nucleus and enlarged ventricles.

Common interventions

There is no known treatment for HD. The following pharmacologic agents may be used to control choreiform movements and alleviate depression: antipsychotics to block dopamine receptors (haloperidol [Haldol], fluphenazine [Prolixin]); drugs that deplete monoamine stores (reserpine); and antidepressants (imipramine [Tofranil]).

Nursing interventions

Physical priorities of care include the respiratory, musculoskeletal, and nutrition status. (*See* Overview and Chapters 2 and 14.)

Physical 1. Assess for evidence of respiratory complications.
2. Assess and record changes of motor functioning.
3. Assist with activities of daily living.
4. Encourage the patient to ambulate as much as possible.
5. Provide a wheelchair if the patient is unable to ambulate.
6. Administer drugs as ordered and monitor for side effects, such as extrapyramidal syndromes and orthostatic hypotension.
7. Provide a high-caloric diet and supplemental feedings to prevent weight loss.
8. Supervise the patient closely during meals to prevent choking or aspiration.
9. Provide a pureed diet when swallowing becomes difficult.
Psychosocial 10. Encourage the patient and family to seek psychologic counseling as appropriate.
11. Observe and report suicidal behavior.
12. Administer drugs as ordered to alleviate depression.
Educational 13. Advise the patient to wear an identification bracelet.
14. Instruct the patient and family regarding voluntary agencies (e.g., Committee to Combat Huntington's Disease, Hereditary Disease Foundation, and National Huntington's Disease Association).

15. Encourage the patient and family to seek genetic counseling.

Prevention 16. Refer the patient and family for genetic counseling and alternatives to childbearing, e.g., adoption or artificial insemination.

Evaluation criteria. *See* Overview. Changes of motor status documented and reported, and proper intervention carried out; patient verbalizes hazards of smoking; patient ambulates independently or with assistance as condition deteriorates; speech improved; better control of involuntary movements. No evidence of suicidal ideation, patient and family seek genetic counseling.

CHAPTER 21

ALTERED HEMATOPOIETIC AND HEPATIC FUNCTIONING

Mary Alice Higgins Donius

HEMATOPOIESIS

OVERVIEW

The hematopoietic system performs and maintains most of the vital functions of the body. Disorders of the blood and blood-forming organs result in widespread adverse systemic effects. Therefore, nursing care and treatment is complex because of the nature of the disease and patient needs.

This first section of this chapter focuses on the function and diseases of the hematopoietic system. It includes a brief description of the anatomy and physiology of the hematopoietic system, the procedures for general assessment, and the interventions most commonly used. The diseases and conditions discussed include leukemias, anemias, clotting disorders, and hemorrhage.

Anatomy and physiology review

The blood is a specialized type of connective tissue that is made up of plasma and cellular components. The cellular components of the blood include RBCs, WBCs, platelets, and chylomicrons (fat droplets). WBCs include nongranulocytes (lymphocytes and monocytes) and granulocytes (neutrophils, eosinophils, and basophils). Plasma components include a fluid component or ground substance, a fibrous component that appears at clotting, and proteins and other solids.

The functions of the blood include the distribution of heat; the transportation of respiratory gases, nutrients, and waste products; selective reaction to factors present in specific tissues, such as osmotic tension, pH, temperature, and hormonal levels; the transportation of cellular components among hematopoietic tissues, connective tissues, and other tissue and organs; and control of the effects of infection and tumors. The formation of blood cells (hematopoiesis) normally occurs in the bone marrow, but may also occur in the lymph nodes or liver and spleen (rarely). The stem cells are the multipotential primitive cells, capable of self-replication and cell differentiation. Ultimately, they produce four types of blood cells. The erythroid committed cell goes through the following stages: erythroblast, reticulocyte, and RBC. The megakaryoid committed cell becomes a megakaryoblast, megakaryocyte, and platelet. The myeloid committed cell becomes a myeloblast, promyelocyte, and granulocyte (basophil, eosinophil, or neutrophil). Or the myeloid committed cell may go through the stages of lymphoblast and lymphocyte (B cell or T cell).

The primary function of the RBC is the transportation of oxygen to tissues via the protein and iron molecule, Hb. Control of the production of RBCs occurs in the following steps: (1) a decreased oxygen supply to the tissues causes hypoxia; (2) the kidneys secrete erythropoietin in response to the hypoxia; (3) erythropoietin travels in the bloodstream to the bone marrow and stimulates production of RBCs.

The primary function of platelets is to assist in clot formation, thereby maintaining hemostasis. The process of platelet functioning is as follows: (1) the adhesion and aggregation of platelets to form a plug at the site of the injured vessel; (2) the release of serotonin and epinephrine to cause vasoconstriction; (3) the release of phospholipid to stimulate the cofactor necessary for coagulation; and (4) the formation of a fibrin clot and clot retraction.

The primary functions of WBCs are (1) defense against bacterial infection (monocytes, neutrophils, eosinophils, and basophils), (2) defense against bacterial and viral infection by means of lymphocytes (B cell immunity), (3) defense against viral, fungal, and parasitic infection, cancer cells, and foreign tissue by means of lymphocytes (T cell immunity), and (4) anticoagulation, i.e., the secretion of heparin (basophils).

Plasma proteins include (1) albumin, which contributes to maintenance of the osmotic pressure of the blood, (2) globulins, which act as transporters for various substances in the blood, and (3) fibrinogen, which, when catalyzed by thrombin, forms the fibrin necessary for clot formation. (There are three types of globulins – alpha, beta, and gamma – the last of which is necessary for antibody production.) Other important substances found in plasma include (1) nonprotein nitrogen, which helps to maintain protein balance in the blood, (2) glucose, which supplies energy to the cells, and (3) electrolytes, which maintain the fluid and acid-base balance.

The lymphatic system is the part of the circulatory system that transports fluids and solutes from interstitial spaces into the blood. The components of the lymphatic system are (1) the lymphatic vessels (capillaries, collecting vessels, and trunks, i.e., the right lymphatic ducts and the thoracic duct), (2) lymphatic tissue, which contains lymphocytes and is found in lymph nodes, mucous membranes, the thymus, spleen, and bone marrow, and (3) lymph. The functions of the lymphatic system are (1) the return of fluid and proteins from interstitial fluid to the blood, (2) filtration and phagocytosis, and (3) the formation of nongranular WBCs in the lymph nodes (i.e., monocytes and lymphocytes).

General assessment

The **health history** includes current health status (nutrition, especially iron, vitamin B_{12}, and folates), past health history (bleeding tendencies or dysfunction, immune diseases, and tumors), the family history (bleeding tendencies), a social history (exposure to radiation, toxic chemicals, or drugs), and a review of systems, which focuses on general status (chronic fatigue and weight loss), the mouth and throat (sores on the mouth and tongue), the respiratory system (dyspnea), the GI system (anorexia and indigestion), the musculoskeletal system (bone pain), immunologic system (increased susceptibility to infection), and mental status (depression).

The **physical exam** includes an integumentary assessment for evidence of bleeding in the skin, mucous membranes, or any body orifice (petechiae, ecchymosis, purpura, epistaxis, hemoptysis, hematemesis, melena, hematuria, hemarthrosis, and hematomas), as well as for evidence of decreased tissue perfusion or oxygenation (heart, lungs, kidneys, bowels, peripheral areas), and evidence of jaundice. The abdomen is assessed for hepato- and splenomegaly. In addition, the patient is assessed for evidence of anemia, leukopenia, and thrombocytopenia.

Laboratory tests are used to determine RBC, WBC, and platelet structure and functioning. The tests for RBC structure and functioning include (1) a CBC, which involves an RBC, Hb level, Hct level, reticulocyte count, and erythrocyte sedimentation rate (ESR), (2) a bone marrow biopsy exam, which determines the number, size, shape, and maturational progress of blood cells, (3) a blood film, which identifies variations and abnormalities in RBC size, shape, and Hb content, (4) RBC indices, which measure RBC mean cell volume, Hb, and Hb concentration (MCV, MCH, and MCHC), (5) an erythrocyte fragility test, which measures the rate at which RBCs become fragile, and (6) an erythrocyte life-span determination, used as a differential diagnosis for anemias. The tests for WBC structure and functioning include (1) a CBC, which involves a WBC differential of granulocytes (basophils, neutrophils, and eosinophils) and nongranulocytes (lymphocytes and monocytes), and (2) a bone marrow biopsy exam, which determines the number, size, shape, and maturational progress of WBCs. The tests for platelet structure and functioning include a platelet count, bleeding time, partial thromboplastin time (PTT), prothrombin time (PT), coagulation time, thrombin time, fibrinogen level, clot retraction, and bone marrow exam, which determines the number, size, shape, and maturational progress of platelets.

Common interventions

Four common interventions are blood transfusion, bone marrow transplant, bone marrow aspiration, and splenectomy.

Blood transfusion. A blood transfusion is the IV introduction of whole blood or blood components (serum, plasma, RBCs, and platelets) for replacement and therapeutic purposes, such as to restore blood volume, prevent shock, or treat severe chronic anemia. **Nursing** responsibilities and interventions include the following:

Physical 1. Check the label and identification form for corresponding information: the patient's name, room number, hospital number, package number, the patient's blood group and Rh status, and the donor's blood group and Rh status.
  2. *Do not administer blood if the information does not correspond.*
  3. Remove the blood from the refrigerator 1 hr before administration.
  4. Identify the patient.
  5. Stabilize the patient's arm on an arm board.
  6. Administer very slowly for the first 15 min.
  7. If there is no reaction, increase the rate of flow.
  8. Administer rapidly if there is shock or hemorrhage.
  9. Assess for signs of transfusion reactions (*see below*).
  10. If there is a reaction, discontinue the blood immediately, notify a physician, send the blood and a sample of the recipient's blood to the blood bank, and administer fluids and medications as ordered.
Educational 11. Teach the patient to tell health professionals, on future hospitalizations or when donating blood, about the transfusion and the presence or absence of complications.

Hemolytic transfusion reaction: The hemolysis (breakdown) of RBCs is the most severe reaction and occurs in ~1 out of 5,000 transfusions. It is due to an ABO or Rh incompatibility. *Symptoms* include chills, fever, hematuria, oliguria, jaundice, headache, backache, dyspnea, cyanosis, and chest pain. *Complications* include renal failure and shock. *Diagnosis* is based on the etiology and symptoms. **Treatment** includes IV fluids, O_2 therapy, sedation, and treatment and prevention of shock. **Nursing** interventions are as follows:

Physical 1. Discontinue the transfusion.
  2. Administer fluids and medications as ordered.
  3. Administer O_2 therapy.
  4. Monitor vital signs q 15 to 30 min.
  5. Assess and prevent hypotension and shock.
  6. Record accurate intake and output.
  7. Assess for the side effects of medication.
Psychosocial 8. Provide emotional support for the patient and family during and after the emergency.

Educational. 9. Advise the patient of the reaction and of the importance of reporting it before future transfusions.

Bacterial transfusion reaction: Bacterial reactions are rare, but result from the administration of blood contaminated by pathogenic organisms. In general, blood newly contaminated with gram-negative bacteria produces the most severe (and even fatal) reactions. The *symptoms* include fever, chills, lumbar pain, headache, malaise, hematemesis, diarrhea, and warm, dry, and pinkish skin. *Complications* include shock and death. *Diagnosis* is based on symptoms and examination of the remaining blood. **Treatment** includes IV fluids, medications (vasopressors, corticosteroids, and antibiotics), and treatment and prevention of shock. **Nursing** interventions are the same as for hemolytic reaction (*see above*). In addition, fever must be reduced; O_2 therapy is not usually necessary.

Allergic transfusion reaction: Hypersensitivity to the blood received is not uncommon. Its cause is unknown. *Symptoms* of a mild reaction include mild edema, hives, bronchial wheezing, itching, and fever. A severe reaction may cause bronchospasm and severe dyspnea. *Complications* include anaphylactic shock and death. *Diagnosis* is based on symptoms. **Treatment** for a mild reaction includes antihistamines and antipyretics. Severe reactions are treated with epinephrine, vasopressors, and corticosteroids. Both types of reaction require IV fluids and respiratory therapy. **Nursing** interventions are as follows:

Physical 1. Discontinue the transfusion if the reaction is severe; slow the rate if the reaction is mild.
2. Administer IV fluids as ordered.
3. Administer medications as ordered.
4. Monitor vital signs q 15 to 30 min.
5. Assess and prevent complications.
6. Assess for the side effects of medication.
7. Refer to hemolytic reaction for other nursing interventions (*see above*).

Circulatory overload: Excessive fluid volume in the blood vessels is more common in elderly and debilitated patients and those with a low cardiac reserve. It is caused by the infusion of fluid in too great a quantity or at too rapid a rate. *Symptoms* include cough, dyspnea, edema, tachycardia, hemoptysis, and frothy, pink-tinged sputum. *Complications* include pulmonary edema and left-sided heart failure. *Diagnosis* is based on etiology and symptoms. **Medical** treatment includes digitalization; **surgical** treatment includes phlebotomy. **Nursing** interventions are as follows:

Physical 1. Discontinue the transfusion.
2. Administer digitalis preparations as ordered.
3. Assess for side or toxic effects.
4. Prepare for phlebotomy procedure.
5. Refer to hemolytic reaction for other nursing interventions (*see above*).

Bone marrow transplant. Bone marrow transplant is the surgical transfer of bone marrow from a healthy to an ill individual. It is a procedure used in the treatment of leukemia. **Nursing** responsibilities and interventions include the following:

1. Before the transplant:
   a. Explain the procedure and treatments to the patient and family.
   b. Prepare the patient for massive chemotherapy and total body irradiation to kill all leukemic cells.
   c. Administer IV fluids for hydration before and after chemotherapy.
   d. Assess daily weight, serum creatinine, the ECG, and central venous pressure (CVP).
   e. Maintain isolation.
2. During the transplant, assess for volume overload, allergic reaction, and signs of pulmonary emboli.
3. After the transplant:
   a. Maintain reverse isolation.
   b. Administer antibiotic therapy.
   c. Administer antibiotic cream to body orifices qid.
   d. Administer pHisoHex bath and shampoo bid.
   e. Obtain a daily CBC.
   f. Administer blood and platelet transfusions as ordered (daily).
   g. Obtain bone marrow aspirations and biopsies as ordered (weekly).
   h. Observe for complications (rejection, leukemic relapse, and graft-versus-host reaction).

Bone marrow aspiration. The needle aspiration of bone marrow to examine RBCs, WBCs, and platelets as they evolve through the stages of maturation is diagnostic for most blood dyscrasias. **Nursing** responsibilities and interventions include the following:

1. Before the procedure:
   a. Explain the procedure to the patient.
   b. Be sure the consent is signed.
   c. Administer sedation as ordered.
   d. Position the patient for the procedure (if sternal, on the back; and if iliac crest, on the opposite side).
   e. Shave and cleanse the site with an antiseptic solution.
2. After the procedure:
   a. Apply a sterile dressing.
   b. Relieve pain.
   c. Position the patient comfortably.

Splenectomy. Removal of the spleen may be performed because of (1) rupture of the spleen due to trauma, surgery, or disease, and (2) hypersplenism (excessive destruction of the elements of the blood), as in anemia, splenomegaly, leukopenia, Hodgkin's disease, non-Hodgkin lymphomas,

TB, portal hypertension, and idiopathic thrombocytopenic purpura (ITP). **Nursing** responsibilities and interventions include the following:

1. Provide preoperative care (*see* Chapter 9).
2. Provide postoperative care (*see* Chapter 11).
3. Observe for signs of hemorrhage, shock, fever (not related to infection), and abdominal distension and discomfort.
4. Apply an abdominal binder, if ordered.
5. Monitor platelet counts.
6. Protect the patient from trauma and bruising.

Evaluation criteria. Absence or reduction of symptoms. Absence or early detection and treatment of complications. Blood values and vital signs within normal limits. Control of underlying pathology. Patient and family verbalize health teaching and participate in self-care.

HEMORRHAGE

Hemorrhage is a profuse blood loss resulting from a disruption in the continuity of one or more blood vessels. Predisposing factors include a congenital weakness of the blood vessels and aging. The causes include traumatic injury to the vessel walls (surgical, physical, chemical, or drug-related), a weakening of the vessel walls, (arterial aneurysms, venous varicosities, or vitamin C deficiency), GI bleeding (stress ulcers, esophageal varices, severe burns, or diverticulitis), hemolytic disorders (hemophilia, impaired coagulability of the blood, anticoagulant therapy, or thrombocytopenia), gynecologic disorders (postpartum hemorrhage, abortion, or menorrhagia), cancer, epistaxis, disseminated intravascular coagulation, hepatic or splenic disorders, leukemia (acute and chronic), and cardiac tamponade. The *symptoms* result from the effects on the organ or tissue in which the bleeding occurs and/or those which usually receive blood from the area of hemorrhage. The severity of the symptoms is determined by the site of blood loss or pooling and the rate and volume of blood loss. Symptoms related to the organ and tissue involved include bleeding from an accessible organ, cavity, or orifice (including an incision), increased intracranial pressure, blood in the CSF, epistaxis, hemoptysis, hematemesis, hematuria, blood in the stool, menorrhagia, and pain. The signs of hypovolemia and hypoxia include a weak, rapid, thready pulse; rapid respirations (deep at first, then shallow); fall in the BP; cool and clammy skin; diaphoresis; pallor; vertigo or faintness; apprehension; and thirst. *Complications* include shock and death. *Diagnosis* is based on the health history, physical exam, and laboratory tests.

Common interventions

The goals of treatment are to stop the hemorrhage and to replace the blood volume. **Medical** interventions include applying pressure as appropriate, administering vitamin K therapy, administering a blood transfusion, checking the specific site of bleeding, and treating the patient for shock. **Surgical** treatment includes repair of the vessel or organ or cauterization of the vessel.

Nursing interventions

Physical 1. Monitor vital signs q 15 min.
  2. Place the patient in Trendelenburg's position.
  3. Assess for the origin of the bleeding.
  4. Assess for the signs of hypovolemia, hypoxia, and shock.
  5. Treat any complications.
  6. Maintain fluid and blood replacement as ordered.
  7. Administer medication as ordered.
  8. Assess for signs of transfusion reaction: vital signs (especially elevated temperature, tachycardia, dyspnea, and decreased BP), chills, itching, urticaria, nausea/vomiting, pain, and apprehension.
  9. If a transfusion reaction occurs, stop the transfusion, notify the physician, administer fluids and medications as ordered, reduce fever, and return the blood to the blood bank. A report detailing the specifics of the transfusion reaction should be sent to the blood bank with the blood and blood samples to be analyzed for incompatibility and bacterial contamination.
Psychosocial 10. Provide emotional support for the patient and family during the emergency.
  11. Reassure the patient and family after the emergency.
Educational 12. Advise the patient as to the source of the hemorrhage.
  13. Teach the patient how to assess hemorrhage.
  14. Teach the patient precautions that help avoid hemorrhage.
  15. Teach the patient and family emergency procedures for treating hemorrhage.

Evaluation criteria. *See* Overview.

ACUTE LEUKEMIA

Acute leukemia is the proliferation of abnormal immature WBCs. Acute lymphoblastic leukemia (ALL) is the proliferation of predominantly lymphoblasts; acute myelogenous leukemia (AML) is the proliferation of predominantly myeloblasts. Acute leukemia occurs primarily in children under the age of 5 yr. Potential causes include genetic predisposition, radiation, chemicals and drugs, viruses, and marrow hypoplasia. (For the classifications, *symptoms*, *complications*, and *diagnosis* of ALL and AML, refer to Table 21-1).

Common interventions

The types of treatment are remission induction therapy (initial treatment), consolidation therapy (initial treatment is continued or modified), and

TABLE 21-1
Acute Lymphoblastic Leukemia and Acute Myelogenous Leukemia

ALL	AML
Classification	
L_1: small and homogeneous lymphoblasts.	M_1: no maturation of myeloblasts.
L_2: heterogeneous lymphoblasts.	M_2: maturation to or beyond promyelocyte stage.
L_3: homogeneous lymphoblasts appear like Burkitt's lymphoma cells.	M_3: variant, with hypergranular promyelocytes and Auer bodies.
Symptoms/complications	
Subtle onset (pallor, anorexia, irritability, and malaise).	Subtle onset of generalized symptoms over longer period of time.
Low-grade fever with intermittent marked temperature elevations, with or without infection.	Preceded by a hematologic defect, most often anemia ("preleukemia").
Bleeding tendencies (petechiae, ecchymosis, and mucous membranes) and anemia.	Mild bleeding tendencies (petechiae and mucous membranes).
	Severe bleeding (GI and GU tracts, and CNS hemorrhage).
Thrombocytopenia, lymph node enlargement, spleno- and hepatomegaly, bone and joint pain, increased susceptibility to infection, meningeal leukemia (headache, nausea, and intracranial pressure), GU manifestations (hematuria, cystitis, and pyelonephritis), and death.	Thrombocytopenia, lymph node enlargement, spleno- and hepatomegaly, bone and joint pain, increased susceptibility to infection, meningeal leukemia (headache, nausea, and intracranial pressure), GU manifestations (hematuria, cystitis, and pyelonephritis), and death.
Diagnosis	
Health history and physical exam.	Health history and physical exam.
Blood studies: anemia, granulo- and thrombocytopenia, elevated WBC with leukemic blast cells or leukopenia, increased uric acid, BUN, and LDH.	Blood studies: anemia, Auer bodies, macrocytic anemia, thrombocytopenia, leukopenia, hypergammaglobulinemia, and increased uric acid.
Bone marrow: leukemia lymphoblast cells.	Bone marrow: leukemia myeloblast cells.

ALL, acute lymphoblastic leukemia; AML, acute myelogenous leukemia; LDH, lactic dehydrogenase.

maintenance therapy (decreasing treatment). **Medical** interventions include chemo-, radio-, and immunotherapy, the treatment and prevention of infection, and supportive care therapy, including platelet and WBC transfusion. **Surgical** treatment includes bone marrow transplant.

Nursing interventions

Physical 1. Refer to nursing interventions for anemia (*see below*).
2. Assess symptoms.
3. Provide measures to control pain, including analgesics.
4. Provide adequate dietary intake and mouth care.
5. Prevent infection.
6. Provide symptomatic relief.
7. Protect the patient from injury and trauma.
8. Assess, treat, and prevent complications of involved organs.
9. Assess, treat, and prevent complications related to therapy.
10. Reduce fever.
11. Provide adequate rest.
Psychosocial 12. Provide emotional support for the patient and family related to terminal illness.
13. Provide assistance for long-term care.
14. Discuss the feelings of the patient and family.
15. Provide information about support groups, if indicated.
16. Provide emotional support related to medical therapy (i.e., chemotherapy and radiation therapy), as well as to diagnostic tests.
Educational 17. Teach the patient and family health care related to the medical regimen, decreasing incidence of complications, and the prevention of complications.

Evaluation criteria. See Overview. Patient and family verbalize feelings related to chronic/terminal illness.

[Chronic lymphocytic and myelocytic leukemia are contrasted in Table 21-2. Nursing interventions and evaluation criteria are the same as for acute leukemia.]

MULTIPLE MYELOMA

Multiple myeloma is a neoplasm of the plasma cells. Its incidence, 2 to 3 per 100,000 individuals, increases with age and is somewhat more common in males. Of unknown etiology, it is *characterized* by malignant cells within the bone marrow, bony lesions produced by tumors, and the presence of abnormal proteins. *Symptoms* include repeated infection, weakness, fatigue, weight loss, increased ESR, increased susceptibility to infection (due to defective antibody synthesis, increased rate of gamma-globulin catabolism, and severe granulocytopenia), hypercalcemia, and the symptoms of anemia. Skeletal lesions produce edema, localized tenderness, unrelenting pain, and pathologic fracture. *Complications* include chronic renal failure, thrombocytopenia, hypercalcemic encephalopathy, infection, polycythemia,

TABLE 21-2
Chronic Lymphocytic Leukemia and Chronic Myelocytic Leukemia

CLL	CML
Definition	
A possible clonal disorder that allows for the production of an excessive number of small lymphocytes.	A clonal disorder of the stem cell, which is allowed to proliferate in preference to normal stem cells.
Incidence	
Uncommon in people <30 yr; increases as age increases. More common in males and whites; rare in Orientals.	Occurs at any age, but most commonly in young or middle-aged adults. More common in males.
Etiology	
Unknown. Same causative factors as ALL, except radiation.	Unknown. Same causative factors as AML.
Symptoms	
Slow onset, anemia, enlarged lymph nodes, spleno- and hepatomegaly, and fever.	Insidious onset, anemia, abdominal fullness, easy bruising and bleeding, massive spleen, fever, very little enlargement of the lymph nodes, and diaphoresis.
Complications	
Infection, hemolytic anemia, and hypogammaglobulinemia.	Infection, thrombocytopenia anemia, thromboembolism, and hemorrhage.
Diagnosis	
Health history and physical exam.	Health history and physical exam.
Blood studies: normal WBCs, decreased RBCs, normal platelet count and blood smears.	Blood studies: increased WBCs, decreased RBCs, increased platelet count, LAP, and blood smears.
Bone marrow exam.	Bone marrow exam.
Medical interventions	
Chemotherapy (alkylating agents), immunotherapy, radiation therapy, treatment of anemia and thrombocytopenia, and treatment and prevention of infection.	Chemotherapy, radiation therapy, radioisotope therapy, treatment of symptoms, and treatment and prevention of infection.
Surgical intervention	
Splenectomy.	

ALL, acute lymphoblastic leukemia; AML, acute myelogenous leukemia; CLL, chronic lymphocytic leukemia; CML, chronic myelocytic leukemia; LAP, leukocyte alkaline phosphatase.

and spinal cord compression. *Diagnosis* is based on the health history, physical exam, and blood studies that reveal moderate to severe anemia, increased ESR, increased rouleau formation of blood smears because of increased amounts of globulin in the plasma, a normal or low platelet count, and hypercalcemia. In addition, leukopenia may be present. Bone marrow aspirations reveal myeloma cells. Protein studies reveal the secretion of abnormal monoclonal serum protein, IgG, IgA, and Bence Jones proteins.

Common interventions

The methods of treatment include chemotherapy, radiation therapy, the treatment of pain, the treatment and prevention of infection, and the treatment of hypercalcemia, renal failure, anemia, and spinal cord compression.

Nursing interventions

Physical 1. Assess symptoms.
2. Provide control of pain, including the administration of analgesics.
3. Prevent infection and pathologic fractures.
4. Assess, treat, and prevent complications related to the disease process (i.e., anemia, hypercalcemia, and renal failure).
5. Assess, treat, and prevent complications related to treatment.
6. Prevent immobility.
Psychosocial 7. Provide emotional support related to terminal illness to the patient and family.
8. Provide emotional support related to diagnostic procedures and medical management (especially chemotherapy and radiation).
Educational 9. Teach the patient and family health care related to the medical regimen, including the administration of medications and the control and prevention of complications.

Evaluation criteria. See Overview. Patient and family verbalize feelings related to chronic/terminal illness.

NON-HODGKIN LYMPHOMAS

Non-Hodgkin lymphomas are malignancies of the lymphoid tissues other than Hodgkin's disease. They are more common in males, and are estimated to constitute 2.5% of all malignancies (excluding nonmelanotic skin cancer and cervical carcinoma in situ). Causes include RNA viruses, genetic factors, immunodeficiencies and immunostimulation, immunosuppressive agents, and high-dose radiation exposure. Tumors may be classified (Rappaport) according to nodular architecture (i.e., nodular or diffuse) or cellular histology (i.e., well-differentiated lymphocytic nodes, poorly differentiated lymphocytic nodes, histiocyte lymphocytic or mixed nodes, histiocytic nodes, or undifferentiated nodes). *Symptoms* include enlarged, painless lymph nodes, usually in the primary sites of the cervical or supracervical areas; lymphadenopathy at another primary site; and fatigue, malaise, GI symptoms, weight loss, fever, infection, bone pain, and possible splenomegaly. *Complications* are related to associated organ involvement (liver, spleen, the parenchyma of the lungs, and the kidneys). Infection is also a complication. *Diagnosis* is based on the health history, physical exam, chest x-ray (mediastinal and hilar nodes), skeletal x-ray (bone nodes), and laboratory data: CBC is usually normal at diagnosis; uric acid may be increased; calcium may be increased if bone is involved; and albumin may be decreased as the disease advances.

Common interventions

Treatment includes radiation therapy to the involved areas, radioisotopes, and chemotherapy.

Nursing interventions

Physical 1. Assess symptoms.
2. Provide adequate rest.
3. Reduce fever.
4. Control pain, including administering analgesics.
5. Prevent infection.
6. Administer medications as ordered.
7. Maintain hydration.
8. Assess, treat, and prevent complications related to the disease process (e.g., anemia, pulmonary edema, ascites).
9. Assess, treat, and prevent complications related to medical treatment.
Psychosocial 10. Provide emotional support for the patient and family related to terminal illness.
11. Provide emotional support for the patient and family related to diagnostic procedures, medical treatment, and complications.
Educational 12. Teach the patient basic pathophysiology related to the disease process and treatment.
13. Teach the patient health care related to the medical regimen, including administration of medication, assessment of side effects and complications, and control and prevention of complications.

Evaluation criteria. *See* Overview. Patient and family verbalize feelings related to chronic/terminal illness.

HODGKIN'S DISEASE

Hodgkin's disease is a chronic and progressive tumor of the lymphatic system. It is most common between the ages of 20 and 40, and more common in males. Causes include viral infections, immunologic dysfunction, and tumor. Histologic classification is based on the presence of Reed-Sternberg cells (diagnostic) or on lymph nodes with a diffuse and mixed infiltration of lymphocytes. The clinical staging is as follows. Stage I includes single lymph node involvement and single extralymphatic organ or site involvement. In stage II, two or more lymph node areas on the same side of the diaphragm are involved, or an extralymphatic organ or site and one or more lymph node areas on the same side of the diaphragm are involved. In stage III, the lymph node areas on both sides of the diaphragm are involved. This stage may or may not be accompanied by extralymphatic organ or site involvement, spleen involvement, or both. Stage IV is marked by diffuse involvement of one or more extralymphatic organs or tissues, with or without associated lymph node involvement. Subclassifications include patients with or without generalized symptoms.

Symptoms of Hodgkin's disease include a painless enlarged mass or swelling (e.g., cervical area), generalized pruritus with rash, symptoms related to the obstruction or pressure of affected lymph node areas and organs, generalized lymphadenopathy, unexplained fever, night sweats, and unexplained weight loss ($>10\%$ in 6 mo). *Complications* are related to organ and tissue involvement, in addition to anemia, pulmonary edema as a result of fluid backup in the lymph system, and ascites.

Diagnosis is based on the health history, physical exam, lymph node biopsy of the cervical node that usually reveals Reed-Sternberg cells (diagnostic), liver and spleen scans, lymphangiography (diagnostic), bone marrow biopsy (bone marrow infiltration), chest x-ray to determine mediastinal involvement, and skeletal x-ray to detect bone involvement. Laboratory tests include CBC (anemia and leukocytosis), serum alkaline phosphatase (elevated with liver or bone involvement), and liver function tests.

Common interventions

Medical treatment includes radiation therapy, chemotherapy, or a combination of the two. **Surgical** treatment includes the removal of tumors (which may be pressing on a nerve or organ).

Nursing interventions

1. Refer to non-Hodgkin lymphomas (*see above*).
2. Prepare the patient for diagnostic procedures.
3. Provide pre- and postoperative care, as indicated (*see* Chapters 9 and 11).

Evaluation criteria. *See* Overview. Patient and family verbalize feelings related to chronic/terminal illness.

ANEMIA

Anemia, a reduction in the concentration of circulating Hb or RBCs, results from the reduced production of RBCs, reduced synthesis of Hb by RBC precursors, increased destruction of RBCs, and loss of RBCs from the circulation.

The symptoms of anemia result from the reduced capacity of the blood to carry O_2, the change in total blood volume, the rate at which these have occurred, the associated manifestations of an underlying disorder, and decreased cardiovascular and pulmonary compensation capacity. Nonspecific symptoms are fatigue, irritability, and a vague sense of the loss of well-being. Specific *symptoms* include pallor of the skin and mucous membranes, tachycardia, systolic flow murmurs, dyspnea, peripheral edema, anorexia, nausea/vomiting, flatulence, abdominal discomfort, constipation, diarrhea, weight loss, headache, vertigo, tinnitus, faintness, chills, feeling of cold, inability to concentrate, drowsiness, restlessness, increased basal metabolic rate, proteinuria and mild fever (with marked anemia), increased susceptibility to bruising and bleeding (petechiae, ecchymosis, purpura, and retinal hemorrhage), scleral icterus, pancytopenia (reduction in RBCs, WBCs, and platelets), and symptoms related to the underlying pathology. *Complications* include myocardial ischemia, left-sided heart failure, renal failure, shock, and the complications related to the underlying pathology.

Diagnosis is based on the health history, physical exam, CBC, blood smears for specific morphology, and urinalysis.

Common interventions

Treatment includes iron supplements, blood transfusions, a well-balanced diet, vitamins, O_2 therapy, and treatment of the underlying pathology and complications.

Nursing interventions

Physical 1. Assess the symptoms of anemia.
2. Maintain blood transfusions as ordered (*see above*).
3. Assess for transfusion reactions (*see above*).
4. Administer medications as ordered (iron supplements and vitamins).
5. Provide a well-balanced diet, high in protein, iron, and vitamins.
6. Assess and prevent complications.
7. Treat the underlying pathology.
8. Assess for the side effects of medication.
9. Provide for periods of rest after activity.
10. Plan for progressive activity.
11. Provide mouth care.
12. Prevent infection.
13. Administer O_2 therapy.
14. Protect the patient from chills.
Psychosocial 15. Provide emotional support related to the debilitating effects of anemia and/or the chronicity of the disease.
16. Provide support related to the underlying pathology.
17. Provide a calm, quiet atmosphere.
Educational 18. Teach the patient and family about medical regimens (proper use of medication, side effects of medication, and proper dietary intake).
19. Teach the patient and family to avoid injury and trauma.
20. Instruct the patient to have periodic blood tests.
21. Teach the patient and family health maintenance related to the underlying pathology.

Evaluation criteria. See Overview.

IRON DEFICIENCY

Iron deficiency, the depletion of the total body iron content, is the most common form of nutritional deficiency and the most common cause of anemia. It occurs most often in children <2 yr of age and in premenopausal women. Causes include inadequate dietary intake, impaired iron absorption, increased iron loss through bleeding (acute or chronic or persistent hemorrhage), and by increased requirements for iron (e.g., during pregnancy, lactation, or infancy).

Symptoms include fatigue, irritability, palpitations, dizziness, breathlessness, headache, and epithelial abnormalities of the nails, tongue, hypopharynx (associated with dysphagia), stomach (associated with gastritis), and nose (associated with ozena [intranasal crusting, discharge, and odor] or atrophy of the nasal mucosa), and pica. Possible symptoms are menorrhagia, neuralgic pains, vasomotor disturbances, numbness, and tingling.

Diagnosis is based on the health history, physical exam, and the following laboratory data: decreased serum levels of Hb, MCV, MCH, and MCHC; normal or decreased levels of reticulocytes and WBCs; an increased platelet count; and a possibly increased total iron binding capacity (TIBC). A blood smear shows decreased Hb in each RBC, with central pallor. The degree of change and the number of RBCs affected will increase with the severity of the disease. Bone marrow aspiration reveals erythroid hyperplasia.

Common interventions

Medical interventions include treatment of the underlying pathology and the prescribing of iron supplements via medications and diet. **Surgical** treatment attempts to resolve the underlying pathology. The **nursing** interventions are the same as for anemia (*see above*).

MEGALOBLASTIC MACROCYTIC ANEMIA

Megaloblastic macrocytic anemia refers to disorders in which the RBC is increased in size and the macrocyte is thicker than normal. It is caused by defective DNA synthesis, and may be inherited or drug-induced. It is associated with vitamin B12 deficiency related to the following factors: decreased dietary intake of B12 (rare), pernicious anemia, gastrectomy, obstruction of the gastric mucosa, small bowel bacterial overgrowth, diseases affecting the ileum, chronic pancreatic disease, congenital malabsorption, and fish tapeworm. Or it may be associated with a folate deficiency related to the following factors: dietary intake, alcoholic cirrhosis, pregnancy, infancy, hematologic illness characterized by rapid cellular proliferation of RBCs or other marrow elements, congenital or drug-induced deficiencies, malabsorption, tropical sprue, celiac disease, regional jejunitis, and small bowel resection.

The *symptoms* and *complications* associated with vitamin B12 deficiency include paresthesias, weakness, incoordination, unsteady gait, inability to perform fine motor skills, personality changes, confusion, and psychosis. Symptoms associated with folate deficiency include poor dietary intake, glossitis, anorexia, dyspepsia, flatulence, and diarrhea. Other symptoms relate to anemia in general (*see above*) and/or are associated with the underlying pathology of vitamin B12 or folate acid deficiency.

Diagnosis is based on the health history, physical exam, and the following laboratory data: blood studies reveal a normal MCHC in macrocytic and normochromic anemia; normal MCHC and an MCV increased in proportion to the severity of the disease; decreased RBC, Hb, and Hct; normal or low WBC; decreased platelet count; prolonged bleeding time; and decreased reticulocyte count. A blood smear reveals erythropoiesis of macrocytic RBCs of a distinctly oval shape. Bone marrow aspiration reveals marrow that is cellular and hyperplastic with characteristic megaloblasts. The Schilling test is normal in pernicious anemia and abnormal in B12 malabsorption.

Common interventions

Treatment includes vitamin B12 therapy, folate therapy, and treatment of the underlying pathology.

Nursing interventions

Physical 1. Administer vitamin B12 and folates as ordered.
2. Provide nursing care related to the specific underlying pathology.
3. Provide nursing care related to anemia (*see above*).
4. Provide nursing care related to diagnostic procedures.
5. Provide safety measures if the patient is experiencing neurologic symptoms.
Psychosocial 6. Provide emotional support related to a genetic and chronic disease and to neurologic symptoms.
Educational 7. Provide genetic counseling.
8. Teach the patient and family about long-term care (*see* anemia *above*).

Evaluation criteria. See Overview.

HEMOLYTIC ANEMIA

Hemolytic anemia results from an increased rate of RBC destruction. The bone marrow is unable to increase the rate of RBC production to compensate sufficiently. Hemolytic anemias are either inherited or acquired disorders. The *symptoms* and *complications* of chronic congenital hemolytic anemia are jaundice, "crisis" periods of asymptomatic disease with episodic symptomatic disease, splenomegaly, cholelithiasis, leg ulcers, severe skeletal abnormalities during growth and development, and symptoms associated with the underlying pathology. Those for acquired hemolytic anemia are rapid onset; aching pains of the back, abdomen, and limbs; headache, malaise, vomiting, fever, and chills; other symptoms of generalized anemia (*see above*); symptoms associated with the underlying pathology; and shock. (If the onset is insidious, symptoms are the same as for congenital hemolytic anemia [*see above*].)

Diagnosis is based on the health history, physical exam, and laboratory data, which indicate decreased RBC survival rate, increased serum bilirubin (unconjugated), increased lactic dehydrogenase, hemoglobinemia, absence of haptoglobin with increased hemoglobinuria, leukocytosis, thrombocytosis, and specific morphologic abnormalities (smear). Bone marrow aspiration reveals hyperplasia.

Common interventions

Treatment depends on the specific diagnosis. **Medical** interventions include making a differential diagnosis, relieving shock, and administering blood transfusions. **Surgical** treatment includes splenectomy.

Nursing interventions

1. Provide care related to anemia (*see above*).
2. Provide pre- and postoperative care if a splenectomy is performed (*see* Chapters 9 and 11).
3. Treat the specific cause and symptoms.
4. Provide genetic counseling, if indicated.

Evaluation criteria.   *See* Overview.

SICKLE CELL ANEMIA

Sickle cell anemia is an inherited condition of abnormal Hb synthesis. It occurs almost exclusively in blacks, and is due to the homozygous inheritance of Hb S, which substitutes valine for glutamic acid in position 6 of the beta chain. The sickling phenomenon occurs when the altered Hb molecules with prolonged deoxygenation aggregate into rigid, liquid crystals and distort the cell into the characteristic sickle shape. This results in increased RBC fragility and permeability. Reversal to the normal shape occurs after oxygenation, but cells with the highest concentration of Hb S sickle irreversibly. Repeated sickling and unsickling decrease the cell's ability to return to normal. Hemolysis takes place both intra- and extravascularly, causing occlusion in the microcirculation.

The *symptoms* and *complications* include a history of chronic hemolytic anemia with jaundice (usually beginning in childhood), recurrent abdominal and limb pain, recurrent pneumonialike symptoms from infections and vascular occlusive episodes, possible delayed skeletal and sexual maturation, cardiomegaly, heart murmurs, dyspnea on exertion, palpitations, pleurisy, episodic abdominal pain, hepatomegaly (without tenderness), altered splenic functioning, splenomegaly, the inability to concentrate urine, hematuria, conjunctival vessel changes, repeated vitreous hemorrhages, susceptibility to infections, and leg ulcers.

Diagnosis is based on the health history, physical exam, and the following laboratory data: blood studies reveal a normal RBC (usually), increased or reduced MCV, decreased ESR, morphologic distortions (poikilocytosis, anisocytosis, and the presence of target cells and Heinz bodies), elevated plasma proteins, and possible elevated WBC and platelet count. Bone marrow aspiration reveals an increased erythroid mass. Sickling tests induce the sickling phenomenon, identify Hb S, and screen the trait.

Common interventions

Medical treatment for an acute episode involves a blood transfusion with normal RBCs, O_2 therapy, analgesics, antibiotics, management of acidosis, treatment and control of complications, and administration of urea. In addition, genetic counseling is provided.

Nursing interventions

Physical 1. Refer to nursing interventions for generalized anemia (*see above*).
2. Maintain the patient on bed rest.
3. Maintain the transfusion and IV therapy.
4. Prevent dehydration.
5. Maintain O_2 therapy.
6. Assess and prevent or treat specific symptoms of disease-related complications, especially respiratory infections, cardiac arrhythmias, and leg ulcers.
7. Assess and prevent complications and pathologic fractures.
8. Prepare the patient for cholecystectomy, if indicated.
9. Screen the family members for the sickle trait.
Psychosocial 10. Provide the patient and family with emotional support related to chronic illness, genetic disease, and crises.
Educational 11. Provide genetic counseling.
12. Teach the patient and family how to deal with crises and prevent complications.

Evaluation criteria. *See* Overview. Increased intervals between crises; evidence of genetic screening and counseling.

HEMOPHILIA

Hemophilia is a hereditary clotting disorder that causes severe hemorrhagic diathesis. It is subdivided into types A and B. Type A is the most common coagulation disorder, and it affects males with a genetic aberration. Type B is less common than type A, and it improves with increasing age. The genetic cause of both types is an X-linked recessive trait that produces a deficiency of factor VIII in type A and a deficiency of factor IX in type B. The classification and *symptoms* for both types are as follows. In "subhemophilia," 25 to 50% of the factor is present, and moderate bleeding follows trauma or surgery. In the mild stage, 5 to 25% of the factor is present, and unsuspected and serious bleeding occurs from trauma or surgery. In the moderate stage, 2 to 5% of the factor is present, and infrequent spontaneous bleeding and hemarthrosis occur, as well as serious bleeding from trivial injuries. In the severe stage, 0 to 2% of the factor is present, and severe, frequent bleeding and hemarthrosis occur. Crippling is common in this stage. The symptoms of hemarthrosis include pain, limited range of motion of the affected joint (which may be flexed, but may be warm, distended, and discolored), muscle spasm, thickening of the synovia, and crippling. Other *complications* include SC and IM hematomas, with resultant increased pressure on vital organs and nerves (e.g., retroperitoneal hemorrhage); acute or chronic GI or GU bleeding; delayed bleeding, occurring hours or days after trauma or injury; hemophilic cysts; poor wound healing; and exsanguination.

The *diagnosis* for type A is based on the health history, physical exam, and the following laboratory data. The coagulation time is prolonged in the severe stage, normal in other stages. The prothrombin coagulation test is abnormal in the severe stage, variable in the moderate stage, and normal in other stages. The PT is normal. The PTT is prolonged in the severe stage and the moderate stage, variable in the mild stage, and usually normal in sub-hemophilia. Thrombocytosis is related to acute or chronic hemorrhage. A factor VIII assay also is performed. The tests for type B are the same as for hemophilia A, except that a factor IX assay is performed.

Common interventions

For type A hemophilia, replacement therapy involves the IV administration of factor VIII in the form of blood or blood products, including cryoprecipitate and purified or fresh frozen citrated plasma. Additional interventions include the treatment and prevention of hemoarthrosis and bleeding. For type B hemophilia, replacement therapy involves the IV administration of factor IX in the form of blood or blood products, including citrated plasma and purified "prothrombin complex." Additional interventions are the same as for hemophilia A.

Nursing interventions

Physical 1. Stop superficial bleeding by applying ice, pressure, and topical thrombin or other medications as ordered.
2. Administer replacement therapy as ordered.
3. Administer analgesics and steroids as ordered.
4. Relieve pain.
5. Encourage bed rest but maintain movement of the joints.
6. Assess and treat continued bleeding and complications.
7. Assess the side effects of therapy.
8. Prevent injury or trauma to the patient and maintain safety.

Psychosocial 9. Provide emotional support to the patient and family during episodic bleeding.

10. Provide emotional support to the patient and family related to genetic disease, chronic illness, and a debilitating disease process.

11. Identify and discuss with the patient and family necessary adaptations in life-style to prevent complications.

12. Provide Medic-Alert identification.

Educational 13. Teach the patient and family the basic pathophysiology related to the disease process and its complications.

14. Teach the patient and family measures to avoid the causes and sources of bleeding and complications, especially trauma and elective surgery.

15. Teach the patient and family the assessment of bleeding.

16. Instruct the patient to inform physicians and dentists about the condition.

17. Obtain genetic counseling for the patient and family.

18. Have the family members screened for the genetic trait.

Evaluation criteria. *See* Overview. Evidence of genetic counseling and family screening.

HYPERSPLENISM

Hypersplenism is the exaggeration of normal splenic activities. In primary hypersplenism, the underlying pathology is not determined. In secondary hypersplenism, the underlying pathology includes infectious, parasitic, or storage diseases, leukemia, lymphosarcoma, and congestive splenomegaly.

Symptoms include anemia, leukemia, and thrombocytopenia (either singly or in combination), cellular bone marrow, splenomegaly, and hypervolemia. Hemorrhage is a *complication*. *Diagnosis* is based on the health history, physical exam, and laboratory data, including chromium-51 (^{51}Cr)-labeled RBCs measuring RBC mass, survival in blood, and rate of mixing in the spleen, and ^{51}Cr-labeled platelets measuring their accumulation in the spleen. In addition, splenic puncture, selected angiography, and spleen scanning are used.

Common interventions

Medical interventions involve treatment of the underlying pathology. Splenectomy is the **surgical** treatment.

Nursing interventions

Physical 1. Assess anemia, leukopenia, and thrombocytopenia and prevent related complications.

2. Prepare the patient for the surgical procedure, if appropriate (*see* Chapters 9 and 11).

Psychosocial 3. Provide emotional support related to the underlying pathology.

4. Allay fear and anxiety related to the surgery.

Educational 5. Instruct the patient on pre- and postoperative management (*see* Chapters 9 and 11).

6. Instruct the patient about the underlying pathology.

Evaluation criteria. See Overview.

SPLENOMEGALY

Splenomegaly is enlargement of the spleen. Inflammatory splenomegaly is caused by acute infection and/or inflammation of the spleen and by chronic infections. Congestive splenomegaly is caused by cirrhosis of the liver and by conditions that cause occlusion of the portal and/or splenic vein. Hyperplastic splenomegaly is caused by hemolytic or chronic anemias, thrombocytopenic purpura, Graves' disease, polycythemia vera, and primary splenic neutropenia. Infiltrative splenomegaly is caused by Gaucher's disease, Niemann-Pick disease, amyloidosis, diabetic lipemia, and gargoylism. In addition, splenomegaly may be caused by benign, malignant, or metastatic tumors, or by leukemias and Hodgkin's disease. The *symptoms* and *complications* are similar to those of hypersplenism, but will pertain to the specific causes. The *diagnosis* is made on the same basis as hypersplenism (*see above*). The **medical**, **surgical**, and **nursing** interventions are the same as for hypersplenism (*see above*).

IDIOPATHIC THROMBOCYTOPENIC PURPURA (ITP)

ITP is a condition that produces thrombocytopenia without apparent exogenous etiologic factors. It is the most common form of thrombocytopenia, and occurs most frequently in children and young adults. Its etiology is unknown, but immunologic factors are suspected. Acute ITP occurs in children of 2 to 6 yr of age, is preceded by infection (1 to 3 wk), and is marked by the abrupt onset of bleeding and a low platelet count. It lasts 4 to 6 wk, and remits spontaneously. Chronic ITP occurs in young adults of 20 to 40 yr of age, and is marked by the insidious onset of bleeding and a decreased platelet count. It may last months or years, and its course fluctuates. *Symptoms* include fever, mild to moderate bleeding (petechiae of the skin and mucous membranes, superficial ecchymosis, bleeding from superficial cuts, excessive bleeding after trauma, vesicles or bullae of the mouth, epistaxis, and GI and GU bleeding), intracranial hemorrhage, aplastic anemia, and mild splenomegaly. The *diagnosis* is based on the health history, physical exam, and laboratory data. Platelets may be found to be totally absent or only slightly decreased in number. They are abnormal in size, morphology, and functioning. Anemia is proportional to blood loss. Blood coagulation tests reveal a prolonged bleeding time, absent or abnormal clot retraction, and an abnormal prothrombin consumption time (PCT). Bone marrow aspiration reveals megakaryocytes and hyperplasia, if blood loss is great.

Common interventions

Medical interventions include steroid therapy and the treatment of bleeding symptoms and their complications. Splenectomy is the **surgical** treatment.

Nursing interventions

Physical 1. Assess for signs of bleeding.
2. Stop the bleeding.
3. Administer steroid therapy and assess for the side effects of medication.
4. Prevent infection and trauma or injury to the patient.
5. Maintain safety measures.
6. Assess and treat the symptoms and complications.
7. Prepare the patient for diagnostic procedures, especially the bone marrow exam.
8. Assess and prevent bleeding after diagnostic procedures.
9. Prepare the patient for splenectomy.
10. Assess and prevent bleeding postoperatively.
11. Provide Medic-Alert identification.

Psychosocial 12. Provide emotional support to the patient and family during the acute phase.
13. Provide emotional support related to chronic illness, if appropriate.
14. Allay fear and anxiety related to the diagnosis and prognosis.
15. Provide support for the patient related to the appearance of superficial bleeding.
16. Provide care before and after diagnostic procedures and surgical treatment.

Educational 17. Teach the patient and family the basic pathophysiology related to the disease process, complications, and medical management.
18. Teach the patient and family the proper administration and side effects of medication.
19. Teach the patient and family how to prevent infection, and how to assess bleeding signs and control bleeding.

Evaluation criteria.   See Overview.

DISSEMINATED INTRAVASCULAR COAGULATION

Disseminated intravascular coagulation (DIC) is a syndrome that produces an accelerated turnover of various coagulation factors in the blood, resulting in diffuse coagulation within the arterioles and capillaries. Causes include obstetric conditions, infections, neoplasms, hematopoietic dysfunction, vascular disorders, and massive tissue injury. DIC is *characterized* by diffusion of fibrin deposits within the arterioles and capillaries, diffuse clotting, and hemorrhage from the kidneys, brain, adrenals, heart, and other organs. Acute *symptoms* include abrupt, severe bleeding and thromboembolic manifestations. Chronic symptoms are superficial, but extensive ecchymosis, recurrent episodes of bleeding, thrombophlebitis at unusual sites, and the symptoms of the underlying pathology. *Complications* include hypovolemia with decreased perfusion to vital organs, acute renal failure, and shock. *Diagnosis* is based on the health history, physical exam, and the following laboratory data: plasma fibrinogen level, thrombin time, low platelet count and high increase in fibrinolysis, possible increase in fibrinogen degradation products (FDP), and prolonged PTT and PT.

Common interventions

Treatment includes the administration of anticoagulants and the replacement of platelets and coagulation factors.

Nursing interventions

Physical 1. Assess bleeding and the amount of blood loss.
2. Assess, treat, and/or prevent complications.
3. Administer anticoagulants as ordered.
4. Administer replacement therapy.
5. Protect the patient from trauma or injury and maintain safety measures.
Psychosocial 6. Provide emotional support for the patient and family related to the disease pathology and prognosis.
7. Provide Medic-Alert identification.
Educational 8. Teach the patient and family the basic pathophysiology related to the disease process, complications, and management.
9. Teach the patient to administer medication, if appropriate.
10. Teach the patient to observe for the side effects of medication.
11. Teach the patient to assess for bleeding and complications and how to manage them.

Evaluation criteria. *See* Overview.

POLYCYTHEMIA VERA

Polycythemia vera is an increased production of RBCs, resulting in an expanded blood volume. It is comparatively common in Jews, and more common in males. Its etiology is unknown. *Symptoms*, which occur insidiously, include polycythemia rubra vera, headache, dizziness, tinnitus, visual disturbances, dyspnea, weakness, ascites, and pruritus. *Complications* include hypertension, CHF, increased potential for respiratory infections, decreased peripheral vascular circulation, bleeding into the skin and mucous membranes, GI and GU bleeding, spleno- and hepatomegaly, and thrombus formation with occlusion of vessels in the heart (MI), lower extremities (gangrene), lungs (pulmonary embolism), and brain (cerebrovascular accident). *Diagnosis* is based on the health history, physical exam, bone marrow aspiration (dark red and hyperplasia of all elements), blood studies (increased RBC, Hb, WBC, platelets, and total blood volume; decreased MCV, MCH, and MCHC), and urinalysis (albuminuria).

Common interventions

Treatment includes venesection or phlebotomy, irradiation of bones, chemotherapy, and treatment of the symptoms and complications.

Nursing interventions

Physical 1. Assess the symptoms, the sites of bleeding, and the amount of blood loss.
2. Administer medications as ordered and assess for side effects.
3. Assess for complications, including cerebrovascular accident, MI, pulmonary emboli, and gangrene.
4. Prevent and/or treat complications.
5. Prepare the patient for phlebotomy.
6. Assess for side effects of irradiation.
7. Force fluids.
8. Maintain accurate intake and output records.
Psychosocial 9. Provide emotional support to the patient and family related to the diagnosis, crises, and prognosis.
10. Provide Medic-Alert identification.
Educational 11. Teach the patient and family the basic pathology related to the disease process and treatment.
12. Teach the patient to assess bleeding, prevent complications, and manage them.
13. Teach the patient to avoid trauma, injury, and elective surgery.
14. Teach the patient to advise physicians, dentists, and nurses about the disease.

Evaluation criteria. See Overview.

THE LIVER

OVERVIEW

The liver is a complex organ that is responsible for many regulatory, digestive, and other biochemical functions in the body. Diseases and disorders of the liver and the hepatic system have local (e.g., enlargement and portal hypertension) and general systemic effects (e.g., altered blood coagulation and utilization of nutrients).

This section focuses on the function and diseases of the hepatic system. It includes a brief description of the anatomy and physiology of the liver, the procedures for general assessment of the hepatic system, and the interventions most commonly used. The diseases and conditions discussed include inflammatory and infectious diseases, neoplasms, cirrhosis, and emergency conditions due to trauma or toxicity.

Anatomy and physiology review

The normal liver lies directly beneath the diaphragm in the upper right quadrant of the abdomen. Most of the liver is covered by a thin fibrous capsule. The surfaces of the liver include the convex diaphragmatic surface: the anterior, superior, right, and posterior surfaces. The visceral or inferior surface includes the posteroinferior surface. The ligaments of the liver connect it to the diaphragm and anterior abdominal wall and hold it in place. They include the coronary, left triangular, right triangular, falciform, and round ligaments. Traditionally, the four main lobes of the liver include the right and left lobe, divided by the falciform ligament, the caudate lobe, and the quadrate lobe (Fig. 21-1).

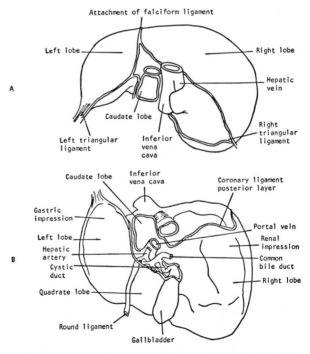

Figure 21-1. Anatomy of the liver. A, Superior aspect; B, inferior surface. *Reprinted with permission from* Orr, M. E. Acute Pancreatic and Hepatic Dysfunction. John Wiley & Sons, Inc., New York. 1981. p. 116.

Blood supply for the liver has both venous and arterial sources. The portal vein transports blood and nutrients from the digestive system. The hepatic artery carries oxygenated blood from the aorta through the celiac artery. The nerve supply is derived from the left vagus nerve and the sympathetic celiac plexus. The porta hepatis runs between the two main lobes of the liver on the inferior surface and contains (1) the right and left branches of the hepatic artery, portal vein, and hepatic ducts, (2) lymphatic vessels, and (3) nerves. The anatomic and functional units of the liver are called lobules (Fig. 21-2). Each lobule contains (1) a central vein (or tributary of the hepatic vein) that passes through the center of each lobule and transports blood to the hepatic vein and, eventually, to the inferior vena cava, (2) hepatic cellular plates, which are two liver cells thick and lie between the biliary canaliculi, which transport bile from the liver cells to the larger bile ducts known as intralobular ducts, (3) hepatic sinusoids, which transport blood from the portal venules and hepatic arterioles to the central vein and contain two types of cells (endothelial cells, which allow for diffusion of plasma proteins, and reticuloendothelial cells, known as Kupffer cells, which are phagocytic), and (4) terminal lymphatics. The intralobular septa contain intralobular ducts, which eventually merge to form two main bile ducts, one from each main lobe of the liver. These two join to form the hepatic duct. In addition, the septa contain portal venules, which transport blood from the portal vein, and hepatic arterioles, which transport blood from the hepatic artery.

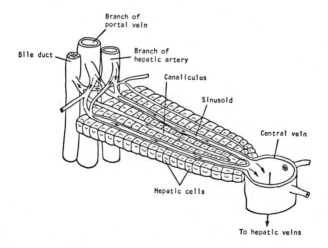

Figure 21-2. Schematic representation of a liver lobule. *Reprinted with permission from* Orr, M. E. Acute Pancreatic and Hepatic Dysfunction. John Wiley & Sons, Inc., New York. 1981. p. 118.

The functions of the liver include carbohydrate metabolism (storing glycogen, converting galactose and fructose to glucose, glyconeogenesis, and forming chemical compounds), fat metabolism (forming acetoacetic acid, lipoproteins, cholesterol, and phospholipids, and converting carbohydrates and fats to proteins), protein metabolism (deamination of amino acids, forming urea and plasma proteins, and synthesizing amino acids and chemical compounds from them), bile formation and excretion, vitamin storage (i.e., A, D, and B complex), iron storage, and the formation of coagulation factors (fibrinogen, prothrombin, acceleration globulin, and factor VII).

General assessment

The **health history** includes an assessment of current health status (nutrition, elimination, and use/abuse of drugs or alcohol), the past health history (liver disease, disorder, or infection, and bleeding tendencies or disorders), the family history (alcoholism, blood disorders, jaundice, and anemia), and the social history (contact with chemicals or other toxic agents). The **physical exam** includes skin, abdominal, cerebral, and neurologic assessment. The skin is assessed for jaundice, noting color of the skin, sclera, and mucous membranes. Several factors can cause jaundice: destruction of RBCs, causing excessive bilirubin production; hepatic dysfunction, in which the liver is unable to conjugate bilirubin; and obstruction, in which conjugated bilirubin is not able to be excreted. In addition, the skin is assessed for evidence of bleeding (petechiae, ecchymosis, purpura, or bleeding from any orifice). The abdomen is assessed for ascites (daily weights, accurate intake and output records, and daily measurements of abdominal girth), hepato- and splenomegaly, and hepatojugular reflex. Cerebral assessment for hepatic encephalopathy includes level of consciousness (mild confusion to deep coma), personality changes, and changes in memory, attention span, and the ability to concentrate. In addition, the EEG may show delta waves. Neurologic assessment includes changes in fine motor skills and flapping tremor or asterixis.

Diagnosis is based on the health history, physical exam, and the following elevated laboratory values: bilirubin (direct or conjugated and indirect or unconjugated), urine or fecal urobilinogen, serum enzymes (SGOT, SGPT, alkaline phosphatase), PT, lipids, cholesterol, and blood ammonia levels. Other important tests in the diagnostic work-up include hepatic scanning (to denote the normal contour and condition of the liver and to detect masses, cysts, and abscesses), ultrasound studies of the liver (to denote lesions and abscesses), percutaneous needle liver biopsy (to test the pathologic and microscopic status of liver cells), and hepatic angiography (to visualize the liver's arterial blood supply). In addition, certain antigen studies are helpful in diagnosing liver disease: hepatitis B surface antigen (HBsAg), which indicates the presence of hepatitis B infection; hepatitis B surface antibody (anti-HBs), which is indicative of passive immunity to hepatitis B; and e antigen, which may indicate chronic active hepatitis.

Common interventions

Medical treatment includes adequate rest, proper diet, and avoidance of hepatotoxic medications. **Surgical** interventions include paracentesis, liver biopsy, and shunts.

Paracentesis.   A paracentesis is the aspiration of accumulated fluid from the peritoneal cavity for the purposes of fluid analysis and relief of abdominal pressure caused by excessive fluid. **Nursing** interventions for this procedure include the following:

1. Before the procedure, advise the patient of the procedure and obtain written consent, have the patient void immediately before the procedure, position the patient sitting upright with feet and back supported, cleanse the skin with antiseptic solution, and assess base-line vital signs.
2. During the procedure, monitor vital signs, assess for signs of hypovolemia and shock, and reassure the patient.
3. After the procedure, monitor vital signs, assess peripheral vascular circulation, apply a sterile pressure dressing to the puncture site, administer salt-poor albumin if ordered, and check the dressing for drainage or bleeding.

Liver biopsy.   A liver biopsy is a surgical procedure in which liver tissue is obtained percutaneously for microscopic examination. **Nursing** responsibilities and interventions include the following:

1. Before the procedure, explain what is to be done, obtain written permission for the exam, obtain and evaluate the PT, administer vitamin K as ordered, obtain base-line vital signs, keep the patient NPO, administer sedation, cleanse the skin with an antiseptic solution, and position the patient supine.
2. During the procedure, instruct the patient to hold his breath while the needle is inserted, when the tissue is obtained, and when the needle is removed.
3. After the procedure, maintain the patient on bed rest, position the patient on the right side, monitor vital signs, and check the dressing for bleeding.

Shunts.   Shunts are the surgical diversion of blood from its usual to an alternative route. Their purposes are to decrease the work of the liver by decreasing the volume of blood brought to the liver, to decrease portal hypertension by decreasing congestion, and to relieve the distension of esophageal varices. Three types of shunts are currently performed. The portacaval shunt is a side-to-side or end-to-side anastomosis of the portal vein to the inferior vena cava. The splenorenal shunt is an end-to-side anastomosis of the splenic vein, following splenectomy, to the renal vein. The mesocaval shunt is an end-to-side anastomosis of the inferior vena cava to the superior mesenteric vein. Complications of these procedures include thrombosis, fluid and electrolyte imbalance, shock, metabolic and respiratory alkalosis, hepatic encephalopathy, delirium tremens, and seizures. Pre-operative **nursing** interventions are the same as for those for the patient undergoing any surgical procedure (*see* Chapter 9). Interventions specific to the patient with liver disease include the following:

1. Maintain blood transfusions before surgery if the patient is anemic.
2. Provide nursing care related to the medical management of ascites (*see below*).
3. Administer diuretics, albumin, and vitamin K as ordered.

Postoperative interventions are the same as for general postoperative care (*see* Chapter 11). Specific interventions include the following:

1. Maintain blood transfusions and IV therapy as ordered.
2. Maintain O_2 therapy.
3. Assess for signs of hypovolemia.
4. Assess for signs of decreasing portal hypertension (absence of ascites, decreased esophageal varices, and decreased evidence of anemia, leukopenia, and thrombocytopenia).
5. Assess for signs of hepatic encephalopathy (*see below*).
6. Teach the patient and family the components of the diet.
7. Reinforce the need to avoid or minimize alcohol intake.
8. Teach the patient to avoid hepatotoxic drugs.
9. Teach the patient and family the signs and symptoms of encepha-lopathy.

Evaluation criteria. Absence or reduction of symptoms. Absence or early detection and treatment of complications. Blood values, vital signs, and level of consciousness within normal limits. Control of underlying pathol-ogy. Patient and family verbalize health teaching and adaptation of life-style as appropriate. Patient and family participate in follow-up care.

PORTAL HYPERTENSION

Portal hypertension is an elevated pressure gradient throughout the portal (hepatic) venous system. Its physiologic causes are increased resistance to hepatic blood flow and increased splanchnic (abdominal) blood flow. Con-tributing factors are cirrhosis, tumors, local inflammation (hepatitis, pancreatitis, or abscess), schistosomiasis, arteriovenous fistulas, and hematologic disorders (e.g., polycythemia vera, lymphoma, or leukemia).

Signs and symptoms include splenomegaly, increased collateral circula-tion as evidenced by varices and caput medusa (engorged tortuous veins radiating from the umbilicus), ascites, and a venous hum at the umbilicus. *Complications* include rupture of the esophageal, gastric, or hemorrhoidal varices. *Diagnosis* is based on the health history, physical exam, laboratory tests for hypoalbuminemia, and the presence of increased portal pressure.

Common interventions

Medical interventions treat the underlying problem(s). **Surgical** treatment involves the use of shunts (*see above*). **Nursing** interventions are the same as for ascites (*see below*), paracentesis, and shunts (*see above*).

ASCITES

Ascites is fluid (lymph) collection in the peritoneal cavity. It is most commonly seen with cirrhosis. The primary causes are decreased plasma colloidal osmotic pressure (hypoalbuminemia), elevated hydrostatic pressure in the hepatic sinusoids, and increased permeability of the peritoneal capillaries (in neoplastic and inflammatory diseases). Contributing causes are portal hypertension and increased plasma aldosterone due to increased renal secretion of aldosterone in response to renin-angiotensin stimulation as well as reduced metabolism by the liver. Ascites results from the increased transudation of lymphatic fluid due to changes in pressure or permeability of the vessels. *Signs and symptoms* include abdominal distension, dullness on percussion, fluid waves on tapping, elevated diaphragm, increasing weight, and decreasing urine output. *Diagnosis* is based on the health history, physical exam, and the following laboratory data: (1) hypoalbuminemia, and (2) decreased sodium and increased potassium in the urine.

Common interventions

Medical treatment includes a low-sodium diet, fluid restriction, albumin, and diuretics. **Surgical** treatment includes paracentesis and hepatic shunts.

Nursing interventions

Physical 1. Maintain diet and fluid restrictions.
2. Administer medications as ordered.
3. Assess and report the side effects of medications.
4. Monitor intake and output accurately.
5. Weigh the patient daily.
6. Measure abdominal girth every shift.
7. Elevate the head of the bed (semi- to high-Fowler's position).
8. Turn and position the patient q 2 hr.
9. Assess and treat the skin for breakdown.
10. Prepare for procedures (*see above*).
Psychosocial 11. Encourage verbalization of fears and concerns.
12. Reinforce the expected effects of the treatment plan.
13. Inform the patient about the positive responses to treatment (e.g., decreased weight and abdominal girth).
Educational 14. Explain the rationale for the treatment plan.
15. Teach the patient about the procedures.

16. Teach the patient and family about the low-sodium diet and fluid restrictions, the need for and side effects of medications, measuring abdominal girth, daily weights, and reporting any unexpected changes to a physician immediately.

Evaluation criteria.   *See* Overview.

HEPATIC ENCEPHALOPATHY

Hepatic encephalopathy is disordered brain functioning as a result of metabolic changes. Causative factors include severe liver dysfunction, portal collateral circulation through the peripheral circulation, and disturbances of ammonia metabolism. Contributing factors are hypoxia, electrolyte and acid-base imbalance, infection, and depressant drugs.

Symptoms include disturbances of consciousness, changes in personality (depression, irritability, anxiety, paranoia, and the loss of concern for person and/or property), mental confusion (memory loss and an inability to concentrate), slow and slurred speech, changes in fine motor skills, asterixis or "liver flap" (a flapping tremor of hand when extended), increased muscle tone, clonus (rapid flexion and extension of the muscles), and ataxia. *Complications* include convulsions, coma, and death. *Diagnosis* is based on the health history, physical exam, and an elevated serum ammonia level.

Common interventions

Medical treatment involves reducing protein and ammonia levels, and maintaining the fluid and electrolyte balance.

Nursing interventions

Physical 1. Provide a diet low in protein.
2. Administer cathartics and enemas to help eliminate protein.
3. Administer neomycin as ordered to help eliminate the bacteria that produce ammonia in the intestines.
4. Prevent hypovolemia by assessing fluid status, intake and output, and weight, and by maintaining fluid balance (PO and IV).
5. Monitor vital signs and CVP.
6. Monitor electrolytes.
7. Assess and prevent hypoxia.
8. Administer O_2 therapy as ordered.
9. Avoid all medications that may be hepatotoxic or that detoxify in the liver.
10. Prevent infection.
11. Avoid depressant drugs.
Psychosocial 12. Provide emotional support to the patient and family.
13. Allay fears and anxiety related to the changes produced by hepatic encephalopathy.

14. Reassure that the symptoms may be reversible with treatment.
Educational 15. Teach the patient about the underlying pathology.
16. Teach the patient to avoid contributing factors.
17. Teach the patient to monitor fluid balance.
18. Teach the patient to avoid infection.

Evaluation criteria. See Overview.

TRAUMA

Injury to the liver constitutes 30 to 35% of all abdominal injuries. These injuries may be open (penetrating) or closed (blunt). *Symptoms* of open injury include evidence of penetration and signs of hemorrhage and shock. The symptoms of closed injury are pain and tenderness in the upper right quadrant, ascites, and signs of hemorrhage and shock. *Complications* of liver trauma include hemorrhage and shock. *Diagnosis* is based on the health history, physical exam, and laboratory data of standard liver function studies (*see above*).

Common interventions

Emergency surgery involves the repair of vessels and tears, liver resection, and the insertion of a drain.

Nursing interventions

Physical 1. Monitor vital signs and intake and output.
2. Assess for signs of hemorrhage and shock.
3. Relieve pain (including the administration of analgesics as ordered).
4. Preoperative interventions are the same as those presented in Chapter 9. (Use preoperative medications cautiously.)
5. Postoperative interventions are the same as those presented in Chapter 11.
6. Assess for signs of postoperative complications, including jaundice, portal hypertension, hemolysis, hepatic toxicity from the anesthesia, hemorrhage, and infection.
Psychosocial 7. Allay the fears and anxieties of the patient and family related to the emergency situation.
8. Provide emotional support pre- and postoperatively.
9. Provide emotional support for the patient and family related to the origin of the trauma or injury.

Evaluation criteria. See Overview.

ESOPHAGEAL VARICES

Esophageal varices are swollen, dilated esophageal veins that result from increased pressure on the collateral portal channels in the esophagus. They are complications of cirrhosis and portal hypertension from any cause. The bleeding is induced by direct trauma or irritation to the esophagus from food and gastric juices, increased intra-abdominal pressure, and increased thoracic pressure. *Symptoms* include sudden and profuse bright red blood from the esophagus, liver dysfunction, and increased bleeding tendencies. *Complications* include rupture of the varices and hemorrhage. *Diagnosis* is based on the health history, physical exam, and laboratory data of standard liver function studies (*see above*).

Common interventions

Medical treatment involves the insertion of a Sengstaken-Blakemore (S-B) tube, in which inflated balloons apply pressure to stop the bleeding. (Ice may also be circulated through the tube.) **Surgical** treatment may involve a shunt procedure (*see above*).

Nursing interventions

Physical 1. Assist in the insertion of the S-B tube.
2. Maintain the ice circulation if ordered.
3. Use the suction range for the amount of blood.
4. Monitor vital signs, including CVP.
5. Keep the patient NPO.
6. Maintain IV therapy as ordered (fluid and blood replacement).
7. Provide mouth care and oral suctioning.
8. Provide care to the nasal mucosa.
9. Deflate the balloon as ordered and assess for bleeding.
10. Administer sedation as ordered.
Psychosocial 11. Provide emotional support to the patient and family during hemorrhaging, S-B tube insertion, and afterward.
12. Provide a calm and quiet atmosphere.
Educational 13. Teach the patient and family the signs of hemorrhage.
14. Teach the patient and family that the patient should avoid aspirin, alcohol, constipation, heavy lifting, and exertive coughing.
15. Teach the patient to chew food well and use antacids.

Evaluation criteria. See Overview.

HEPATIC TOXIC STATUS

Hepatic toxic status results from the inability of the liver to detoxify exo- and endogenous substances. Causes include exposure to toxic chemicals, excessive ingestion of hepatotoxic drugs or chemicals, excessive ingestion of alcohol over time, and hypersensitive reactions. *Symptoms* — which result from necrosis of the liver cells, interference with normal liver cellular functioning, and changes in bile formation — resemble those of acute viral hepatitis without fever (*see below*). Other symptoms are augmented and prolonged drug action, and endocrine disorders from altered metabolic functioning. Irreversible liver damage is a *complication*. *Diagnosis* is based on the health history, physical exam, a liver biopsy, and the following laboratory data: abnormal liver function studies (*see* viral hepatitis *below*) and increased serum level of drugs or anesthetics.

Common interventions

Medical treatment involves removing hepatotoxins from the GI tract and avoidance of contact (if possible), administering antidotes (if known), maintaining the patient on bed rest, treating complications, reducing dietary protein, and maintaining fluid and electrolyte balance.

Nursing interventions

Physical 1. Maintain the patient on bed rest.
2. Do not administer medicines that detoxify in the liver.
3. Assess liver functioning, including jaundice, ascites, hemolysis, and hepatic encephalopathy.
4. Maintain adequate nutrition but low dietary protein.
5. Treat and prevent complications, including immobility.
6. Identify the sources of toxicity.
7. Prevent bleeding and bruising.
8. Assess level of consciousness or coma.
9. Assess and maintain respirations.
Psychosocial 10. Allay fear and anxiety related to acute toxicity.
11. Help the patient to identify the sources of toxicity.
12. Help the patient to identify ways to avoid toxic substances.
13. Provide support for adaptations in life-style necessary to avoid toxic agents.
14. Provide counseling, if appropriate.
15. Identify support groups.
Educational 16. Teach the patient the basic pathophysiology related to toxicity and liver function.
17. Teach the patient ways in which to avoid toxic substances.

Evaluation criteria. *See* Overview.

VIRAL HEPATITIS

Viral hepatitis is an infection of the liver by either of two types of viruses: Type A (acute infectious hepatitis) which has a short incubation period of 2 to 6 wk; or type B (serum hepatitis) which has a long incubation period of 6 wk to 6 mo. Type A is endemic or epidemic; type B shows an increasing prevalence over type A. The etiologic factors of hepatitis A and B are presented in Table 21-3.

The *symptoms* of acute viral hepatitis are the same for types A and B. The symptoms of the anicteric phase are similar to those of other viral infections, and are identified only with an epidemic outbreak. Symptoms of the pre-

TABLE 21-3
Etiologic Factors of Hepatitis A and B

Factor	Hepatitis A	Hepatitis B
Virus	Hepatitis A	Hepatitis B
Source	Poor sanitary conditions (e.g., contaminated feces, water, or shellfish).	Contaminated blood.
Transmission	Usually, fecal-oral route; occasionally parenteral route.	Usually, parenteral route: (1) blood transfusion; (2) inadequately sterilized needles, syringes, and other equipment; or (3) nosocomial/accidental exposure of hospital personnel who handle blood products (e.g., OR/dialysis unit staff and laboratory technicians). Occasionally, fecal-oral route. Insect vectors (mosquitoes and bedbugs) in endemic areas (e.g., West Africa).

icteric phase include fever, anorexia, headache, myalgia, pain and tenderness in the upper right quadrant, joint pains, rashes, abrupt onset with type A, and vague onset with type B. The symptoms of the icteric phase are increasing GI symptoms (anorexia, nausea, and vomiting), increasing upper right quadrant pain and tenderness, increasing jaundice, hepatomegaly, splenomegaly, dark urine, and pale stools. The symptoms of the convalescent phase are variable tiredness and malaise and mild hepatic tenderness (both may be precipitated by unaccustomed activity). *Complications* are the same for types A and B: hepatitis with predominant cholestasis, massive hepatic necrosis (fulminant hepatitis), submassive hepatic necrosis (subacute hepatic necrosis), prolonged or recurrent hepatitis, and chronic, aggressive hepatitis. With type A, there is active immunity after infection. With type B, there is passive immunity with anti-HBs immune globulin and active immunity after infection.

Diagnosis is based on the health history, physical exam, and the following laboratory data: blood studies (normal to mild decrease in Hb and Hct, normal to reduced WBC, mild reduction in RBC, and slight increase in ESR) and urinalysis (increased urobilinogen and bilirubin and mild proteinuria).

In the icteric phase, there is increased direct and indirect bilirubin, serum transaminase, alkaline phosphatase, and sulfobromophthalein (BSP) retention.

Common interventions

Prophylactic measures for hepatitis A include proper sanitation and hand washing, careful screening of food handlers, avoidance of areas known to have endemic or epidemic hepatitis A, and administration of immune serum globulin (ISG). Preexposure administration of ISG is recommended for individuals planning to reside in tropical or developing countries. Post-exposure administration of ISG is recommended within 2 wk for individuals having close personal contact with an infected patient. It is not recommended for contacts in schools or hospitals unless an outbreak of hepatitis A is evidenced.

Prophylactic measures for hepatitis B include screening of blood donors, proper sterilization of equipment used in transfusions and surgery, safe handling of blood products by hospital personnel, and administration of ISG or hepatitis B immune globulin (HBIG). Preexposure prophylaxis is recommended for individuals having repeated exposure to hepatitis B virus (HBV) (e.g., patients and staff in hemodialysis units). Postexposure prophylaxis is recommended for persons accidentally punctured by contaminated needles and for spouses of patients with HBV.

Therapeutic measures for hepatitis include the avoidance of fatigue (bed rest in the early symptomatic stage, and limited activity for the patient who is jaundiced but otherwise asymptomatic) and adequate nutrition (low-fat, high-protein, and high-carbohydrate diet; IV glucose supplements as necessary; and vitamin therapy as necessary). Limited use of medications and the avoidance of hepatotoxic drugs (e.g., sedatives [except oxazepam] and narcotics) is also advised. Steroids are not recommended in acute hepatitis. In chronic active hepatitis, steroids (e.g., prednisone) and antimetabolites (e.g., azathioprine [Imuran]) may be helpful. Surgery should be avoided.

Nursing interventions

Physical 1. Assess for ascites, jaundice, hemolysis, hepatic encephalopathy, and bleeding.
  2. Prevent fatigue by maintaining the patient on complete bed rest during the early symptomatic phase and by limiting activity when the patient is asymptomatic except for jaundice.
  3. Maintain isolation as indicated (stool precautions with separate bathroom/commode facilities, syringe and needle precautions, linen precautions, gown and gloves worn by staff having direct patient contact, disposable dishes, and scrupulous hand washing).
  4. Maintain the patient on a balanced diet with small, frequent feedings.
  5. Do not administer drugs that detoxify in the liver or are hepatotoxic.

6. Prevent infection, bleeding, and bruising.
7. Provide good skin care.
8. Prevent complications related to prolonged bed rest.

Psychosocial 9. Provide emotional support related to prolonged bed rest and isolation.

10. Provide emotional support to the patient and family related to the disease process and prognosis.

Educational 11. Teach the basic pathophysiology related to the disease process and medical management.

12. Teach the patient and family the need for, and the techniques of, proper hand washing, hygiene, and care of linens.
13. Teach the patient to increase activity progressively and to rest frequently or when tired.
14. Reinforce patient avoidance of preparing meals or handling food if he is discharged with active hepatitis.
15 Teach the patient the correct administration and side effects of medications received for chronic hepatitis.
16. Reinforce the need for the patient to inform physicians and dentists of the hepatitis, to avoid being a blood donor, and to avoid or limit the use of alcohol.

Evaluation criteria. See Overview.

PARASITISM

Parasitism, a result of seeding ova in the portal areas, causes an inflammatory response with resulting fibrotic changes in the liver. Its incidence is higher in tropical climates, but is increasing in the USA because of rapid air travel. (Specific infections vary with geographic locales.) Causes include amoebas (*Entamoeba histolytica* or malarial parasites), schistosomes (*Schistosoma mansoni*), flukes (*Clonorchis sinensis* or *Fasciola hepatica*), and tapeworms (*Echinococcus granulosus*). *Symptoms* are the same as for acute viral hepatitis (*see above*). In the later stages, there is evidence of portal hypertension (ascites, splenomegaly, esophageal and gastric varices, hemorrhoids, and venous hum). *Complications* include rupture of the esophageal varices and infection of other organs. *Diagnosis* is based on the health history, physical exam, liver and rectal biopsies to detect the presence of ova, and the following laboratory data: elevated alkaline phosphatase and BSP, normal liver function tests, and the presence of ova in the stools.

Common interventions

Medical treatment is the same as for hepatitis (*see above*). In addition, medications that are specific for the causative microbe are given. **Surgical** treatment includes a portacaval shunt to reduce portal hypertension and complications.

Nursing interventions

Physical 1. Refer to nursing interventions for hepatitis *(see above)*.
2. Administer medications as ordered.
3. Assess for the side effects of medication.
4. Assess for signs of portal hypertension.
5. Treat and prevent complications.
6. Culture stools, sputum, and urine.
7. Provide pre- and postoperative care for shunts *(see above)*.
Psychosocial 8. Provide emotional support related to bed rest, isolation, and surgery.
9. Identify the sources of the microbes.
10. Help the patient to identify the life-style adaptations necessary to avoid parasites.
Educational 11. Teach the patient the proper administration of medications and their side effects.
12. Teach the patient to avoid contact with the sources of the microbes.

Evaluation criteria. *See* Overview.

CANCER OF THE LIVER

Malignant tumors of the liver cells or bile ducts may be either primary or metastatic. They are more common in males and in Orientals. The average age of development is 60 to 70 yr. Factors associated with liver cancer are prolonged postnecrotic cirrhosis, hemochromatosis, and intestinal parasites. *Symptoms* include initial weight loss followed by increased weight due to ascites and fluid retention, weakness, cachexia, anemia, abdominal pain, fever, obstructive jaundice and pruritus, abnormal liver function tests, splenomegaly, hepatomegaly with palpable tumor nodules, and a bruit or venous hum over the liver. *Complications* include bruising, bleeding, portal hypertension (with CHF, renal failure, GI bleeding, esophageal varices, and pericarditis), hepatic encephalopathy and coma, feminization in males, and masculinization in females. *Diagnosis* is based on the health history, physical exam, laboratory data (increased alkaline phosphatase, BSP test, and serum proteins), liver scan (which denotes neoplasms), and liver biopsy (needle aspiration or exploratory laparotomy).

Common interventions

Medical treatment includes chemotherapy and adjunctive or palliative radiation therapy. **Surgical** treatment for a nonmetastatic, localized tumor includes subtotal hepatectomy and lobectomy.

Nursing interventions

Physical 1. Relieve pain (including the administration of analgesics that are not hepatotoxic).

2. Position the patient comfortably and so as to assist with breathing.
3. Provide a diet low in sodium and protein.
4. Monitor fluid intake and output carefully.
5. Treat the side effects of chemotherapy and radiation therapy.
6. Provide good skin care.
7. Assess and treat complications, including ascites, anemia, bleeding, and hepatic encephalopathy.
8. Provide pre- and postoperative care (see Chapters 9 and 11).

Psychosocial 9. Provide emotional support for the patient and family related to terminal illness.
10. Provide emotional support related to altered body image from an endocrine disorder.
11. Provide emotional support related to the side effects of chemotherapy and radiation therapy.
12. Provide counseling or support groups, if appropriate.

Educational 13. Teach the patient health care related to the symptomatic relief and management of side effects.
14. Teach the patient the signs and symptoms that need immediate attention.
15. Teach the patient appropriate diet and meal planning.
16. Teach the patient to monitor his own intake and output.

Evaluation criteria. See Overview.

CIRRHOSIS

Cirrhosis results from changes in the liver architecture characterized by the nodular regeneration of parenchymal cells and the proliferation of connective tissue. The major classifications are Laennec's, biliary, and postnecrotic cirrhosis. The incidence of Laennec's cirrhosis parallels the consumption of alcohol. Biliary cirrhosis occurs most frequently in women between 40 and 60 yr of age and is more common than postnecrotic cirrhosis. Laennec's (or portal) cirrhosis is caused by alcoholism and possibly by genetic and dietary factors. Postnecrotic (posthepatic and idiopathic) cirrhosis is caused by toxic or viral hepatitis, but it may occur in the absence of a history of toxic or chronic hepatitis. Primary cirrhosis is of unknown etiology, but it may be a result of chronic intrahepatic cholestasis. Secondary biliary cirrhosis is due to chronic duct obstruction. (An infection is not always present.) Cardiac cirrhosis results from chronic CHF. Metabolic cirrhosis is due to hemochromatosis (large deposits of iron in the parenchymal tissue) or Wilson's disease, an inherited, autosomal disorder that involves degeneration of the basal ganglia and liver. Schistosomal cirrhosis is caused by flukes found in the fresh water of Africa, Asia, the Caribbean, and South America. (The *symptoms*, *complications*, *diagnosis*, and **medical** interventions for Laennec's, postnecrotic, and biliary cirrhosis are presented in Table 21-4.)

TABLE 21-4
Laennec's, Postnecrotic, and Biliary Cirrhosis

Laennec's	Postnecrotic	Biliary
Symptoms		
Insidious onset of anorexia, fatigue, and weakness.	Malaise, weakness, anorexia, jaundice, low-grade fever, spider angioma, ascites, and peripheral edema.	Early: pruritus, jaundice, dark urine, and pale stools.
Abdominal pain from hepato-megaly, gastritis, or pancreatitis. Vomiting with or without hematemesis. Gradual jaundice and ascites.		Later: cutaneous xanthoma, symptoms of cholestasis, and ascites.
Possibly symptoms of alcohol withdrawal.		
Fever, dehydration, and coma.		
Complications		
Bleeding from esophageal varices, sudden onset of ascites, hepatic encephalo-pathy and coma, signs of hepatic carcinoma, portal hypertension, anemia, and malnutrition.	Hepatic coma and bleeding from esophageal varices.	Bleeding and patho-logic fractures.
Diagnosis		
Health history and physical exam: firm and enlarged liver.	Health history and physical exam: very tender and shrunken liver; splenomegaly (mild or massive); endocrine disorders (gynecomastia and absence of axillary and pubic hair).	Health history and physical exam: firm and enlarged liver and splenomegaly.
Laboratory data		
Serum levels: increased conjugated bilirubin, increased transaminase, variable alkaline phospha-tase, decreased potassium, increased uric acid, and anemia.	Serum levels: same as for Laennec's cirrhosis; may mimic biliary cirrhosis.	Serum levels: same as for cholestasis; rising or decreased serum bilirubin.
Liver biopsy: bile stasis and parenchymal cells that are distended with fat droplets contain hyaline-eosinophilic cytoplasmic inclusions, and are infiltrated with inflammatory cells.	Liver scan: macro-nodular liver.	

Laennec's	Postnecrotic	Biliary
Medical interventions		
Cessation of alcohol intake, adequate rest, and adequate diet (high in calories and vitamins).	Limited physical activity and steroid therapy.	Supplements of fat-soluble vitamins K, A, and D, and calcium supplement.
Treatment and prevention of complications, especially bleeding, ascites, and hepatic encephalopathy and coma.	Treatment and prevention of complications.	Treatment and prevention of complications.

Nursing interventions

Physical 1. Maintain the patient on bed rest or minimal activity.
2. Relieve pain.
3. Administer medications as ordered.
4. Assess for the side effects of medications.
5. Do not administer medications that may be hepatotoxic or that detoxify in the liver.
6. Provide adequate nutrition in small, frequent feedings.
7. Administer vitamin supplements as ordered.
8. Prevent infection.
9. Provide good skin care.
10. Prevent bleeding and bruising.
11. Provide safety measures.
12. Assess and treat complications, including ascites, jaundice, hemolysis, dehydration, hepatic coma, esophageal varices, and pathologic fractures.
13. Assess and treat the underlying pathology.
14. Prevent complications related to bed rest.
15. For the postnecrotic regimen, administer steroid therapy as ordered and prevent the side effects of therapy.
Psychosocial 16. Provide emotional support for the patient and family related to the diagnosis and prognosis of the disease.
17. Provide emotional support related to prolonged bed rest.
18. Identify the sources of the underlying pathology.
19. Identify the changes in life-style needed to prevent the recurrence of cirrhosis.
20. Provide counseling or a support group for the patient and family, if appropriate.
Educational 21. Teach the patient the basic pathophysiology related to the disease process, prognosis, and management.

22. Teach the patient the proper administration and side effects of medication.
23. Teach the patient and family diet and nutritional meal planning.
24. Teach the patient and family to avoid infection.
25. Teach the patient and family to assess the signs of complications and to administer emergency treatment.

Evaluation criteria.   *See* Overview.

CHAPTER 22

ALTERED ENDOCRINE AND METABOLIC FUNCTIONING

Caroline Camuñas

OVERVIEW

A vast amount of knowledge concerning glandular functioning and metabolism exists and is increasing rapidly as research produces new discoveries. However, in many areas, knowledge is at best fragmentary and signs and symptoms of glandular disorders cannot be explained.

Endocrine diseases are often familial and are generally characterized by hormone production that is excessive, inadequate, or inappropriate. They may arise from failure of target tissue to respond normally (e.g., nephrogenic diabetes insipidus) and are increasingly recognized as being related to brain functioning. Releasing and inhibitory hypothalamic factors have been found to have important effects on the pituitary. Many patients who were once thought to have pituitary failure are now diagnosed as having a defect in hypothalamic functioning. Endocrine diseases tend to have multisystemic symptoms and can usually be treated and managed effectively. If permanent control is achieved, the patient still requires long-term follow-up.

Symptoms of endocrine diseases tend to be subtle. Changes may develop so slowly that the patient is unaware of differences in his appearance. Eventually, profound changes in appearance may result. Metastasis of cancer from nonendocrine organs to an endocrine gland can produce hypofunctioning if tissue destruction is extensive. Endocrine disorders can occasionally produce emergencies. Emergency situations include diabetic acidosis, hypoglycemia, pituitary apoplexy, thyroid storm, and myxedema coma. These conditions are difficult to treat, and their mortality rate is often high.

Anatomy and physiology review

There are two kinds of glands — exocrine and endocrine. Exocrine glands have ducts through which their secretions are released. These include the liver, part of the pancreas, and the intestinal, mammary, prostate, lacrimal, salivary, sebaceous, and sweat glands.

The secretions (hormones) of endocrine glands are released directly into the bloodstream and control the different metabolic functions of the body: the rate of chemical reactions in cells; the transport of substances across cell membranes; and other aspects of cellular metabolism, such as growth and secretion. The rate of action is variable, ranging from seconds to days and longer.

The release of hormones from glands is regulated by chemical and neurologic stimuli. Negative feedback is, in part, the chemical control for hormonal blood levels. Therefore, a rise or fall in the blood level of one hormone influences the blood level of another hormone.

Hormonal regulation is also achieved by the ANS and CNS. The CNS reacts to internal and external stimuli, which activate the hypothalamus, which, in turn, activates the pituitary. The pituitary secretions then activate the appropriate gland, e.g., the adrenal medulla or the posterior pituitary.

The ANS controls or modulates involuntary functions such as BP, heart rate, glandular secretions, and the release of renin. The CNS sends impulses to the sympathetic and parasympathetic systems, where synapses are formed at autonomic peripheral ganglia before innervating target tissue. The adrenal medulla, which is derived from embryonic tissue as autonomic ganglia (neural crest), releases epinephrine into the circulation after stimulation.

Hormones affect a wide variety of body functions. Because hormones regulate intermediary metabolism, endocrine disorders can be viewed as disturbances of regulation. Many effects of each hormone have been described. Identification of primary vs. derivative effects is difficult, since it is believed that the initial action of a hormone is amplified many times in succeeding reactions.

Altered endocrine and metabolic functioning results from hormonal imbalance. These disorders may occur by a variety of mechanisms: primary hypofunction, primary hyperfunction, secondary failure, functional disorders, end-organ failure, production of an abnormal or unusual hormone — inborn errors of metabolism, ectopic secretion of hormones, prostaglandins, and iatrogenic endocrine disease.

Specific anatomy, physiology, and assessments will be reviewed as each gland is discussed.

Common interventions

Medical treatment consists of drug and diet therapy. Drug therapy is directed toward correcting the underlying hypo- or hyperfunctioning. Diet therapy is directed toward correcting nutrient and electrolyte imbalance. **Surgery** can be performed to remove hyperfunctioning glands that do not respond to chemotherapy. Hormonal supplements may be prescribed post-operatively to correct hypofunctional states created by surgery.

Nursing interventions

Nursing interventions are varied because the patient with altered endocrine functioning has many needs. Changes in metabolism bring with them changes in appearance, personality, energy levels, and ability to cope with the stresses of daily life. In addition, some patients must have major surgery; others must modify their life-style. The nurse has four major functions in caring for the patient with endocrine disorders: provision of emotional support, accurate collection of specimens for diagnostic tests, administration of hormones, and teaching the patient to live with the disease in the best way possible.

Physical 1. Assess the patient continuously for any changes in signs or symptoms.
2. Report changes to the physician.
3. Collect specimens for laboratory tests.
   a. Begin and end all tests on time.
   b. Preserve specimens correctly.
   c. Instruct the patient and personnel about collection of the specimens.
4. Administer hormones.
   a. Know the symptoms of underdosage and overdosage.
   b. Give medications on time.
Psychosocial 5. Provide emotional support for the patient and significant others; especially consider the following: changes in appearance and personality; changes that result in exhaustion, debilitation, and inability to cope with stresses; stresses that accompany diagnostic tests and major surgery; and changes that necessitate permanent modifications in life-style, diet, or daily activities.
6. Use available resources (hospital and community) to assist the patient and family in dealing with the situation.
Educational 7. Teach for lifelong self-care (dietary requirements, administration of drugs, personal hygiene, indications of hormonal imbalance, the need for follow-up, and when to call the physician).

Evaluation criteria

Symptoms are absent or minimized. Changes in mental status are assessed. Medications are received on time. Specimens are collected appropriately. Laboratory data are within normal limits. Complications are avoided. The patient/family verbalize components of ongoing care and actively participate in care. Appointments are kept. The physician is called when problems occur.

DEVIATIONS

PITUITARY DISORDERS

In the past, the pituitary has been called the master gland because of its effect on body functioning. It is now known that the pituitary is controlled by the hypothalamus. The hypothalamus, the highest integrative center for the endocrine system and ANS, controls endocrine glands by both neural and hormonal pathways.

The pituitary, or hypophysis, is a small endocrine gland that weighs <0.5 g and is <1 cm in diameter. The gland lies in the sella turcica, at the base of the brain, and is connected to the hypothalamus by the hypophyseal stalk. The gland consists of two distinct parts: the anterior pituitary, or adenohypophysis; and the posterior pituitary, or neurohypophysis.

The hypothalamus, which secretes releasing and inhibiting factors that reach the pituitary by way of the portal vessels in the hypophyseal stalk, is mainly responsible for controlling pituitary functioning. Each pituitary hormone may have both a releasing and an inhibiting factor.

The pituitary hormones and their functions are listed in Table 22-1. Although stimulation regulates most pituitary hormones, prolactin and melanocyte-stimulating hormone (MSH) are regulated predominantly by inhibition. *General assessment* includes the health history, physical exam, and diagnostic tests. The past health history should include questions about slow growth in childhood and endocrine disorders. A review of body systems should include the integument (changes in pigmentation and excessive dryness or perspiration), head (headaches in >50% of patients with pituitary tumors), eyes (visual field defects in <50% of patients), and GU tract (loss of sexual functioning, decrease or loss of libido, and amenorrhea). Physical examination findings include changes in cranial nerve (3rd, 4th, 6th) signs in ~5% of patients. Laboratory tests include plasma prolactin, plasma for follicle-stimulating hormone (FSH) and luteinizing hormone (LH), plasma thyroxine (by radioimmunoassay [RIA] or column), plasma cortisol, and 24-hr urine for 17-ketogenic steroids and 17-ketosteroids. Skull x-rays and pneumoencephalogram or CAT scan are also used. Visual field testing is used if there is evidence of sella turcica enlargement. Other tests are employed for specific evaluation of hormones.

Common interventions

Ablation (removal) of the pituitary may be accomplished by partial or total hypophysectomy (transcranial or transsphenoidal). Radiation implanta-

TABLE 22-1
Pituitary Hormones and Their Functions

Hormone	Function
Anterior lobe	
Growth hormone or somatropin (GH)	Promotes growth of bones and muscles (linear growth in children). Promotes cell division. Promotes nitrogen retention. Regulates rate of protein synthesis. Facilitates conversion of amino acids into protein.
Thyrotropin or thyroid-stimulating hormone (TSH)	Promotes growth of thyroid. Promotes synthesis and release of thyroid hormones.
Adrenocorticotropin (ACTH)	Regulates growth. Regulates secretion activity of adrenal cortex.
Prolactin (LTH)	Governs growth and development of the breasts. Controls lactation.
Melanocyte-stimulating hormone (MSH)	Assists in regulation of skin pigmentation.
Gonadotrophins	Regulate growth, development, and functioning of ovaries and testes.
Follicle-stimulating hormone (FSH)	In females: Matures ovarian follicles. Stimulates estrogen secretion. In males: Stimulates spermatogenesis.
Luteinizing hormone (LH)	In females: Provokes ovulation. Stimulates formation of corpus luteum. Stimulates secretion of progesterone.
Interstitial cell-stimulating hormone (ISCH)	In males: Stimulates secretion of testosterone.
Posterior lobe	
Oxytocin	Stimulates contraction of the uterus toward the end of pregnancy. Causes expression of milk from mammary glands in response to sucking.
Antidiuretic hormone (ADH)	Promotes reabsorption of water from renal tubules, decreasing excretion of water. Causes vasoconstriction in large pharmacologic amounts (therefore, also called vasopressin).

tion (transsphenoidal) employs ^{90}yttrium or ^{32}P. Transcutaneous radiation includes x-ray and heavy particles (protons). Thermal procedures (stereo-taxic, transsphenoidal) consist of radiofrequency coagulation (heat) and cryosurgery (freezing). Replacement of the hormones secreted by target organs includes corticosteroids for correction of secondary adrenocortical insufficiency, thyroid hormone for treatment of myxedema, sex hormones to correct hypogonadism, and human growth hormone (HGH) to correct hypophyseal dwarfism. **Nursing** interventions are described in the Overview.

ANTERIOR PITUITARY DISORDERS

Hyperpituitarism involves oversecretion of one or more of the pituitary hormones. The cause is usually a benign adenoma arising from one of the three basic cell types of the pituitary (i.e., eosinophils, basophils, and chromophobes).

Growth hormone (GH) is hypersecreted in 10 to 15% of pituitary tumors. **Acromegaly** and **gigantism** are rare diseases caused by GH hypersecretion arising from an eosinophilic tumor. Gigantism begins before epiphyseal closure and causes proportional growth of all body tissues. Children grow as much as 15 cm (6 in.)/yr. Acromegaly begins after epiphyseal closure, causes bone thickening and transverse growth, and occurs equally among men and women between the ages of 30 and 50 yr.

Local *signs and symptoms* of tumor growth include an enlarged sella turcica in 80 to 93% of patients, headache in 75 to 87% of patients, and visual field impairment in <50 to 62% of patients. Systemic signs and symptoms include coarsening of facies, enlargement of the hands and feet in essentially all patients, excessive sweating, hypertrichosis (excessive hair), arthritic complaints, visceromegaly (enlargement of the body organs), weight gain, goiter (usually nontoxic nodular), impaired carbohydrate tolerance, clinical diabetes mellitus, galactorrhea (excessive flow of milk) with or without prolactin, increased prolactin secretion in ~40% of patients, and decreased gonadal functioning in ≥25% of patients.

Diagnosis is based on the health history, physical exam, and measurement of GH during an oral glucose tolerance test. Specimens are obtained at 0, ½, 1, and 2 hr. The criterion for acromegaly is failure to suppress GH to <5 at some time during the test. *Treatment* consists of reduction of the secretion of GH by pituitary ablation and reduction of the stress response and edema with cortisone.

Nursing interventions

Physical 1. Assess the patient for skeletal changes (arthritis), signs of hyperglycemia, and visual defects.
2. Administer medications.
3. Assist the patient with range-of-motion (ROM) exercises.
4. Assist weak patients with activities of daily living in the late stage of acromegaly.

Preoperative 5. Explain that brain damage will not be sustained and that the patient will feel relatively well during the postoperative period and will get better each day.

6. Explain that surgery prevents permanent soft-tissue deformities but that bone changes that have occurred will not change.

7. Teach measures to prevent CSF leakage.
   a. Encourage frequent deep breathing to prevent complications of anesthesia. Do not encourage coughing.
   b. Advise the patient to avoid constipation, bending at the waist, and sneezing. (Pressure on the inner aspect of both sides of the nose or upper lip beneath the separation of the nostrils helps control sneezing.)

8. Discuss diabetes insipidus, e.g., the presence of polyuria and polydipsia (usually temporary), medication for control, and the need for accurate measurement of intake and output.

9. Discuss mouth care. (Brushing of teeth is not allowed until the incision is healed, up to 10 days; mouthwash and dental floss are used.)

Postoperative 10. Check visual acuity, vital signs, and neurologic status.

11. Maintain fluid balance. (Intake: usually discontinue the IV the first morning after surgery, usually start fluids PO within 6 hr after surgery, and proceed to regular diet on the first day postoperatively. Output: insert a straight catheter and remove it after the bladder is drained if the patient is unable to void 6 to 8 hr after surgery. Measure urinary sp gr each voiding. It can approach 1.000).

12. Administer vasopressin.
   a. Give 5 to 10 U of aqueous vasopressin when output is >800 to 900 ml in 2 hr or when sp gr is <1.004.
   b. Give every 3 to 4 hr prn.
   c. Give only after a careful assessment of fluid balance.
   d. Prevent output from exceeding 7,000 ml/24 hr.
   e. Assess for signs of water intoxication such as drowsiness, listlessness, and headache; prevent convulsions and terminal coma.
   f. Reduce incidence and severity of side effects (blanching of skin, abdominal cramps, and nausea) by giving a full glass of water with the drug.

13. Relieve pain or discomfort.
   a. Elevate the head of the bed to a 30-degree angle at all times to decrease pressure on the sclla turcica and alleviate headache.
   b. Give analgesics for headache resulting from surgical approach and packing (low doses of meperidine or codeine during the first 24 hr, aspirin or acetaminophen after 24 hr).
   c. Report any headache that becomes sharp or changes in character — may be caused by intracranial air. Anteroposterior and lateral skull films confirm the diagnosis; air will be absorbed in 1 to 2 wk.

14. Provide activity.
    a. Elevate the head of the bed 30 degrees; higher for meals.
    b. Allow bathroom privileges on the day of surgery, if able.
    c. Ambulate on the first postoperative day.
15. Observe the patient for Addisonian crisis.
    a. Assess for the development of generalized weakness, orthostatic hypotension, dizziness, fever, and nausea proceeding to coma, shock, and death.
    b. Treat with appropriate steroids.
16. Observe the patient for diabetes insipidus.
    a. Assess for dehydration or water intoxication.
    b. Treat with vasopressin, fluids, and electrolytes.
17. Observe the patient for CSF leak.
    a. Report any complaint of postnasal drip or runny nose, or persistent and severe, generalized, or supraorbital headache, which may indicate a CSF leak into the sinuses.
    b. Test any clear drainage for glucose (CSF contains glucose).
    c. Treat with bed rest for 72 hr, spinal taps to reduce CSF pressure and to allow the fossa to heal if the leak persists or is severe, and IV antibiotics.
18. Observe the patient for meningitis with or without a CSF leak (caused by organisms introduced at the time of surgery; may be normal flora in the sinuses of the particular patient; treated with IV antibiotics).
19. Observe the patient for intracranial complications, which are serious and frequently result in death. Such complications may be caused by direct trauma, secondary vascular effects, previous craniotomy causing anatomic changes, and very large tumors.

Psychosocial 20. Provide emotional support to help the patient cope with a grotesquely altered body.
21. Explain that mood changes are a result of the disease and that they will decrease with treatment.
22. Explain that surgery prevents permanent soft-tissue deformities. Bone changes that have occurred will not change.

Educational 23. Teach the patient the need for and method of administration of vasopressin (if diabetes insipidus persists) and/or of steroid and thyroid replacement.
24. Explain that there may be changes in reproductive and sexual functioning (sterility and possible impotence in men; testosterone may be given; human pituitary gonadotrophin may restore fertility in some women).
25. Explain to female patients that they may experience atrophy of the vaginal mucosa (estrogen may be given; a lubricant may be needed for intercourse; some women may be newly fertile and need a contraceptive).

26. Explain the need to report changes in sexual functioning and libido, which may indicate tumor regrowth.
27. Explain the necessity for lifelong follow-up care.

Evaluation criteria.   *See* Overview.

CUSHING'S SYNDROME

Cushing's syndrome is a condition involving excessive secretion of glucocorticoids, primarily as a result of hypersecretion of ACTH. The condition is called Cushing's disease when a pituitary disorder (usually a basophilic tumor) causes excessive ACTH secretion. This rare disease has its peak incidence between the ages of 30 and 40 yr and is considerably more common in women than in men, with a ratio of 4:1.

Increased secretion of ACTH may result from an ACTH-secreting tumor of the anterior pituitary, an ectopic ACTH-secreting malignant tumor, or nodular dysplasia. Excessive cortisol secretion also may result as a consequence of adrenal carcinoma or adenoma. Iatrogenic causes include long-term use of ACTH and steroids.

Great emotional trauma often precedes the onset of Cushing's syndrome by several weeks. Systemic *signs and symptoms* resulting from excessive secretion of cortisol consist of abnormal fat distribution (moon face, central obesity marked by a pendulous abdomen and thin extremities, no real change in total body weight, and a dorsal fat pad and supraclavicular fossae fat pads forming the distinctive "buffalo hump"), increased protein catabolism (thin, paperlike skin easily penetrated by venipuncture needles or torn by adhesive tape; capillary fragility, characterized by ecchymoses over the arms and legs; red or purple striae over the abdomen, buttocks, breasts, and thighs; osteoporosis; impaired wound healing; muscle wasting and atrophy, most marked in the extremities and associated with muscle weakness, which may also result from hypokalemia; hypercalciuria [occasionally accompanied by renal calcinosis or lithiasis]), diabetes mellitus (often present because of increased gluconeogenesis and also secondary to antagonism by hydrocortisone or circulating insulin levels), neural hyperexcitability leading to a variety of neurotic and psychotic symptoms not specific to Cushing's syndrome, hypertension (possibly caused by increased sensitivity of the peripheral vessels to catecholamines), leukopenia and eosinopenia, and hyperpigmentation caused by excessive ACTH and MSH levels (not present in patients with adrenal neoplasms). Signs and symptoms resulting from excessive secretion of adrenal androgens include excessive hair growth over the face and body (chin, sideburn area, cheeks, upper lip, between the breasts, upward extension of pubic hair in women), deepening of the voice in women, acne, loss of scalp hair in the temporal areas and over the crown of the head, erythrocytosis, increased libido (especially in women), abnormal menses, an enlarged clitoris, and the anabolic effect of adrenal androgens. When these hormones are present in excess, the catabolic effects of cortisol may be masked, distorting the typical clinical picture of Cushing's syndrome to resemble primary characterization of virilization.

Diagnosis is based on the health history, physical exam, and laboratory tests. Urinary steroids disclose that urinary 17-hydroxycorticosteroids are elevated. The normal circadian cycle and characteristic patterns of urinary cortisol excretion are absent. Some patients with mixed syndrome have normal output of 17-hydroxycorticosteroids. Plasma tests show plasma cortisols in the high-normal to distinctly elevated range. Diurnal variation is absent. The dexamethasone suppression test is used to differentiate between Cushing's syndrome (caused by an adrenal tumor), Cushing's disease (caused by a pituitary oversecretion of ACTH), and ectopic ACTH syndrome (caused by an ectopic ACTH-secreting tumor). The rapid dexamethasone suppression test is a more reliable indicator. The level of 17-hydroxycortico-steroids is >10 mg/100 ml. This suggests nonsuppressibility of ACTH and is diagnostic of Cushing's syndrome. Estrogen raises the transcortin level, producing high levels of plasma hydroxycorticosteroids; therefore, the patient on estrogen-containing birth control pills must have levels measured the day before and day after dexamethasone administration. Normal patients show a very marked suppression of cortisol levels on the second day. The ratio of urinary corticosteroid:creatinine can be used in place of plasma cortisol determinations to indicate suppression by dexamethasone. The metyrapone (Metopirone) test assesses pituitary as well as adrenal functioning. A marked increase in urinary corticosteroids indicates Cushing's syndrome. Levels do not increase in Cushing's syndrome if the disorder is caused by autonomously functioning adrenal cortical adenomas. This test also detects inadequate pituitary reserve. X-rays of the sella turcica and other bones may disclose pathologic fractures or osteoporosis. Arteriograms and venograms of the adrenal glands may also be useful.

Common interventions

Medical therapy is used when Cushing's syndrome is the result of an inoperable carcinoma of the adrenal cortex with metastasis. Otherwise, **surgery** is the treatment of choice. Table 22-2 discusses treatment of the various aspects of Cushing's syndrome.

Nursing interventions

Physical 1. Assess the patient for hypertension.
   a. Check vital signs.
   b. Check for headache.
2. Assess the patient for infection and inflammation (glucocorticoids suppress immune responses; in a severe infection, symptoms may be slight).
3. Protect the patient from infections.
4. Assess the patient for hyper- or hypoglycemia.
   a. Test the patient's urine for glucose and acetone.
   b. Check lab data for blood glucose values.

TABLE 22-2
Treatment for Cushing's Syndrome

Condition	Etiology	Treatment
Cushing's syndrome	Unilateral or bilateral adrenal cortex tumors (benign or malignant).	Unilateral or bilateral adrenalectomy.
	Adrenal carcinoma with widespread metastasis.	Metyrapone, aminoglutethimide, mitotane (Lysodren).
Cushing's disease	Hypersecretion of ACTH by a normal pituitary in response to hypothalamic stimulation, or by a basophilic tumor of the pituitary.	Pituitary ablation, bilateral adrenalectomy to correct adrenal hyperplasia caused by excessive ACTH stimulation.
Ectopic ACTH syndrome	Extra-adrenal malignant tumor secreting ACTH. Usually oat cell carcinoma of the lung; also occurs with tumors of the parotid, liver, pancreas, thymus, thyroid, esophagus, and the adrenal medulla.	Surgical removal of tumor and chemotherapy; chemotherapy palliative.

5. Assess the patient for edema and heart disease.
   a. Weigh the patient at the same time each day and on the same scale.
   b. Check for dyspnea.
   c. Keep an intake and output record.
6. Administer medications.
   a. Give sedatives or hypnotics if necessary.
   b. Give corticosteroids before surgery as ordered if the patient has been treated with cortisol inhibitors.
7. Assist weak patients with activities of daily living.
8. Protect the patient from falls and other trauma.
   a. Keep the bed in a low position.
   b. Keep the side rails up if the patient is restless or disturbed.
9. Administer postoperative care (*see* Chapter 11).
   a. Assess the patient for shock (take and record vital signs q 10 to 15 min; measure and record hourly urine output).
   b. Administer medications (IV solutions, vasopressors, corticosteroids, antiemetics, analgesics).
   c. Prevent infection (patients are especially prone to fungus infections) by encouraging the patient to cough, deep breathe, and turn hourly and by using meticulous sterile technique when changing or reinforcing the dressing.
   d. Control nausea and vomiting (keep the nasogastric [NG] tube to suction, and maintain its patency by irrigation).
   e. Provide activity (elevate the head of the bed as tolerated; turn the patient hourly; assist the patient out of bed to a chair on the first day postoperatively, if ordered).
   f. Observe the patient for withdrawal symptoms (fever; fatigue, weakness, lethargy; dizziness, orthostatic hypotension; depression; psychosis) when corticosteroids are tapered (sudden withdrawal may be fatal).
   g. Observe the patient for complications (infection, cardiovascular problems, renal failure).
Psychosocial 10. Provide emotional support to help the patient cope with altered body appearance.
11. Explain that the appearance of the body will gradually return to normal with treatment.
12. Explain that mood changes are a result of the disease and that they will decrease with treatment.
Educational 13. Teach the patient the need for and method of administration of lifelong steroid replacement if bilateral adrenalectomy was performed (IM as well as PO; conditions requiring increased steroids).
14. Teach the patient the need for and administration of steroid replacement temporarily if unilateral adrenalectomy was performed.

15. Explain that the patient may experience changes in reproductive and sexual functioning (atrophy of the vaginal mucosa may require estrogen therapy and a lubricant during intercourse).
16. Instruct the patient to report any changes in sexual functioning or libido because these changes may indicate tumor growth.
17. Instruct the patient that lifelong follow-up care is necessary (10 to 15% of patients who have had a bilateral total adrenalectomy for Cushing's syndrome resulting from adrenal hyperplasia develop an ACTH-secreting chromophobe adenoma of the pituitary ~3 yr after surgery).
18. Instruct the patient to wear a medical alert identification bracelet.

Evaluation criteria.   *See* Overview.

HYPOPITUITARISM

Hypopituitarism is a rare deficiency of one or more of the anterior pituitary hormones. Panhypopituitarism is the failure of both the anterior and the posterior lobes to secrete hormones. Primary disease may be a result of hypophysectomy, nonsecreting pituitary tumors (nonfunctioning chromophobe adenoma, craniopharyngioma), pituitary dwarfism caused by a deficiency of GH at birth, postpartum pituitary necrosis (which develops after postpartum hemorrhage and circulatory collapse and results from tissue anoxia), functional disorders resulting in inadequate nourishment of the gland (starvation, anorexia nervosa, severe anemia, inadequate absorption of nutrients because of GI disorders), and sexual and reproductive disorders. Secondary disease involves a deficiency of releasing factors produced by the hypothalamus, possibly resulting from infection, trauma, or tumor.

Signs and symptoms develop slowly and usually do not appear until 75% of the pituitary becomes nonfunctioning. The patient's age at onset and specific hormone deficiencies affect symptomatology. LH and FSH deficiency can produce sterility, decreased libido, and decreased secondary sex characteristics. Women develop infertility and amenorrhea. Men have decreased spermatogenesis and testicular atrophy. Hypothyroidism may cause fatigue, lethargy, sensitivity to cold, and menstrual disturbances. Adrenocortical insufficiency may involve hypoglycemia, anorexia, nausea, abdominal pain, and hypotension. Postpartum necrosis of the pituitary (Sheehan's syndrome) may cause failure of lactation and menstruation, decreased growth of pubic and axillary hair, adrenocortical failure, and diabetes insipidus. GH failure may result in growth failure if it is present at birth. Failure of development of secondary sex characteristics may also occur. Males may have small testes and experience impotence. Females may have immature development of the breasts, sparse or absent pubic and axillary hair, and primary amenorrhea. Panhypopituitarism involves symptoms such as lethargy, psychosis, orthostatic hypotension, bradycardia, and anorexia.

Diagnosis is based on the health history, physical exam, and a variety of tests. Evaluation of the hormonal deficiency requires assessment of impairment or destruction of the pituitary or impairment of target organs or the hypothalamus. Provocative tests include PO administration of metyrapone (blocks cortisol synthesis, which, in turn, stimulates pituitary secretion of ACTH), insulin-induced hypoglycemia (stimulates ACTH secretion), and measurement of GH in the blood after administration of regular insulin (to induce hypotension) in order to provoke increased secretion of GH. Persistently low GH levels confirm GH deficiency. Intra- or extracellar tumors may be visible on CAT scan, pneumoencephalogram, or cerebral angiography.

Common interventions

Medical therapy consists of replacement of the hormones secreted by the target organs. Corticosteroids are used for treatment of adrenocortical insufficiency; thyroid hormone, for treatment of myxedema; androgens or estrogen, for treatment of hypogonadism; and HGH, for treatment of hypophyseal dwarfism.

Nursing interventions

Physical 1. Assess the patient for signs of hormone deficiency (thyroid deficiency: increasing lethargy; adrenal deficiency: weakness, orthostatic hypotension, hypoglycemia, fatigue, weight loss; gonadal deficiency: decreased libido, lethargy, apathy; panhypopituitarism: anorexia).

2. Provide the patient with adequate nutrition (palatable diet, favorite foods, appropriate calories).

3. Weigh the patient daily.

4. Prevent infection.
    a. Provide meticulous skin care (use bath oil instead of soap and apply lotion for dry skin).
    b. Provide adequate clothing and covers if the body temperature is low.

5. Administer medications.

6. Assist the patient with activities of daily living if necessary.

Psychosocial 7. Explain that mood changes are a result of the disease and that they will decrease with treatment.

8. Explain that the changed body appearance will gradually return to normal with treatment.

Educational 9. Teach the patient the need for and method of administration of hormones.

10. Teach the need for wearing a medical alert bracelet.

11. Explain changes in reproductive functioning.

12. Explain the necessity of lifelong follow-up.

Evaluation criteria. *See* Overview.

POSTERIOR PITUITARY DISORDERS

The posterior lobe is rarely destroyed by disease. If it is destroyed or damaged, hormonal disease does not occur because oxytocin and ADH are synthesized by the hypothalamus. If the hypothalamus is damaged, hormonal deficiency will occur even if the posterior lobe is intact.

Diabetes insipidus is an uncommon disease of ADH deficiency characterized by polydipsia and polyuria. It may arise slowly or appear suddenly and occurs equally among men and women, usually between the ages of 10 and 20 yr. Factors affecting ADH secretion are listed in Table 22-3. Vasopressin deficiency is responsible for primary diabetes insipidus, which accounts for 50% of cases. Secondary diabetes insipidus results from destruction of the pituitary by tumors, trauma, infection, vascular accidents, or metastases from breast or lung tumors. Nephrogenic diabetes insipidus is an inherited defect in which renal tubules are unable to absorb water; it occurs secondary to potassium depletion or pyelonephritis. Major *signs and symptoms* of diabetes insipidus are polyuria and polydipsia. The patient may drink and excrete 4 to 40 liters of fluid a day. Urinary sp gr ranges between 1.001 and 1.006. Dehydration and hypovolemic shock may occur. Fatigue may result from inadequate rest because of frequent voiding and excessive thirst.

Diagnosis is based on the health history, physical exam, and laboratory tests. Vasopressin deficiency may be demonstrated during a water restriction test. After obtaining base-line vital signs, weight, and urine and plasma osmolalities, fluids are withheld. Hourly vital signs, weight, and urine

TABLE 22-3
Factors Affecting ADH Secretion

Factors	Examples
Factors that increase ADH secretion	
Increased plasma osmolality and decreased blood volume	Hemorrhage, decreased CO, dehydration, hypoalbuminemia
Limbic stimulation	Pain, fear, anxiety, major trauma
Pharmacologic agents	Nicotine, morphine, barbiturates, general anesthetics, beta-adrenergic agents, clofibrate (Atromid-S), vincristine, cyclophosphamine (Cytoxan), carbamazepine (Tegretol), chlorpropamide
Factors that decrease ADH secretion	Ethanol, diphenylhydantoin, hyposmolality, morphine antagonists, total body immersion, hypervolemia

osmolality or sp gr are measured. This procedure continues until the patient loses 3% of his body weight or until severe postural hypotension occurs. Aqueous vasopressin, 5 U, is given SC. Patients with diabetes insipidus have a decreased urine output and increased sp gr. Patients with nephrogenic diabetes insipidus show no response to vasopressin.

Common interventions

Medical treatment consists of replacement of ADH with vasopressin tannate IM or SC or lypressin intranasally. Benzothiadizine diuretics are used alone or in combination with sulfonylurea to reduce polyuria by possibly releasing ADH or potentiating its effects. **Surgical** resection is necessary if the cause is a tumor.

Nursing interventions

Physical 1. Assess the patient's fluid balance.
- a. Maintain a record of intake and output.
- b. Weigh the patient daily.
- c. Measure and record urine sp gr.
2. Provide for adequate fluid intake.
3. Assess for dehydration and hypovolemic shock.
- a. Measure vital signs at regular intervals.
- b. Observe skin turgor.
- c. Observe mucous membranes for dryness.
- d. Assess for constipation and provide food high in roughage, fruit, fruit juices, and laxatives if necessary.
- e. Observe for dizziness.
4. Assess for signs of hypoglycemia if the patient is receiving chlorpropamide.
- a. Ensure adequate caloric intake.
- b. Keep orange juice or other simple carbohydrate available.
5. Administer medications.
- a. Assess urinary output, sp gr, and fluid intake between doses.
- b. Ensure that the hormone is adequately suspended in oil before injecting (warm the solution by rotating it between the hands if it is cold; shake the bottle well).
- c. Identify all patients with cardiovascular disease before administering medications (vasopressin constricts vessels).
Psychosocial 6. Explain to the patient that the prognosis is good in uncomplicated diabetes insipidus. (Patients can usually lead normal lives. The prognosis varies if the disease is caused by metastasis.)
7. Explain that lifelong follow-up is necessary.
Educational 8. Teach the patient the need for and proper administration of medications.
- a. Explain that medication should be taken at the onset of polyuria, not before.

    b. Explain that weight gain (fluid retention) indicates that the dosage is too high.

    c. Explain that polyuria indicates that the dosage is too low.

9. Instruct the patient regarding signs of hypoglycemia and its treatment if the patient is taking chlorpropamide.

10. Instruct the patient regarding the need to wear a medical alert bracelet.

11. Instruct the patient to carry the medication at all times.

Evaluation criteria. *See* Overview.

ADRENAL DISORDERS

The adrenal glands are two small structures located on the tops of the kidneys. These glands are composed of the adrenal cortex and the adrenal medulla.

The adrenal cortex produces steroid corticoid hormones and adrenocortical hormones (without which, death occurs within a few days). Its secretory activity is regulated by the anterior pituitary hormone ACTH. The adrenal medulla secretes the hormones epinephrine and norepinephrine. It is part of the sympathetic nervous system and is controlled by the hypothalamus. The adrenal hormones and their functions are listed in Table 22-4.

General assessment includes the health history, physical exam, and diagnostic tests. The past health history should include questions about endocrine disorders and hypertension. The review of body systems should focus on integumentary (skin: changes in pigmentation, thinness, fragility, easy bruisability, red or purple straie, impaired wound healing, and acne; hair: changes in growth and loss of scalp hair), cardiovascular problems (hyper- or hypotension), GI tract (constipation, diarrhea, nausea, vomiting, anorexia, and abdominal pain), GU tract (changes in libido and abnormal or absent menses), musculoskeletal abnormalities (muscle wasting, atrophy, and osteoporosis), neurologic signs (neural hyperexcitability), and endocrine disturbances (diabetes mellitus and abnormal fat distribution, e.g., moon face, central obesity, distinctive dorsal and supraclavicular fat pads).

Laboratory tests consist of assay of plasma catecholamines, IV ACTH test, plasma cortisol response to the ACTH test, water excretion tests, 24-hr urine for metanephrines and vanillylmandelic acid (VMA), and serum electrolytes. X-rays and radiologic studies may include IV pyelogram (IVP), arteriography, venography, CAT scan, and chest x-ray.

Interventions and evaluation criteria are as described in the Overview.

ADRENAL CORTEX DISORDERS

Hyposecretion of the adrenal cortex hormones is due to primary disease of the adrenal glands, deficiency of pituitary ACTH secondary to pituitary disease, and prolonged suppression of pituitary and adrenal hormones by chronic treatment with natural or synthetic adrenal hormones.

TABLE 22-4
Adrenal Hormones and Their Functions

Hormone	Function
Adrenal cortex	
Mineralocorticoids (aldosterone,* desoxycorticosterone, corticosterone)	Conserve sodium, maintain blood and ECF volume, maintain normal BP and CO.
Glucocorticoids (cortisol,† cortisone, corticosterone§)	Regulate glucose metabolism, regulate protein metabolism, maintain fluid and electrolyte balance, regulate inflammatory and immune responses, provide for resistance and adjustment to stress.
Sex hormones (androgens, estrogens)	Govern certain secondary sex characteristics, secrete smaller amounts of hormones than do the gonads, affect sodium and water balance.
Adrenal medulla	
Epinephrine	Constricts peripheral blood vessels; raises BP; increases CO; increases pulse greatly; constricts spleen, putting stored RBCs into circulation; increases respiratory rate and depth of respirations; dilates bronchi; stimulates CNS, producing feeling of alertness, fright, impending doom; dilates pupils; inhibits GI tract; converts glycogen to glucose; increases metabolism; increases nonesterified fatty acid level of the blood.
Norepinephrine	Constricts all blood vessels, increases peripheral resistance, causes marked hypertension, decreases CO because of increased peripheral resistance, increases pulse, dilates pupils, inhibits GI tract, increases metabolism slightly, increases nonesterified fatty acid level of the blood.

*The principal mineralocorticoid.
†The principal glucocorticoid.
§Also a mineralocorticoid.

Addison's disease is a primary adrenal disease resulting in insufficient secretion of adrenal cortex hormones. It is a rare disorder (occurring in 1 out of every 100,000 persons) that affects all age groups and both sexes. Approximately 70% of cases are considered idiopathic and may have an autoimmune basis. Less common causes include bilateral TB of the adrenals, amyloidosis, metastatic disease, and histoplasmosis.

Systemic *signs and symptoms* resulting from mineralocorticoid deficiency include hypotension (especially when standing), hyponatremia, lethargy, easy fatigability, vertigo, syncope, and dehydration. Symptoms of glucocorticoid deficiency include weakness, fatigue, weight loss, hypoglycemia, hyperpigmentation, and emotional disturbances. Androgen deficiency results in the absence of pubic and axillary hair in women, but causes no symptoms in men.

Diagnosis is based on the health history, physical exam, and laboratory tests, including an 8-hr IV ACTH test (urinary steroid output does not rise after ACTH stimulation because of gland atrophy in primary Addison's disease, but urinary steroid output gradually rises if the test is repeated over several days in hypofunction secondary to pituitary insufficiency). However, plasma cortisol response to ACTH is more reliable and faster than the 8-hr IV ACTH test. A water excretion test reveals that adrenocortical insufficiency reduces the ability to handle water load. Less water than normal will be excreted. Other laboratory studies involve blood chemistry evaluation (low serum sodium, high serum potassium, low fasting blood glucose, decrease in CO_2-combining power, and elevated BUN) and hematology tests (elevated Hct, low WBC, relative lymphocytosis, and increased eosinophils). X-rays reveal a small heart, calcifications in the adrenals, and renal and pulmonary TB.

Common interventions

Medical treatment involves replacement of glucocorticoids and mineralocorticoids daily *without exception.*

Nursing interventions

Physical 1. Assess fluid balance.
   a. Record intake and output.
   b. Force fluids until drug replacement is effective and hydration is normal.
   c. Weigh the patient daily.
2. Assess for hypotension.
   a. Check vital signs on a regular basis.
   b. Report drops in BP to the physician.
3. Protect the patient against infections.
   a. Assess for infections.
   b. Report symptoms to the physician.
   c. Increase steroids to cope with the stress of infections.
4. Observe the patient for sodium and potassium imbalance and monitor laboratory reports. (Sodium loss and potassium retention will continue if steroid replacement is inadequate; sodium and water retention will be excessive, and large amounts of potassium will be excreted if steroid replacement is too high.)

5. Provide for nutritional replacement.
   a. Encourage a high-carbohydrate, high-protein diet.
   b. Encourage a diet that provides adequate sodium and potassium.
   c. Provide between-meal snacks or 6 small meals a day to ensure adequate intake.
6. Assess the patient for hyper- or hypoglycemia.
   a. Test the urine for glucose and acetone.
   b. Monitor laboratory reports.
   c. Adjust insulin if necessary because of steroid replacement.
   d. Keep orange juice, etc., available for the patient in case hypoglycemia occurs.
7. Administer medications.
   a. Give oral cortisol preparations with meals or antacids to decrease gastric irritation and to prevent the development of peptic ulcer.
   b. Administer parenteral cortisol preparations deep into the gluteal muscle. (Do not inject into the deltoid muscle as this drug causes sterile abscesses, atrophy of tissue, and abnormalities of pigmentation when injected into SC tissue.)
8. Assist weak patients with activities of daily living.

Psychosocial 9. Explain to the patient that mood changes are a result of the disease and that they will decrease with treatment.

10. Explain that, with treatment, listlessness and exhaustion will be replaced by physical vitality and emotional well-being.

Educational 11. Teach the patient self-care regarding adrenocortical drug replacement.
   a. Teach the patient the need for and proper administration of life-long steroid replacement either PO or IM.
   b. Teach the patient the actions of the drugs prescribed and signs of underdosage or overdosage.
   c. Teach the patient which situations require an increase in dosage of glucocorticoids (emotional upheavals, upper respiratory tract infections, dental extractions, minor as well as major surgery) or mineralocorticoids (fever, infections, strenuous physical exertion, hot weather).

12. Instruct the patient that information and supplies for emergency use should always be carried.
   a. Encourage the patient to obtain an identification bracelet and inscribe it with his own name, the names and telephone numbers of the doctor and a person to contact in an emergency, and the statement "I have adrenal insufficiency. In any emergency involving injury, vomiting, or loss of consciousness, the hydrocortisone in my possession should be injected under my skin and my physician notified."
   b. Encourage the patient to obtain an emergency kit containing hydrocortisone, 100 mg, kept in a prepared syringe, sterile

alcohol sponges, and information about drug prescription and dosage schedules.

Evaluation criteria. *See* Overview.

ADDISONIAN CRISIS

Addisonian crisis involves acute adrenal insufficiency manifested by a critical deficiency of glucocorticoids, severe hypotension, hyperkalemia, and vascular collapse requiring rapid and vigorous treatment. It is a rare condition that results from stress from infection, trauma, diaphoresis, etc. Refer to Addison's disease (*see above*) for methods of diagnosis and laboratory evaluation. Treatment may be initiated before confirmation of laboratory tests because of the emergency nature of the situation.

Common interventions

Medical treatment consists of glucocorticoid replacement (hydrocortisone 100 to 250 mg IV as a bolus; then hydrocortisone 50 to 100 mg IM or IV in a normal saline infusion until the condition is stable; then hydrocortisone is gradually reduced). Cardiovascular support may include fluid replacement with normal saline (5 liters may be required during the acute stage), plasma expanders, vasopressors, and oxygen. Other causes of the crisis are treated (e.g., antibiotics for infection). With rapid and aggressive treatment, Addisonian crisis usually resolves within a few hours. The condition stabilizes and convalescence begins.

Nursing interventions

Physical 1. Monitor BP and vital signs; observe for shock.
2. Administer medications and IV solutions.
3. Observe the patient for and report overdosage of glucocorticoids and overhydration (generalized edema, hypertension, psychoses, flaccid paralysis resulting from hypokalemia, loss of consciousness).
4. Monitor fluid balance.
   a. Assess intake hourly.
   b. Measure and record urine output and sp gr hourly; report oliguria.
Psychosocial 5. Prevent further physical or emotional stress to the patient.
6. Refer to Addison's disease (*see above*) for educational nursing interventions and evaluation criteria.

PRIMARY HYPERALDOSTERONISM

Primary hyperaldosteronism is hypersecretion of aldosterone because of a lesion of the adrenal cortex. Its incidence is unknown, but 8 to 20% of all patients with hypertension may be affected. It is the most frequently diagnosed functioning tumor of the adrenal glands and is twice as frequent in females as in males, usually occurring between the ages of 30 and 50 yr. Bilateral tumors occur in ≤5% of affected patients. Primary hyperaldosteronism usually results from a single, benign aldosterone-secreting adrenal adenoma and occasionally is a consequence of adrenocortical carcinoma. *Signs and symptoms* include hypertension (frequently mild) and sodium retention accompanied by headache, cardiac enlargement, and edema (rare). Hypokalemia is also common and is associated with muscle weakness and paralysis, tetany, paresthesias and muscle cramps, and hypokalemic renal damage (polyuria, polydipsia, nocturia, proteinuria).

Diagnosis is based on the health history, physical exam, and various tests. Laboratory tests aid in establishing the presence of hyperaldosteronism (Table 22-5) and in differentiating between primary and secondary hyperaldosteronism (Table 22-6). Adrenal scan is also used. Chest x-ray may demonstrate cardiac hypertrophy from chronic hypertension. ECG may reveal changes resulting from hypokalemia.

Common interventions

Medical treatment consists of administration of the aldosterone antagonist spironolactone (Aldactone), which does not alter production of aldosterone by the adrenals. Potassium salts are administered to correct hypokalemia. **Surgical** removal of an aldosterone-secreting tumor may be required.

Nursing interventions

Physical 1. Administer medications as ordered.
2. Monitor and record fluid balance (intake, output, daily weights).
3. Monitor serum electrolytes.
4. Monitor and record BP as ordered.
5. Observe for signs and symptoms of hypocalcemia.
6. Provide a low-sodium, high-potassium diet.
7. Administer pre- and postoperative care as for adrenalectomy (*see below*), if surgery is performed.
Psychosocial 8. Explain that lifelong follow-up care is needed for control of hypertension.
9. Explain that the fatigue and weakness are symptoms of the disease and will disappear with treatment.

Evaluation criteria. See Overview.

PHEOCHROMOCYTOMA

Pheochromocytoma is a functional tumor of chromaffin tissue of the adrenal medulla that produces severe symptoms and can cause sudden death. It is usually benign; <5% are malignant. Its incidence is estimated at 0.4 to 2.0% of all hypertensive patients, or 600 to 800 new cases/yr in the USA.

TABLE 22-5
Diagnostic Tests for Aldosteronism

Test	Primary	Secondary	Normal or essential hypertension
Serum potassium	≤3 mEq/100 ml	≤3 mEq/100 ml	>3 mEq/100 ml
Serum sodium	High-normal or high	Normal or low	Normal
Urine potassium on high-sodium diet	Often exceeds intake <20 mEq/day rules out >30 mEq/day likely >50 mEq/day diagnostic	20-40 mEq/day	Less than intake (usually <20 mEq/day)
Urine potassium on low-sodium diet	Falls	Falls	Increases
Aldosterone excretion in urine	>10 μg/day (often 15-50 μg/day)	>10 μg/day (often 25-100 μg/day)	≤10 μg/day
Aldosterone secretion rate	>170 μg/day	>170 μg/day	60-170 μg/day
Spironolactone test	Use in serum K >1 mEq/liter	Rise in serum K >1 mEq/liter	Low K does not rise

TABLE 22-6
Tests to Differentiate Primary from Secondary Hyperaldosteronism

Test	Primary	Secondary	Normal or essential hypertension
Plasma renin on high-sodium diet	Low or absent	High	Normal
Plasma renin on low-sodium diet	Low or absent	Very high	High
Aldosterone response to DCA administration	No change	Falls	Falls
Renal vein renin	Low	High	Normal
Adrenal vein aldosterone	High on side with tumor	High on both sides	Normal
Renal arteriography	Normal	Arterial lesion	Normal
Adrenal angiography	Tumor present	No tumor	No tumor
Angiotensin infusion	BP rises	No BP changes	BP rises

DCA, deoxycorticosterone acetate.

It occurs most often between 40 and 60 yr of age, but patients range in age from 5 mo to 82 yr. One fifth of the reported cases have been children. Some cases have a hereditary basis. Attacks may be spontaneous or precipitated by changes in posture, physical exertion, emotional upsets, urination, tyramine-containing foods, trauma, pregnancy, anesthesia, monoamine oxidase-inhibiting drugs, and surgery. Abrupt attacks may last for a few minutes to a few hours. Attacks are infrequent early in the disease; the frequency and severity of the attacks tend to increase over time.

Symptoms depend on whether the secretion of hormones (epinephrine or predominantly norepinephrine) is continuous or intermittent. Hypertension, the most common symptom, may be paroxysmal or sustained. (In children, hypertension is more often sustained.) Hyperglycemia, glucosuria, and albuminuria may occur during an attack. Attacks often end with a feeling of fatigue and prostration. BP may rise to 200 to 300/150 to 175 mmHg during an attack. Severe headache may occur, as well as diaphoresis, anxiety, palpitations, dizziness, peripheral vasoconstriction, nausea, vomiting, precordial pain, hot flashes, visual disturbances, and trembling. *Complications* include permanent cardiovascular damage and death from pulmonary edema, ventricular fibrillation, or cerebral hemorrhage.

Diagnosis is based on the health history, physical exam, and other tests. Results of 24-hr urine tests for VMA and catecholamines are elevated. Results of direct assay of catecholamines in the blood are elevated. Radiologic studies and CAT scan are used to confirm the diagnosis and to localize the tumor for surgery. These studies include a CAT scan of both adrenal glands, IVP with nephrotomograms, abdominal arteriograms, and selective venography.

Common interventions

Medical therapy involves control of the symptoms with the use of oral phentolamine or longer-acting adrenergic-blocking agents. **Surgical** removal of the tumor is usually required.

Nursing interventions

1. Administer the following care during the acute attack:
   Physical a. Encourage bed rest.
   b. Elevate the head of the bed to a 45-degree angle to take advantage of orthostatic reduction of BP.
   c. Give phentolamine (Regitine) 2 to 5 mg IV q 5 min until hypertension is controlled.
   d. Give phentolamine 2 to 5 mg IV q 2 to 4 hr to maintain control of BP.
   e. Monitor the patient for life-threatening arrhythmias.
   f. Give propranolol (Inderal) 1 to 2 mg IV over 5 to 10 min for severe sinus tachycardia and atrial or ventricular arrhythmias (Inderal is later given PO).

g. Assess for slow pulse rate, because ~20% of patients have bradycardia during an attack.

Psychosocial h. Reassure the patient that necessary medications and interventions to control the symptoms will be given.

i. Provide any support necessary to allay fear of impending death.

2. Administer preoperative (**adrenalectomy**) care.

Physical a. Give alpha-blocking agents (titrated to the individual patient's requirement) for 10 to 14 days preoperatively as ordered — phentolamine 50 to 100 mg PO 4 to 6 times a day or phenoxybenzamine (Dibenzyline) 10 mg PO initially, then increased by 10 mg q 4 d to a maximum dosage of 60 mg/day.

b. Give beta-blocking agents (titrated to the individual patient's requirement) to control tachycardia and arrhythmias. (The indication for beta blockade is tachycardia of ≥ 100 bpm and arrhythmias. Do not give a beta-blocker unless an alpha-blocker is also ordered. Beta blockade alone will cause an unopposed alpha effect, leading to severe hypertension.)

c. Give propranolol 20 mg tid for 4 days before surgery.

d. Give drugs (e.g., alpha-methylparatyrosine [AMPT]) that decrease catecholamine synthesis, as ordered, in a dose titrated to the individual and ranging from 500 mg to 2 g qd with a half-life of ~12 hr. The last dose is given at midnight before surgery.

Psychosocial e. Assure the patient that all available techniques will be used to reduce the risks of the procedure.

f. Recognize that patients experience considerable anxiety because the exact localization of the tumor often is not possible until the operation.

3. Administer postoperative (adrenalectomy) care.

Physical a. Monitor IV fluids (large amounts of colloid and crystalloid solutions are given as replacement for third space losses).

b. Monitor hypotension because of low blood volume resulting from peripheral vasoconstriction.

c. Assess for sudden peripheral vasodilation, which occurs when the tumor is excised.

d. Assess the effects of phenoxybenzamine and AMPT given preoperatively (residual effects last 36 hr).

e. Measure and record urinary output with every voiding.

f. Measure urine sp gr every voiding.

g. Give corticosteroids as ordered.

h. Provide general postoperative care (*see* Chapter 11).

Educational i. Teach the patient the need for and method of administration of steroids, if necessary.

j. Teach the patient the need for lifelong follow-up (10 to 13% recurrence rate after successful surgery).

k. Teach the patient the need for genetic counseling and family planning if the disease is familial.

Evaluation criteria.   *See* Overview.

THYROID DISORDERS

Thyroid diseases are usually characterized by multiorgan involvement. Symptoms may be subtle. Organs differ in their sensitivity to thyroid hormones; sensitivity is related to the patient's age in some cases. The thyroid gland synthesizes and secretes three hormones: thyroxine (T_4), tri-iodothyronine (T_3), and thyrocalcitonin. Thyroid hormones influence growth and development and regulate a wide variety of metabolic processes in a specific way, as described in Table 22-7. Although a variety of effects of thyroid hormones have been described, the mechanism of action is unknown.

This shield-shaped gland is located in the anterior neck below the larynx. Synthesis and release of the thyroid hormones is controlled by thyrotropin, or thyroid-stimulating hormone (TSH), which is released by specific thyrotropic cells of the anterior pituitary. The secretion of TSH is under the control of hypothalamic thyrotropin-releasing hormone (TRH).

The thyroid, the anterior pituitary, and the hypothalamus function together in a negative-feedback loop to control thyroid hormone synthesis and release. Increased secretion of TSH results in increased synthesis and release of thyroid hormones, which feed back on the anterior pituitary to shut off further TSH release. It is not clear that thyroid hormones directly regulate TRH synthesis and release. There is no long-term suppression of the hypothalamic-pituitary-thyroid axis. After withdrawal of exogenous thyroid hormones, the hypothalamic-pituitary-thyroid axis recovers quickly and functions normally within 6 wk.

Thyroid hormones are poorly soluble in aqueous solutions and are transported in the blood attached to binding proteins: thyroxine-binding globulin, thyroxine-binding prealbumin, and albumin. T_3 is less firmly bound to plasma proteins than T_4. The protein-bound T_3 and T_4 are physiologically inert and exist with minute amounts of free hormone, which can cross cell membranes and interact with intracellular receptor sites. The free hormone concentration accurately reflects thyroid status. Because thyroid hormones are bound to protein carriers, they are cleared from the circulation more slowly than other hormones. The half-life of parathyroid hormone is <1 min; cortisol, ~1 hr; T_3, 1 to 2 days; and T_4, 6 to 7 days. T_4 has a longer half-life because it binds more tightly to plasma proteins. T_3 is three to four times more active than T_4 and supplies $\sim90\%$ of thyroid hormone activity. T_4 is converted to T_3 mainly in the liver and the kidneys. Of the circulating T_3, 80% is derived from conversion of T_4, and only 20% is normally secreted directly from the thyroid. T_3 is not converted to T_4.

General assessment includes the health history, physical exam, and diagnostic tests. The past health history should include questions about heat or cold intolerance, weight loss or gain, and exposure to ionizing radiation. The review of body systems should include integumentary (skin: changes in temperature, texture, dryness, sallow complexion; hair: changes in texture and amount, e.g., scalp alopecia), eyes (proptosis/exophthalmos − protrusion of the eyeball, extraocular muscle involvement, corneal changes, and loss of vision because of optic nerve involvement), ears (decreased hearing), mouth and throat (decreased taste), neck (presence or absence of goiter and nodules), respiratory changes (increased susceptibility to pneumonia and pleural effusion), cardiac abnormalities (tachycardia, bradycardia, palpitations, increased pulse pressure, and CHF), GI tract (increased or decreased bowel motility and malabsorption), GU tract (polyuria and oligomenorrhea − scanty menstruation), neurologic signs (general: coma; motor: tremor, muscle weakness, myalgias, myopathy), endocrine disturbances (hypoglycemia, hypercholesterolemia, galactorrhea, and precocious puberty). Mental status is assessed for lethargy, apathy, psychosis, and emotional lability.

Diagnostic laboratory tests include serum T_3 or T_4 resin uptake and free thyroid hormones. Other tests include protein-bound iodine and butanol, extractable iodine (rarely used today because of lack of specificity), plasma thyrotropin, TRH and TSH stimulation, ^{131}I uptake, serum cholesterol, basal metabolic rate, and Achilles tendon reflex.

Common interventions

Medical treatment involves hormonal replacement. **Surgical** therapy includes subtotal or total thyroidectomy.

Nursing interventions

Physical 1. Refer to thyroidectomy for pre- and postoperative care (*see below*).
2. Administer medications as prescribed and note effects.
3. Maintain nutrition and fluid balance.
4. Assess tissue breakdown.
5. Maintain environmental temperature.
6. Monitor the patient's cardiac status.
7. Pace activities.
8. Avoid sedation.
9. Monitor physical and mental activity.
10. Assist the patient with activities of daily living.
11. Support vital functions during crisis/coma.
Psychosocial 12. Explain changes in body image and activity, and expected changes with therapy.
13. Provide a calm environment.

TABLE 22-7
Thyroid Hormones and Their Functions

Hormone	Function
Thyroxine (T_4)	Regulates body metabolism. Aids in regulating growth and development (physical and mental). Is involved in carbohydrate, protein, and fat metabolism.
Triiodothyronine (T_3)	Assists in reproduction. Governs vitamin requirements. Assists in resistance to infection.
Thyrocalcitonin	Regulates serum calcium and phosphorus.

Educational 14. Explain the nature of the condition and the need for follow-up as necessary.
15. Teach about the signs and symptoms of exacerbation as appropriate.
16. Teach about nutritional needs and caloric intake.

Evaluation criteria. See Overview.

GRAVES'S DISEASE

Graves's disease (toxic diffuse goiter) is characterized by hypersecretion of thyroid hormone accompanied by hyperthyroidism, enlargement of the thyroid (goiter), and exophthalmos. Graves's disease is highly prevalent, affects women four times as often as men, and usually occurs between the ages of 20 and 40 yr. The cause is unknown, but may involve either an autoimmune, cell-mediated, delayed hypersensitivity induced by thymic-dependent lymphocytes situated in the thyroid or an intrinsic thyroid cellular disorder with secondary autoimmune phenomena as contributory factors.

Local *signs and symptoms* consist of a symmetrically enlarged thyroid (three to four times normal size), rare obstructive symptoms related to the size of the gland or encroachment on the trachea or esophagus, and a normal-size thyroid in ~3% of patients. Systemic signs and symptoms are numerous and varied and include heat intolerance (increased calorigenesis); weight loss (increased calorigenesis, malabsorption); warm, smooth skin resulting from the decreased keratin layer and increased blood flow; increased sweating; fine, thin hair that readily falls out with combing; and exophthalmos (protruding eyes, fixed stare, inability to close the lids in severe cases). Other symptoms include cardiac (tachycardia, palpitations, increased pulse pressure, CHF, atrial fibrillation); increased GI motility causing diarrhea, malabsorption, and increased excretion of calcium; softening and increased fragility of the nails and separation of the distal margins from the nail bed; gynecomastia; oligomenorrhea or amenorrhea with increased libido, reduced fertility, and high rate of miscarriage; and hypercalcemia/hypercalciuria with no increased incidence of renal calculi and decreased bone density. Neuromuscular symptoms include tremor, muscle wasting, muscle weakness, and fatigue that are most prominent in the proximal limb muscles and affect men more frequently than women; hyperactive Achilles tendon reflex; and hyperkinesia. (The clinical picture may be confused because hyperthyroidism occurs in 3 to 6% of patients with myasthenia gravis.) Mental status changes include emotional lability and insomnia.

Diagnosis is based on the health history, physical exam, elevated serum thyroid levels, 24-hr radioactive iodine uptake, thyroid scan, and depressed serum cholesterol levels.

Common interventions

Medically, antithyroid drug therapy is used to block hormone synthesis for patients <18 yr and for pregnant women. ^{131}I therapy is used for middle-aged and elderly patients. **Surgical** treatment, thyroidectomy, is used for fairly young patients who do not have conditions that make them poor operative risks.

Nursing interventions

Physical 1. Assess the patient's cardiac status.
   a. Monitor vital signs and BP frequently, especially if the pulse is >100 bpm.
   b. Check for dyspnea.
   c. Monitor urinary output.
2. Maintain nutrition and promote weight gain.
   a. Provide a balanced, high-carbohydrate, high-protein diet.
   b. Discourage foods that increase peristalsis, such as highly seasoned, bulky, fibrous foods.
   c. Provide between-meal snacks or 6 meals/day to satisfy the patient's hunger.
   d. Provide a low-sodium diet.
   e. Weigh the patient daily and report a loss of >2 kg (~4½ lb).
   f. Obtain an order for supplemental vitamins, especially B complex, if nourishment does not improve.
3. Provide a cool environment.
   a. Omit a plastic draw sheet.
   b. Use only a lightweight sheet for a top cover.
   c. Change linens as frequently as needed if the patient is diaphoretic.
   d. Encourage the use of light, loose bedclothes.
4. Provide a restful environment.
   a. Assign the patient to a private room if possible.
   b. Keep the room quiet and dark.

5. Administer medications.
   a. Give sedatives as necessary.
   b. Give iodine with milk to prevent gastric irritation, hydrate the patient, and mask the very salty taste.
   c. Give iodine through a straw to prevent tooth discoloration.
   d. Give adrenergic-blocking agents as ordered to control over-activity of the sympathetic nervous system and lessen tachycardia, nervousness, and tremor.
6. Assist weak patients with activities of daily living.
7. Reduce eye discomfort and prevent corneal ulceration and infection.
   a. Encourage the patient to wear dark glasses.
   b. Encourage the patient to avoid dust and dirt.
   c. Tape the lids closed at night if needed.
   d. Relieve edema in the eye area by elevating the head of the bed and restricting salt intake.
   e. Instruct the patient to exercise the extraocular muscles daily (direct eyes from upper right to upper left to lower right to lower left several times a day).
   f. Administer methylcellulose eye drops qid.

Preoperative 8. Prevent the intraoperative and postoperative complications of **thyroidectomy**.
   a. Check that the thyroid test results are within the normal range.
   b. Check that the signs of hyperthyroidism are diminished or absent; the patient appears rested and relaxed.
   c. Check that nutritional status is normal and weight lost has been regained.
   d. Check that cardiac functioning is within normal limits.
9. Conduct preoperative teaching.
   a. Explain to the patient that pillows and sandbags will be used to support the head and neck and that they will limit movement.
   b. Instruct the patient not to extend or hyperextend the neck.
   c. Teach the patient how to support the head and neck when sitting up, moving in bed by placing the hands at the back of neck when flexing his neck or moving.
10. Provide other preoperative care (*see* Chapter 9).
11. Assemble the necessary equipment at the bedside before the patient returns from the OR (tracheotomy set, oxygen, humidifier, calcium gluconate, and other routine equipment).

Postoperative 12. Maintain a patent airway.
   a. Assess the patient frequently for respiratory distress resulting from edema of the glottis, bilateral laryngeal nerve damage, or tracheal compression from hemorrhage.
   b. Report signs of airway obstruction immediately (e.g., increasing restlessness, tachycardia, apprehension, cyanosis, crowing respirations, retraction of the neck muscles).

13. Assess the patient for hemorrhage.
    a. Check the dressing for increasing tightness or blood.
    b. Check the back of the neck for blood.
14. Assess the patient for hypocalcemia resulting from inadvertent removal of the parathyroid glands.
    a. Check for positive Chvostek's sign.
    b. Check for positive Trousseau's sign.
    c. Check serum calcium levels on the evening of surgery and daily thereafter (may develop 1 to 7 days after surgery).
    d. Report muscular spasm or twitching.
    e. Have calcium gluconate available.
15. Assess for laryngeal nerve injury.
    a. Check for hoarseness or weakness of the voice.
    b. Check for voice changes q 30 to 60 min.
    c. Discourage unnecessary talking to avoid prolonging hoarseness.
    d. Reassure the patient that hoarseness and weakness will subside in a few days.
16. Relieve pain or discomfort.
    a. Use semi-Fowler's position.
    b. Support the head and neck with sandbags or pillows.
    c. Give analgesics for pain in the throat area, usually meperidine 50 to 100 mg IM q 3 to 4 hr prn.
17. Maintain fluid balance.
    a. Provide fluids PO as soon as the patient is fully conscious.
    b. Discontinue IV fluids as soon as the patient tolerates fluids.
    c. Provide a soft diet on the afternoon of the first day after surgery.
    d. Observe for difficulty in swallowing.
    e. Reassure the patient that difficulty in swallowing lasts only 1 to 2 days.
    f. Measure and record intake and output for 24 to 48 hr postoperatively.
    g. Weigh the patient daily.
18. Observe for signs of thyroid storm.
    a. Take rectal temperature q 4 hr for 24 hr; orally thereafter.
    b. Report any elevation over 37.8°C (100°F) rectally or 37.2°C (99°F) orally.
    c. Report signs of extreme restlessness, agitation, and tachycardia.
Psychosocial 19. Explain that bizarre, difficult behavior is a result of the disease and should steadily improve with treatment.
20. Attempt to remain calm and understanding when working with the patient.
21. Accept outbursts and irritation as manifestations of the disease.
22. Explain that the appearance of the body will gradually return to normal (exophthalmos does not necessarily regress with treatment).
Educational 23. Instruct the patient in ROM exercises postoperatively to prevent contractures.

    a. Obtain the surgeon's permission after the sutures are removed.
    b. Explain that the exercises are to be performed several times a day
       (flex the head forward and laterally, hyperextend the neck, turn
       the head from side to side).
24. Apply a moisturizer to the incision after the sutures are removed to
    decrease scarring.
25. Teach the patient the need for and proper administration of thyroid
    medications.
26. Instruct the patient that lifelong follow-up care is necessary.

Evaluation criteria. *See* Overview.

THYROIDITIS

Thyroiditis is an inflammation of the thyroid that can be either acute (rare), subacute, or chronic. **Chronic thyroiditis** (Hashimoto's disease) occurs most commonly, affecting women (usually during menopause) four to five times as frequently as men. Its etiology is thought to be an auto-immune basis or a genetic predisposition. *Signs and symptoms* include enlargement of the neck, pain and tenderness in the thyroid region, difficulty in breathing and swallowing, cough and shortness of breath, increasing fatigue, and increase in weight.

Diagnosis is based on the health history, physical exam, and the following laboratory test results: ^{131}I uptake may be elevated, thyroidal uptake and T_4 are subnormal as the disease progresses, thyroid function tests and clinical manifestations are suggestive of euthyroid state in a majority of patients, high titers of thyroid antibodies (agglutination of tanned RBCs), and needle biopsy to confirm diagnosis.

Common interventions

Medical treatment involves suppressive doses of thyroid hormone. **Surgical** therapy includes a subtotal thyroidectomy and clearing around the trachea if there are symptoms of marked pressure, a malignant tumor is suspected, or for cosmetic purposes, if the gland is extremely enlarged. Postoperatively, thyroid hormones are administered as suppressive therapy.

Nursing interventions

Physical 1. Monitor vital signs.
2. Provide a liquid diet if dysphagia is present.
3. Measure and record the circumference of the patient's neck daily (if
    his neck is swollen).
4. Administer medications as ordered.
5. Assess for signs of hypothyroidism.
Psychosocial 6. Explain that mood changes are a result of the disease
    and should improve with treatment.
Educational 7. Teach the patient to observe for signs of thyroid
    dysfunction.

8. Instruct the patient that follow-up care is necessary.
9. Reinforce the need for and administration of medications.

Evaluation criteria. *See* Overview.

NONTOXIC GOITER

Nontoxic goiter is an enlargement of the thyroid in response to hormonal deficiency. It may be endemic, sporadic, or familial in nature. Endemic goiter most frequently occurs in winter and fall and during times of growth spurts (adolescence, pregnancy, lactation). It is more prevalent in areas that have a deficiency of iodine in the water and soil, and it affects men and women equally. Sporadic goiter affects more women than men in a ratio of 8:1. Endemic goiters may result from iodine deficiency or the ingestion of goitrogens. Genetic factors may have a contributory role. Sporadic goiters may result from (1) a possible compensatory response to impaired efficiency of the thyroid, (2) hypersecretion of TSH-stimulating glandular growth and morphologic changes, or (3) ingestion of goitrogens (Table 22-8). Familial goiters are rare, may be caused by an inborn error of metabolism, and are usually associated with hypothyroidism. They are generally inherited as an autosomal recessive train, but occasionally may be a dominant trait.

Most patients with endemic goiter are asymptomatic and do not consult a physician. *Symptoms* consist of increasing neck size or the presence of a mass (most common symptom), respiratory embarrassment, dysphagia, distension of the jugular veins, and sudden pain resulting from a rapid increase in the size of the goiter. This increase may be caused by hemorrhage into part of the goiter or a cyst or degenerating lesion. Symptoms usually subside spontaneously, and the gland reverts to its previous size. In rare cases, hemorrhage may be life threatening because of obstruction of the airway.

TABLE 22-8
Goitrogens* (Agents That Inhibit Thyroxine Production)

Foods containing goitrogenic glycosides	Medications containing goitrogenic substances
Rutabaga	Thioureas (propylthiouracil)
Cabbage	Thiocarbamides (aminothiazole, tolbutamide)
Soybeans	Iodine-containing solutions
Peanuts	Para-aminosalicylic acid
Peaches	Lithium
Peas	
Strawberries	
Radishes	

*Substances may cross the placental barrier and affect the fetus.

Complications of longstanding goiter include thyrotoxicosis in 60% of the patients (average duration of goiter before onset is 17 yr), CHF, and atrial fibrillation.

Diagnosis is based on the health history and physical exam, which may reveal a palpable mass that moves on swallowing. Failure of the thyroid to move during swallowing may indicate a goiter with intrathoracic extension, carcinoma of the thyroid with invasion of surrounding tissues, or thyroiditis extending into the adjacent structures. Laboratory data show normal levels of thyroid ^{131}I uptake, T_3, and T_4 in most patients. X-rays of the chest and neck may assist in the diagnosis, as well as barium swallow if dysphagia is present. Needle biopsy may also be performed.

Common interventions

Medical treatment involves replacement of iodine or thyroid hormone or discontinuation of the offending drug, if the condition is drug induced. If continuation of the drug is required, administration of thyroxin is recommended. Endemic goiter may be prevented by the use of iodized salt. **Surgery** may be required if the signs and symptoms are related to pressure, if pain and rapid increase in the size are related to intraglandular bleeding, or for cosmetic reasons. **Nursing** interventions are similar to those for thyroidectomy, as described under Graves's disease (*see above*).

CANCER OF THE THYROID

Malignant tumors of the thyroid may be caused by exposure to ionizing radiation during childhood, although one exact etiology is unknown. Types of tumors, their clinical manifestations, treatment, and prognosis are discussed in Table 22-9. **Nursing** interventions are the same as for thyroidectomy, as described under Graves's disease (*see above*).

HYPOTHYROIDISM

Hypothyroidism is a hypoactive, hypometabolic state associated with deficiency of either T_3 or T_4 or both. Hypothyroidism in children, or **cretinism**, is caused by a deficiency of thyroid hormone during fetal life or may result from functional failure of the thyroid soon after birth. It is a severe condition requiring immediate treatment. **Myxedema** is caused by a deficiency of thyroid hormone in the adult. It is a rare disease, usually affecting older people. Of the adults with hypothyroidism, 80% are women. Primary hypothyroidism (caused by pathologic changes within the thyroid) possibly occurs on an autoimmune basis, e.g., during the course of chronic (Hashimoto's) thyroiditis. It may be an iatrogenic result of the treatment of hyperthyroidism. Other causes include thyroidectomy with insufficient thyroid replacement, destruction of the thyroid by ^{131}I therapy, or overuse of antithyroid drugs. Secondary hypothyroidism may follow the development of destructive pituitary tumors, pituitary insufficiency, or postpartum necrosis of the pituitary.

TABLE 22-9
Thyroid Tumors

Class	Incidence	Clinical manifestations	Treatment	Prognosis
Papillary carcinoma	Most common malignant tumor of thyroid. Usually affects people in 30s and 40s. Occurs 3 times more frequently in women than in men.	Asymptomatic nodule. Enlargement of regional lymph nodes. Fixation of thyroid. Pressure on adjacent structures. Distant metastasis occurs late.	Surgical excision, lobectomy, isthmectomy, or total thyroidectomy (choice of procedure depends upon extent of lesion).	Excellent 1-yr survival (84-90%).
Follicular carcinoma	One quarter of malignant thyroid tumors. Usually affects people in 50s. Occurs 3 times more frequently in women than in men.	Many patients have long history of goiter with recent change. Pain and invasion of adjacent structures occurs late. Lungs and bones most frequent sites of metastases.	Same as for papillary carcinoma. May regress with suppressive thyroid hormone.	10-yr survival (no invasiveness) 86%. 10-yr survival (with invasiveness) 44%.

Medullary (solid) carcinoma	Comprises 7-10% of malignant thyroid tumors. Usually occurs after age of 50 yr. Slightly more common in women than men. Associated with other endocrine abnormalities, especially pheochromocytoma.	Hard nodular mass in thyroid. Enlargement of lymph nodes. Pain and tenderness may be severe. Lymph node metastases in over half of patients.	Pheochromocytomas, if present, are removed first. Total or near-total thyroidectomy and modified.	10-yr survival 61%.
Anaplastic carcinoma	10% of malignant lesions of thyroid. Usually occurs after age of 50 yr. Ratio of men to women is 1.3:1.0. 50% are in 70s to 80s.	Painful enlargement of thyroid. Thyroid often fixed; moves poorly when swallowing. Lymph nodes frequently enlarged. Signs and symptoms from pressure common. Metastases usually in lungs.	Total thyroidectomy and modified neck dissection. Lesion is not resectable in many patients.	Extremely rapid course. 75% of patients die within 1 yr.

Systemic *symptoms* include cold intolerance (decreased calorigenesis); weight gain; dry, flaky, atrophic, inelastic, cool skin; sallow complexion caused by decreased conversion of carotene to vitamin A; thick, coarse hair; alopecia of the scalp; diminished ability to sweat; hypothermia (may mask an infection); and dangerously increased sensitivity to narcotics, barbiturates, and anesthetics. Neurosensory deficits such as decreased hearing and blunted taste acuity may also occur. Respiratory symptoms consist of alveolar hypoventilation (CO_2 narcosis and hypoxia), increased susceptibility to pneumonia, and pleural effusion. Cardiac symptoms include pericardial effusion (low-voltage ECG, distant sounds), decreased contractility, and bradycardia. GI symptoms involve decreased bowel motility (constipation), malabsorption, and ascites with high protein content. GU symptoms consist of azotemia, hyponatremia (inability to excrete a water load), bladder atony (frequent urinary tract infections), infertility, decreased libido, and menorrhagia. Musculoskeletal aberrations such as myalgias, myopathy, and delayed relaxation time of reflexes (especially the Achilles tendon) also occur. Neurologic signs include coma and high CSF protein. Hematopoietic symptoms include iron deficiency, folate deficiency, coexistent pernicious anemia, leukopenia, and decreased aggregation of platelets. Endocrine symptoms include hypoglycemia, hypercholesterolemia, increased prolactin (galactorrhea), low urine 17-ketogenic steroids (decreased turnover of cortisol metabolites), and precocious puberty (Van Vyk-Grumbach syndrome). Mental status changes include lethargy and psychosis ("myxedema madness") characterized by paranoia and delusions.

Diagnosis is based on the health history, physical exam, and laboratory findings, e.g., abnormally low serum thyroid hormone levels and markedly elevated serum cholesterol.

Treatment consists of replacement of thyroid hormone.

Nursing interventions

Physical 1. Monitor cardiac status.
   a. Observe and report signs and symptoms of heart failure.
   b. Observe and report signs and symptoms of MI.
2. Maintain nutrition and fluid balance.
   a. Assess the patient's appetite.
   b. Force fluids to combat constipation if cardiac status allows.
   c. Provide a high-roughage diet to combat constipation.
   d. Provide a low-calorie diet to promote weight loss.
   e. Measure and record urine output.
   f. Observe for edema of tissues.
   g. Observe for decreasing output, indicating heart failure.
   h. Weigh the patient daily.
   i. Observe for significant weight loss with increased activity, decreased edema.
3. Monitor physical and mental activity.

a. Assist the patient with activities of daily living as necessary, especially if cardiac complications are present.

b. Assess energy levels and interest in the surroundings as an indication of the effectiveness of therapy.

4. Provide a warm environment. Give extra clothing. Give warm blankets. Monitor temperature frequently until it is stable.

5. Administer medications.

a. Give small doses of thyroid hormone initially if cardiac complications are present (large doses can precipitate cardiac failure).

b. Notify the physician immediately if cardiac symptoms appear; do not give the hormone until the patient's condition is reassessed.

c. Assess progress frequently to prevent complications; response to replacement therapy is dramatic.

d. Observe the patient for symptoms of hyperthyroidism (restlessness, nervousness, sweating, excessive weight loss).

e. Avoid sedating the patient if possible. If sedatives are given, administer no more than one half to one third the usual dose and observe carefully for signs of respiratory depression or coma.

f. Administer a stool softener or cathartics if the patient is constipated.

6. Support vital functions during myxedema coma.

a. Monitor BP and vital signs.

b. Administer IV levothyroxine and hydrocortisone to correct possible pituitary or adrenal insufficiency.

c. Provide respiratory support with oxygen and mechanical ventilation, if necessary.

d. Monitor fluid replacement.

e. Monitor fluid balance and serum electrolytes.

f. Administer antibiotics if infection is present.

g. Prevent complications of immobility.

h. Observe for and report hypertension or CHF.

i. Monitor arterial blood gases for hypoxia, respiratory acidosis, or the need for ventilatory assistance.

j. Check for possible sources of infection.

Psychosocial 7. Explain that lethargy and apathy are the results of the disease and will disappear with therapy.

8. Explain that the appearance of the body will gradually return to normal.

Educational 9. Explain the need for and method of administration of thyroid hormones.

10. Provide a written list of symptoms of thyroid deficiency or excess.

11. Instruct the patient that lifelong follow-up care is necessary.

12. Instruct the patient that if medication is taken daily, the depressed hypometabolic state of myxedema should not recur.

Evaluation criteria. *See* Overview.

PARATHYROID DISORDERS

The parathyroid glands are primarily involved with calcium regulation. However, parathyroid disorders are usually characterized by multiorgan involvement. The symptoms may be subtle.

The parathyroid glands are four small glands attached to, near to, or embedded in the thyroid; sometimes they are found in the mediastinum. Parathyroid hormone (PTH), the hormone secreted by the gland, controls calcium and phosphorus metabolism, maintains normal serum calcium levels by regulating metabolism of bone (resorption), controls excitability of nerves and muscles by calcium and phosphorus levels, increases degradation of collagen, and increases urinary hydroxyproline excretion. Its release is dependent on a feedback relationship between the serum calcium level and the serum PTH level. Elevated serum calcium causes decreased PTH secretion and results in decreased mobilization of calcium from bone and a lowering of serum calcium. Low serum calcium causes increased PTH secretion and results in increased mobilization of calcium from bone and an increase in serum calcium. Other substances related to bone resorption and nerve excitability are summarized in Table 22-10.

TABLE 22-10
Substances (Other Than PTH) Related to
Bone Resorption and Nerve Excitability

Substance	Function
Calcium	Determines excitability of nerve function and contractility of skeletal cardiac muscle. Forms structure and assists in function of cell membranes and organs, and in cell metabolism including hormone release.
Phosphorus	Assists in maintenance of acid-base balance. Combines with calcium in the formation and strengthening of bones. Functions in many metabolic processes in a way that makes it the most important mineral constituent for cellular activity (is an essential constituent of nucleic acids and nucleoproteins, assists in oxidation of carbohydrates, regulates hormone activity, and determines permeability of cell membranes).
Magnesium	Catalyzes many intracellular reactions. Determines excitability of nerves and contractility of skeletal muscle.
Vitamin D (cholecalciferol)	Mobilizes calcium from bone. Enhances intestinal absorption of calcium. Acts as a physiologic hormone.

The disease is found early because of the laboratory tests now available. As a result, patients generally are not as sick (the disease has not progressed) as in the past.

General assessment includes the health history, physical exam, and diagnostic tests. Past health and family histories are important. (However, the patient may be asymptomatic, and abnormal calcium may be found incidentally on laboratory study.) The review of systems should include inspection, palpation, and percussion of the integument (pruritus, mucocutaneous candidiasis), eyes (conjunctival calcification, band keratopathy — abnormal gray band around the cornea, cataracts), mouth (abnormal tongue movements, loose teeth, loss of lamina dura), cardiovascular system (hypertension, anemia), GI tract (peptic ulcers, pancreatitis, nausea, vomiting, constipation, weight loss), GU tract (nephrolithiasis, nephrocalcinosis — calcium deposits in the renal tubules, mild renal tubular acidosis, renal insufficiency, decreased ability to concentrate urine), musculoskeletal system (easy fatigability, proximal muscle weakness, hypotonia, bone cysts, brown tumors, fractures, bone pain, resorptive changes in distal phalanges, thinning of distal clavicles, gout, pseudogout), CNS (increased neuromuscular irritability, positive Chvostek's and Trousseau's signs, calcification of basal ganglia), endocrine system (pituitary and/or pancreatic adenomas — multiple endocrine neoplasia type I — pheochromocytoma and/or medullary thyroid carcinoma), and mental status (decreased memory, lethargy, depression, personality disturbances, decreased level of consciousness).

Diagnostic tests may include bone x-rays or biopsy and laboratory data. Blood is evaluated for serum calcium, phosphorus, alkaline phosphatase, and plasma calcitonin concentrations; tubular resorption of phosphate (TRP); and BUN and creatinine levels. The Ellsworth-Howard test is used for measurement of cyclic AMP. Urine tests are for qualitative and quantitative urinary calcium, hydroxyproline excretion, and cyclic AMP. RIA of plasma PTH concentration is also used.

Common interventions

Medical treatment with vitamin D and calcium is used for hypocalcemia. Medications used to lower serum calcium in hypercalcemia are discussed in Table 22-11. **Surgical** removal of the diseased gland may be advisable.

Nursing interventions

Physical 1. Refer to preoperative and postoperative teaching for thyroidectomy (*see above*).
2. Assess the patient for hormonal imbalance or hypocalcemia (mild tetany is expected; tingling of the hands and around the mouth is usually transient; if symptoms are persistent or severe, administer IV calcium gluconate).

TABLE 22-11
Drugs Used to Lower Serum Calcium

Drug	Dosage/route	Complications
Sodium chloride solution (isotonic)	1 liter IV q 3-4 hr	Pulmonary edema.
Sodium sulfate solution (isotonic)	3 liters IV over 9 hr	Pulmonary edema, hypernatremia.
Furosemide	100 mg/hr IV	Volume depletion hypokalemia.
Ethylenediamine-tetraacetate	50 mg/kg body wt IV over 4-6 hr	Renal failure, hypotension.
Cortisone	PO or parenteral 150 mg/day	Hypercorticism.
Mithramycin	25 mg/kg body wt IV	Hemorrhage, thrombocytopenia, nausea, vomiting.
Phosphate	1 mM/kg body wt IV over 6-8 hr 1-2 mM/kg body wt PO daily	Extraskeletal calcification, hypocalcemia.
Calcitonin	1-5 MRC units/kg body wt/day parenterally	Nausea, vomiting.

MRC, Medical Research Council.

3. Prevent patients with bone disease from becoming hypocalcemic (reduction of bone resorption and rapid rebuilding of bone causes "bone hunger").
   a. Monitor serum calcium levels.
   b. Encourage foods high in calcium.
   c. Administer oral calcium preparations if ordered.
   d. Encourage ambulation.
4. Refer to nursing interventions for thyroid disorders (*see above*) for psychosocial and educational measures.

Evaluation criteria. See Overview.

ACUTE HYPERCALCEMIC CRISIS

Elevated serum calcium may result in an acute hypercalcemic crisis, a serious and potentially lethal complication of many diseases. An understanding of the underlying disease is necessary to determine if an emergency exists. Individual patient tolerance to hypercalcemia varies and reflects the rate at which serum calcium rises. Patients with primary hyperparathyroidism may be asymptomatic with serum calcium levels of 15 mg/100 mg. Patients with rapidly progressive cancer may be moribund with serum calcium levels of 12 mg/100 mg. The incidence of hypercalcemic crisis is variable and is dependent on etiology. It is equally common in males and females and is most likely to occur if severe renal damage is present. It may appear as a complication of primary hyperparathyroidism, vitamin D intoxication, metastatic carcinoma (especially of the breast, kidneys, lungs, thyroid, prostate), multiple myeloma, sarcoidosis, or Paget's disease of the bone.

In crisis, *symptoms* of hypercalcemia (*see below*) rapidly progress to lethargy and drowsiness, confusion, severe muscle weakness, prostration, coma, severe dehydration, and oliguria.

Diagnosis is based on the health history, physical exam, and laboratory findings (e.g., elevated serum calcium).

Common interventions

Medical therapy consists of restoration of ECF volume by isotonic sodium chloride IV and reduction of serum calcium with IV fluids and drugs (*see* Table 22-11). Treatment of the underlying disorder may require radiation therapy; cytotoxic drugs; corticosteroids; and withdrawal of milk, alkali, estrogens, thiazides, and vitamin D. **Surgical** removal of neoplasms after control of hypercalcemia is established may be advisable.

Nursing interventions

Physical 1. Observe the patient for signs of pulmonary edema.
2. Observe for signs of complications related to drugs.
3. Observe for signs of changes in serum calcium levels (*see below*).

HYPERPARATHYROIDISM

Hyperparathyroidism is a syndrome caused by hypersecretion of PTH by one or more of the parathyroid glands. Primary hyperparathyroidism is a generalized disorder of calcium, phosphate, and bone metabolism characterized by excessive and incompletely regulated secretion of PTH from the parathyroid gland. Secondary hyperparathyroidism is a compensatory hypersecretion of PTH in response to a lowered serum calcium level that is a result of another disorder such as renal disease or malabsorption syndromes leading to calcium wasting or poor calcium absorption from the intestines (rickets, osteomalcia). Primary hyperparathyroidism was previously considered a rare disease, but its incidence is now estimated to be as high as 1 in 1,000 persons/yr (0.1 to 0.5% of the general population) because of increased technology using multichannel autoanalyzers for blood. It most commonly occurs between the ages of 30 and 60 yr and is more common in women than in men, with a ratio of 2:1. Most cases (75 to 85%) of primary hyperparathyroidism are caused by a single parathyroid adenoma;

15 to 20% result from multiple hyperplastic glands. Parathyroid carcinoma is rare (1%). Familial factors are assumed to be autosomal dominant with incomplete penetrance. Secondary hyperparathyroidism is more common than the primary disease and may be associated with rickets, abnormal vitamin D metabolism, chronic renal failure, and osteomalacia due to phenytoin or laxative abuse.

Signs and symptoms related to hypercalcemia include renal damage (colic, azotemia with increased serum phosphate and hypocalcemia, especially with chronic renal failure), mental changes (depression, fatigue, listlessness, confusion, delirium, coma), musculoskeletal changes (bone pain, general muscle weakness, hypotonia, hyperactive reflexes), GI changes (loss of appetite and weight, nausea, vomiting, abdominal pain, constipation, peptic ulcer, pancreatitis, gastric disturbances), eye changes (band keratitis, calcium in palpebral tissue), cardiovascular changes (hypertension, ECG changes – short Q-T interval and nearly absent ST segment), and fever. Signs and symptoms related to increased urinary calcium include thirst, polyuria, polydipsia, and hypokalemia. Signs and symptoms related to hypomagnesemia are paresthesias and hyperreflexia. Signs and symptoms related to direct action of PTH consist of demineralization of the skeleton because of bone resorption (bone pain, cysts, tumors, fractures) renal damage, peptic ulcer, and pancreatitis. Signs and symptoms related to renal damage (30% of patients) include hypertension, renal stones, nephrocalcinosis, and cardiac failure. Less than 5% of parathyroid adenomas can be palpated. In patients with hypercalcemia crisis, the tumor is normally very large and can be palpated in 40% of the cases. The most acute *complication* is hypercalcemic crisis.

Diagnosis is based on the health history, physical exam, and laboratory findings that include elevated serum calcium, chloride, and PTH levels; low serum phosphorus levels; and hyperchloremic metabolic acidosis. Calcium infusion and TRP tests are also diagnostic. A PTH infusion test may be carried out in conjunction with TRP and is performed only when the patient is not azotemic. X-rays of the skull show a typical "moth-eaten" appearance.

Common interventions

Medical treatment involves the reduction of hypercalcemia with drugs and sodium chloride 0.9% IV (*see* Table 22-7). The underlying disease in secondary hyperparathyroidism is treated as appropriate. **Surgical** removal of the diseased glands is usually advised. If all four parathyroid glands are diseased, three and one half glands are usually removed. The remaining one half gland is usually sufficient to maintain normal levels of PTH.

Nursing interventions

Physical 1. Reduce serum calcium level.
    a. Force fluid intake to at least 3,000 ml/day.
    b. Maintian IVs.

    c. Increase urine acidity by giving cranberry or prune juice (calcium is more soluble in acid urine).

    d. Provide a low-calcium diet.

    e. Ambulate the patient as early as possible (stress of muscle on bone decreases calcium loss in bone).

2. Monitor cardiopulmonary status.

    a. Record intake and output.

    b. Observe for signs of pulmonary edema.

    c. Monitor vital signs.

    d. Monitor carefully if the patient is on digitalis (calcium and digitalis have a synergistic effect on the myocardium and conducting system; toxic symptoms may develop quickly).

3. Administer medications.

    a. Give medications as ordered to reduce serum calcium.

    b. Give stool softeners or laxatives as needed.

    c. Give antacids as needed for peptic ulcer.

4. Observe for renal stones.

    a. Strain all urine.

    b. Save abnormal specimens for the physician to examine.

5. Assist weak patients with activities of daily living.

6. Protect the patient from pathologic fractures if skeletal involvement exists.

    a. Keep the bed in a low position.

    b. Use side rails.

    c. Assist the patient with ambulation.

    d. Move weak, immobile patients carefully.

    e. Check x-rays to determine which bones are the weakest.

7. Provide pre- and postoperative care (*see* thyroidectomy *above*).

Psychosocial 8. Explain that the mental symptoms are a result of the disease and should return to normal once the hyperparathyroidism is corrected (for most but not all patients).

9. Explain that the chance for recovery is good if the patient was surgically treated early in the course of the illness.

10. Explain that bone pain may disappear by the third postoperative day and that bone lesions may heal completely.

11. Provide support if renal damage is serious.

Educational 12. Teach the need for and correct administration of medications.

13. Teach the patient to maintain a low-calcium diet as necessary.

14. Instruct the patient that lifelong follow-up care is necessary.

Evaluation criteria. *See* Overview.

HYPOPARATHYROIDISM

Hypoparathyroidism results from hyposecretion of PTH by the parathyroid glands, causing low serum calcium levels and high serum phosphate levels. Its most common occurrence is after thyroid surgery (2 to 3% of patients). Idiopathic primary hypoparathyroidism is extremely rare and is usually seen in patients under the age of 16 yr. Iatrogenic causes involve accidental removal of the parathyroid glands during thyroidectomy, infarction of the parathyroid glands during surgery because of interference with the blood supply, or trauma to the glands. Idiopathic causes include autoimmune disease, congenital abnormality, or multiple end-organ endocrine failure.

Signs and symptoms are caused by hypocalcemia. Acute hypoparathyroidism (iatrogenic) is associated with painful muscle spasm, grimacing, tetany, positive Chvostek's and Trousseau's signs, tingling of the fingers and circumoral area, laryngospasm, arrhythmias (prolongation of the Q-T interval), irritability, tonic and clonic convulsions, and anxiety. Symptoms of chronic hypoparathyroidism (idiopathic) include lethargy, thin and patchy hair, brittle nails, dry and scaly skin, cataracts, calcification of the basal ganglia, personality changes, psychosis, organic brain syndrome, arrhythmias leading to heart failure, increased deep tendon reflexes, abdominal pain, weakened tooth enamel, chronic tetany (possibly leading to laryngospasm), and tonic and clonic convulsions. Signs and symptoms are always more severe in the presence of an elevated serum pH (alkalosis).

Diagnosis is based on the health history, physical exam, and laboratory findings that reveal low serum calcium, high serum phosphate, and decreased plasma PTH. Urinary calcium is low or absent. X-rays reveal increased bone density and calcifications of the basal ganglia.

Common interventions

Acute hypoparathyroidism with acute tetany is life threatening. It is essential to elevate serum calcium levels as quickly as possible. Administration of 10% calcium gluconate is given IV. Mild respiratory acidosis is initiated by having the patient rebreathe his own CO_2 from a paper bag. It is essential to prevent or treat convulsions, control laryngospasm, and maintain a patent airway. Chronic hypoparathyroidism is managed by elevating serum calcium to normal levels through diet (high calcium, low phosphorus) and medications (calcium salts — calcium gluconate, calcium lactate, or calcium chloride; and vitamin D).

Nursing interventions

Physical 1. Assess the patient for signs and symptoms of tetany.
2. Maintain a patent IV.
3. Keep a tracheostomy tray and endotracheal tubes available.
4. Keep IV calcium gluconate at the bedside.
5. Administer medications as ordered.
6. Monitor patients on digitalis carefully (dosage may need to be adjusted; calcium and digitalis have a synergistic effect on the myo-

cardium and conducting system; toxic symptoms may develop quickly).
7. Assess for signs of heart block and decreasing CO.
8. Assist with activities of daily living as necessary.
9. Provide a high-calcium, low-phosphorus diet.

Psychosocial 10. Explain that full recovery from the effects of hypo-parathyroidism can be expected.

11. Provide support if serious, irreversible complications such as cataracts and brain calcifications have formed (such complications are irreversible).

Educational 12. Teach the patient about the need for and method of administration of calcium salts and vitamin D.

13. Teach the patient about the need for having the serum calcium level checked at least 3 times/yr for life.

14. Provide a written list of symptoms of hypercalcemia and hypocalcemia.

15. Instruct the patient that normal serum calcium levels must be maintained to prevent complications.

16. Instruct the patient that medication must be taken daily.

17. Provide the patient with a written high-calcium, low-phosphorus diet.

Evaluation criteria. *See* Overview.

PANCREATIC DISORDERS

The pancreas plays a major role in the digestion and metabolism of carbohydrates (CHO), proteins, and fats through its secretion of enzymes and hormones. CHO are the preferred and most immediate source of energy. When CHO are not available or cannot be properly utilized, proteins and fats are used for energy. The pancreas is a solid, slender organ divided into three parts (head, body, and tail), extending transversely across the upper abdomen behind the stomach. Its main duct (pancreatic duct of Wirsung) joins with the common bile duct at the ampulla of Vater to enter the duodenum. Acinar cells secrete enzymes for digestion of CHO, proteins, and fats. Centroacinar cells produce sodium bicarbonate and water and neutralize the acid pH of chyme. The endocrine function of the pancreas involves the secretion of hormones that regulate CHO (and some protein and fat) metabolism. Alpha, beta, and delta cells are scattered throughout the pancreas in the islets of Langerhans. Alpha cells produce glucagon, which elevates intracellular phosphorylase, enhances gluconeogenesis and keto-genesis, causes glycogenolysis in the liver, and releases glucose into the bloodstream. Beta cells produce insulin. The various actions of this hormone are described in Table 22-12. Delta cells produce gastrin, which (1) stimulates the release of gastric acid, pepsin, and an intrinsic factor by the stomach; (2) stimulates growth of the stomach, exocrine pancreas, and

TABLE 22-12
Actions of the Hormone Insulin

Area of action	Major action
Muscle	Facilitates glucose transport into cells. Facilitates conversion of glucose to glycogen. Facilitates oxidation of glucose to pyruvate and lactate. Facilitates oxidation of glucose to CO_2 and H_2O. Enhances amino acid uptake into cells. Inhibits uptake of FFA.
Adipose tissue	Facilitates glucose transport. Stimulates conversion of glucose to fat (lipogenesis). Enhances FFA uptake into cell. Enhances activity of lipoprotein lipase. Inhibits lipolysis by providing more a-glycerol phosphate and inhibiting lipase.
Liver	Promotes glucose uptake. Inhibits hepatic glucose output. Enhances glycogen production. Decreases gluconeogenesis. Stimulates FFA synthesis. Enhances triglyceride formation. Promotes synthesis of specific proteins such as enzymes. Effects protein synthesis generally.

FFA, free fatty acid.

mucosa of the small intestine and colon; (3) decreases absorption of nutrients from the gut; and (4) stimulates pancreatic secretion. Other nonpancreatic hormones that help regulate CHO metabolism are listed in Table 22-13.

General assessment includes the health history, physical exam, and diagnostic tests. Key areas for assessment are the current health status (nutrition history, alcohol intake), past health/family history (endocrine disorders, jaundice), and a review of the following body systems: integumentary (jaundice, moistness or dryness, skin turgor, infections), eyes (changes in vision, retinopathy), cardiovascular (macrovascular changes, microvascular changes, peripheral vascular disease), GI tract (nausea, vomiting, distension, abdominal pain), and GU tract (polyuria, urinary tract infections, nephropathy, changes in sexual functioning). Blood tests include fasting blood glucose, 2-hr postprandial glucose, glucose tolerance test, and serum electrolytes and amylase. Urine is evaluated for glucose, acetone, and amylase. X-rays may include oral or IV cholecystogram and chest and abdomen.

Common interventions

Medical treatment includes increased or decreased CHO diet and medications, e.g., insulin, hypoglycemics, pancreatic enzymes, or others, as indicated. **Surgical** procedures include partial pancreatectomy, Whipple's procedure, or removal of a tumor.

TABLE 22-13
Regulation of Carbohydrate Metabolism by Other Hormones

Hormone	Function	Stimulus
ACTH (gluco-corticoids)	Converts fats and protein to glucose.	Stress, abnormally low blood glucose.
Epinephrine	Converts glycogen to glucose.	Stress.
Thyroid hormone	Promotes utilization of glucose for energy.	Normal conditions.
	Promotes conversion of fats and proteins to glucose for energy.	Starvation.

Nursing interventions

Physical 1. Administer medications and fluids as ordered.
2. Monitor vital signs.
3. Assess endocrine functioning.
   a. Check urinary glucose and acetone.
   b. Monitor blood glucose.
   c. Assess for signs and symptoms of hypoglycemia or hyperglycemia.
4. Monitor intake and output.
5. Provide a stable internal environment for preoperative insulin-dependent diabetic patients.
   a. Administer adequate fluids to prevent severe fluid loss brought about by osmotic diuresis caused by hyperglycemia.
   b. Administer insulin appropriately to prevent ketosis.
   c. Prevent hypoglycemia and insulin shock.
6. Prepare the patient on the day of surgery.
   a. Omit food, water, insulin, and oral hypoglycemics.
   b. Schedule surgery as early in the morning as possible.
   c. Assess preoperative laboratory tests (fasting and postprandial blood sugars, urine tests for glucose and acetone, CO_2-combining power, BUN, ECG, chest x-ray).
   d. Ensure that blood glucose is obtained and that the results are reported to the surgeon within 1 hr of the operation.
   e. Administer 5% glucose in water IV, with insulin as ordered.
7. Provide postoperative care.
   a. Administer IV 5% glucose in water until the patient is able to take PO nourishment and the IV is discontinued.

    b. Monitor diabetic control (test urine for glucose and acetone at least q 6 hr; check blood glucose results — usually ordered tid during the initial postoperative period).

    c. Administer insulin as necessary (regular insulin is given until diabetic control is reestablished; then return to preoperative insulin type).

    d. Prevent infection by changing dressings with meticulous sterile technique and maintaining bladder functioning (avoid distension or retention; use nursing techniques to ensure emptying of bladder; avoid indwelling catheterization; catheterize intermittently if necessary).

Psychosocial 8. Provide emotional support for the patient and significant others living with a chronic illness that requires changes in living habits.

Educational 9. Teach the patient and family about the nature of the disease, its signs and symptoms, treatment, complications, the need for lifelong treatment and follow-up care, the need for and provision of adequate nutrition, ways of adapting life-style with minimum interruptions, sources of information and community resources, and the need to carry a medical alert card and/or bracelet.

Evaluation criteria. *See* Overview.

HYPOGLYCEMIA

Hypoglycemia is characterized by low blood glucose levels that may lead to coma, permanent brain damage, and death if left untreated. Its occurrence is common in insulin-dependent diabetics, who usually experience hypoglycemia at some time. Attacks may be precipitated by an overdose of insulin (or rarely, a sulfonylurea), skipped meals or decreased food intake, increased exercise or exertion without increased intake of CHO, or nausea and vomiting leading to fluid and nutritional imbalance.

Early *symptoms* consist of headache, weakness, irritability, poor muscular coordination, apprehension, and diaphoresis. Later symptoms include pallor, bradycardia, bradypnea, visual disturbances, alteration in level of consciousness, memory loss or confusion, hallucinations, generalized or focal seizures or status epilepticus, primitive movements (sucking, lip smacking, positive Babinski's sign), and coma.

Diagnosis is based on the health history, physical exam, and low blood glucose (≤ 60 mg/100 ml), which is the single best indicator of the disorder.

Common interventions

Treatment of mild hypoglycemia consists of orange juice or other simple sugar PO. Severe hypoglycemia usually requires an immediate IV of 20 to 50 ml of 50% glucose. Oral glucose is given to raise blood glucose after consciousness is regained. Other medications include glucagon, 1 mg IV or SC, and epinephrine, 0.5 to 1.0 ml of 1:100 SC.

Nursing interventions

Physical 1. Establish and maintain a patent airway.
2. Start an IV if the patient is unconscious.
   a. Use a 16- or 18-gauge catheter.
   b. Draw blood for glucose testing.
   c. Ask the lab for the blood glucose report as rapidly as possible.
3. Give 50 ml of 50% DW IV after blood glucose is drawn (most patients wake up during or after the first dose of 50% DW; some patients may require a second dose).
4. Maintain IV with 5 to 10% DW.
5. Monitor cardiac status; obtain a 12-lead ECG.
6. Monitor blood glucose; repeat testing in 1 to 2 hr.
Psychosocial 7. Provide reassurance that appropriate care is being given.

Evaluation criteria. *See* Overview.

KETOACIDOSIS

Ketoacidosis (coma) is the excessive accumulation of ketone bodies leading to acidosis and a decreased level of consciousness. It is a fairly common occurrence in persons who take too little insulin, omit doses of insulin, or have an increased need for insulin because of surgery, trauma, fever, or pregnancy. Insulin resistance may also be a factor. As a result of hyperglycemia, water shifts from intracellular to extracellular space to maintain osmotic equilibrium (sufficient insulin is necessary for glucose to permeate cell membranes). Osmotic diuresis occurs, and water and electrolytes, as well as glucose, are excreted in the urine. Plasma sodium concentration is usually low because of the osmotic effect of glucose and because of increased water intake provoked by intense thirst. Water and electrolyte depletion occurs. Circulatory insufficiency with azotemia and hypotension may occur with subsequent catecholamine discharge. Ketosis develops because the catabolism of protein and fat is enhanced by a deficiency of insulin. Excessive quantities of ketones are produced by the liver, and the body is unable to metabolize or excrete them. Renal excretion of ketones is depressed in severe volume depletion with circulatory insufficiency. Blood pH eventually decreases. Acidosis and/or ketones tend to interfere with the action of insulin used in treatment.

Polyuria and polydipsia are early *symptoms* of ketoacidosis. Other symptoms include nausea, vomiting, and dehydration accompanied by weight loss, dry mucous membranes, hot and flushed skin, and soft eyeballs. Hypotension, shock, oliguria, and anuria are late symptoms. Abdominal pain, Kussmaul's respiration, an acetone odor on the breath, weakness, paralysis, paresthesia, and coma or stupor (late symptoms) may also occur.

Diagnosis is based on the health history, physical exam, and laboratory studies that are used to determine if the coma is caused by hypo- or hyperglycemia: CBC, blood glucose, BUN, electrolytes, ketones, osmolarity, arterial blood gases, and evaluation of the urine for glucose, ketones, and protein.

Common interventions

Treatment includes providing exogenous insulin to promote CHO utilization and lipogenesis and to inhibit lipolysis; restoring normal blood volume; correcting fluid and electrolyte imbalance; correcting precipitating factors; and correcting severe acidosis by administering sodium bicarbonate.

Nursing interventions

Physical 1. Establish and maintain a patent airway.
2. Administer O_2.
3. Ensure that a large-bore IV is started.
4. Ensure that blood is drawn before medication is given.
5. Insert a Foley catheter.
   a. Test the urine for sugar, ketones, and protein.
   b. Send specimens to the laboratory for urinalysis, culture, and sensitivity tests.
6. Monitor arterial blood gases.
7. Begin continuous cardiac monitoring.
8. Keep the patient NPO.
9. Monitor fluid balance.
   a. Administer 0.90 or 0.45% sodium chloride.
   b. Measure and record output hourly.
10. Ensure that x-rays are taken as ordered.
11. Observe for signs of hyperkalemia (bradycardia, weakness, flaccid paralysis, oliguria, cardiac arrest).
12. Observe for signs of hypokalemia (weakness, flaccid paralysis, paralytic ileus, cardiac arrest).
13. Prevent hypoglycemia.
    a. Administer 5% glucose in water after blood glucose has decreased to 300 mg/100 ml (usually within 4 to 6 hr after insulin therapy is begun).
    b. Monitor laboratory reports.
Psychosocial 14. Provide reassurance that appropriate care is being given.

Evaluation criteria. *See* Overview.

PANCREATITIS

Pancreatitis is an inflammatory process of the pancreas with varying degrees of pancreatic edema, fat necrosis, or hemorrhage. It may be acute or chronic or may exist in combination forms. Pancreatitis is a fairly common but potentially fatal process. Alcohol abuse is the most common cause (70% of patients). Clinical pancreatitis becomes evident after only 6 to 8 yr of heavy alcohol ingestion. Pathogenesis is uncertain. Cholelithiasis is present in 16% of patients. Postoperative pancreatitis may occur after abdominal (especially gastric and biliary) surgery. Direct injury may be the cause but pathogenesis is unclear. Other etiologies include hyperlipoproteinemia, hypercalcemia, viral infection, pregnancy, and drugs (corticosteroids, thiazide diuretics, sulfonamides, and toxins such as methyl alcohol, zinc oxide, and cobaltous chloride).

Symptoms include pain that usually begins suddenly, but may start gradually. It frequently is located in the midepigastrium and often radiates to the back. Pain is extremely variable in character and ranges from a steady knifelike distress to agonizing intermittent cramping. It may occur in the left or right upper quadrants when it is caused by severe involvement of the head or tail of the pancreas. Nausea, extreme retching, and vomiting are common and usually occur with an empty stomach. Vomiting may be repeated but usually is not copious in volume. The character of the vomitus is unremarkable, consisting of gastric or duodenal contents, and is not feculent. Other symptoms include fever, tachycardia, leukocytosis, extreme malaise and restlessness, shock (depending on the amount of fluid and blood lost in the retroperitoneal area and perotoneal cavity as well as from vomiting), mild jaundice (occurs in 20 to 30% of patients), and carpopedal spasm resulting from hypocalcemia. Upper abdominal tenderness and guarding may be present. The abdomen is moderately distended. Moderate muscle spasm is usual; true rigidity is infrequent.

Diagnosis is based on the health history, physical exam, and laboratory tests. Serum amylase is elevated, which in itself is not diagnostic of pancreatitis and may also occur in other conditions. One third of patients with proven pancreatitis have values <200 Somogyi units, one third have values between 200 and 500 units, and one third have values >500 units. Two-hour urine for amylase is often high. Elevated levels of amylase may be found in the pleural fluid. Oral cholecystogram frequently fails to produce visualization of the biliary tree even when it has been completely normal for as long as 6 wk after an attack. IV cholecystogram is useful in differentiating acute pancreatitis from acute cholecystitis. X-rays of the chest and abdomen reveal pleural effusions, loss of the psoas muscle outlines, laziness of the epigastric region, distortion fo the gastric air bubble, increased gastrocolic separation, duodcnal or segmental small intestine ileus, and dilation of the transverse colon. Laparotomy may be necessary on occasion to avoid misdiagnosing a strangulating obstruction of the small intestine or other dangerous condition.

Common interventions

Medical therapy consists of replacement and maintenance of colloid, fluid, and electrolytes; alleviation of pain; reduction of pancreatic stimulus; and prevention or treatment of hyperglycemia. **Surgery** may be performed for a biliary tract disorder, when the diagnosis is doubtful, or for drainage of a pseudocyst. In severe pancreatitis, total pancreatectomy may be necessary when alternatives are unsuccessful.

Nursing interventions

1. *See* Overview.
Physical 2. Maintain circulatory volume; replace fluid and electrolyte loss.
   a. Monitor the central venous pressure hourly.
   b. Monitor urinary output hourly.
   c. Measure urine sp gr.
   d. Monitor intake and output.
   e. Monitor serum electrolyte balance.
   f. Administer fluids, albumin, blood, and electrolytes as ordered.
   g. Monitor vital signs and assess for shock.
3. Reduce pancreatic stimulus.
   a. Maintain constant NG suction.
   b. Keep the patient NPO.
   c. Maintain bed rest.
4. Administer analgesics (meperidine is usually given; morphine and its derivatives are avoided because they increase spasm of the sphincter of Oddi; morphine is given in extreme cases).
5. Administer other medications as ordered.
   a. Give antacids or cimetidine to prevent bleeding from acute gastroduodenal ulceration.
   b. Give calcium gluconate for hypocalcemia.
   c. Avoid anticholinergics, especially if tachycardia and fever are present.
6. Provide nutritional support.
   a. Begin IV hyperalimentation as soon as practicable in patients with severe pancreatitis.
   b. Keep the patient NPO for 24 to 48 hr after NG suction is discontinued.
   c. Provide low-fat PO feedings when tolerated.
7. Assess the patient for altered endocrine pancreatic functioning (hyper- or hypoglycemia).
   a. Monitor blood glucose levels.
   b. Check the urine for glucose and acetone.
   c. Assess for other signs and symptoms.
8. Assess the patient for hypocalcemia and hypomagnesemia.
   a. Assess for signs of tetany.
   b. Monitor serum calcium levels.
   c. Administer calcium gluconate.
9. Assess the patient for cardiovascular failure.

       a. Assess for hypotension, tachycardia, and decreased CO.
       b. Monitor ECG changes.
10. Assess the patient for respiratory complications (cyanosis, restlessness, tachypnea, pulmonary infiltrates, atelectasis, and pleural effusions).
11. Assess for renal and hepatic failure.
12. Assess for local sequelae (paralytic ileus; duodenal obstruction; biliary obstruction; pseudocysts — most common complication — usually occur after the 2nd wk; pancreatic abscess — rare, mortality close to 100% if the cause is clostridial, occurs after the 3rd wk).
13. Assess for sequelae of repeated attacks, which are more common in alcoholic pancreatitis and rare in gallstone pancreatitis (pancreatic calcification, secondary diabetes mellitus, steatorrhea).
14. Encourage the patient to avoid alcohol.

Evaluation criteria. See Overview.

PSEUDOCYSTS OF THE PANCREAS

Pseudocysts of the pancreas have a fibrous lining and are filled with a collection of pancreatic juice and necrotic or suppurative pancreatic tissue. They are more common than true cysts (more than three-fourths of all cystic lesions are pseudocysts), occur most often in the fourth and fifth decades of life, and are more common in men than women. They may result from alcoholic pancreatitis or trauma.

Signs and symptoms include persistent pain, fever, and ileus appearing 2 to 3 wk after an attack of pancreatitis or trauma. Symptoms usually appear after several attacks of pancreatitis. A nontender mass, nausea, vomiting, and anorexia occur in 20% of patients. *Complications* include GI hemorrhage from esophageal varices resulting from compression of the portal venous system and jaundice caused by narrowing of the common bile duct. Accentuation of fever and toxicity at least 3 wk after the onset of pancreatitis indicates the development of pancreatic abscess.

Diagnosis is based on the health history, physical exam, continued elevation of serum amylase, high amylase content of the ascitic fluid, and x-rays. Upper GI series shows an extrinsic mass displacing the stomach. A barium enema may show displacement of the colon. The presence of gas bubbles on x-ray of the abdomen and positive blood culture indicate abscess.

Common interventions

Medical treatment of acute pancreatitis should be continued and the patient should be observed for several weeks if the condition remains satisfactory. **Surgical** correction may be necessary if the mass becomes larger, if the condition worsens, or for such frequent complications as secondary infection, severe hemorrhage, rupture into the adjacent viscus (organ) or into the free peritoneal cavity. Once a thick fibrous wall has developed, lesions rarely resolve. **Nursing** interventions are the same as for carcinoma of the pancreas (*see below*).

CARCINOMA OF THE PANCREAS

Carcinoma of the pancreas is a malignancy that affects males more frequently than females. Patients are of all races and have an average age of 60 yr. Approximately 3% of all cancers are pancreatic malignancies. The cause is unknown, but biliary lithiasis has been suspected as the cause of carcinoma of the common bile duct. Pancreatic malignant tumors occur at least twice as frequently in diabetic as in nondiabetic patients, but diabetes is rarely the first sign of pancreatic cancer.

Weight loss is the most common *symptom*. Pain is extremely frequent (70 to 80%), is dull and aching, and is most often confined to the midepigastrium. It may radiate to the back and is relieved by sitting in a hunched position, is accentuated by lying supine, and aggravated by eating. Other symptoms include jaundice, anorexia and weakness (~50%), pruritus, a palpable liver in 50 to 70% with carcinoma of the head of the pancreas, and a palpable gallbladder in 25 to 30% of cases.

Diagnosis is based on the health history, physical exam, x-rays for abnormalities, and laboratory tests for obstructive jaundice. Serum bilirubin almost never rises >30 to 35 mg/100 ml; alkaline phosphatase almost always is increased; fecal urobilinogen is <5 mg/24 hr; and serum transaminase often rises to >1,000 U.

Common interventions

Medical treatment includes adequate nutrition and correction of anemia as quickly as possible to prepare for surgery. Preoperative evaluation of renal functioning is valuable because postoperative renal failure is common in severely jaundiced patients. Adequate hydration before surgery helps to prevent renal failure. **Surgical** resection, the only definitive and potentially curative treatment, involves Whipple's procedure. Chemotherapy and radiotherapy are not useful. The 5-yr survival rate after resection for carcinoma of the head of the pancreas is ~18%.

Nursing interventions

Physical 1. Refer to Chapter 9 for preoperative care and Chapter 11 for postoperative care.
2. Assess the patient for renal failure.
3. Monitor fluid balance hourly (assess intake, measure output, measure sp gr, measure CVP, and monitor serum electrolytes).
4. Observe for pancreatic fistula (third most common complication);

generally closes in 2 to 3 wk if adequate nutrition and electrolyte balance are maintained).
   a. Observe the dressing.
   b. Report drainage.
   c. Ensure that the sump drainage is working once the complication is diagnosed and treatment has begun.
   d. Measure and record sump drainage.
   e. Protect the skin from drainage.
5. Assess for diabetes.
   a. Monitor blood chemistry.
   b. Check urinary glucose and acetone.
   c. Administer glucose or hypoglycemic agents as necessary.
6. Assess the patient's nutritional status.
   a. Weigh the patient daily.
   b. Measure abdominal girth.
7. Provide adequate nutrition.
   a. Give 2,500 calories IV, PO, or via NG tube.
   b. If ascites is present, provide a low-sodium diet.
   c. Serve small, frequent meals.
   d. Administer pancreatic enzymes at mealtime.
8. Provide skin care.
   a. Assess jaundice.
   b. Keep the skin clean and dry.
   c. Prevent excoriation if pruritus is severe by clipping the nails and providing light cotton gloves.
9. Assess for signs of GI bleeding.
   a. Hematest stools and enuresis.
   b. Monitor Hb and Hct.
   c. Administer antacids as ordered.
Psychosocial 10. Assist the patient and family to cope with the diagnosis of cancer and deal with impending death (as appropriate) and chronic illness (iatrogenic diabetes mellitus and pancreatic enzyme replacement).
Educational 11. Teach the patient and family about the need for and method of administration of medications (enzyme replacement, analgesics, glucose, and hypoglycemic agents) and about the management of diabetes mellitus (*see below*).
12. Teach the patient about the need for lifelong maintenance and follow-up.
13. Teach the patient about the need for and provision of adequate nutrition.
14. Teach the patient about the available resources (visiting nurse referral and other community agencies).

Evaluation criteria. See Overview.

DIABETES MELLITUS

Diabetes mellitus is a chronic familial disorder of CHO metabolism resulting from a relative or absolute lack of insulin, characterized by hyperglycemia. It affects ~2% of the USA population (5 million people). Its incidence increases with age, affecting >6% of persons over the age of 65 yr, men and women equally. In maturity (adult)-onset nonketotic diabetes, inheritance plays a strong role. Juvenile insulin-dependent diabetes may arise from an inherited predisposition with environmental triggering events (probably viral).

Insulin deficiency results in wasting of tissue because of a negative nitrogen balance (protein stores are used for energy). Ketosis may result from fat breakdown (fat stores are used for energy). Hyperglycemia causes cellular and extracellular dehydration and glycosuria.

Symptoms of insulin deficiency include weight loss, polyuria, polydipsia, and polyphagia. *Complications* are many and varied. Macrovascular disease involves atheromatous changes in the large vessels and medial calcification. The vessels of the heart, brain, and legs are especially at risk. These changes occur earlier and are more extensive in diabetic patients than in normal persons. Microvascular disease involves accelerated thickening of the basement membrane of the capillaries and arterioles. Glomerular capillaries of the kidneys and eyes are particularly susceptible, but the skin, skeletal muscle, adipose tissue, and peripheral nerves may also be affected. Related vascular diseases are numerous. Nephropathy is manifested by diffuse glomerulosclerosis, nodular intracapillary glomerulosclerosis, and vascular lesions affecting all vessels. Tubular and interstitial changes develop in about one third of diabetics, begin ~15 yr after onset (highly variable), and cause death in about one fifth of diabetics. Marked acceleration of diabetic complications occurs with increasing renal failure. Retinopathy is discussed in Chapter 13. Cardiovascular/coronary artery disease, the leading cause of death (50%) in diabetics, is 2 to 4 times more common, is more severe, and occurs at a younger age in diabetic patients than in normal individuals. Hypertension, obesity, and hyperlipidemia increase the risk, but these factors are not the total etiology. Excessive platelet aggregation and reduced fibrinolysis also play a role in its development. Advanced vascular disease in the lower legs is common, severe, and often gangrenous; amputations are often necessary. Neuropathies include segmental demyelination of nerves and dysfunction of the brain, spinal cord, and peripheral nerves (as a primary metabolic lesion or secondary to vascular disease). Peripheral neuropathy is the most common lesion. Mononeuropathy, polyneuropathy, amyotrophy, and autonomic dysfunction are common. Infection is common in poorly controlled diabetics. The most common infections are cutaneous staphylococcus, vaginal and intertrigal (skin folds) *Candida*, and bacteria in the urinary tract. Less common infections include TB, gas gangrene, and mucormycosis (Mucorales fungal disease).

Diagnosis is based on the health history, physical exam, and laboratory tests of the blood and urine, e.g., fasting blood glucose, 2-hr postprandial glucose, glucose tolerance test, blood ketone bodies, glucosuria, and ketonuria.

Common interventions

Medical treatment of diabetes mellitus involves diet modifications, medications (insulin and oral hypoglycemic agents), and exercise.

Nursing interventions

Physical 1. Administer medications on time.
   2. Provide diet as ordered.
   3. Have orange juice or other simple sugar available in case hypoglycemia occurs.
   4. Test the urine and blood.
   5. Assess the patient for complications of insulin therapy.
      a. Assess for hypoglycemia (altered consciousness, tachycardia, diaphoresis).
      b. Assess for hyperglycemia (polyuria, nocturia, ketoacidosis, hyperosmolar coma).
      c. Assess for tissue hypertrophy or atrophy (lipodystrophy — localized disturbance of fat metabolism involving thickening of subcutaneous tissues at injection sites; either a lumpy and hard or soft and spongy mass; dimpling of tissues or extensive depressed areas; altered absorption of insulin; associated with the use of cold insulin, failure to rotate injection sites, injection of insulin into fat, and allergic or immune mechanisms).
      d. Avoid injection in the damaged areas until healing is complete.
      e. Assess for insulin reaction (hypoglycemia, trembling, headache, irritability).
      f. Have orange juice available.
   6. Assess the patient for erratic insulin action caused by the following factors.
      a. Improper diet habits (overeating, eating free sugar or at irregular intervals, omitting snacks).
      b. Incorrect injection techniques (*see above*).
      c. Chronic overdosages of insulin (Somogyi effect).
      d. Intermittent use of drugs that affect blood sugar (aspirin, butazolidin, steroids, oral contraceptives, thiazides, alcohol).
      e. Irregular exercise or rest.
      f. Emotional or psychiatric conflicts.
Psychosocial 7. Stress that compliance with the program of care is essential for long-term health.

8. Provide support for living with a long-term chronic illness with many complications.
9. Encourage the patient to live as near a normal life as possible.
10. Provide support for the patient and significant others; especially consider changes that necessitate permanent modification in diet or life-style.
11. Suggest obtaining additional support from organizations (American Diabetes Association or Juvenile Diabetes Foundation).

Educational 12. Teach factual material to the patient and family.
   a. Stress that compliance is essential.
   b. Educate the patient about the nature of the disease, its treatment and complications.
   c. Emphasize the need for and provision of adequate nutrition, especially the relationship to activity; distribution of protein, CHO, and fat; and the necessity of three meals a day (with between-meal snacks if insulin is used).
13. Emphasize the following dietary guidelines:
   a. Make the diet interesting and palatable by varying foods.
   b. Do not add sugar, honey, or sweeteners to foods.
   c. Use only water-packed fruits, artificially sweetened desserts, beverages, sodas.
   d. Avoid fruit "drinks" or "cocktails."
   e. Avoid the use of pure canned or frozen fruit juice.
   f. Avoid excessive amounts of coffee (caffeine causes blood glucose to increase).
   g. Use alcohol in moderation (maximum of 2 oz./day with water or unsweetened mixtures, if the physician approves).
   h. Eat all the foods prescribed (make up calories and nutrients at a later time if unable to finish a meal, drink milk or eat a cracker if a meal is delayed).
   i. Avoid gravies, casseroles, fried food, and sweetened desserts when dining out.
   j. Use polyunsaturated fats whenever possible.
14. Instruct the patient to maintain correct body weight.
   a. Weigh self 2 to 3 times a week on the same scale at the same time of day, wearing the same amount of clothing.
   b. Report fluctuations of >2 kg (4.4 lb) to the physician.
15. Stress the need for and proper administration of medications (insulin and oral hypoglycemics).
16. Teach procedures for insulin administration, urine testing, and blood glucose testing.
17. Stress proper care of the feet (good hygiene, treatment of corns, calluses, and abrasions, avoiding cold feet).
18. Teach proper care of the skin.
   a. Prevent excoriation.
   b. Obtain care for even slight injuries (e.g., scratches, hangnails).

     c. Use heat lamps or heating pads, with caution.
     d. Protect the hands with gloves when using cleaning agents.
19. Report serious injuries and infections to the physician immediately.
20. Instruct the patient to modify activity and life-style as appropriate.
     a. Explore the life-style and suggest areas that should be modified.
     b. Make recommendations regarding adjustment of the treatment to fit personal needs and preferences.
     c. Plan treatment to conform as closely as possible with activities of daily living.
21. Instruct the patient that information and supplies for emergency use should always be carried.
22. Instruct the patient that lifelong follow-up care is necessary.
23. Provide information for care during the illness:
     a. Notify the physician if an illness lasts >72 hr.
     b. Continue insulin despite other illnesses.
     c. Call the physician if vomiting or diarrhea is present.
     d. Take oral agents as usual but stop taking them if unable to eat.
     e. Go to bed and keep warm and have someone who knows what to do in case of an insulin reaction stay with them.
     f. Test the urine for glucose and acetone, using second voided specimens, checking at least qid and q 2 to 4 hr if a juvenile or brittle diabetic.
     g. Replace hourly any fluids lost in vomiting, diarrhea, or fever.
     h. Replace the prescribed diet with liquid and semiliquid (CHO) foods if unable to eat; if unable to eat after replacing 4 to 5 meals with liquid or semiliquid CHO, call the physician.
24. Encourage genetic counseling for young diabetics who are planning families.

Evaluation criteria. *See* Overview.

HYPERGLYCEMIC, HYPEROSMOLAR NONKETOTIC COMA

Hyperglycemic, hyperosmolar nonketotic coma (HHNK) is a hyperosmolar state characterized by extremely elevated blood glucose levels without ketosis. It usually occurs in elderly patients with relatively mild, maturity-onset diabetes. Stress appears to be a precipitating factor. Associated factors include infection, pancreatitis, cardiovascular problems, TPN (hyperalimentation), and dialysis (if solutions containing large amounts of glucose are used). *Symptoms* are similar to those of ketoacidosis without Kussmaul's respiration, unless significant lactoacidosis is present. Serum and urine ketones are not elevated. *Diagnosis* is based on the health history, physical exam, and extremely elevated blood sugar. **Medical** treatment is the same as for ketoacidosis (*see above*), but administration of sodium bicarbonate usually is not necessary because ketosis is not present. **Nursing** care is the same as for ketoacidosis (*see above*).

[For a discussion of cystic fibrosis, *see* Chapter 14.]

APPENDIX A: ABBREVIATED OUTLINE OF A HEALTH HISTORY*

The purpose of the health history is to have a permanent record of the past and present total state of health (including health-related practices) of an individual that can be used by any health team member in planning or implementing care. The health history consists of the following factors:

I. Reason for Contact
   A. Brief statement, by the individual/significant other, describing why health care (hospitalization) was sought.

II. Biographical Data
   A. Basic information identifying the individual: complete name, address, phone number, age, and date and place of birth.
   B. Sex.
   C. Ethnic group and religious affiliation.
   D. First/major language spoken.
   E. Marital, educational, occupational status.
   F. Source and policy number of health insurance.
   G. Social Security number.
   H. Parent's names (mother's maiden name).

III. Current Health Status
   A. Specific complaint (in detail).
   B. Patterns of personal behavior (usual habits and any recent changes).
      1. Physiologic: e.g., diet, bowel and bladder elimination, hygiene and sleep practices, use of drugs (including tobacco and alcohol), sexuality.
      2. Recreational (including exercise).

---

*Adapted with permission from Mahoney, E., and L. Verdisco. How to Collect and Record a Health History. J. B. Lippincott Co., Philadelphia. 1982. Second edition.

IV. Past Health History
   A. Developmental data: current status, appropriateness, any problems.
   B. Promotive and preventive practices, including nature, frequency, dates of immunizations.
   C. Restorative interventions (nature of problem; dates, places, and kinds of treatment).
   D. Obstetric history.
   E. Allergies, including manifestations and treatment.
   F. Foreign travel (dates and places, including other areas of the USA).
 V. Family History
   A. Composition and relationships among members.
   B. Health status of members, including recent illnesses or stressors.
   C. Familial illnesses.
VI. Social History
   A. Relationships (in general).
   B. Occupation/school (current and past), nature of position, environmental conditions, satisfaction, finances, etc.
   C. Environment (housing and community).
VII. Review of Systems (by interview)
   A. General status.
   B. Body systems (individual's description of pain, discomfort, and/or alteration in functioning).
      1. Integumentary (skin, hair, nails).
      2. Head.
      3. Eyes.
      4. Ears.
      5. Nose and sinuses.
      6. Mouth and throat.
      7. Neck.
      8. Breast.
      9. Respiratory.
      10. Cardiovascular.
      11. Gastrointestinal.
      12. Genitourinary.
      13. Musculoskeletal.
      14. Neurologic.
      15. Hematopoietic.
      16. Endocrine.
      17. Allergies and immunologies.
   C. Mental status (including appearance, emotional state, thought processes, orientation, and intellectual functioning).

APPENDIX B: LABORATORY TESTS

Normal Values for Various Laboratory Tests

Test	Definition, function, and/or purpose	Normal value*	Clinical implication/significance Elevated	Clinical implication/significance Lowered
Blood Chemistry				
ACTH	Governs secretion of glucocorticoids and the sympathetic response to stress from the adrenal glands.	15–70 pg/ml	Primary adrenal deficiency Ectopic ACTH producing tumors Pituitary adenomas	Adrenocortical tumor Adrenal insufficiency due to hypopituitarism
Albumin, quantitative	Responsible for ~ 80% of colloid oncotic pressure in serum.	3.2–4.5 g/dl (salt fractionation) 3.2–5.6 g/dl (electrophoresis)	Myeloproliferative diseases: multiple myeloma, Hodgkin's disease, leukemia Chronic granulomatous infections: TB, brucellosis, chronic active hepatitis, collagen diseases, sarcoidosis Shock	Chronic liver disease Malnutrition Nephrotic syndrome Malabsorption syndrome Burns Hemorrhage
Amylase	Digestive enzyme for carbohydrate.	4–25 U/ml	Acute pancreatitis Biliary tract disease Mumps Renal insufficiency	Chronic pancreatitis Cirrhosis
Base excess (BE)	Refers to bicarbonates and other bases in the blood.	Male: −3.3 to 1.2 Female: −2.4 to 2.3	Metabolic alkalosis	Metabolic acidosis
Bicarbonate (HCO3)	Alkaline substance in the blood.	21–28 mM/liter	Metabolic alkalosis	Metabolic acidosis

791

Test	Definition, function, and/or purpose	Normal value*	Clinical implication/significance	
			Elevated	Lowered
Bilirubin	Chief bile pigment in man; derived principally from the breakdown of Hb. Is bound to albumin in the circulation.	Direct: ≤0.3 mg/dl Indirect: 0.1–1.0 mg/dl Total: 0.1–1.2 mg/dl	Hemolytic jaundice Hepatic jaundice Obstructive jaundice	
Blood gases				
pH	Indicates net acid-base status of blood.	Arterial: 7.35–7.45 Venous: 7.36–7.41	Alkalemia: may be respiratory, metabolic, or both in origin	Acidemia: may be respiratory, metabolic, or both in origin
PCO₂	Measures adequacy of alveolar ventilation.	Arterial: 35–40 mmHg Venous: 40–45 mmHg	Pulmonary disease COPD Diffuse interstitial and alveolar lung disease (restrictive lung disease) Alveolar hypoventilation	Hyperventilation
PO₂	Gives estimate of pulmonary O₂ transport functioning.	Arterial: 95–100 mmHg		Pulmonary disease COPD Restrictive lung disease Pulmonary embolism
Calcium	Mineral that affects neuromuscular excitability and cellular and capillary permeability necessary for blood coagulation.	4.8–5.8 mEq/liter	Hyperparathyroidism Sarcoidosis Multiple myeloma Malignancies with or without metastasis to the bone Thyrotoxicosis Bone fractures Paget's disease	Hypoparathyroidism Diarrhea Osteomalacia Malabsorption syndrome Acute pancreatitis Pregnancy Diuretics (Furosemide) Respiratory alkalosis

Test	Significance	Normal Value		
Carbon dioxide (CO$_2$ content)	Measures total carbonic acid (H$_2$CO$_3$) and bicarbonate (HCO$_3$) in plasma.	24–30 mM/liter	Milk-alkali syndrome Hypervitaminosis D Diuretics (chlorothiazide)	Uremic acidosis Diabetic ketoacidosis Lactic acidosis Respiratory alkalosis (hyperventilation syndrome)
Chloride	Influences acid-base balance and osmotic pressure.	95–103 mEq/liter	Tetany COPD Intestinal obstruction Vomiting Serum alkalosis and intracellular acidosis associated with hypokalemia and hypochloremia Renal tubular acidosis Iatrogenic due to tube feedings and inappropriate IV fluids Anemia Cardiac decompensation	Diabetic ketoacidosis Uremic acidosis Renal tubular acidosis Lactic acidosis Hyperventilation syndrome Diarrhea Anesthesia Potassium-saving diuretics Hypokalemic-chloremic alkalosis Burns Diarrhea Diabetes Intestinal obstruction
Cholesterol	Used in the body to form cholic acid in the liver, which in turn produces bile salts needed to digest fat.	150–250 mg/dl (varies with diet and age)	Liver disease with biliary obstruction Nephrotic stage of glomerulonephritis Familial hypercholesterolemia Possible relationship with atherosclerosis and coronary artery disease Hypothyroidism	Malnutrition Hyperthyroidism Anemia Severe infection
Creatine phosphokinase (CPK)	Enzyme released by heart, skeletal muscle, and brain in response to damaged tissue.	Male: 5–35 U/ml Female: 5–25 U/ml	MI Skeletal muscle disease Cerebral infarctions Vigorous exercise	

Test	Definition, function, and/or purpose	Normal value*	Clinical implication/significance Elevated	Lowered
Creatinine	Waste product of creatine that is present in skeletal muscle (creatine phosphate). Tests for renal functioning by reflecting balance between its production and filtration by renal glomerulus.	0.6–1.2 mg/dl	Kidney disease when ≥50% of nephrons are destroyed	
Glucose (fasting)	Product of carbohydrate metabolism.	70–110 mg/dl	Diabetes mellitus Cushing's syndrome (hyperadrenalism) Cushing's disease (secondary hyperadrenalism) Hyperthyroidism Acute stress Pheochromocytoma Diuretics (especially thiazide diuretics) Pancreatic insufficiency (acute and chronic)	Pancreatic islet cell tumor Pituitary hypofunctioning Addison's disease (adrenocortical hypofunctioning) Extensive liver disease Tumors of nonpancreatic origin (e.g., large retroperitoneal sarcomas or large hepatomas) Severe vomiting
Immunoglobulins IgG IgA IgM IgD IgE	Components of gamma globulin that are involved in antigen-antibody reactions to protect the body from infectious organisms.	800–1,600 mg/dl 50–250 mg/dl 40–120 mg/dl 0.5–3.0 mg/dl 0.01–0.04 mg/dl	Multiple myeloma Macroglobulinemia Autoimmune diseases	

Test	Description	Normal Values	Increased	Decreased
Iron (serum) Iron binding capacity	Element that is mainly contained in Hb (essential iron). Also found in bone marrow, spleen, liver, and muscle.	50–150 μg/dl 250–450 μg/dl	Pernicious, aplastic, and hemolytic anemia	Iron deficiency anemia
Lactic dehydrogenase (LDH)	Enzyme that catalyzes the reversible oxidation of lactic acid to pyruvic acid. Present in most metabolizing cells, especially the heart, liver, brain, kidney, skeletal muscle, and RBCs.	80–120 Wacker units 71–207 IU/liter 150–450 Wroblewski units	MI Hemolytic disorders (pernicious anemia) Chronic viral hepatitis Pneumonia Pulmonary emboli Malignancies of skeletal muscle, liver, brain, kidney, and heart Renal infarcts Cerebrovascular accidents	
Magnesium	Intracellular cation that is essential for neuro-muscular integration.	1.5–2.5 mEq/liter 3.0 mg/dl	Parathyroidectomy	Malnutrition Chronic alcoholism Chronic nephritis Prolonged diarrhea Long-term IV therapy without Mg^{++} replacement Intestinal malabsorption Prolonged diuretic therapy
Phosphatase (acid, total)	Enzyme present in serum that catalyzes the cleavage of phosphatase esters.	0–1.1 U/ml (Bodansky) 1–4 U/ml (King-Armstrong)	Carcinoma of the prostate Paget's disease Hyperparathyroidism	
Phosphatase (alkaline)	Enzyme present in serum. Function not understood.	1.5–4.5 U/dl (Bodansky) 4–13 U/dl (King-Armstrong)	Hyperparathyroidism Osteomalacia Rickets Healing fractures Pregnancy Some drugs (e.g., allopurinol, oral contraceptives) can cause false positives	

Test	Definition, function, and/or purpose	Normal value*	Clinical implication/significance Elevated	Lowered
Phosphorus	Mineral of which 85% is combined with calcium in the skeleton. Is involved in almost all metabolic processes.	1.8–2.6 mEq/liter 3.0–4.5 mg/dl	Chronic glomerular disease Hypoparathyroidism	Hyperparathyroidism Osteomalacia Renal tubular acidosis Malabsorption syndrome
Potassium	A major cation of ICF that functions in ECF. Influences acid-base balance, cellular membrane potential, and osmotic pressure.	3.5–5.0 mEq/liter	Renal failure Addison's disease Massive tissue destruction	Chronic diuretic therapy Cushing's syndrome Diabetic acidosis Primary and secondary hyperaldosteronism with chronic CHF Liver disease with ascites Excessive licorice ingestion (hypertension) Anti-inflammatory drugs (indomethacin, steroids) Malignant hypertension, hypertensive disease Poor diet, crash diets Chronic stress Chronic diarrhea Malabsorption syndrome Diaphoresis Chronic fever Renal tubular acidosis Vomiting

Proteins Total Albumin Globulin (Total protein and A/G ratio)	Organic substance composed of carbon, hydrogen, oxygen, and nitrogen. Serves as source of rapid replacement of tissue proteins, buffers in acid-base balance, and transporters of constituents of blood. Albumin constitutes 52–68% of total protein. Responsible for ~ 80% of the colloid oncotic pressure in serum.	Total: 6.0–7.8 g/dl Albumin: 3.2–4.5 g/dl Globulin: 2.3–3.5 g/dl	Hemoconcentration Shock Chronic liver disease Myeloproliferative diseases: multiple myeloma, Hodgkin's disease, leukemia Chronic granulomatous infections: TB, collagen diseases, chronic active hepatitis, sarcoidosis	Malnutrition Hemorrhage Burns Proteinuria Chronic liver disease Nephrotic syndrome Malabsorption syndrome
Renin activity	Peptide substance secreted by kidney in response to decreased intravascular volume.	Upright: 1.9 ± 1.7 ng/ml/hr Supine: 2.7 ± 1.8 ng/ml/hr	High renin essential hypertension (vaso-constriction) Hypertension due to renal artery stenosis Low-salt diet Diuretic therapy Hemorrhage	Low renin essential hypertension (sodium retention) Primary aldosteronism
Sodium	Major cation of ECF that plays important part in acid-base balance, guarding against excessive fluid loss, and preserving normal functioning of muscle tissue.	136–142 mEq/liter	Iatrogenic via administration of excessive IV sodium Hypothalamic lesions Head trauma Dehydration Excessive steroid administration Nephritis Hemoconcentration	Addison's disease Chronic sodium-losing nephropathy Vomiting Diarrhea Tube drainage Diaphoresis Burns Diuretics (mercurial and chlorothiazide) Chronic renal insufficiency with acidosis Starvation with acidosis Diabetic acidosis

Test	Definition, function, and/or purpose	Normal value*	Clinical implication/significance	
			Elevated	Lowered
				Dilution hyponatremia: secondary hyperaldosteronism, hepatic failure with ascites, CHF, acute or chronic renal failure, lobar pneumonia Bronchogenic carcinoma Pulmonary infections Porphyria
Thyroid hormone T₃ (resin uptake) T₄ (Murphy-Pattee) Thyroid-stimulating (TSH)	Principle hormones secreted by the thyroid (T₃, triiodothyronine; T₄, thyroxine). Both hormones help regulate lipid and carbohydrate metabolism and are necessary for normal growth and development. TSH is secreted by the anterior pituitary.	T₃: 25–38 relative % uptake T₄: 6.0–11.8 µg/dl TSH: 0.5–3.5 µU/ml	Graves's disease (diffuse toxic goiter) Hyperthyroidism	Nontoxic goiter Hypothyroidism Nephrotic syndrome
Transaminases	Enzymes that are liberated from destroyed cells.			
SGOT	Found in skeletal and cardiac muscle and in liver tissue.	8–33 U/ml	Liver disease Cardiac disease: MI, pericarditis Generalized infection: mononucleosis	
SGPT	Found mainly in liver tissue.	1–36 U/ml	Same diseases as SGOT, but increase of SGPT is more marked in liver disease than is SGOT	

Triglycerides	Blood lipids that are bound to protein in the plasma.	10–190 mg/dl	Coronary artery disease Alcoholism Pancreatitis	Tryptophan-specific malabsorption syndrome
Urea nitrogen (BUN)	End product of protein metabolism. Formed in liver, excreted in urine.	8–25 mg/dl	Acute or chronic renal failure Acute glomerulonephritis Prostatic enlargement with urinary obstruction Nephrotic syndrome	Severe hepatic failure
Uric acid	End product of purine metabolism that is cleared from plasma by kidneys.	3.0–7.0 mg/dl	Gouty arthritis Acute leukemia Chronic renal failure Lymphomas treated by chemotherapy	Malabsorption
Vitamin B12	Extrinsic factor found in meat, eggs, and milk that is necessary for formation of RBCs.	Male: 200–800 pg/ml Female: 100–650 pg/ml	Myeloproliferative disorders (myeloid leukemia) with liver damage	Pernicious anemia Alcoholism Ileal resection Total or partial gastrectomy
Hematology Coagulation tests Bleeding time (Ivy) Bleeding time (Duke)	Measure rate of platelet clot formation.	1–6 min 1–3 min	Purpura Vascular abnormalities Thrombocytopenia Excessive aspirin ingestion	
Partial thromboplastin time (PTT)	Test for normalcy of the coagulation process. Useful in identifying deficiencies of coagulation factors, prothrombin, and fibrinogen. Used for control of anticoagulation with heparin.	60–70 sec	Coagulation disorder due to deficiency of a coagulation factor (e.g., hemophilia)	

Test	Definition, function, and/or purpose	Normal value*	Clinical implication/significance	
			Elevated	Lowered
Prothrombin time (PT)	Determines activity and interaction of factors V, VII, X, prothrombin, and fibrinogen. Used to determine dosages of oral anticoagulant medications.	12–14 sec	Anticoagulation therapy Indicates low fibrinogen concentration, impaired prothrombin activity, deficiency of factors V, VII, X Cirrhosis Hepatitis	
Venous clotting time	Measures coagulation time in venous blood. Used to regulate heparin dosages.	5–15 min	Hemorrhagic disease Coagulation factor deficiencies Heparin administration	
Complete blood count (CBC) Hct	Determines volume percentage of packed RBCs in whole blood.	Male: 40–54% Female: 38–47%	Polycythemia vera Hemoconcentration resulting from fluid loss and dehydration	Severe anemia Massive blood loss
Hb	Oxygen-carrying pigment of RBCs.	Male: 13.5–18.0 g/dl Female: 12.0–16.0 g/dl	Polycythemia COPD CHF with hypoxemia	Anemia Hypochromic microcytic anemia: iron deficiency, sickle cell Macrocytic anemia: folic acid deficiency, vitamin B12 deficiency (pernicious anemia)
RBC	Cell formed in red bone marrow. Contains Hb (iron and protein), which functions to transport oxygen to the tissues and carry carbon dioxide to the lungs.	Male: $4.6–6.2 \times 10^6/\mu l$ Female: $4.2–5.4 \times 10^6/\mu l$	Polycythemia vera COPD Severe diarrhea Dehydration Pulmonary fibrosis	Anemia Leukemia

Test	Description	Normal value	Increased in	Decreased in
WBC	Cell involved in protecting the body from infection. WBCs are either granular (basophils, neutrophils, and eosinophils) or nongranular (lymphocytes and monocytes). Formed in lymph nodes, thymus, or red bone marrow.	4,500–11,000/µl	Infectious diseases (usually bacterial) / Severe sepsis / Acute leukemia / Collagen diseases	Aplastic anemia / Agranulocytosis
Differential WBC Neutrophils	Granulocytic. Have phagocytic action.	Mean %: 56	Bacterial infections / Inflammatory disorders / Tumors / Stress	Benign neutropenia (familial) / Acute viral infections / Anorexia nervosa / Drug induced
Eosinophils	Granulocytic, phagocytic antigen-antibody complexes.	Mean %: 2.7	Allergic disorders / Parasitic disease / Leukemia / Collagen diseases	Acute or chronic stress / Endocrine causes
Basophils	Granulocytic. Contain heparin. Role uncertain.	Mean %: 3	Myeloproliferative disease	Anaphylactic reaction / Acute hypersensitive reactions / Hyperthyroidism / Radiation therapy / Acute and chronic infection
Lymphocytes	Nongranular. T cells are derived from thymus. Protect body from infection.	Mean %: 34	Chronic lymphatic leukemia / Infectious diseases: infectious mononucleosis / Viral infections / Chronic infections / Thyrotoxicosis / Adrenal insufficiency	
Platelet count	Cells important in blood coagulation.	200,000–350,000/mm	Polycythemia / Chronic granulocytic leukemia	Aplastic anemia / Thrombocytopenic purpura / Acute leukemia

Test	Definition, function, and/or purpose	Normal value*	Clinical implication/significance	
			Elevated	Lowered

Sedimentation rate (ESR)	Nonspecific test that measures the speed at which RBCs settle in uncoagulated blood. Used as a screening test. Has no organ or disease specificity.	Males <50 yr: <15 mm/hr
		        >50 yr: <20 mm/hr
		Females <50 yr: <20 mm/hr
		        >50 yr: <30 mm/hr
			Rheumatic fever (follow progress in)
			Inflammation	

Urine Acetone	A ketone. Class of organic compound having one oxygen atom.	Negative	Diabetes mellitus Starvation	
Albumin	Protein. Not usually contained in urine.	Negative	Renal vein abnormality Hypertension	
Bence Jones protein	Protein substance excreted in urine of persons with certain malignancies.	Negative	Multiple myeloma Bone tumors	
Bilirubin	Chief bile pigment in man mainly derived from breakdown of Hb.	Negative	Jaundice (hemolytic, hepatic, or obstructive)	
Blood, occult	Blood that is not visible to the eye.	Negative	Hemorrhagic cystitis Calculi in renal pelvis TB Tumors of renal system	
Catecholamines	Term that refers to epinephrine and norepinephrine.	Epinephrine <20 μg/24 hr Norepinephrine <100 μg/24 hr	Pheochromocytoma Shock	

			Tubular or glomerular disease	
Casts	Formed elements that result from agglutination of protein in the kidneys.	None		
Creatinine	Endogenous waste product of creatine from skeletal muscle. Estimates GFR.	15–25 mg/kg of body wt/ 24 hr	Acute and chronic glomerulonephritis SLE Nephritis Tetanus	Anemia Leukemia Advanced degeneration of kidneys
Glucose (glucosuria)	Indicates point of blood sugar level at which kidney begins to excrete glucose.	Negative	Diabetes mellitus Pancreatic disorders Stress Pituitary disorders	Low renal threshold for glucose resorption
Ketone bodies	End product of fat metabolism.	Negative	Uncontrolled diabetes Fasting Severe infections accompanied by vomiting and diarrhea	
pH	Refers to acidity or alkalinity.	4.6–8.0	Metabolic acidosis Uncontrolled diabetes	Metabolic alkalosis Alkalizing medications Renal tubular acidosis
Specific gravity (concentration)	Indicates the concentration of urine. Can be used to estimate hydration status.	1.002–1.035	Dehydration Post x-ray procedures due to contrast medium Substances (protein, glucose) in urine	Overhydration Tubular disease Endocrine disease
WBCs	*See above*	0–4	Infectious process in urinary tract (kidney infection, bladder infection)	

Test	Definition, function, and/or purpose	Normal value*	Clinical implication/significance	
			Elevated	Lowered
Blood: miscellaneous Carcinoembryonic antigen (CEA)	Nonspecific antigen for carcinoma. Used for follow-up of cancer patients.	0–2.5 ng/ml 97% healthy nonsmokers	Carcinoma (highest titers found in carcinoma of colon and pancreas)	
Antinuclear antibodies (ANA)	Immunoglobulins that react with nuclear component of leukocytes.	Positive if detected in serum that has been diluted 1:10	SLE Rheumatoid antibodies	
Venereal disease research laboratory test (VDRL)	Nonspecific antibodies.	Nonreactive	Syphilis False-positives seen with acute febrile illnesses, heroin users, after smallpox vaccination, in collagen vascular disease, and auto-immune disease	
Cerebrospinal fluid (CSF) Albumin		10–30 mg/dl	Neurologic disorders (e.g., brain tumors)	
Cell count (WBC and and RBC)		0–8 cells/µl	Infection in the CNS (viral infection, TB, bacterial meningitis) Hemorrhage in CNS	
Chloride		100–130 mEq/liter	Uremia	Bacterial infections (acute generalized meningitis, tubercular meningitis)

Glucose	45–75 mg/dl	Diabetes mellitus Diabetic coma Uremia Epidemic encephalitis	Bacterial infections (meningococcal meningitis, *Hemophilus influenzae* meningitis, or any bacterial meningitis) Insulin shock
Protein	15–45 mg/dl	Aseptic meningitis caused by a virus or collagen disease Guillain-Barré syndrome Poliomyelitis Neurosyphilis	

*Various texts and manuals may list differing laboratory values. Therefore, the nurse must be familiar with those values used in individual institutions. The basic reference for the values given in this appendix is Tilkian, S., M. Conover, and A. Tilkian. Clinical Implications of Laboratory Tests. C. V. Mosby Co., St. Louis. 1980. Second edition. Secondary references for these values are Brunner, L., and D. Suddarth. Textbook of Medical-Surgical Nursing. J. B. Lippincott Co., Philadelphia. 1980. Fourth edition; Luckmann, J., and K. C. Sorensen. Medical-Surgical Nursing. W. B. Saunders Co., Philadelphia. 1980. Second edition; and Windmann, F. Clinical Interpretation of Laboratory Tests. F. A. Davis Co., Philadelphia. 1979. Eighth edition.

BIBLIOGRAPHY

Chapter 1

Bell, J. Stressful life events and coping methods in mental illness and wellness behaviors. *Nursing Research* (March-April 1977). 136-141.

Boland, M., R. B. Murray, and N. Nolan. Application of adaptation theory to nursing. *In* Murray, R. B., and J. P. Zentner, editors. Nursing Concepts for Health Promotion. Prentice-Hall, Inc., Englewood Cliffs, N. J. 1979. Second edition.

Brallier, L. Stress management as a path toward wholeness. *In* Krieger, D., editor. Foundations for Holistic Health Nursing Practices: The Renaissance Nurse. J. B. Lippincott Co., Philadelphia. 1981.

Claus, K. E., and J. T. Bailey. Living with Stress and Promoting Well Being: A Handbook for Nurses. C. V. Mosby Co., St. Louis. 1980.

Elliott, G., and C. Eisdorfer, editors. Stress and Human Health. Springer Publishing Co., New York. 1982.

Henderson, G., and M. Primeaux. Transcultural Health Care. Addison-Wesley Publishing Co., Menlo Park, Calif. 1981.

Holmes, T., and R. M. Rahe. The social readjustment rating scale. *Journal of Psychosomatic Research* (August 1967). 213-218.

Peplau, H. A working definition of anxiety. *In* Bird, S., and M. Marshall, editors. Some Clinical Approaches to Psychiatric Nursing. MacMillan Publishing Co., Inc., New York. 1963.

Rahe, R. H., J. L. Mahan, and R. J. Arthur. Prediction of near-future health change from subjects preceding life changes. *Journal of Psychosomatic Research* (December 1970). 401-406.

Selye, H. The Stress of Life. McGraw-Hill Book Co., New York. 1976. Revised edition.

Selye, H. Stress Without Distress. J. B. Lippincott Co., Philadelphia. 1974.

Chapter 2

Ewald, E. B. Recipes for a Small Planet. Ballantine Books, Inc., New York. 1973.

Guyton, A. C. Textbook of Medical Physiology. W. B. Saunders Co., Philadelphia. 1981. Sixth edition.

Lappé, F. M. Diet for a Small Planet. Ballantine Books, Inc., New York. 1976.

Lewis, C. M. Nutrition: Nutritional Considerations for the Elderly. F. A. Davis Co., Philadelphia. 1978.

Lewis, C. M. Nutrition: The Basics of Nutrition. Family Nutrition. F. A. Davis Co., Philadelphia. 1978.

Lewis, C. M. Nutrition: Vitamins and Minerals. Sodium and Potassium. F. A. Davis Co., Philadelphia. 1978.

Lewis, C. M. Nutrition: Weight Control. F. A. Davis Co., Philadelphia. 1978.

Luckmann, J., and K. C. Sorensen. Medical-Surgical Nursing. W. B. Saunders Co., Philadelphia. 1980. Second edition.

Tilkian, S., M. Conover, and A. Tilkian. Clinical Implications of Laboratory Tests. C. V. Mosby Co., St. Louis. 1979. Second edition.

Williams, S. R. Essentials of Nutrition and Diet Therapy. C. V. Mosby Co., St. Louis. 1978. Second edition.

Chapter 3

Bates, B. A Guide to Physical Examination. J. B. Lippincott Co., Philadelphia. 1979. Second edition.

Bricker, N. S., editor. The Sea Within Us. Searle & Co., San Juan, P. R. 1975.

Guyton, A. C. Textbook of Medical Physiology. W. B. Saunders Co., Philadelphia. 1981. Sixth edition.

Isselbacher, K. J., R. D. Adams, E. Braunwald, R. G. Petersdorf, and J. D. Wilson, editors. Harrison's Principles of Internal Medicine. McGraw-Hill Book Co., New York. 1980. Ninth edition.

Luckmann, J., and K. C. Sorensen. Medical-Surgical Nursing. W. B. Saunders Co., Philadelphia. 1980. Second edition.

Metheny, N. M., and W. D. Snively, Jr. Nurses' Handbook of Fluid Balance. J. B. Lippincott Co., Philadelphia. 1979. Third edition.

Phipps, W. J., B. C. Long, and N. F. Woods, editors. Medical-Surgical Nursing. Concepts and Clinical Practice. C. V. Mosby Co., St. Louis. 1979.

Porth, C. Pathophysiology: Concepts of Altered Health States. J. B. Lippincott Co., Philadelphia. 1982.

Smith, L. H., and S. O. Thier. Pathophysiology: The Biological Principles of Disease. W. B. Saunders Co., Philadelphia. 1982.

Chapter 4

Boguslawski, M. Therapeutic touch: a facilitator of pain relief. *Topics in Clinical Nursing* (April 1980). 27-37.

Brown, D. Neurosciences for Allied Health Therapies. C. V. Mosby Co., St. Louis. 1980.

McCaffery, M. Nursing Management of the Patient with Pain. J. B. Lippincott Co., Philadelphia. 1979. Second edition.

Melzack, R. The Puzzle of Pain: Revolution in Theory and Treatment. Basic Books, Inc., New York. 1973.

Simonton, C., S. Matthews-Simonton, and J. L. Creighton. Getting Well Again: A Step-by-Step Self-Help Guide to Overcoming Cancer for Patients and Their Families. Bantam Books, Inc., New York. 1978.

Young, W., and J. Hisgen. Pain clinics. *Health Education* (November-December 1980). 16-18.

Chapter 5

Davis-Sharts, J. Mechanisms and manifestations of fever. *American Journal of Nursing* (November 1978). 1874-1877.

DeLapp, R. D. Taking the bite out of frostbite and other cold weather injuries. *American Journal of Nursing* (January 1980). 56-60.

Dinarello, C. A., and S. M. Wolff. Pathogenesis of fever in man. *New England Journal of Medicine* (March 16, 1978). 607-612.

Guyton, A. C. Textbook of Medical Physiology. W. B. Saunders Co., Philadelphia. 1981. Sixth edition.

Hayter, J. Hypothermia/hyperthermia in older persons. *Journal of Gerontological Nursing* (February 1980). 65-68.

Miller, J. W., F. Danzl, and D. Thomas. Urban accidental hypothermia. *Annals of Emergency Medicine* (September 1980). 456-461.

Myers, A. M., J. S. Britten, and R. A. Cowley. Hypothermia: quantitative aspects of therapy. *Journal of the American College of Emergency Physicians* (December 1979). 523-527.

O'Keefe, K. M. Accidental hypothermia: a review of 62 cases. *Journal of the American College of Emergency Physicians* (November 1977). 491-496.

Rae, D. Accidental hypothermia: emergency rewarming techniques. *Canadian Nurse* (February 1980). 28-30.

Tate, G. V., C. Gohrke, and L. W. Mansfield. Correct use of electric thermometers. *American Journal of Nursing* (September 1970). 1898-1899.

Chapter 6

Bellanti, J. A. Immunology II. W. B. Saunders Co., Philadelphia. 1980. Second edition.

Friedman, S. O., and P. Gold. Clinical Immunology. Harper & Row, Publishers, Inc., New York. 1976. Second edition.

Fudenberg, H. H., D. P. Stites, J. L. Caldwell, and J. V. Wells. Basic and Clinical Immunology. Lange Medical Publications, Los Altos, Calif. 1978. Second edition.

Gordon, B. L., and D. K. Ford. Essentials of Immunology. F. A. Davis Co., Philadelphia. 1972. Second edition.

Harvey, A. M., R. J. Johns, V. A. McKusick, A. H. Owens, and R. S. Ross. The Principles and Practice of Medicine. Appleton-Century-Crofts, East Norwalk, Conn. 1980. Twentieth edition.

Luckmann, J., and K. C. Sorensen. Medical-Surgical Nursing. W. B. Saunders Co., Philadelphia. 1980. Second edition.

Chapter 7

Agris, J., and M. Spira. Pressure ulcers: prevention and treatment. *Clinical Symposia.* (1979). 1-32.

Berecek, K. Etiology of decubitus ulcer. *Nursing Clinics of North America* (March 1975). 157-170.

Boroch, R. Elements of Rehabilitation in Nursing. C. V. Mosby Co., St. Louis. 1976.

Carnevali, D., and S. Brueckner. Immobilization reassessment of a concept. *American Journal of Nursing* (July 1970). 1502-1507.

Chodil, J., and B. Williams. The concept of sensory deprivation. *Nursing Clinics of North America* (September 1975). 453-465.

Deitrick, J. The effect of immobilization on metabolic and physiological functions of normal men. *American Journal of Medicine* (1948). 364-375.

Kottke, F., and R. Blanchard. Bedrest begets bedrest. *Nursing Forum* (1964). 57-72.

Meissner, J. Which patient on your unit might get a pressure sore? *Nursing* (June 1980). 64-65.

Mikulic, M. Treatment of pressure ulcers. *American Journal of Nursing* (June 1980). 1125-1128.

Sorensen, K. C., and J. Luckmann. Basic Nursing. W. B. Saunders Co., Philadelphia. 1979.

Chapter 8

Bouchard-Kurtz, R., and N. Speese-Owens. Nursing Care of the Cancer Patient. C. V. Mosby Co., St. Louis. 1981. Fourth edition.

Copenhaver, W. M. Bailey's Textbook of Histology. Williams & Wilkins Co., Baltimore. 1978. Seventeenth edition.

Dietz, K. A. Programmed instruction: radiation therapy. *Cancer Nursing* (April 1979). 129-138.

Harvey, A. M., R. J. Johns, V. A. McKusick, A. H. Owens, and R. S. Ross. The Principles and Practice of Medicine. Appleton-Century-Crofts, East Norwalk, Conn. 1980. Twentieth edition.

Kruse, L. C., J. L. Reese, and L. K. Hart. Cancer: Pathophysiology, Etiology, Management. C. V. Mosby Co., St. Louis. 1979.

Luckmann, J., and K. C. Sorensen. Medical-Surgical Nursing. W. B. Saunders Co., Philadelphia. 1980. Second edition.

Marino, L. B. Cancer Nursing. C. V. Mosby Co., St. Louis. 1981.

Oncology Nursing Society and American Nurses' Association Division on Medical-Surgical Nursing Practice. Outcome Standards for Cancer Nursing Practice. American Nurses' Association, Kansas City, Mo. 1979.

Silverberg, E. Cancer Statistics, 1982. American Cancer Society, New York. 1982.

Weisman, A. D. Coping With Cancer. McGraw-Hill Book Co., New York. 1979.

Chapter 9

Brunner, L. S., and D. S. Suddarth. Medical-Surgical Nursing. J. B. Lippincott Co., Philadelphia. 1980. Fourth edition.

Dziurbejko, M. M., and J. C. Larkin. Including the family in preoperative teaching. *American Journal of Nursing* (November 1978). 1892-1894.

Luckmann, J., and K. C. Sorensen. Medical-Surgical Nursing. W. B. Saunders Co., Philadelphia. 1980. Second edition.

Moidel, H. C., E. C. Giblin, and B. M. Wagner, editors. Nursing Care of the Patient with Medical-Surgical Disorders. McGraw-Hill Book Co., New York. 1976. Second edition.

Phippen, M. L. Nursing assessment of preoperative anxiety. *(AORN) Association of Operating Room Nurses Journal* (May 1980). 1019-1026.

Redman, B. K. The Process of Patient Teaching in Nursing. C. V. Mosby Co., St. Louis. 1980. Fourth edition.

Seropian, R., and B. M. Reynolds. Wound infection after preoperative depilatory vs. razor preparation. *American Journal of Surgery* (March 1971). 251-254.

Chapter 10

AORN Standards of Practice. Association of Operating Room Nurses, Inc., Denver. 1978.

Brooks, S. M. Fundamentals of Operating Room Nursing. C. V. Mosby Co., St. Louis. 1975.

Drain, C., and S. Shipley. The Recovery Room. W. B. Saunders Co., Philadelphia. 1979.

Dripps, R., J. Eckenhoff, and L. Vandam. Introduction to Anesthesia. W. B. Saunders Co., Philadelphia. 1977. Fifth edition.

Gruendemann, B. J., S. B. Casteron, S. C. Hesterly, B. B. Minckley, and M. G. Shetler. The Surgical Patient: Behavioral Concepts for the Operating Room Nurse. C. V. Mosby Co., St. Louis. 1977. Second edition.

MacClelland, D. C. Test your knowledge. *(AORN) Association of Operating Room Nurses Journal* (February 1979). 332.

Nursing Care of the Patient in the O.R. Ethicon, Inc., Somerville, N. J. 1975.

Rhodes, M. J., B. J. Gruendemann, W. F. Ballinger, and V. Friedman. Alexander's Care of the Patient in Surgery. C. V. Mosby Co., St. Louis. 1978. Sixth edition.

Chapter 11

Cooper, D. M., and D. Schumann. Postsurgical nursing intervention as an adjunct to wound healing. *Nursing Clinics of North America* (December 1979). 713-725.

Croushore, T. M. Postoperative assessment: the key to avoiding the most common nursing mistakes. *Nursing 79* (April 1979). 47-51.

Hercules, P. R. Nursing in the postoperative care unit: a review. Part 1: respiratory complications. *(AORN) Association of Operating Room Nurses Journal* (December 1978). 1042-1048.

Hercules, P. R. Nursing in the postoperative care unit: a review. Part 2: other complications. *(AORN) Association of Operating Room Nurses Journal* (December 1978). 1049-1052.

Lemaitre, G. D., and J. A. Finnegan. The Patient in Surgery: A Guide for Nurses. W. B. Saunders Co., Philadelphia. 1980. Fourth edition.

Libman, R. H., and J. Keithley. Relieving airway obstruction in the recovery room. *American Journal of Nursing* (April 1975). 603-605.

Luckmann, J., and K. C. Sorensen. Medical-Surgical Nursing. W. B. Saunders Co., Philadelphia. 1980. Second edition.

Metheny, N. Preoperative fluid balance assessment. *(AORN) Association of Operating Room Nurses Journal* (January 1981). 51-56.

O'Byrne, C. Clinical detection and management of postoperative wound sepsis. *Nursing Clinics of North America* (December 1979). 727-742.

Smith, B. J. Safeguarding your patient after anesthesia. *Nursing 78* (October 1978). 53-56.

Chapter 12

American Cancer Society. How to Examine Your Breasts. American Cancer Society, Inc., New York. 1977.

Bates, B. A Guide to Physical Examination. J. B. Lippincott Co., Philadelphia. 1979. Second edition.

Brunner, L. S., and D. S. Suddarth. Lippincott Manual of Nursing Practice. J. B. Lippincott Co., Philadelphia. 1978. Second edition.

Nursing Photobook Series. Dealing with Emergencies. Intermed Communications, Inc., Horsham, Pa. 1981.

Luckmann, J., and K. C. Sorensen. Medical-Surgical Nursing. W. B. Saunders Co., Philadelphia. 1980. Second edition.

National Cancer Institute. The Breast Cancer Digest. U. S. Department of Health, Education and Welfare, Bethesda, Md. DHEW publication no. (NIH) 79-1691. 1979.

Parrish, J. A. Dermatology and Skin Care. McGraw-Hill Book Co., New York. 1975.

Plewig, G., and A. M. Kligman. Acne: Morphogenesis and Treatment. Springer-Verlag New York, Inc., New York. 1975.

Rubin, A. Black skin. *RN* (March 1979). 31-35.

Sauer, G. C. Manual of Skin Diseases. J. B. Lippincott Co., Philadelphia. 1980. Fourth edition.

Chapter 13

DeWeese, D. D., and W. H. Saunders. Textbook of Otolaryngology. C. V. Mosby Co., St. Louis. 1982. Sixth edition.

Havener, W. H. Synopsis of Ophthalmology. C. V. Mosby Co., St. Louis. 1979. Fifth edition.

Lee, K. J., editor. Essential Otolaryngology. Medical Examination Publishing Co., Inc., Garden City, N.Y. 1977. Second edition.

Lee, K. J. Differential Diagnosis in Otolaryngology. Arco Publishing, Inc., New York. 1978.

Saunders, W. H., W. H. Havener, C. F. Keith, and G. Havener. Nursing Care in Eye, Ear, Nose and Throat Disorders. C. V. Mosby Co., St. Louis. 1979. Fourth edition.

Schwartz, S., and T. Shires. Principles of Surgery. McGraw-Hill Book Co., New York. 1979. Third edition.

Silverberg, E. Cancer statistics, 1983. *Ca-A Cancer Journal for Clinicians* (January-February 1983). 9-25.

Smith, J. F., and D. P. Nachazel. Ophthalmologic Nursing. Little, Brown & Co., Boston. 1980.

Vaughan, D., and T. Asbury. General Ophthalmology. Lange Medical Publications, Los Altos, Calif. 1980. Ninth edition.

Wyngaarden, J. B., and L. H. Smith. Cecil Textbook of Medicine. W. B. Saunders Co., Philadelphia. 1982. Sixteenth edition.

Chapter 14

Borg, N., D. Nikas, J. Stark, and S. Williams, editors. Core Curriculum for Critical Care Nursing. W. B. Saunders Co., Philadelphia. Second edition. 1981.

Emanuelsen, K. L., and M. J. Densmore. Acute Respiratory Care. John Wiley & Sons, Inc., New York. 1981.

Isselbacher, K. J., R. D. Adams, E. Braunwald, R. G. Petersdorf, and J. D. Wilson, editors. Harrison's Principles of Internal Medicine. McGraw-Hill Book Co., New York. 1980. Ninth edition.

Loebl, S., G. Spratto, and E. Heckheimer. The Nurse's Drug Handbook. John Wiley & Sons, Inc., New York. 1983. Third edition.

Luckmann, J., and K. C. Sorensen. Medical-Surgical Nursing. W. B. Saunders Co., Philadelphia. 1980. Second edition.

Price, S. A., and L. M. Wilson. Pathophysiology: Clinical Concepts of Disease Processes. McGraw-Hill Book Co., New York. 1982. Second edition.

Robbins, S. L., M. Angell, and V. Kumar. Basic Pathology. W. B. Saunders Co., Philadelphia. 1981. Third edition.

Shibel, E. M., and K. M. Moser, editors. Respiratory Emergencies. C. V. Mosby Co., St. Louis. 1977.

Stephens, G. J. Pathophysiology for Health Practitioners. Macmillan Publishing Co., Inc., New York. 1980.

Chapter 15

Alpert, J. S., and J. M. Rippe. Manual of Cardiovascular Diagnosis and Therapy. Little, Brown & Co., Boston. 1980.

Dietrich, E. B. Advances in Cardiovascular Nursing. Robert J. Brady Co., Bowie, Md. 1980.

Disch, J. M. Diagnostic Procedures for Cardiovascular Disease. Appleton-Century-Crofts, East Norwalk, Conn. 1979.

Hurst, J. W., editor. The Heart. McGraw-Hill Book Co., New York. 1978.

Luckmann, J., and K. C. Sorensen. Medical-Surgical Nursing. W. B. Saunders Co., Philadelphia. 1980. Second edition.

Pinneo, R. Congestive Heart Failure. Appleton-Century-Crofts, East Norwalk, Conn. 1978.

Rubin, M. B. Nursing Care for Myocardial Infarction. Warren H. Green, Inc., St. Louis. 1977.

Sokolow, M., and M. B. McIlroy. Clinical Cardiology. Lange Medical Publications, Los Altos, Calif. 1981. Third edition.

Summerall, C., J. Mangearscena, and J. McNeely. Monitoring Heart Rhythm. John Wiley & Sons, Inc., New York. 1976.

Wenger, N. K., J. W. Hurst, and M. C. McIntyre. Cardiology for Nurses. McGraw-Hill Book Co., New York. 1980.

Chapter 16

Bates, B. A Guide to Physical Examination. J. B. Lippincott Co., Philadelphia. 1979. Second edition.

Guyton, A. C. Textbook of Medical Physiology. W. B. Saunders Co., Philadelphia. 1981. Sixth edition.

Holland, J. F., and E. Frei, III. Cancer Medicine. Lea & Febiger, Philadelphia. 1982. Second edition.

Lewis, C. M. Nutrition: The Basics of Nutrition. Family Nutrition. F. A. Davis Co., Philadelphia. 1977.

Luckmann, J., and K. C. Sorensen. Medical-Surgical Nursing. W. B. Saunders Co., Philadelphia. 1980. Second edition.

Roberts, S. L. Behavioral Concepts and the Critically Ill Patient. Prentice-Hall, Inc., Englewood Cliffs, N. J. 1976.

Shipman, J. J. Mnemonics and Tactics in Surgery and Medicine. Year Book Medical Publishers, Inc., Chicago. 1978.

Sorensen, K. C., and J. Luckmann. Basic Nursing. W. B. Saunders Co., Philadelphia. 1979.

Tilkian, S. M., M. B. Conover, and A. G. Tilkian. Clinical Implications of Laboratory Tests. C. V. Mosby Co., St. Louis. 1979.

Williams, S. R. Nutrition and Diet Therapy. C. V. Mosby Co., St. Louis. 1981. Fourth edition.

Chapter 17

Beeson, P. B., W. McDermott, and J. Wyngaarden. Cecil Textbook of Medicine. W. B. Saunders Co., Philadelphia. 1979. Fifteenth edition.

Brenner, B. M., and F. C. Rector, Jr. The Kidney. W. B. Saunders Co., Philadelphia. 1981, Second edition.

Brundage, D. J. Nursing Management of Renal Problems. C. V. Mosby Co., St. Louis. 1980. Second edition.

Denniston, D. J., and K. T. Burns. Home peritoneal dialysis. *American Journal of Nursing* (November 1980). 2022-2026.

Innes, B., and M. Bruya. Post-operative voiding patterns and contributing factors. *Washington State Journal of Nursing* (Summer-Fall 1977). 13-25.

Kagen, L. W. Renal Disease: A Manual of Renal Problems. McGraw-Hill Book Co., New York. 1979.

Smith, D. R. General Urology. Lange Medical Publications, Los Altos, Calif. 1981. Tenth edition.

Sontag, J. M. Experimental identification of genitourinary carcinogens. *Urologic Clinics of North America* (October 1980). 803-814.

Tobiason, S. J. Benign prostatic hypertropy. *American Journal of Nursing* (February 1979). 286-290.

Chapter 18

Benson, R. C. Handbook of Obstetrics & Gynecology. Lange Medical Publications, Los Altos, Calif. 1980. Seventh edition.

Bouchard-Kurtz, R., and N. Speese-Owens. Nursing Care of the Cancer Patient. C. V. Mosby Co., St. Louis. 1981. Fourth edition.

Brunner, L. S., and D. S. Suddarth. Medical-Surgical Nursing. J. B. Lippincott Co., Philadelphia. 1980. Fourth edition.

Hawkins, J. W., and L. P. Higgins. Maternity and Gynecological Nursing. J. B. Lippincott Co., Philadelphia. 1981.

Hogan, R. Human Sexuality: A Nursing Perspective. Appleton-Century-Crofts, East Norwalk, Conn. 1980.

Mims, F. H., and M. Swenson. Sexuality: A Nursing Perspective. McGraw-Hill Book Co., New York. 1980.

Murray, R. B., and J. P. Zenter. Nursing Assessment and Health Promotion Through the Life Span. Prentice-Hall, Inc., Englewood Cliffs, N. J. 1979.

Smith, E. D. Maternity Care: A Guide for Patient Education. Appleton-Century-Crofts, East Norwalk, Conn. 1981.

Tortora, G. J., R. L. Evans, and N. P. Anagnostakos. Principles of Human Physiology. Harper & Row, Publishers, Inc., New York. 1982.

Woods, N. F. Human Sexuality in Health and Illness. C. V. Mosby Co., St. Louis. 1979.

Chapter 19

Anthony, C. P., and G. A. Thibodeau. Textbook of Anatomy and Physiology. C. V. Mosby Co., St. Louis. 1979. Tenth edition.

Bradford, D. S., R. R. Foster, and H. L. Nossel. Coagulation alterations, hypoxemia, and fat embolism in fracture patients. *The Journal of Trauma* (1970). 316-318.

Hilt, N. E., and S. B. Cogburn. Manual of Orthopedics. C. V. Mosby Co., St. Louis. 1980.

Keim, H. Low back pain. *In* Clinical Symposia (vol. 25, no. 3). Ciba-Geigy, Summit, N. J. 1973.

816   Handbook of Medical-Surgical Nursing

Levine, R. R. Pharmacology: Drug Actions and Reactions. Little, Brown & Co., Boston. 1978. Second edition.

Marmor, L. Arthritis Surgery. Lea & Febiger, Philadelphia. 1976.

Matsen, F. A., III. Compartmental Syndromes. Grune & Stratton, Inc., New York. 1980.

Rockwood, C. A., and D. P. Green. Fractures. J. B. Lippincott Co., Philadelphia. 1975.

Steward, J. D. M. Traction and Orthopaedic Appliances. Churchill Livingston, Inc., New York. 1978.

Verdisco, L. Nursing care of patients with fractured hips. *From* Course presentation outline AAOS continuing education course: *What's Happening in the Joints.* 1982. p. 22-26.

Chapter 20

Adams, R. D., and M. Victor. Principles of Neurology. McGraw-Hill Book Co., New York. 1981. Second edition.

Erickson, R. Essentials of Neurological Examination. SmithKline Corp., Philadelphia. 1974.

Gilman, A. G., L. S. Goodman, and A. Gilman, editors. Goodman and Gilman's The Pharmacological Basis of Therapeutics. Macmillan, Inc., New York. 1980. Sixth edition.

Hickey, J. The Clinical Practice of Neurological and Neurosurgical Nursing. J. B. Lippincott Co., Philadelphia. 1981.

Merritt, H. H. A Textbook of Neurology. Lea & Febiger, Philadelphia. 1979. Sixth edition.

Mitchell, P., and N. Mauss. Intracranial pressure: fact and fancy. *Nursing 76* (June 1976). 53-57.

Noback, C. R., and R. J. Demarest. The Human Nervous System. McGraw-Hill Book Co., New York. 1980. Second edition.

Plum, F., and J. Posner. The Diagnosis of Stupor and Coma. F. A. Davis Co., Philadelphia. 1980. Third edition.

Salcman, M., editor. Neurologic Emergencies: Recognition and Management. Raven Press, New York. 1980.

Solomon, G. E., and F. Plum. Clinical Management of Seizures: A Guide for the Physician. W. B. Saunders Co., Philadelphia. 1976.

Chapter 21

Baldonado, A., and D. A. Stahl. Cancer Nursing: A Holistic Multidisciplinary Approach. Medical Examination Publishing Co., Inc., Garden City, N. Y. 1978.

Eastman, R. D. Clinical Haematology. John Wright & Sons, Ltd., London. 1977. Fifth edition.

Guyton, A. C. Textbook of Medical Physiology. W. B. Saunders Co., Philadelphia. 1981. Sixth edition.

Hashkell, C. M., editor. Cancer Treatment. W. B. Saunders Co., Philadelphia. 1980.

Luckmann, J., and K. C. Sorensen. Medical-Surgical Nursing. W. B. Saunders Co., Philadelphia. 1980. Second edition.

Mourant, A. E., A. C. Kopec, and K. Domaniewska-Sobezak. Blood Groups and Disease. Oxford University Press, New York. 1978.

Sabiston, D. C., editor. Davis-Christopher Textbook of Surgery. W. B. Saunders Co., Philadelphia. 1981. Twelfth edition.

Sherlock, S. Diseases of the Liver and Biliary System. Blackwell Scientific Publications, Oxford. 1975. Fifth edition.

Weiss, L. The Blood Cells and Hematopoietic Tissues. McGraw-Hill Book Co., New York. 1977.

Wyngaarden, J. B., and L. H. Smith. Cecil Textbook of Medicine. W. B. Saunders Co., Philadelphia. 1982. Sixteenth edition.

Chapter 22

Beazley, R. M., and I. Cohn. Pancreatic cancer. *Cancer Journal for Clinicians* (November-December 1981). 346-364.

Gann, D. S. Symposium on endocrine surgery. *Surgical Clinics of North America* (April 1974). 277-469.

Goldman, L., G. S. Gordon, and B. S. Roof. The parathyroids: progress, problems and practice. *Current Problems in Surgery* (August 1971). 3-64.

Harrison, T. S., and N. W. Thompson. Multiple endocrine adenomatosis: I and II. *Current Problems in Surgery* (August 1975). 7-51.

Javadpour, N., E. A. Woltering, and M. F. Brennan. Adrenal neoplasms. *Current Problems in Surgery* (January 1980). 5-52.

Ranson, J. H. C. Acute pancreatitis. *Current Problems in Surgery* (November 1979). 5-83.

Schwartz, S., and T. Shires. Principles of Surgery. McGraw-Hill Book Co., New York. 1979. Third edition.

Silverberg, E. Cancer Statistics, 1983. *Cancer Journal for Clinicians* (January-February 1983). 9-25.

Van Way, C. W., III, H. W. Scott, D. L. Page, and R. K. Rhamy. Pheochromocytoma. *Current Problems in Surgery* (June 1974). 4-59.

Wyngaarden, J. B., and L. H. Smith. Cecil Textbook of Medicine. W. B. Saunders Co., Philadelphia. 1982. Sixteenth edition.

INDEX

A

Abdomen
  and diet, 20, 25
Abdominal
  adhesions, 465
  aneurysm, 429
  angina, 453
  -perineal resection, 457
Abducens nerve
  function of, 616
Abnormal responses
  to stress, 5
ABO antigens, 116
Abortion, 539
  discussion of, 514
Abscess
  and rectal fistula, 467
  of brain, 646
  of breast, 239
  rectal, 460
Absence seizures, 662, 665
Absolutistic position, 501
Absorption
  of nutrients, 15
Acetaminophen
  and pain, 90
Acetylcysteine
  and respiratory care, 324
Acid
  eructation, 442
  in body fluids, 47
Acid-ash diet, 483
Acid-base balance, 47
  regulation of, 49
Acid-base imbalance
  signs and symptoms, 56
Acidemia, 48, 52
Acidosis
  metabolic, 48, 49
  respiratory, 49, 52
  signs and symptoms, 56
Acini, 235
Acne vulgaris, 213
Acoustic nerve
  function of, 616
Acoustic neuroma, 651
Acquired agammaglobulinemia, 117
Acquired immunity, 114
Acromegaly, 732
ACTH
  and homeostasis, 38

ACTH production
  and immobility, 135
Active immunity, 114
Active transport, 37
  in cells, 141
Activity
  and respiratory care, 338
  and temperature, 103
Acute airway obstruction, 344
Acute arterial occlusion, 424
Acute fevers, 110
Acute gastritis, 442
Acute leukemia, 690
Acute pain, 82
  symptoms of, 84
Acute renal failure, 477
Acute rheumatic fever, 401
Acute stress ulcer
  postoperative, 202
Acyclovir, 522
Adam's apple, 304
Adaptation, 1
  syndromes, 4
  to stress, 1
Addiction
  and pain, 81, 82
Addisonian crisis, 747
Addison's disease, 744
Adenine arabinoside, 645
Adenitis, 215
Adenocarcinoma, 365
  classification of, 148
Adenofibroma, 240
Adenoma
  classification of, 148
  pituitary, 651
ADH
  and homeostasis, 38
ADH secretion
  and immobility, 133, 135
  factors affecting, 741
Adhesions
  abdominal, 465
Adrenal
  cortex, 743
  disorders, 743
  hormone functions, 744
Adrenalectomy
  patient care, 752
Adrenergic fibers, 386

Adrenocorticosteroids
  and respiration, 326
Adrenocorticotropin, 731
Adult primary glaucoma, 266
Adult respiratory distress syndrome, 347
Aerophagia, 436
Affect theory
  of pain, 74
Agammaglobulinemia, 117
Agglutins, 116
Aging
  and diet, 18, 19
Air embolus
  and hyperalimentation, 30
Airway
  artificial, 190
  obstruction, 344
Akinetic seizures, 662, 665
Alarm stage
  to stress, 4
Alcoholism
  and hypothermia, 111
Aldosterone
  and homeostasis, 38
  and immobility, 135
  function of, 744
Aldosteronism
  and hypertension, 428
  diagnosis of, 749
Alkalemia, 51, 54
Alkali
  in body fluids, 47
Alkaline-ash diet, 483
Alkalosis
  metabolic, 49, 51
  respiratory, 49, 54
  signs and symptoms, 56
Allergic
  asthma, 121
  rhinitis, 121
  transfusion reaction, 687
Allergy, 113, 121
  and diet, 25
Allografts, 211
Alopecia, 206
  care of, 158
Altered antigen theory, 123
American Foundation for the Blind, 253
American Nurses' Association
  cancer outcome standards, 154
Aminophylline
  and respiratory care, 325
Amnesia, 667
Amputation, 422
Amyloidosis, 704
Amyotrophic lateral sclerosis, 678
Analgesics
  and musculoskeletal system, 567
  and pain, 87, 90, 91
Anaphylactic reactions
  care of, 160
Anaphylactic shock, 121
Anaphylaxis
  slow reactive substance of, 121
Anaplastic carcinoma, 763

Anastomosis
  ureterovesicular, 485
Anatomy
  and fluids and electrolytes, 34
  and immunity, 115
  and nutrition, 14
  and sensations, 72
  and stress, 3
  and temperature, 102
  female reproductive, 502, 504
  male reproductive, 502, 508
  of breasts, 235
  of ears, 273
  of eyes, 246
  of glands, 728
  of heart, 383
  of hematopoiesis, 683
  of kidneys, 470
  of liver, 708
  of lower GI tract, 439, 451
  of lungs, 311
  of metabolism, 728
  of mouth, 293
  of neck, 303
  of nervous system, 611
  of noise, 283
  of skeletal system, 547
  of skin, 203, 205
  of throat, 293
  of upper GI tract, 438, 439
  vascular, 420
Androgens, 503
  function of, 744
Anemia, 696
  and diet, 25
  and renal failure, 488
  care of, 157
  hemolytic, 699
  megaloblastic, 698
  patient teaching, 161
  sickle cell, 700
Anesthesia
  advantages and disadvantages, 176,
    177
  and surgery, 174, 175
  assessment, 164
  stages of, 175
Anesthetic agents
  types of, 176, 177
Aneurysm, 428
  clipping of, 661
Aneurysmal bone cyst, 595
Angina, 95·
  abdominal, 453
Angina pectoris, 419
Angiography
  and nervous system, 628
  renal, 478
Angioma
  spider, 723
Angioplasty, 391
Angiosarcoma
  classification of, 148
Anions, 35
Ankles

assessment of, 563
Anorexia, 20, 25
    and immobility, 134
    and renal failure, 476
    nervosa, 447
Anoscopy, 452
Anosmia, 632
Anoxia, 126
ANS, 613
    and stress, 3
Antibiotics
    and respiration, 325
Antibodies, 116
Anticholinergics
    and urinary retention, 475
Anticipatory planning
    and stress, 8
Anticonvulsants
    purpose of, 630
Antidepressants
    and pain, 88, 90
Antidiuretic hormone, 731
Antienzymes, 116
Antigens, 115
Antigen theories, 123
Antihistamines
    and respiration, 325
Antimicrobials
    renal, 480
Antirabies, 648
Antistreptolysin O titer, 491
Antitoxins, 116
Antitussives
    and respiration, 324
Anus
    excision of, 457
Anxiety
    and immobility, 136
    and pain, 73, 79
    and stress, 4
    and surgery, 165, 178
    reduction of, 178
Aorta
    normal BP, 421
Aortic valve diseases
    comparison of, 403
Apathy
    and diet, 201
Aphthous stomatitis, 297
Apocrine glands, 205
Apoplexy, 655
Appendectomy, 455
Appendicitis, 459
Appendix
    rupture of, 454
Appetite, 17
    how to increase, 27
Aqueduct of Sylvius, 612
Arbovirus encephalitis, 645
ARDS, 347
Arterial
    acute occlusion, 424
Arterial blood
    changes in, 49
Arterial leg ulcers, 230

Arteries
    role of, 421
Arteriosclerosis, 430
    coronary, 418
Arthritis, 95
    degenerative, 591
    hypertrophic, 591
    rheumatoid, 586
Arthrography
    discussion of, 565
Artificial airway, 190, 318
    illustration of, 319
Asbestos
    and cancer, 147
Ascaris, 461
Ascites, 713
Asepsis
    and hyperalimentation, 30
Aspiration
    bone marrow, 688
    during surgery, 182
    pneumonia, 354
Aspirin
    and pain, 90
Assault
    sexual, 507
Assessment
    cardiac, 387
    circulatory and casts, 575
    dietary, 21, 24, 25
    nutritional, 24, 25
    of acute pain, 82
    of electrolyte status, 39
    of fluid status, 39
    of mobility, 126
    of musculoskeletal sytem, 552
    of reproduction, 501
    of respiratory system, 313
    of stress, 6
    of temperature, 104
Assessment tool, 85
Asthma, 372
    allergic, 121
    cardiac, 396
Astrocytoma, 650
Ataxia, 647
Atelectasis, 377
Atheroma formation, 428
Atherosclerosis, 428
    and heat injuries,
    coronary, 418
Athlete's foot, 223
Atopic dermatitis, 122, 225
ATP
    and active transport, 37
Atrial
    fibrillation, 413
    premature contraction, 416
Atrophic vaginitis, 525
Atrophy
    and cells, 143
    and immobility, 128
Auer bodies, 691
Aura, 667
Autografts, 211

Autohypnosis
    and stress, 8
Autoimmune diseases, 123
Autonomic nervous system, 613
    divisions of, 617
Axilla
    and temperature, 106, 107
Axons, 611
Azure A, 440
Azuresin, 440

B

Babinski reflex
    test for, 627
Babinski's sign, 776
Back
    assessment of, 563, 564
    care of, 606-610
    problems, 604
Bacteria
    on skin, 205
Bacterial
    pneumonia, 354
    transfusion reaction, 687
Bacteriologic studies
    urinary, 473
Bacteriolysins, 116
Bacteroides, 646
Balanced suspension
    care of, 577
Balkan frame
    and hip fractures, 588
Barium enema, 452
Baroreceptor reflexes, 386
Bartholin's cyst, 527
Bartholin's glands
    function of, 504
Basal cell carcinoma
    classification of, 148
Basal cell epithelioma, 228
Basal metabolic rate, 135
Basic food groups, 9, 13
Basic four food groups, 13
Basic six food groups, 13
Baths
    and skin, 207
B cells, 115
Bedsore, 126
Behavior
    sexual, 501
Belching
    relief of, 436
Bence Jones proteinuria, 119
Benign neoplasms
    definition of, 145
Benzonatate
    and respiratory care, 324
Beriberi, 24
Bicarbonate buffer system, 47
Biliary cirrhosis, 723
Binge-purge disease, 448
Binocular vision, 246

Biofeedback
    and stress, 8
Biopsy
    breasts, 237
    Craig needle, 596
    liver, 711
    renal, 478
Blackheads, 213
Bladder
    anatomy of, 470
    cancer, 493
    neurogenic, 475, 498
Blastomyces dermatitidis, 364
Blastomycosis, 363
Bleeding disorders
    and temperature monitoring, 106
Blenderized foods, 28
Blepharitis, 262
Blindness, 271
Blood
    altered functioning of, 683
    and the CNS, 612
    flow, 421
    transfusions, 686
Blood clots
    and immobility, 129 130
Blood supply
    and immobility, 126
Blood test
    and nutrition, 22
Blunt injuries
    thoracic, 349
Body
    fluid and solid composition, 34
    fluids, 33
Body calcium
    forms of, 61
Body jacket, 572
Body temperature
    core, 101
Boils, 217
Bone
    aneurysmal cyst, 595
    cancellous, 548
    compact, 548
    depressions, 549
    discussion of, 547
    landmarks, 549
    marrow aspiration, 566, 688
    marrow cells, 142
    marrow transplant, 688
    projections, 549
    repair process of, 548
    resorption, 766
    scan, 565
Bone marrow depression
    care of, 156
    patient teaching, 161
Bones
    and immobility, 128
Boredom
    and immobility, 136
Bottle systems, 329
    illustration of, 330

Bouginage, 446
Bovine TB, 360
Bowed legs
    and diet, 20, 25
Bowlegs, 567
Bowman's capsule, 471
Bradycardia, 411
Brain
    abscess, 646
    and sensations, 73
    functions of, 614, 615
    lobes, 614
    structures of, 614, 615
Breast
    abscess, 239
    anatomy, 235
    complications, 234
    examination, 236-238
Breathing exercises
    and respiratory care, 338
Bricker procedure, 484
Brittle hair
    and diet, 20
Brompheniramine maleate
    and respiratory care, 325
Brompton's mixture, 88, 91
Bronchiectasis, 358
Bronchitis, 356
Bronchodilators
    and respiration, 325
Bronchography
    purpose of, 315
Bronchopneumonia, 354
Bronchoscopy
    purpose of, 315
Brudzinski's sign, 643, 659
Bruise, 583
Bryant's traction
    and compartmental syndrome, 579
Buck's extension, 576
    and hip fractures, 589
Buerger's disease, 431
Buffalo hump, 735
Buffer systems, 47
Bulbourethral glands
    function of, 509
Bulbs of Krause, 72
Bulimia, 448
Bulk
    and diet, 15, 16
Bunions, 601
Bupivacaine
    and surgery, 177
Burkitt's lymphoma, 691
Burns
    and fluid imbalance, 33
    chemical, 256
    degrees of, 210
    flash, 256
    of the skin, 209
    thermal, 257
Bursa of Fabricius, 115
Bypass
    femoral-popliteal, 423

C

Cachexia
    and diet, 20
Caffeine
    and pain, 90
Calcium
    deficit, 61
    excess, 63
    forms of, 61
    imbalance, 61
Calcium RDAs, 11
Calculi, 443
Callosal commisurotomy, 663
Calorie-free foods, 13, 16
Calyces
    of kidneys, 470
Cancellous bone, 548
Cancer, 301
    and diet, 16
    and indigestion, 435
    cervical classification, 532
    concepts, 147
    death rate, 146
    definition of, 145
    etiology, 145
    gastric, 445
    general treatment of, 151-154
    goals of care, 152
    incidence of, 146
    invasive, 150
    of bladder, 493
    of colon, 463
    of larynx, 307
    of liver, 721
    of prostate, 491, 494
    of thyroid, 761
    pancreatic, 782
    quiescent, 150
    rectal, 464
    risk factors, 147
    sigmoid, 464
    stomach, 445
    testicular, 537
    warning signs, 150
Candida, 784
Candida albicans
    and vaginitis, 525
Candidiasis, 525
Canker sores, 297
Cantor tube, 453
Capillaries
    role of, 421
Carbetapentane citrate
    and respiratory care, 324
Carbohydrates, 9, 12
    in cells, 139, 140
Carbonic acid buffer system, 47
Carcinogenesis
    definition of, 145
Carcinoma
    cervical, 531, 532
    definition of, 145
    endometrial, 534

ovarian, 535
uterine, 533
Cardiac (*see also* Heart)
  compensatory mechanisms, 408
  overloading, 408
  pressure overloading, 408
  volume overloading, 408
Cardiac arrest, 392
  during surgery, 182
Cardiac asthma, 396
Cardiac disease
  and fluid imbalance, 33
Cardiac output
  definition of, 387
Cardiac tamponade, 398
  and pericardial effusion, 407
Cardiac work load
  and immobility, 130
Cardiogenic shock, 395
  postoperative, 201
Cardiovascular
  postoperative complications, 197
Cardiovascular system (*see also* Heart)
  altered functioning of, 383
  and homeostasis, 37
  and immobility, 129
Caries, 298
  and diet, 20
Carpal tunnel syndrome, 602
Cartilage, 548
Casts
  and pressure, 574
  care of, 569
  complications, 574
  types of, 572, 573
Cataract, 269
Catheterization
  renal vein, 479
Cations, 35
CAT scan, 629
Cecostomy, 454
Celiac disease
  and malabsorption, 436
Cell
  cycle, 141, 142
  death, 127
  division, 142
  growth, 142
  life-span, 155
  -mediated immunity, 114
  membrane, 140
  special units, 142
  tissue, 142
Cellular
  composition, 139
  death, 155
  function, 140
  growth, 139
  immunity, 115
  necrosis, 155
  structure, 140
Cellulitis, 217, 425
Central
  nervous system, 612
  pain, 77, 78

Cerebellar functioning
  assessment of, 623
Cerebellum
  function of, 614
Cerebral functioning
  examination of, 618
Cerebral hemorrhage, 656
Cerebral ischemic attack, 656
Cerebrovascular accident, 655
Cerebrum
  function of, 614
Cervical
  cancer classification, 532
  carcinoma, 531, 532
  intraepithelial neoplasia classification, 531
  smears, 523
Chaddock reflex
  test for, 627
Chalazion, 262
Chemical burns
  of eyes, 256
Chemical substances
  and stress, 6
Chemoreceptor reflexes, 386
Chemotherapy, 119
  discussion of, 151
  side effects of, 156-160
Chest
  flail, 350
  injuries, 349
Chest deformity
  and diet, 20
Chest expansion
  and immobility, 132
Chest percussion
  positions for, 341
Chest tube systems, 329
Chest x-rays
  purposes of, 315
CHF, 407
  renal signs of, 474
Children
  RDAs, 10, 11
Chill phase
  of fever, 110
Chlorpheniramine maleate
  and respiratory care, 325
Cholangiography, 440
Cholecystitis, 444
Cholecystography, 440
Choledocholithiasis, 443
Cholelithiasis, 443
Cholesterol
  in cells, 140
Cholinergic fibers, 385
Cholinergics, 480
Chondroma, 595
  classification of, 148
Chondrosarcoma, 596
  classification of, 148
Chordotomy, 97
Choriocarcinoma
  classification of, 149
Chorionepithelioma

classification of, 149
Chromophobic adenoma, 657
Chromosomes, 141
Chronic gastritis, 443
Chronic
  gastritis, 443
  obstructive pulmonary disease, 371
  pain, 95
  renal failure, 494
  valvular disease, 400
Chvostek's sign, 772
Circadian temperature rhythm, 102
Circulation
  and back problems, 609
  coronary, 384, 385
  pulmonary, 383
  systemic characteristics, 421
Circulatory overload, 687
Cirrhosis, 722
Climacteric
  female, 502
  male, 503
Clinics
  for pain, 98
Clitoris
  function of, 504
Clonal selection theory, 116
Clone
  theory, 123
Clonorchis sinensis, 720
Closed-angle glaucoma, 266
Closed head injury, 637
CNS, 612
  and stress, 3
  and temperature control, 103
Coagulation
  disseminated intravascular, 705
Cocaine
  and surgery, 177
Coccidioides immitis, 364
Coccidioidomycosis, 363
Codeine
  and pain, 91
  and respiratory care, 324
Cognitive response
  to pain, 73
Coitus interruptus
  effectiveness of, 512
Cold
  and pain, 87
Cold injuries, 111
Colectomy, 457
Colitis
  ulcerative, 456
Colloids
  role in body, 34
Colon
  excision of, 457
  neoplasms of, 463
Clonoscopy, 452
Colorectal cancer
  and diet, 16
Colostomy, 454, 463
Colporrhaphy, 485
Coma, 777

description of, 619
  hyperglycemic, hyprosmolar
    nonketotic, 787
Comedones, 213
Commercially prepared supplements,
    28, 29
Commisurotomy
  callosal, 663
Common warts, 221
Communication
  and pain, 85
Compact bone, 548
Compartmental syndrome, 579
Complete abortion, 540
Compresses
  and skin, 207
Concentration
  effect on diffusion, 36
Condom
  effectiveness of, 513
Conducting system, 311
Conduction, 385, 387
Conduction (of heat), 103
Condyle, 549
Condyloma acuminata, 221
Congential agammaglobulinemia, 117
Congestive heart failure, 407
Conjunctivitis, 262
Connective tissue, 142
Conn's syndrome, 438
Consciousness
  altered states of, 619
Constipation
  and colon cancer, 463
  and diet, 20, 25
  and immobility, 134
  discussion of, 436, 437
  postoperative, 199
Constrictive pericarditis, 406
Consults
  and surgery, 165, 166
Contactants, 121
Contact dermatitis, 226
Continent ileostomy
  care of, 457
Continuous mechanical ventilation, 322
Contraception
  types of, 512
Contraction
  premature atrial, 416
  premature ventricular, 417
Contracture
  Dupuytren's, 602
Contusion, 583
Convection (of heat), 103
Convulsive disorders, 662
Cooper's ligaments, 235
COPD, 371
Coping mechanisms, 2
Core body temperature, 101
Corneal arcus, 24
Coronary
  arteriosclerosis, 418
  artery bypass graft, 390
  atherosclerosis, 418

circulation, 384, 385
heart disease, 418
sinus, 386
veins, 386
Corticosterone
function of, 744
Cortisol
function of, 744
CO₂ narcosis
and immobility, 132
Coughing
and respiratory care, 338
and surgery, 169
Counseling
and stress, 8
Countertraction, 571
Cowper's glands
function of, 509
Craig needle biopsy, 596
Cranial nerves, 613, 616
assessment of, 620-622
deficit, 632
functions of, 616
Craniotomy, 661
Creatine phosphokinase-myocardial
band
and MI, 393
Crescendo angina, 419
Cretinism, 761
Crohn's disease, 438
and enteritis, 455
and ulcerative colitis, 456
Crust, 204
Crutchfield tongs, 640
Cryosurgery, 732
Cryptitis, 460,467
Curling's ulcer, 450
Cushing's disease
and hypertension, 428
and osteoporosis, 597
Cushing's syndrome, 735
Cushing's ulcer, 450
Cyclopropane
and surgery, 176
Cyst
aneurysmal bone, 595
Bartholin's, 527
Graafian, 529
lutein, 529
ovarian, 529
pilonidal, 462
sebaceous, 227
Cystadenoma
classification of, 148
Cystectomy, 484
Cystic fibrosis, 379
Cystitis, 481
signs of, 474
Cystogram
voiding, 479
Cystolithomy, 485
Cystometrogram, 479
Cystoscopy, 479
Cystostomy, 477
Cytologic studies

urinary, 473
Cytology
of breasts,237
Cytomorphosis, 155
Cytoplasm, 140, 141
Cytotoxins, 116

D

Deafness, 273, 281
Death
and stress, 6
Debridement
and cancer, 155
Deconditioning
physiologic, 125, 126
Decortication
purpose and care, 334
Decubitus ulcers, 126, 230
stages of, 128
Deep breathing
and surgery, 169
Deep pain, 77, 78
Defervescence
during fever, 110
Deficient response
to stress, 5
Deficit
calcium, 61
magnesium, 65
potassium, 57
Dehiscence
postoperative, 196
Dehydration
and heat injuries, 105
and immobility, 129
signs of, 474
Déjà vu phenomenon, 667
Demyelination, 670
Dendrites, 611
Dennis tube, 453
Dental caries, 298
Depression
and immobility, 136
Dermatitis, 224
atopic, 122
venenata, 226
Dermis, 204, 205
Dermoid cyst
classification of, 149
Desoxycorticosterone
function of, 744
Detrussor
of bladder, 470
Deviated septum, 292
Devine tube, 453
Dextromethorphan hydrobromide
and respiratory care, 325
Diabetes
and heat injuries, 105
Diabetes insipidus, 741
Diabetes mellitus, 784
and renal disease, 475
and sexual functioning, 516

Diabetic retinopathy, 264
Diagnostic tests
  special, 566
Dialysis, 481
  patient care during, 489
Diaphragm
  effectiveness of, 513
Diarrhea
  and diet, 20, 25
  and fluid imbalance, 33
  discussion of, 436, 437
Diascopy, 207
Diastolic click, 389
Diencephalon
  function of, 615
Diet, 9
  and fluid imbalance, 33
  an renal disorders, 482, 483
  and respiratory functioning, 326
  and temperature, 103
  elemental, 26
Diethylstilbestrol
  and cancer, 147
  and prostatic cancer, 494
Diffusion, 35
  in cells, 141
Digestion, 15
Digestive process, 293
Dilation and currettage, 530
Diplococcus pneumoniae, 354, 643
Disaccharides
  and cellular growth, 140
Disc
  herniated, 604
Discoloration
  and diet, 24, 25
Discrimination
  tactile, 72
  two-point, 71
Disease
  Addison's, 744
  and diet, 17
  autoimmune, 123
  binge-purge, 448
  celiac, 436
  Crohn's, 455, 456
  Cushing's, 735
  Gaucher's, 704
  Graves's, 755
  Hashimoto's, 759
  Hodgkin's, 648, 695
  Huntington's, 680
  iron deficiency, 698
  Lou Gehrig, 678
  Mucorales, 784
  Niemann-Pick, 704
  organ-specific, 124
  Paget's, 598
  Parkinson's, 671
  pelvic inflammatory, 523
  renal, 494
  systemic, 124
  tests for, 791-805
Discoloration, 584
Disorientation

  and acid-base imbalances, 56
Disposable unit systems, 329
  illustration of, 331
Dissecting aneurysm, 428
Disseminated intravascular coagulation, 705
Disseminated sclerosis, 670
Distended abdomen
  and diet, 20, 25
Distorted anticipatory response
  to stress, 5
Distraction
  and pain relief, 95, 97
Disuse atrophy, 143
Disuse phenomena, 125
Diuretics, 480
Diverticulitis, 458
  and constipation, 437
Diverticulosis, 458
  and diet, 16
Diverticulum
  and stress, 6
DNA, 140, 141
Documentation
  during surgery, 181
Doppler examination
  of the heart, 388
Doppler ultrasonography, 654
Double-barreled colostomy, 463
Drainage
  postural, 339, 341
Draping
  during surgery, 179
Dressings
  and skin, 207
  and surgery, 170, 181
Drooling
  and diet, 24
Drowning, 342
Drug infiltration
  care for, 153
Drugs
  and respiration, 324
Dry-drowning, 342
Dry skin, 208
Duchenne's dystrophy, 676
Duodenal ulcer, 450
Dupuytren's contracture, 602
Dwarfism, 739
Dyplopia, 632
Dysentery, 461
Dyspepsia, 435
  discussion of, 436
Dysuria, 474

E

Ear
  altered functioning of, 273
  cross section of, 275
  functions, 274
  loss of hearing, 281
  obstruction of, 276
  structures, 274

swimmer's 277
Eccrine glands, 205
ECF
  role in body, 34
ECG
  and heart block, 414, 415
  conduction tracing, 385
  tracing implications, 390
Echinococcus granulosus, 720
Ecology
  and stress, 4
Eczema, 122, 224
Edema
  and diet, 20, 24
  and fluid imbalance, 33
  laryngeal, 305
  pulmonary, 395
EEG, 629
Effusion
  pericardial, 406, 407
Ejaculatory ducts
  function of, 509
Elbow
  assessment of, 559
Elderly
  dietary requirements, 23
Elective surgery, 163
Electrical potential
  effect on diffusion, 36
Electrolyte
  balance, 33
Electrolyte
  composition, 36
  movement, 35
Electrolytes, 35
  in cells, 139, 140
Electromyography, 566
Elemental diets, 26
Ellsworth-Howard test, 767
Embolectomy, 423
Embolic CVA, 655
Embolism
  fat, 582
  pulmonary, 345
Embolus
  and hyperalimentation, 30
Embryonal carcinoma
  classification of, 149
Embryonal sarcoma
  classification of, 149
Emergency surgery, 163
Emphysema, 369
  subcutaneous, 351
Encephalitis, 645
Encephalopathy
  hepatic, 714
Endarectomy, 423
  for TIAs, 654
Endocarditis, 400
Endocrine disorders
  and fluid imbalance, 33
Endocrine system
  altered functioning of, 727
  and homeostasis, 38
  and stress, 3

Endogenous pain control theory, 75, 76
Endometrial
  carcinoma, 534
Endometriosis, 543
Endomysium, 550
Endorphin
  and pain, 75
Endothelioma
  classification of, 148
Endotracheal tubes
  discussion of, 319
Enema
  barium, 452
Enflurane
  and surgery, 176
Entamoeba histolytica, 461, 720
Enteritis, 455
Enterobacteriaceae, 643, 646
Enterobius, 461
Enteroscopy, 452
Environment
  and cancer, 147
Enzymes
  and cellular growth, 140
Eosinophilic adenoma, 651
Ependymoma, 650
Ephedrine sulfate
  and respiratory care, 325
Epidemiology
  and cancer, 146, 147
Epidermis, 204, 205
Epididymis
  functions of, 508
Epididymitis, 528
Epidural anesthesia, 178
Epilepsy, 662
Epimysium, 550
Epinephrine
  and heat production, 102
  and homeostasis, 38
  and stress, 3
  function of, 744
Epispadias
  and infertility, 538
Epistaxis, 288
Epithelial tissue, 142
Epithelioma
  basal cell, 228
Equine encephalitis, 645
Erb's point, 388
Erosion, 204
Eructation, 442
Escherichia coli, 527, 643, 646
Esophageal stricture, 445
Esophageal varices, 715
Esophagitis, 442
Essential hypertension, 426
Estrogen
  and reproduction, 502
Estrogens
  function of, 744
Estrogen tablets
  effectiveness of, 512
Ethambutol hydrochloride
  and TB, 361

Ether
  and surgery, 176
Evaporation
  and loss of heat, 103
Evisceration
  postoperative, 196
Ewing's sarcoma, 597
  classification of, 148
Excess
  calcium, 63
  magnesium, 66
  potassium, 59
  water, 42
Excessive response
  to stress, 5
Exercise
  and rheumatoid arthritis, 587
  breathing, 338
Exhaustion
  heat, 110, 111
Exhaustion stage
  to stress, 5
Exophthalmos, 271
Expectorants
  and respiration, 324
Expiratory volume
  forced, 316
Exploratory thoracotomy
  purpose and care, 334
External otitis, 277
Extracapsular fractures, 585
Extracellular
  solute deficit, 42
  volume excess, 45
  volume depletion, 43
Extraocular muscles, 248
Extrinsic asthma, 121
Eyes
  agencies for, 253
  altered functioning of, 245
  and diet, 20, 24
  cross section of, 246
  functions, 247, 249
  innervation of, 251
  structures, 247, 249

F

Fabricius
  bursa of, 115
Face
  and diet, 20, 24, 25
Face mask, 317
  illustration of, 317
Facial nerve
  function of, 616
Facioscapulohumeral dystrophy, 676
Fallopian tubes
  function of, 504
Fallot
  tetralogy of, 646
Fasciola hepatica, 720
Fat
  embolism, 582

  -soluble vitamin RDAs, 10
Fatigue
  and diet, 20, 24
  and pain, 87
Fats, 9, 12
Fatty acids, 12
Fear
  of pain, 73
Fecal impaction
  and temperature monitoring, 106
Fecolith, 454, 459
Feet
  assessment of, 563
Female RDAs, 10, 11
Femoral hernia, 466
Femoral-popliteal bypass, 423
Fentanyl
  and surgery, 177
Fertility, 503
Fetor
  uremic, 476
Fever, 107, 110
  and fluid imbalance, 33
  phases of, 110
  rheumatic, 399
  risk factors, 105
Fiber
  and diet, 15, 16
Fibrillation
  atrial, 413
  ventricular, 413
Fibrinous pleurisy, 362
Fibrocystic disease, 239
Fibroids
  of the uterus, 530
Fibroma
  classification of, 148
Fibrosarcoma, 596
  classification of, 148
Filtration, 37
  renal, 471
Finger
  trigger, 603
First-degree heart block, 414
Fissure, 204
  -in-ano, 467
  rectal, 467
Fistula
  formation, 485
  -in-ano, 467
  rectal, 467
Flaccid muscles
  and diet, 20
Flail chest, 350
Flap amputations, 422
Flash burns
  of eyes, 256
Flatfoot, 601
Fluid
  balance, 33
  body composition, 34
  movement, 35
  shifts, 67
Flush phase
  of fever, 110

Focal seizures, 662
Folacin RDAs, 11
Follicle-stimulating hormone, 502, 731
Follicular carcinoma, 762
Food
  lack of, 17
Food chain, 16
Food exhange list, 13
Food intake
  inadequate, 16
Foot
  flat, 601
Foramen, 549
  of Monro, 612
Forced expiratory volume
  definition of, 316
Foreign body
  in eyes, 253
  ingestion of, 441
Fossa, 549
  blow-out of orbit, 259
  nasal, 287
  rib 351
Fractured jaw, 295
Frank-Starling law, 386, 408
FTA-ABS test, 521
Fungal infections, 222
  respiratory, 363
Fungal pneumonia, 354
Furuncle, 217
Fusiform aneurysm, 428

G

Gallbladder series, 440
Ganglion, 602
Ganglioneuroma
  classification of, 148
Gangrene
  and arterial occlusion, 424
  and cellulitis, 425
Gardner-Wells tongs, 640
Gargoylism, 704
Gas exchange
  discussion of, 313
Gastrectomy, 450
Gastric cancer, 445
Gastric contents
  analysis of, 440
Gastric gavage, 28
Gastric ulcer, 450
Gastritis
  acute, 442
  and indigestion, 435
  chronic, 443
Gastroenteritis
  and vomiting, 436
Gastrointestinal system
  altered functioning of, 435
Gastrojejunostomy, 450
Gastrostomy feedings, 28, 29
Gate control theory
  of pain, 75, 75

Gaucher's disease, 704
Gavage
  gastric, 28
Gender
  roles, 501
General
  anesthesia, 175.
  enteritis, 455
Generalized seizures, 662, 664-667
Genital
  herpes, 521
Genitalia
  female, 504
  male, 508
Genu valgum, 567
Genu varum, 567
GI disorders
  and fluid imbalance,33
Gigantism, 732
Gingivitis, 296
GI system
  and homeostasis, 38
  and immobility, 134
Gland
  and diet, 20
  apocrine, 205
  Bartholin's, 504, 527
  Bulbourethral, 509
  Cowper's, 509
  eccrine, 205
  functioning, 727
  sebaceous, 205
  Skene's, 504
Glaucoma, 266
  secondary, 268
Glial cells, 611
Glioblastoma
  classification of, 148
  multiforme, 650
Glioma, 650
  classification of, 148
Glomerulus, 470
Glossitis, 296
  and diet, 20, 24
Glossopharyngeal nerve
  function of, 616
Glucocorticoids
  function of, 744
Glycerol, 12
Glyceryl guaiacolate
  and respiratory care, 324
Goiter
  nontoxic, 760
  toxic diffuse, 755
Goitrogens, 760
Gonadotrophins, 731
Gonads
  female, 504
Gonococci
  and urethral stricture, 499
Gonorrhea, 519
Gordon reflex
  test for, 627
Gout, 593
Graafian cyst, 529

Graft
   coronary artery bypass, 390
Grafts
   for burns, 211
Grand mal seizures, 662, 664
Graves's disease, 755
Gravity
   and immobility, 129, 130, 132, 134
Greasy skin
   and diet, 20
Growth hormone, 142, 731
Guaiac test, 452
Guillain-Barré syndrome, 144, 648
Gums
   and diet, 20, 24
Gynecomastia, 241, 723

H

Haemophilus influenzae, 354, 643
Hair, 204, 205
   and diet, 20, 24
Hallucinations
   from immobility, 136
Hallux valgus, 600
Halothane
   and surgery, 176
Halo traction brace, 640
Halter monitoring
   of the heart, 388
Hammer toe, 599
Hands
   assessment of, 558
Haptens, 115
Harris tube, 453
Hashimoto's disease, 759
Hauser procedure
   and compartment syndrome, 579
Head
   altered functioning of, 245
   injury, 637
Health history
   purpose of, 789
Hearing loss, 281
Heart (*see also* Cardiac,
      Cardiovascular)
   altered functioning of, 383
   anatomy and physiology, 383
   block, 412
   clicks, 389
   coronary disease, 418
   exterior view, 384
   failure, 407
   function of, 386
   interior view, 384
   invasive studies, 388
   left-sided failure, 409
   major components of, 384
   noninvasive studies, 388
   normal BP, 421
   right-sided failure, 409
   sounds, 389
Heart block
   types of, 414, 415

Heartburn, 442
Heat
   abnormal loss, 104
   abnormal production, 104
   and pain, 87
   exhaustion, 110, 111
   loss, 102
   production, 102
Heat injuries, 110, 111
   risk factors, 105
Heatstroke, 110, 111
Hedonistic position, 501
Heimlich maneuver, 344
Heinz bodies, 701
Hemangioendothelioma
   classification of, 148
Hemangioma
   classification of, 148
Hematologic abnormalities
   and plasma cell myeloma, 119
Hematoma
   evacuation of, 638
Hematopoietic system
   altered functioning of, 683
Heminephrectomy, 484
Hemispherectomy, 663
Hemodialysis, 481
   patient care during, 490
Hemolysins, 116
Hemolytic anemia, 699
Hemolytic transfusion reaction, 686
Hemophilia, 701
Hemorrhage, 689
   and pain, 83
   cerebral, 656
   postoperative, 197
   subarachnoid, 658
Hemorrhagic CVA, 655
Hemorrhoidectomy, 467
Hemorrhoids, 466
Hemothorax, 350
Henle
   loop of, 471
Hepatic
   toxic status, 716
Hepatic encephalopathy, 714
Hepatic system (*see also* Liver)
   altered functioning of, 683
Hepatitis
   etiology, 718
   viral, 717
Hernia, 465
   hiatus, 446
   volvulus, 453
Herniated
   discs, 604
   nucleus pulposus, 604
Herniorraphy, 466
Herpes, 297
   genitalis, 521
   Resource Center, 523
   simplex, 219
   simplex encephalitis, 645
   zoster, 219
Heterophile antigen theory, 123

Hiatus hernia, 446
Hidradentitis suppurativa, 215
High
  -flow systems, 317
  -nitrogen supplements, 29
  -nutrient-density foods, 27, 28
  -protein supplements, 29
Hilum, 470
Hip
  assessment of, 560
  fracture, 585, 588-590
  spica, 572
Histamine, 121
Histoplasma capsulatum, 364
Histoplasmosis, 363
History
  purpose of, 789
Hives, 121
Hodgkin's disease, 648, 695
Holography
  of breasts, 237
Holter monitoring, 653
Homeostasis
  and immunity, 113
Homeostatic mechanisms, 33, 37
Homonymous hemianopsia, 632, 647, 654
Honeymoon cystitis, 487
Hordeolum, 262
Hormones
  and heat production, 102
  pituitary, 731
Host factors
  of cancer, 147
Hostility
  and immobility, 136
Human TB, 360
Humidification
  and respiratory care, 339
Humoral immunity, 114, 115
Hump back
  and diet, 20
Hunger, 17
Huntington's chorea, 680
Hydatidiform mole
  classification of, 149
Hydrogen ion imbalance, 47
Hydronephrosis, 472
Hydrostatic pressure, 67
Hymen
  function of, 504
Hyperaldosteronism, 747
  diagnosis of, 750
Hyperalimentation, 26, 30
Hypercalcemia, 63
Hypercalcemic crisis, 768
Hypercoagulability
  and immobility, 130
Hyperglycemic, hyperosmolar
  nonketotic coma, 787
Hyperkalemia, 59
Hyperkalemics, 480
Hypermagnesemia, 66
Hypernatremia, 41
Hyperosmolar imbalances, 41

Hyperparathyroidism, 769
  and urolithiasis, 497
Hypersensitivity, 114, 121
Hypersplenism, 703
Hypertension
  and renal disease, 475, 476
  and sexual functioning, 516
  essential, 426
  portal, 712
  primary, 426
  secondary, 428
Hyperthermia
  during surgery, 183
  malignant, 183
Hyperthyroidism
  and diarrhea, 437
Hypertonic
  IV solutions, 26
  solutions, 37
Hypertrophy, 144
  benign prostatic, 491
  female, 240
  male, 241
  ventricular, 408
Hyperuricemia
  and gout, 593
Hypervitaminosis A, 17
Hypervitaminosis D
  and urolithiasis, 497
Hypervolemia, 45
Hypesthesia, 99
Hyphema, 258
Hypocalcemia, 61
Hypogammaglobulinemia, 117
Hypoglossal nerve
  function of, 616
Hypoglycemia, 776
Hypokalemia, 57
Hypokalemics, 480
Hypomagnesemia, 65
Hyponatremia, 42
Hypoosmolar imbalance, 42
Hypoparathyroidism, 771
Hypophysectomy, 730
Hypopituitarism, 739
Hypospadias
  and infertility, 538
Hypostatic pneumonia, 354
Hypotension
  and renal failure, 476
  orthostatic, 129, 130
Hypothalamus
  and homeostasis, 38
  and stress, 3
  and temperature control, 103
  function of, 615
Hypothermia, 111
Hypothyroidism, 761
Hypotonic solutions, 37
Hypovolemia, 43
  and renal failure, 488
Hypovolemic shock
  during surgery, 182
  postoperative, 200
Hysterosalpingography, 523

I

ICF
   electrolyte composition, 36
   role in body, 34
Ictal phase, 664-667
Idiopathic thrombocytopenic purpura,
   704
Ileitis
   terminal, 455
Ileostomy
   for ulcerative colitis, 457
Ileus
   paralytic, 199, 465
Imagery
   and pain relief, 98
Imbalances
   calcium, 61
   fluid and electrolyte, 41
   hydrogen, 47
   magnesium, 65
   potassium, 57
Immobility, 125, 126
Immunity, 113
Immunoglobulins, 116
Immunotherapy
   discussion of, 151
Implants
   and pain relief, 97
Impotence, 541
Impulse
   point of maximal, 388, 389
   transmission, 612
Inadequate food intake, 16
Inappropriate response
   to stress, 5
Inattentiveness
   and diet, 20, 25
Incentive spirometer, 377, 378
Incisional hernia, 466
Incomplete abortion, 540
Increased intracranial pressure, 635
Indigestion, 435
   and diet, 20
Induced abortion, 539
Inevitable abortion, 540
Infant RDAs, 10, 11
Infarction
   myocardial, 393
Infection
   and fever, 105
   at pin sites, 576
   fungal, 222, 363
   of eyes, 262
   of wound, 195
   oral, 296
   parasitic, 461
Infertility, 538
Inflammation
   of eyes, 262
Influenza, 351
Ingestants, 121
Ingestion, 14
Inguinal canal
   function of, 509
Inguinal hernia, 465
Inhalants, 121
Injury
   and stress, 6
Innervation
   of the eye, 246, 251
Insecticides
   ingestion of, 441
Insensible water loss, 35
In situ lesions, 150
Inspiratory capacity
   definition of, 315
Instructive theory of antibody formation,
   116
Insulin
   actions of, 774
Intake
   altered needs, 19
   and surgery, 170
Integument (see also Skin)
   and immobility, 126
Interferon
   as immunotherapy, 119
Interstitial
   fluid shifts, 69
Interstitial cell-stimulating hormone, 503
Interstitial fluid
   role in body, 34
Interventions
   dietary, 23
   fluids and electrolyes, 40
   for temperature alterations, 109
   preoperative, 168
Intestinal
   obstruction, 453
Intracapsular fractures, 585
Intracranial pressure
   increased, 635
Intraoperative needs, 173
Intrarenal failure
   causes of, 488
Intrauterine device
   effectiveness of, 513
Intussusception, 453
Invasive cancers, 150
Iodine RDAs, 11
Ion charge
   effect on diffusion, 36
IPPB, 321
Iron
   deficiency, 698
   RDAs, 11
Irritableness
   and diet, 20, 25
Isoflurane
   and surgery, 176
Isografts, 211
Isoniazid, 361
Isotonic solutions, 37
IV
   and surgery, 175
   for surgery, 169
   postoperative, 187
IVP test, 478

J

Jacksonian seizures, 652, 662, 666
Jaw
  assessment of, 558
  fractured, 295
Jejunoileitis
  granulomatous, 455
Jejunostomy feedings, 28, 29
Joint
  and immobility, 128
  aspiration, 566
  assessment of, 558, 564
  contracture, 569
  definition of, 552
  types of, 554, 555

K

Keloid, 206
Keratitis, 262
Kernig's sign, 643, 659
Ketamine
  and surgery, 177
Ketoacidosis, 77
Ketosis, 18
Kidneys (see also Renal)
  altered functioning of, 469
  and homeostasis, 37
  artificial, 469
  as buffer system, 47
  inflammation of, 488
  polycystic, 495
  transplant, 485
Kinsey
  on impotence, 541
Klebsiella, 643
Klebsiella pneumoniae, 354
Knee
  assessment of, 561, 562
Knock-knees, 567
  and diet, 20
Krause
  bulbs of, 72
Kronlein's operation, 272
KUB test, 478
Kupffer cells, 709
Kussmaul's respiration, 777, 787
  and renal failure, 476
Kussmaul's sign
  and tamponade, 398

L

Labia
  function of, 504
Lacerations
  of eyes, 254
Lactation RDAs, 10, 11
Lactic dehydrogenase
  and MI, 393
Lactose-free supplements, 29
Laennec's cirrhosis, 723

Laminectomy, 640
Landouzy-Déjérine dystrophy, 676
Langerhans
  islets of, 773
Laparoscopy, 523
Lappé, Frances M., 15
Laryngeal
  cancer, 307
  edema, 305
Laryngectomies
  clubs for, 310
Laryngitis, 306
Laryngospasm
  and surgery, 182
Larynx, 303
Lateralization, 621
LeFort III, 295
Left-sided heart failure, 409
Legal blindness, 271
Leiomyoma
  classification of, 148
Leiomyosarcoma
  classification of, 148
Lentigo maligna melanoma, 229
Leptomeningitis, 643
Lesions
  in situ, 150
  integumentary, 204
Lethargy
  description of, 619
Leukemia, 690
  and gout, 593
  classification of, 148
  definition of, 145
Leukopenia
  care of, 156
  patient teaching, 161
Levine tube, 453
Lice, 214, 215
Lidocaine
  and surgery, 177
Life cycle
  of cells, 141, 142
Ligaments
  functions, 551
  skeletal, 549
Ligation
  of hemorrhoids, 467
  saphenous vein, 423
  tubal, 514
Limb-girdle dystrophy, 676
Lip cancer, 301
Lipemia
  diabetic, 704
Lipids, 12
  in cells, 139, 140
Lipodystrophy, 438
Lipoid deposits, 428
Lipoma
  classification of, 148
Liposarcoma
  classification of, 148
Lips
  and diet, 20, 24
Listlessness

and diet, 20, 24
Little stroke, 653
Liver (*see also* Hepatic system)
    altered functioning of, 683
    biopsy, 711
    cancer, 721
    lobule, 709
    trauma to, 715
Lobar pneumonia, 354
Lobular carcinoma, 242
Local anesthesia, 178
Log-rolling, 608
Loop
    colostomy, 463
    diuretics, 480
    of Henle, 471
Lost Chord Club, 310
Lou Gehrig disease, 678
Low back problems, 604
Low-calorie supplements, 29
Lower airway, 312
    functions of, 311
Lowe's syndrome, 269
Low
    -flow systems, 316
    -protein supplements, 29
    -residue supplements, 29
Lumbar puncture, 628
Lumbosacral transitional vertebrae, 604
Lungs
    anatomy of, 312
    and homeostasis, 37
    and immobility, 132
    as buffer system, 47
Lupus, 231
Lutein cyst, 529
Luteinizing hormone, 502, 731
Lymphangioendothelioma
    classification of, 148
Lymphangioma
    classification of, 148
Lymphangiosarcoma
    classification of, 148
Lymphatic leukemia
    classification of, 148
Lymphoblastic leukemia, 691
Lymphocytic leukemia, 693
Lymphoma
    definition of, 145
    non-Hodgkin, 694
Lymphoreticular system, 115
Lymphosarcoma
    classification of, 148

M

Macroglobulinemia, 118
Macronutrients, 14
Macrophages, 116
Macula densa, 471
Macule, 204
Magnesium
    deficit, 65
    excess, 66

imbalances, 65
    RDAs, 11
Malabsorption
    discussion of, 436, 437
Male RDAs, 10,11
Malignant hyperthermia, 183
Malignant lymphoma
    classification of, 149
Malignant melanoma, 229
    classification of, 148
Malignant neoplasms, 242
    definition of, 145
    respiratory, 365
Malnutrition
    and fever, 105
Malpositioned teeth
    and diet, 20, 24
Mammary sarcoma, 242
Mammography, 237
Mandibular fractures, 295
Manual traction, 574
Marriage
    and stress, 6
Marshall-Marchetti procedure, 485
Massage
    and pain, 92
Mastitis, 237
Maxillary fractures, 295
McGivney ligator, 467
Meckel's diverticulum, 458
Median nerve
    and compartmental syndrome, 581
Medications
    and musculoskeletal system, 567
    and rheumatoid arthritis, 587
    and sexual functioning, 510
    and surgery, 170
    and the nervous system, 630
    for skin, 207
    postoperative, 190
    problems of undermedicating, 81, 82
    renal, 480
    to lower serum calcium, 768
Medulla
    function of, 615
Medullary carcinoma, 763
Medulloblastoma, 650
Megaloblastic macrocytic anemia, 698
Megavitamin therapy, 15
Melanocarcinoma
    classification of, 148
Melanocyte-stimulating hormone, 731
Melanoma, 229
Membrane permeability
    effect on diffusion, 35
Memory cells, 117
Ménière's disease, 279
Meningioma, 650
    classification of, 148
Meningitis, 643
Menopause, 502
    and gout, 593
    and osteoporosis, 597
Menstrual cycle, 502, 506
Mental illness

and hypothermia, 111
Mental status
    and acid-base imbalance, 56
Meperidine
    and pain, 88, 91
Mesocaval shunt, 711
Metabolic
    acidosis, 48, 49
    alkalosis, 49, 51
Metabolic system
    altered functioning of, 727
    and immobility, 135
Metabolism
    and diet, 19
    hormone regulation of, 775
Metastasis
    means of, 149
Methoxyflurane
    and surgery, 176
MI, 393
    and renal failure, 488
    and sexual functioning, 517
Micronutrients, 14
Micturition
    usual pattern, 474
Midbrain
    function of, 615
Migraine, 95
Miller-Abbott tube, 453
Mineralocorticoids
    function of, 744
Minerals, 9, 14
    RDAs, 11
Minerva jacket, 572
Miscarriage, 539
Missed abortion, 540
Mitochondria, 141
Mitosis, 142
Mitral valve disease
    comparison of, 402
Mobility, 125
Mobilization
    and surgery, 169
Monilial vaginitis, 525
Moniliasis, 525
Monro
    foramen of, 612
Monro-Kellie hypothesis, 636
Mons pubis
    function of, 504
Mons veneris
    function of, 504
Montgomery's tubercles, 235
Morphine
    and pain, 91
Motor neurons, 611
Motor system
    assessment of, 624
Mouth (see also Oral)
    altered functioning of, 292
    and temperature, 105, 106
    functions, 294
    structures, 294
M protein, 119
Mucorales fungal disease, 784

Multiple myeloma, 596, 692
    classification of, 148
Multiple sclerosis, 670
    and neurogenic bladder, 498
Mumps, 298
Muscles
    and diet, 20, 25
    and immobility, 128
    assessment of, 624
    extraocular, 248
    features of, 552
    fibers, 550
    skeletal, 550
Muscle cells, 142
Muscle tissue, 143
Muscular contraction
    and heat production, 102
Muscular dystrophy, 676
Musculoskeletal
    altered functioning of, 547
Myasthenia gravis, 673
Mycobacterium tuberculosis, 360
Myelocytic leukemia, 693
Myelogram, 629
    discussion of, 565
Myeloma
    and gout, 593
    multiple, 596, 692
    plasma cell, 118
Myocardial infarction, 393
Myocarditis, 405
Myoclonic seizures, 662, 665
Myoma
    uterine, 530
Myxedema, 761
Myxedema madness, 764
Myxoma
    classification of, 148
Myxosarcoma
    classification of, 148

N

Nails, 204
Narcotic antagonists
    and respiration, 326
Narcotics
    and pain, 88, 91
Nasal (see also Nose)
    packing, 285
Nasal cannula, 316
Nasogastric tube, 440
Nasopharyngeal tubes
    illustration of, 319
Natural immunity, 113
Nausea
    discussion of, 436
Near-drowning, 342
Neck
    altered functioning of, 245, 303
    assessment of, 558
    functions, 304
    structures, 304
Negative nutrition, 24, 25

Neisseria gonorrhoeae, 519, 523, 527
Neisseria meningitidis, 354, 643
Neoplasia
  definition of, 145
Neoplasms
  classification of, 148
  definition of, 145
  malignant, 242, 365
  of brain, 649, 651
  of colon, 463
  ovarian, 536
  respiratory, 365
Nephrectomy, 484
Nephritis
  interstitial, 474
Nephrolithotomy, 485
Nephrons, 470
Nephroscopy, 497
Nephrostomy, 484
Nephrotic syndrome, 496
Nephrotoxins
  and renal failure, 494
Nephroureterectomy, 484
Nerve
  blocks, 96
  cells, 142, 611
  excitability, 766
fibers and sensations, 72
  optic, 251
Nerves
  and compartment syndrome, 581
  cranial, 613, 616
  spinal, 613
Nervous sytem
  altered functioning of, 611
  and homeostasis, 38
  diagnostic tests, 628, 629
Nervous tissue, 142
Neurectomy
  and pain relief, 96
Neurilemoma
  classification of, 148
Neurinoma
  classification of, 148
Neuroblastoma
  classification of, 148
Neuroendocrine interactions, 502
Neurofibroma, 651
  classification of, 148
Neurofibrosarcoma
  classification of, 148
Neurogenic bladder, 498
  signs of, 475
Neurogenic sarcoma
  classification of 148
Neuroglia, 612
Neurologic exam
  equipment for, 618
Neuroma
  acoustic, 651
  classification of, 148
Neurons, 611
New Voice Club, 310
Niacin RDAs, 11
Niemann-Pick disease, 704

Nitrogen
  balance, 18, 19
  excretion, 18
Nitrous oxide
  and surgery, 176
Nocturia, 474
Nodular melanoma, 229
Nodule, 204
Non-Hodgkin lymphoma, 695
Nonnarcotics
  and pain, 88, 90
Nonshivering thermogenesis, 102
Nontoxic goiter, 760
Norepinephrine
  and heat production, 102
  and homeostasis, 38
  function of, 744
Nose (*see also* Nasal)
  altered functioning of, 283
  anterior, 293
  functions of 283
Nosebleed, 288
NPO
  and diet, 17
  for surgery, 170
Nucleus
  of cells, 140, 141
Nursing care
  and hyperalimentation, 31
  and pain, 80
  and tube feedings, 31
  believing the patient, 82, 84
  dietary, 27
  fluid and electrolytes, 40
  for respiratory system, 337
  inappropriate judgment, 80
  pain-relief principles, 89
Nutrition, 9
  altered needs, 26
  and musculoskeletal functioning, 567
  lack of, 17
  negative, 24, 25
  positive, 24, 25
  theories, 15
Nystagmus
  and MS, 670

O

Oat cell carcinoma, 365
Obesity, 17, 448
  and colon cancer, 463
Obstruction
  intestinal, 453
  of airway, 344
  of the ear canal, 276
Obtundation
  description of, 619
Occlusion
  acute arterial, 424
Oculomotor nerve
  function of, 616
Odor
  and diet, 24

Olfactory nerve
    function of, 616
Oligodendroglioma, 659
Oncology Nursing Society
    outcome standards, 154
Oophoritis, 523
Open amputations
    reasons for, 422
Open-angle glaucoma, 266
Open head injury, 637
Ophthalmodynamometry, 654
Oppenheim reflex
    test for, 627
Opsonins, 116
Optic nerves, 251
    function of, 616
Oral (*see also* Mouth)
    cancer, 301
    infections, 296
Orchiectomy, 494
Organ-specific disorders, 124
Oropharyngeal tubes
    illustration of, 319
Oropharynx cancer, 301
Orthostatic hypotension
    and immobility, 129, 130
Osmolarity
    normal value, 36
Osmosis, 36
Osmotic
    diuretics, 480
    pressure, 36
Osteoarthritis, 591
Osteoclastoma, 594
Osteogenic sarcoma, 595
    classification of, 148
Osteoid osteoma, 594
Osteoma
    classification of, 148
    osteoid, 594
Osteomalacia, 61
Osteoporosis, 61, 597
    and diet, 25
    from immobility, 128
Otitis
    external, 277
    media, 278
O_2
    extraction, 408
    therapy, 316
Output
    and surgery, 170
Ovarian
    carcinoma, 535
    cycle, 502, 506
    cyst, 529
    neoplasm, 536
Ovaries
    function of, 504
Overhydration
    signs of, 474
Oxygen
    postoperative, 187
Oxytocin, 731

P

Pacemaker
    insertion of, 391
Paget's disease, 242, 598
    and osteogenic sarcoma, 595
Pain
    acute, 82
    and addiction, 81, 82
    and angina, 419
    and surgery, 169
    and the nurse, 80
    attitudes toward, 81
    avoidance of, 73
    center, 73
    chronic, 95
    clinics, 98
    experience, 76
    fear of, 73
    misconception of, 81
    phantom, 75, 77
    principles of relief, 89
    producers of, 83
    psychologic dimension of, 73
    realities of, 81, 82
    receptors, 72
    reporting of, 77, 78, 79
    sensation of, 72
    syndromes, 77
    theories, 74, 75
Pancreas
    cancer of, 782
    disorders of, 773
    pseudocysts of, 781
Pancreatitis, 778
Papillae
    of kidneys, 470
Papillary carcinoma, 762
Papilloma
    classification of, 148
Pap smear, 522
Papule, 204
Para-aminosalicylic acid, 361
Paracentesis
    of liver, 711
Paralysis
    Todd's, 666
Paralysis agitans, 671
Paralytic ileus, 465
    postoperative, 199
Paranasal sinuses
    functions of, 283
Paraplegia
    and sexual functioning, 517
Parasitic infection, 461
Parasitism
    hepatic, 720
Parasympathetic nervous system
    function of, 617
Parathormone
    and homeostasis, 38
Parathyroid
    and homeostasis, 38
    and disorders of, 766

hormone, 766
Parkinson's disease, 671
Paronychia, 216
Parotitis, 298
Partial seizures, 662, 666
Passive immunity, 114
Pathology
 of fluids and electrolytes, 38
Pathophysiology
 and nutrition, 18
 in stress, 5
Pattern theory
 of pain, 74, 75
Pauling, Linus, 15
PCO2
 changes in, 49
Pearson attachment, 577
Pediculosis
 capitis, 214
 corporis, 214
 pubis, 215
Pedunculated polyps, 462
Pelvic inflammatory disease, 523
Pelvis
 renal, 470
Penetrating injuries
 thoracic, 349
Penicillin
 and respiratory care, 325
Penis
 function of, 508
Peptic ulcer, 449
 and diet, 16
 and indigestion, 435
Peptides
 and reproduction, 502
Percussion
 and respiratory care, 339
 positions for, 341
Percutaneous transluminal coronary
 angioplasty, 391
Perforating injuries
 thoracic, 349
Pericardial effusion, 406, 407
Pericarditis, 405
 and renal failure, 476
 constrictive, 406
Perimysium, 550
Peripheral nervous sytem, 613
Periosteum, 548
Peritoneal dialysis, 481
Peritonitis, 459
Peronial nerve
 and compartmental syndrome, 581
Perspiration
 and fluid imbalance, 33
Pes planus, 601
Petechiae
 and diet, 20
Petit mal seizures, 662, 665
pH
 changes in, 49
 normal, 37
Phagocytosis, 114, 141

Phantom pain, 75, 77
Pharyngeal tubes
 discussion of, 319
Pheochromocytoma, 748
 and hypertension, 428
Phlebotomy, 687
Phonation, 303
Phosphate buffer system, 47
Phospholipids
 in cells, 140
Phosphorus RDAs, 11
Photophobia, 643, 659
Physiologic deconditioning, 125, 126
Physiologic factors
 in stress, 2
Physiology
 and fluids and electrolytes, 34
 and immunity, 115
 and nose, 283
 and nutrition, 14
 and sensations, 72
 and stress, 3
 and temperature, 102
 female reproductive, 500, 504
 male reproductive, 502, 508
 of blood, 683
 of ears, 273
 of eye, 246
 of glands, 728
 of heart, 383
 of kidneys, 470
 of liver, 708
 of lower GI tract, 451
 of lungs, 311
 of metabolism, 728
 of mouth, 293
 of neck, 303
 of nervous system, 611
 of skeletal system, 547
 of throat, 293
 of upper GI tract, 438
 vascular, 420
Pigmentation, 205
Pigmented nevus
 classification of, 148
Piles, 466
Pilonidal cyst, 462
Pinocytosis, 141
Pin sites, 576
Pinworms, 461
Pituitary
 adenoma, 651
 and homeostasis, 38
 and pain, 75
 disorders of, 730
 hormone function, 731
Placebos
 and pain, 89
Plaque, 204
Planning
 anticipatory and stress, 8
Plantar warts, 221
Plasma
 cell myeloma, 118

fluid shifts, 68
role in body, 34
Plasmapheresis, 120
Plaster casts
care of, 569
complications of, 574
types of, 572, 573
Pleurae
functions of, 312
Pleurevac, 329
illustration of, 331
Pleurisy, 362
Pleuritis, 362
Plication 451
Pneumoencephalogram, 629
Pneumonia, 353
Pneumothorax, 350
Poikilocytosis, 701
Point of maximal impulse, 388, 389
Poison
ingestion of, 441
Polyarteritis nodosa, 233
Polycystic kidney, 495
Polycythemia vera, 706
and gout, 593
Polymyxin B sulfate
and respiratory care, 325
Polyneuritis
and hypertension, 428
Polyps, 462, 530
Polysaccharides
and cellular growth, 140
Polyunsaturated fats, 12
Pons
function of, 615
Portacaval shunt, 711
Portal hypertension, 712
Positioning
and respiratory care, 338
and surgery, 180
postoperative, 196
Positive nutrition, 24, 25
Postictal phase, 664-667
Postmenopausal vaginitis, 525
Postnecrotic cirrhosis, 723
Postoperative needs, 185
Postovulatory phase, 506
Postrenal failure
causes of, 488
Postural drainage
and respiratory care, 339
positions for, 341
Posture
and diet, 20, 24, 25
Postvaccinal encephalitis, 645
Potassium
deficit, 57
excess, 59
imbalances, 57
-sparing diuretics, 480
Prausnitz-Kustner reaction, 121
Precipitins, 116
Pregnancy
and rape, 518
and stress, 7

RDAs, 10, 11
Preleukemia, 691
Premature
atrial contraction, 416
ventricular contraction, 417
Preoperative needs, 163
Preovulatory phase, 506
Prerenal failure
causes of, 488
Presbycusis, 282
Pressure
and casts, 574
and immobility, 126, 129
and pain relief, 92
and traction, 575
hydrostatic, 67
increased intracranial, 635
osmotic, 36
Pressure gradient
effect on diffusion, 36
Pressure sore, 126
Primary
hyperaldosteronism, 747
hypertension, 426
impotence, 541
P-R interval
implication of, 390
Prinzmetal angina, 419
Procaine
and surgery, 177
Proctoscopy, 452
Proctosigmoidectomy, 464
Prodromal phase
of fever, 110
Progesterone
and reproduction, 502
Progestogen tablets
effectiveness of, 512
Prolactin, 731
Prolonged fevers, 110
Prophylactics
effectiveness of, 513
Proprioception, 71, 72
Proptosis, 271
Prostaglandins, 121
Prostatectomy, 484
Prostate gland
function of, 509
Prostatic hypertrophy, 491
Prostatic surgery
patient care, 492, 493
Prostatitis, 527
signs of, 474
Protein
buffer system, 47
complementarity, 15
fortifiers, 27
M, 119
RDA, 10
role in body, 34
Proteins, 9, 12
and immunity, 113
in cells, 139, 140
Proteus, 497, 646
Proteus mirabilis, 643

Protoplasm
  in cells, 139
Pruritus, 208
Pseudocysts
  pancreatic, 781
Pseudoephedrine hydrochloride
  and respiratory care, 325
Pseudofolliculitis, 206
Pseudohypertrophic dystrophy, 676
Pseudomonas, 643
Pseudomonas aeruginosa, 354
Psoriasis, 226
Psychologic
  pain dimensions, 73
Psychologic factors
  in stress, 2
Psychosomatic illness
  and stress, 5
Psychotropic agents
  purpose of, 630
Puberty, 503
Pulmonary circulation, 383
Pulmonary edema, 395
  phases of, 396
Pulmonary embolism, 345
Pulmonary function studies
  use of, 315
Pulmonary surgery
  purpose and care, 333
Pulmonary trauma, 349
Pulsus paradoxus
  and renal failure, 476
Pustule, 204
P wave
  implication of, 390
Pyelogram, 429, 478
Pyelolithotomy, 485
Pyelonephritis, 488
  signs of, 474
Pyloric ulcer, 450
Pyloroplasty, 451
Pyramids
  renal, 470

Q

QRS complex
  implication of, 390
Quadriplegia
  and sexual functioning, 517
Quiescent cancers, 150

R

Radial nerve
  and compartmental syndrome, 581
Radiation (of heat), 102
Radiation therapy, 119
  discussion of, 151
  patient teaching, 161
Rape, 507
  clinical manifestations, 518
  phases of, 519

Rappaport tumor classification, 694
Raynaud's disease, 431
Reabsorption
  renal, 471
Reaction
  hemolytic transfusion, 686
Readjustment
  rating scale, 6
Reagin, 121
Receding gums
  and diet, 20
Recommended Daily Allowances table, 10, 11
Recording for the Blind, 253
Recovery room 185
Rectal
  abscess, 460
  carcinoma, 464
  fissure, 467
  fistula, 467
Rectal disease
  and temperature monitoring, 106
Rectum
  and temperature, 105, 106
  excision of, 457
Reed-Sternberg cells, 695
Reflex
  baroreceptor, 386
  chemoreceptor, 386
Reflex status
  assessment of, 626, 627
Refraction
  structures of, 250
Regional
  anesthesia, 178
  enteritis, 455
Regurgitation
  and valvular dysfunction, 401
Relativistic utilitarian position, 501
Relaxation techniques, 93, 94, 95
Release of forbidden clone theory, 123
Renal (*see also* Kidneys)
  acute failure, 477
  care of patient, 486, 487
  disease, 494
  failure, 476
  filtration, 471
  pyramids, 470
  reabsorption, 471
  scan, 479
  secretion, 472
  tests, 478, 479
Renal calculi
  and immobility, 133
Renal disorders
  and sexual functioning, 517
Renal pelvis, 470
Renal system
  and immobility, 133
Renal toxicity
  care of, 159
Repetitive thought process
  and pain relief, 94
Reproduction
  discussion of, 501
  medications affecting, 510

Reproductive functioning
    altered, 510
Resection
    abdominal-perineal, 457
    of the colon, 463
    submucous, 286
Resectional surgery
    purpose and care, 334
Residual volume
    definition of, 316
Resistance stage
    to stress, 5
Resolution
    of stress, 2
Respiration
    muscles of, 312
Respiratory
    acidosis, 49, 52, 132
    alkalosis, 49, 54
    postoperative complications, 196
Respiratory system
    altered functioing of, 311
    illustration of, 312
Responses to stress, 4, 5
Restlessness
    and diet, 25
Retention
    urinary, 475
Reticulum cell sarcoma
    classification of, 148
Retinal detachment, 259
Retinopathy
    diabetic, 264
Retirement
    and stress, 7
Rhabdomyoma
    classification of, 148
Rhabdomyosarcoma
    classification of, 148
Rh antigens, 116
Rheumatic fever, 399
    acute, 401
Rheumatoid arthritis, 586
Rhinitis, 289
    allergic, 121
Rhinoplasty, 287
Rhizotomy, 97, 642
Rhythmic breathing
    and pain relief, 94
Rhythm method
    effectiveness of, 512
Rib fractures, 351
Riboflavin RDAs, 10
Rickets, 769
Rifampin
    and TB, 361
Right-sided heart failure, 409
Ringworm, 223, 224
Rinne test, 621
RNA, 140, 141
Roundworms, 461
Ruffini's nerve, 72
Ruptured appendix, 454
Russell traction, 576
    and hip fractures, 589

S

Saccular aneurysm, 428
Sacralization, 604
Salmonella
    and diarrhea, 437
Salpingitis, 523
Saphenous vein ligation, 423
Sarcoblasts, 143
Sarcoidosis, 375
Sarcolemma, 550
Sarcoma
    definition of, 145
    Ewing's, 597
    osteogenic, 595
Satiety, 17
Saturated fats, 12
Scale, 204
Scaly dermis
    and diet, 20
Scan
    CAT, 629
    renal, 479
Scanogram
    discussion of, 565
Schistosoma mansoni, 720
Schwannoma, 651
Scleroderma, 232
Scrotum
    function of, 508
Scurvy, 25
Sebaceous
    cysts, 227
    glands, 205
Seborrhea, 212
Secondary
    glaucoma, 268
    hypertension, 428
    impotence, 541
Second-degree heart block, 414
Secretion
    renal, 472
Seeing Eye, 253
Seizure
    disorders, 662, 664-667
    Jacksonian, 652
Selye, Hans, 3
Semen
    function of, 509
Seminal fluid
    function of, 509
Seminal vesicles
    function of, 509
Sengstaken-Blakemore tube, 716
Senile vaginitis, 525
Senility
    and diet, 25
Sensations, 71
Sensory decision theory
    of pain, 75, 76
Sensory deprivation, 136
Sensory neurons, 611
Sensory response
    to pain, 73
Sensory system

assessment of, 625
Septic shock
  postoperative, 200
Septum
  deviated, 292
Sequesterd antigen theory, 123
Serofibrinous pleurisy, 362
Serotonin, 121
Serous otitis media, 278
Serum calcium
  forms of, 61
Sessile polyps, 462
Sex
  roles, 501
Sexual assault, 507
Sexual behavior, 501
Sexual functioning
  altered, 501
Shaking palsy, 671
Shedding
  viral, 522
Sheehan's syndrome, 438, 739
Shigella, 461
Shingles, 219
Shipman's mnemonic, 438
Shivering
  and heat production, 102
Shock
  anaphylactic, 121
  cardiogenic, 395
  during surgery, 182
  postoperative, 198, 200, 201
  septic, 200
Shoulder
  assessment of, 559
  spica, 572
Shunt
  formation, 485
  liver, 711
Sigmoid carcinoma, 464
Sigmoidoscopy, 452, 457
Simple touch, 72
Sinus
  bradycardia, 411
  coronary, 386
  paranasal, 283
  tachycardia, 411
Sinusitis, 291
Situational impotence, 541
Skeletal
  ligaments, 549
  muscles, 550
Skeletal traction, 575
Skene's glands
  function of, 504
Skin (*see also* Integument)
  altered functioning of, 203
  and diet, 20, 24
  and immobility, 126
  burns, 209
  deviations, 209
  dry, 208
  lesions, 204
  receptors, 72
  traction, 574

ulcers, 230
SLE, 231
  and renal disease, 475
Slow reactive substance of anaphylaxis,
    121
Smoking
  and temperature monitoring, 106
  pack-years, 313
Snake bites
  and compartmental syndrome, 579
Snellen chart, 618
Social readjustment rating scale, 6
Sociocultural factors
  in stress, 2
Sodium
  and water imbalances, 41
Solid
  body composition, 34
Somatropin, 731
Somogyi effect, 785
Specificity theory
  of pain, 74, 75
Specimen care
  during surgery, 181
Speech, 303
Spermatic cord
  function of, 509
Spermatogenesis, 503
Spermicides
  effectiveness of, 513
Spica, 572, 573
Spider angioma, 723
Spina bifida
  and neurogenic bladder, 498
Spinal accessory nerve
  function of, 616
Spinal anesthesia, 178
Spinal cord
  and sensations, 72
  and the CNS, 612
Spinal cord injury, 639
  and urinary retention, 475
Spirometer, 377
  illustration of, 378
Splenectomy, 688
Splenomegaly, 704
Splenorenal shunt, 711
Splint
  Thomas, 577
Splints
  and compartmental syndrome, 579
Spondylolisthesis, 604
Spondylolysis, 604
Spontaneous abortion, 539
Sprain, 584
Sprue
  and malabsorption, 436
Squamous cell carcinoma, 365
  classification of, 148
Stable angina, 419
Stages of anesthesia, 175
Staphylococcus, 523, 646
Staphylococcus aureus, 354, 527, 643
  and cellulitis, 425
  and endocarditis, 400

"Star of good eating," 12
Starvation, 22
Stasis of urine
   and immobility, 133
Steatorrhea, 438
Stenosis
   and valvular dysfunction, 401
Stereognosis, 71
Sterotactic
   ablation, 663
   surgery, 97, 672
Steroids
   and fever, 105
   and reproduction, 502
Stiffness
   from immobility, 128
Stoicism
   and pain, 73
Stomach
   cancer, 445
   plication of, 451
Stomatitis, 296
   care of, 157
Stones
   in gallbladder, 443
Stools
   tarry, 438
Strain
   muscle, 583
Streptococcus, 523, 643, 646
Streptococcus viridans
   and endocarditis, 400
Streptomycin
   and respiratory care, 325
   and TB, 361
Stress, 1, 3
   abnormal responses to, 5
   adaptation process, 2
   normal responses to, 4
   rating, 6
Stressors, 1, 3
Stress ulcer, 450
   postoperative, 202
Striae
   and diet, 24
Stricture
   esophageal, 445
   ureteral, 499
Stroke, 655
   TIA, 653
Strychnine
   ingestion of, 441
ST segment
   implication of, 390
Stupor
   description of, 619
Sty, 262
Subarachnoid hemorrhage, 658
   gradations of, 660
Subcutaneous
   emphysema, 351
   tissue, 204, 205
Subhemophilia, 701
Sublimation
   and stress, 8

Subluxation, 584
Submucous resection, 286
Suctioning
   and respiratory care, 339
Sulfonamides, 480
Sunken chest
   and diet, 20
Superficial pain, 77, 78
Superficial spreading melanoma, 229
Supplements
   commercially prepared, 28, 29
Suppurative otitis media, 278
Suprapubic cystostomy, 484
Supreme Court
   and abortion, 539
Surgery
   and cancer, 157
   and documentation, 181
   and pain relief, 96
   and renal failure, 488
   and respiratory functioning, 326
   and specimen care, 181
   brain, 624
   complications, 182, 184
   elective, 163
   emergency, 163
   postanesthesia assessment, 188
   postoperative assessment, 186
   prostatic, 492, 493
   pulmonary, 333
   renal, 484, 485
   resectional, 334
   risk factors, 164
   stereotactic, 97, 672
   urinary, 484, 485
Surveillance theory
   of cancer, 147
Suspension
   balanced, 577
Swimmer's ear, 277
Swine influenza, 648
Swollen abdomen
   and diet, 20
Swollen gums
   and diet, 20, 24
Sylvius
   aqueduct of, 612
Sympathectomy, 97
Sympathetic nervous system
   function of, 617
Symptoms
   of nutritional deficiency, 19, 20, 24, 25
   of stress, 4
Syndrome
   adult respiratory distress, 347
   carpal tunnel, 602
   compartmental, 579
   Conn's, 438
   Cushing's, 735
   ectopic ACTH, 737
   Guillain-Barré, 648
   nephrotic, 496
   pain, 77
   Sheehan's, 438, 739
   toxic shock, 544

Van Vyk-Grumbach, 764
    Waterhouse-Friderichsen, 643
    Werner's, 269
Synovial sarcoma
    classification of, 148
Synovioma
    classification of, 148
Syphilis, 521
Systemic circulation, 384
    characteristics, 421
Systemic cold injuries, 111
    risk factors, 105
Systemic disorders, 124
Systemic lupus erythematosus, 231
Systolic ejection click, 389

T

Tabes dorsalis
    and neurogenic bladder, 498
Tachycardia
    sinus, 411
    ventricular, 412
Tactile discrimination, 72
Tamponade
    cardiac, 398, 407
Tapeworms, 461, 720
TB
    and pericarditis, 405
T cells, 115
Technology
    and stress, 3
Teeth
    and diet, 20, 24
Temperature
    contraindications to taking, 106
    control, 101
    interventions for, 109
    laboratory tests, 108
    measurement of, 106
    measurement sites, 105, 106
    normal range, 101, 106
    risk factors, 105
    sensation of, 72
Tenckhoff catheter, 481, 485
Tendons, 550
Tenosynovitis, 569
TENS, 96
Tension
    and stress relieving, 8
Teratocarcinoma
    classification of, 149
Terpin hydrate
    and respiratory care, 324
Test
    Ellsworth-Howard, 767
    laboratory, 791-805
    normal laboratory values, 791-805
    renal, 478
    Rinne, 621
    Weber, 621
Testes
    cancer of, 537
    function of, 508

Testosterone, 503
Tetracaine
    and surgery, 177
Tetraiodothyronine
    and homeostasis, 38
Tetralogy of Fallot, 646
Thalamus
    and pain, 75
    function of, 615
Theophylline
    and respiratory care, 325
Theories
    pain, 74, 75
Therapeutic touch
    and pain relief, 95
Thermal burns
    of eyes, 257
Thermogenesis
    nonshivering, 102
Thermomography
    for breasts, 237
Thermoregulation
    impaired, 104
    theories, 104
Thiamin RDAs, 10
Thiazide diuretics, 480
Thiopental sodium
    and surgery, 176
Third-degree heart block, 414
Thomas splints, 577
Thoracentesis
    purpose and care, 332
Thoracic
    aneurysm, 429
    injuries, 349
Thoracoplasty
    purpose and care, 334
Thoracotomy
    exploratory, 334
Threatened abortion, 540
Throat
    altered functioning of, 292
    functions, 294
    structures, 294
Thrombocytopenia
    care of, 156
    patient teaching, 161
Thrombophlebitis, 426
Thrombosis
    at pin sites, 576
Thrombotic CVA, 655
Thrombus
    and immobility, 129, 130
Thymectomy
    for MG, 675
Thyrocalcitonin, 753, 755
Thyroid
    cancer, 761
    disorders, 753
    hormone functions, 755
    -stimulating hormone, 731
    tumors, 762, 763
Thyroidectomy
    patient care, 757
Thyroid enlargement

and diet, 20
Thyroiditis, 759
Thyrotoxicosis, 438
Thyrotropin, 731
Thyroxine, 753, 755
Tidal volume
  definition of, 315
Tinea
  capitis, 222
  pedis, 223
  unguium, 224
Tissue, 142
  subcutaneous, 204, 205
Todd's paralysis, 666
Toe
  hammer, 599
Tomogram
  discussion of, 565
Tongue
  and diet, 20, 24
Tonic-clonic seizures, 662, 664
Tonsillitis, 299
Tooth decay, 298
Tophi
  and gout, 593
Touch
  and pain relief, 95
  sensation of, 72
  simple, 72
Tourniquets
  and compartmental syndrome, 579
Toxic shock syndrome, 544
TPI test, 521
TPN, 26
Trace elements, 14
Tracheostomy
  purpose and care, 326
Traction
  and low back problems, 605
  and pressure, 575
  Bryant's, 579
  care during, 571
  manual, 574
  pelvic, 607
  Russell, 576, 589
  skeletal, 575
  skin, 574
Transfusion
  blood, 686
  reaction, 686
Transient agammaglobulinemia, 117
Transient ischemic attack, 653
Transillumination
  for breasts, 237
Transitional cell carcinoma
  classification of, 148
Transplant
  bone marrow, 688
  kidney, 485
  renal, 495
Transplantation
  renal, 495
Transplant rejection, 114
Transport
  active, 37

Trapeze
  and hip fractures, 588
Trauma
  and immobility, 129, 130
  hepatic, 715
  pulmonary, 349
Treponema pallidum, 521
Trichinella spiralis, 461
Trichomonas vaginalis, 524
Trichomoniasis, 524
Tricuspid valve diseases
  comparison of, 404
Trigeminal nerve
  function of, 616
Trigger finger, 603
Triiodothyronine, 753, 755
  and homeostasis, 38
Trochanter, 549
Trochlear nerve
  function of, 616
Trousseau's sign, 772
T-tube cholangiography, 440
Tubal ligation
  discussion of, 514
Tube feedings, 28
Tuberculosis, 360
Tuberosity, 549
Tubes
  and surgery, 170
Tubule
  renal, 470
Tumor, 145
  and pain, 83
  and renal failure, 488
  brain, 649-651
  effects of, 149
  formation, 147
  spread, 149
  thyroid, 762, 763
Tumor doubling time
  definition of, 147
Turning
  in respiratory care, 338
T wave
  implication of, 390
Twitching
  and diet, 25
Two-point discrimination, 71

U

UGIS, 439
Ulcer, 204, 449
  acute stress, 202
  and diet, 16
  and fluid imbalance, 33
  decubitus, 126
  peptic, 435
  postoperative, 202
  skin, 230
Ulcerative colitis, 456
  and diarrhea, 437
Ulnar nerve
  and compartmental syndrome,
    581

Ultrasound
  for breasts, 237
  renal, 479
Umbilical hernia, 466
Undermedicating
  problems of, 81, 82
Unstable angina, 419
Upper airway, 312
  functions of, 311
Upper GI series, 439
Urban hypothermia, 111
Uremic fetor
  and renal failure, 476
Ureteral stricture, 499
Ureterectomy, 484
Ureterolithotomy, 485
Ureteroneocystostomy, 485
Ureteroplasty, 485
Ureterosigmoidostomy, 494
Ureterostomy, 484
Ureterovesicular anastomsis, 485
Ureters
  anatomy of, 470
Urethra
  anatomy of, 470
  function of, 509
Urethral smears, 523
Urethral stricture, 499
Urgency
  urinary, 474
Uric acid
  and gout, 593
Urinalysis, 473
  and diet, 22
Urination
  and immobility, 133
Urinary (see Kidneys)
  retention, 475
  urgency, 474
Urolithiasis, 497
  and urinary retention, 475
Urticaria, 121
Uterine
  carcinoma, 533
  expulsion, 539
  myoma, 530
Uterus
  function of, 505
UTI
  care of patient, 487
Uveitis, 262
U wave
  implication of, 390

V

Vagina
  function of, 505
Vaginitis, 524
Vagotomy, 450
Vagus nerve
  function of, 616
Valsalva's maneuver
  and hyperalimentation, 30

  and immobility, 130, 131
Valve disease
  aortic, 403
  mitral, 403
  tricuspid, 404
Valvular disease
  chronic, 400
Van Vyk-Grumbach syndrome, 764
Variant angina, 419
Varices
  esophageal, 715
Varicose veins, 432
Vasa recta, 471
Vascular
  anatomy and physiology, 420
Vas deferens
  function of, 508, 509
Vasectomy
  discussion of, 514
Vater
  ampulla of, 773
VD
  and rape, 518
VDRL test, 521
Vegetarian foods, 28
Veins
  coronary, 386
  role of, 421
  varicose, 432
Vena cana
  normal valves, 421
Venereal warts, 221
Venous stasis
  and immobility, 129, 130
  ulcers, 230
Ventilation
  definition of, 313
  mechanical aids to, 321
Ventilatory function studies
  use of, 315
Ventricles
  and the CNS, 612
Ventricular
  fibrillation, 413
  hypertrophy, 408
  premature contraction, 417
  tachycardia, 412
Venules
  role of, 421
Verbalization
  of pain, 74
Verrucae, 221
Vertebrae
  lumbosacral transitional, 604
Vertigo, 273
Vesicant drugs
  infiltration of, 153
Vesicle, 204
Vesicourethral suspension, 485
Vestibule
  function of, 504
Vibration
  and respiratory care, 339
Viral
  hepatitis, 717

pneumonia, 354
shedding, 522
Visually handicapped
    rehabilitation of, 253
Vital capacity
    definition of, 253
Vital signs
    and surgery, 170, 175
    postoperative, 190
Vitamin A, 9
Vitamin RDAs, 10, 11
Vitiligo, 206
Vomiting
    and fluid imbalance, 33
    contraindication to, 441
    discussion of, 436
    during surgery, 182
    postoperative, 198
von Economo's encephalitis, 645
Vulvitis, 526

W

WAISTED
    malabsorption mnemonic, 438
Waldenström's macroglobulinemia,
    118
Warts, 221
Water, 14
    amounts and sources, 35
    and sodium imbalances, 41
    as nutrient, 9
    balance, 35
    excess, 42
    excretion, 35
    insensible loss, 35
    role in body, 34
Waterhouse-Friderichsen syndrome,
    643
Weakness

    and immobility, 128
Weber test, 621
Weight
    and diet, 20, 24, 25
    fluid and solid composition, 34
Wens, 227
Werner's syndrome, 269
Wet compress, 207
Wet dressings, 207
Wet-drowning, 342
Wheal, 204
Whipple's disease, 438
Whipple's procedure, 774, 782
Whiteheads, 213
Wirsung
    duct of, 773
Wood's light, 207
Worms, 461
Wound infection, 195
Wounds
    and fluid imbalance, 33
Wrist
    assessment of, 559

X

Xanthoma, 723
Xeroderma pigmentosum, 229
Xerography, 237
X-rays
    of chest, 315
    special procedures, 565

Z

Zeis's glands, 247
Zenografts, 211
Zinc RDAs, 11
Zovirax, 522